THE ROUTLEDGE HANDBOOK OF PHILOSOPHY OF PUBLIC HEALTH

In comparison to medicine, the professional field of public health is far less familiar. What is public health, and perhaps as importantly, what should public health be or become? How do causal concepts shape the public health agenda? How do study designs either promote or demote the environmental causal factors or health inequalities? How is risk understood, expressed, and communicated? Who is public health research centered on? How can we develop technologies so the benefits are more fairly distributed? Do people have a right to public health? How should we integrate ethics into public health practice?

The Routledge Handbook of Philosophy of Public Health addresses these questions and more, and is the first collection of its kind. Comprising 26 chapters by an international and interdisciplinary team of contributors, the handbook is divided into four clear parts:

- Concepts and distinctions
- Reasons and actions
- Distribution and inequalities
- Rights and duties.

The Routledge Handbook of Philosophy of Public Health is a field-defining and sustained reflection on the various ethical, political, methodological, and conceptual aspects of global public health. As such it is an essential reference source for students and scholars working in political philosophy, bioethics, public health ethics, and the philosophy of medicine, as well as for professionals and researchers in related fields such as public health, health economics, and epidemiology.

Sridhar Venkatapuram is Associate Professor of Global Health and Philosophy at King's College London, UK. He is based at the Global Health Institute, where he is Deputy Director, and Director of Global Health Education. He publishes widely across various disciplines, has helped establish health justice philosophy, and has worked in various ethics advisory roles to public and global health institutions. He is the author of *Health Justice: An Argument from the Capabilities Approach* (2011) and co-editor of *Vulnerable: The Law, Policy and Ethics of Covid-19* (2020). He can be found at @sridhartweet.

Alex Broadbent is Professor of Philosophy of Science at Durham University, UK, and Visiting Professor at the University of Johannesburg, South Africa. His research concerns the philosophy of epidemiology and medicine, causation, counterfactuals, prediction, complexity, conceptual aspects of machine learning, and scientific evidence in law. He is Editor-in-Chief of the journal *Philosophy of Medicine*. He is an Associate Member of Millennium Chambers, The Barrister Network, London.

ROUTLEDGE HANDBOOKS IN APPLIED ETHICS

Applied ethics is one of the largest and most diverse fields in philosophy and is closely related to many other disciplines across the humanities, sciences and social sciences. *Routledge Handbooks in Applied Ethics* are state-of-the-art surveys of important and emerging topics in applied ethics, providing accessible yet thorough assessments of key fields, themes, thinkers, and recent developments in research.

All chapters for each volume are specially commissioned, and written by leading scholars in the field. Carefully edited and organized, *Routledge Handbooks in Applied Ethics* provide indispensable reference tools for students and researchers seeking a comprehensive overview of new and exciting topics in applied ethics and related disciplines. They are also valuable teaching resources as accompaniments to textbooks, anthologies, and research-orientated publications.

ALSO AVAILABLE:

THE ROUTLEDGE HANDBOOK OF THE ETHICS OF CONSENT
Edited by Peter Schaber and Andreas Müller

THE ROUTLEDGE HANDBOOK OF ETHICS AND PUBLIC POLICY
Edited by Annabelle Lever and Andrei Poama

THE ROUTLEDGE HANDBOOK OF ANIMAL ETHICS
Edited by Bob Fischer

THE ROUTLEDGE HANDBOOK OF FEMINIST BIOETHICS
Edited by Wendy A. Rogers, Jackie Leach Scully, Stacy M. Carter, Vikki Entwistle, and Catherine Mills

THE ROUTLEDGE HANDBOOK OF PHILOSOPHY OF PUBLIC HEALTH
Edited by Sridhar Venkatapuram and Alex Broadbent

For more information about this series, please visit: https://www.routledge.com/Routledge-Handbooks-in-Applied-Ethics/book-series/RHAE

THE ROUTLEDGE HANDBOOK OF PHILOSOPHY OF PUBLIC HEALTH

Edited by
Sridhar Venkatapuram and Alex Broadbent

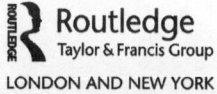

LONDON AND NEW YORK

Cover image: © Getty Images

First published 2023
by Routledge
4 Park Square, Milton Park, Abingdon, Oxon OX14 4RN

and by Routledge
605 Third Avenue, New York, NY 10158

Routledge is an imprint of the Taylor & Francis Group, an informa business

British Library Cataloguing-in-Publication Data
A catalogue record for this book is available from the British Library

Library of Congress Cataloging-in-Publication Data
Names: Venkatapuram, Sridhar, editor. | Broadbent, Alex, 1980- editor.
Title: The Routledge handbook of philosophy of public health / edited by Sridhar Venkatapuram and Alex Broadbent.
Description: Abingdon, Oxon; New York, NY: Routledge, 2023. | Series: Routledge handbooks in applied ethics | Includes bibliographical references and index.
Identifiers: LCCN 2022009628 (print) | LCCN 2022009629 (ebook) | ISBN 9781138938823 (hardback) | ISBN 9781032323879 (paperback) | ISBN 9781315675411 (ebook)
Subjects: LCSH: Public health—Philosophy. | Medical ethics—Philosophy. | Epidemiology—Philosophy.
Classification: LCC RA427 .R68 2023 (print) | LCC RA427 (ebook) | DDC 362.101—dc23/eng/20220628
LC record available at https://lccn.loc.gov/2022009628
LC ebook record available at https://lccn.loc.gov/2022009629

ISBN: 978-1-138-93882-3 (hbk)
ISBN: 978-1-032-32387-9 (pbk)
ISBN: 978-1-315-67541-1 (ebk)

DOI: 10.4324/9781315675411

Typeset in Bembo
by codeMantra

CONTENTS

ACKNOWLEDGMENTS

We, the editors, are extremely grateful to Alison Lockhart, whose exceptional and diverse skills and drive were pivotal in bringing this volume to completion. We are also grateful to all the contributors for their collegiality, for creating original work for this volume and for their painstaking refinements. It is no small matter that they did this all during a pandemic that was directly affecting their daily lives. We are also indebted to Olaf Dammann, Jonathan Fuller, and Daniel Steel for their valuable assistance. We also wish to thank Adam Johnson at Routledge for his assistance and patience as we worked to bring this volume into the world.

CONTRIBUTORS

Avni Amin (https://orcid.org/0000-0002-3136-1218) is Technical Officer, Violence against Women, in the Department of Sexual and Reproductive Health and Research of the World Health Organization, and is based in Geneva, Switzerland.

Mel Bartley (https://orcid.org/0000-0002-5981-0046) is Professor Emeritus of Medical Sociology in the Department of Epidemiology and Public Health, University College London in the United Kingdom, where she was professor from 2001 to 2012. She was co-ordinator of the ESRC Research Priority Network "Capability and Resilience" (2003–2006) and Director of the ESRC International Centre for Lifecourse Studies in Society and Health (2008–2012). She is author of *Health Inequality: An Introduction to Concepts, Theories and Methods*.

Agnès Berthelot-Raffard (https://orcid.org/0000-0003-0896-9847) is a political philosopher. She is Assistant Professor of Health and Critical Disability Studies at York University (Canada). She published papers about the rights of caregivers, and the ethical aspects of caring for the elderly or someone living with a disability, a chronic illness, or a cognitive impairment. She has also published papers on Black feminist epistemology. Through her research in the Canadian context, she is well known as an emerging expert in Black health/ Black disability studies.

Derek W. Braverman (https://orcid.org/0000-0002-7882-2376) is a PhD student in the Department of Philosophy at Washington University in St. Louis, Missouri, in the United States, and an MD student at Johns Hopkins University, Maryland. Previously a fellow in the Department of Bioethics at the National Institutes of Health Clinical Center, Maryland, he works primarily in the philosophy of medicine.

Alex Broadbent (https://orcid.org/0000-0001-5120-3584) is Professor of Philosophy of Science at Durham University, United Kingdom, and Visiting Professor at the University of Johannesburg, South Africa. His research concerns the philosophy of epidemiology and medicine, causation, counterfactuals, prediction, complexity, conceptual aspects of machine learning, and scientific evidence in law. He is Editor-in-Chief of the journal *Philosophy of Medicine*. He is an Associate Member of Millennium Chambers, The Barrister Network, London.

John Coggon (https://orcid.org/0000-0002-6420-8420) is Professor of Law in the Centre for Health, Law, and Society, at the University of Bristol Law School in the United Kingdom. He is also an Honorary Member of the UK Faculty of Public Health. Professor Coggon is author of the monograph *What Makes Health Public?* (Cambridge University Press, 2012) and co-author, with Keith Syrett and A. M. Viens, of the textbook *Public Health Law: Ethics, Governance, and Regulation* (Routledge, 2017).

Olaf Dammann (https://orcid.org/0000-0002-0046-4863) is Professor and Vice Chair of Public Health and Community Medicine at Tufts University School of Medicine in Boston, in the United States. He is a pediatrician, perinatal epidemiologist, and philosopher of science. His most recent book is *Etiological Explanations* (CRC Press, 2020).

Michael Da Silva (https://orcid.org/0000-0002-7021-9847) is the Alex Trebek Postdoctoral Fellow in AI and Health Care and a Research Associate of the Canadian Institutes of Health Research-funded Machine M.D. team in the University of Ottawa Faculty of Law and AI + Society Initiative (Ottawa, Ontario, Canada). He discusses some issues in this chapter in *The Pluralist Right to Health Care: A Framework and Case Study* (Toronto: University of Toronto Press, 2021).

Sara L. M. Davis (https://orcid.org/0000-0003-0914-3529) is a senior researcher leading the Digital Health and Rights Project at the Global Health Center of the Graduate Institute of International and Development Studies in Geneva, Switzerland. She is author of *The Uncounted: Politics of Data in Global Health* (Cambridge University Press, 2020), and co-editor, with Carmel Williams, of the special section "Big Data, Technology, Artificial Intelligence and the Right to Health" of *Health and Human Rights Journal* (2020).

Michael Diamond-Hunter (https://orcid.org/0000-0002-6719-7325) is a Fellow in the Department of Philosophy, Logic, and Scientific Method at the London School of Economics and Political Science in the United Kingdom. His research interests include philosophy of science (including philosophy of biology and philosophy of the social sciences), philosophy of race, and philosophy of language (especially at their intersection). He is particularly interested in the ways that ontological and methodological presuppositions affect empirical projects, and is very keen on making philosophy more collaborative.

Samantha Fritz (https://orcid.org/0000-0001-9452-5892) is a PhD student at the University of Pennsylvania, Philadelphia, in the United States. Her research primarily lies in political philosophy, especially questions surrounding state legitimacy and political obligations.

Kebadu Mekonnen Gebremariam (https://orcid.org/0000-0001-9076-0895) is Assistant Professor of Philosophy at Addis Ababa University in Ethiopia. He teaches social and political philosophy, and serves as graduate programs coordinator. Prior to this, he was a visiting scholar at the Department of Ageing and Life Course at the World Health Organization in Geneva, Switzerland, where he worked with Ritu Sadana on developing the WHO's policy framework for healthy ageing. He has a PhD from the Centre for Ethics of the University of Zurich.

Daniel Goldberg (https://orcid.org/0000-0003-1843-7422) is Core Faculty in the Center for Bioethics and Humanities at the University of Colorado Anschutz Medical Campus (Aurora, Colorado, United States). He holds faculty appointments in the Department of Family Medicine and in the Department of Epidemiology, and is trained as a public health lawyer, a historian, and a public health ethicist. His current work focuses on the social determinants of health, non-communicable disease, stigma, and legal epidemiology.

Thomas Grote (https://orcid.org/0000-0002-9832-6046) is a research fellow at the Ethics and Philosophy Lab of the Cluster of Excellence "Machine Learning: New Perspectives for Science" at the University of Tübingen, Germany. His research focuses on issues in machine learning lying at the intersection of ethics and philosophy of science. In particular, he is interested in problems of interpretability, fairness, and research ethics—with an emphasis on the medical domain.

Chad Harris (https://orcid.org/0000-0002-7763-9107) is Senior Lecturer at the Department of Philosophy, University of Johannesburg, South Africa. He is a member of the African Centre for Epistemology and Philosophy of Science (ACEPS), a research center attached to the department. His primary research interest is in philosophy of science broadly construed, with particular focus on the methodology of social science. At ACEPS his research is conducted under the project "Rationality and Power."

Kristen Hessler (https://orcid.org/0000-0003-2697-8341) is an Associate Professor in the Department of Philosophy at the University at Albany (SUNY) in the United States. Her research is primarily in political philosophy and bioethics, with a focus on human rights and international law. She is currently writing a book on women's human rights.

Stephen John (https://orcid.org/0000-0002-1062-0188) is Hatton Trust Senior Lecturer in Philosophy of Public Health at the Department of History and Philosophy of Science, University of Cambridge in the United Kingdom. His research focuses mainly on the intersection between epistemological and ethical debates in public health policy. He is currently working on a project on philosophical issues in early detection of cancer.

Winnie Ma (https://orcid.org/0000-0001-9027-4459) is a Lecturer in Philosophy at King's College London and a Research Associate at the Sowerby Philosophy & Medicine Project in the United Kingdom. She teaches and works at the intersection of epistemology and ethics, specializing in the ethics of belief of stereotyping and profiling in both medical and non-medical contexts.

Michael Marmot (https://orcid.org/0000-0002-2431-6419) is Director of the Institute of Health Equity (University College London, Department of Epidemiology & Public Health) in the United Kingdom. He has been Professor of Epidemiology at University College London since 1985. He is the author of *The Health Gap: The Challenge of an Unequal World* (Bloomsbury, 2015), and *Status Syndrome: How Your Place on the Social Gradient Directly Affects Your Health* (Bloomsbury, 2004).

Mathew Mercuri (https://orcid.org/0000-0001-8070-9615) is Assistant Professor in the Department of Medicine, McMaster University, and at the Institute of Health Policy, Management and Evaluation, University of Toronto in Canada. He is also a Research Associate at the Institute for the Future of Knowledge, University of Johannesburg, South Africa, and Editor-in-Chief of the *Journal of Evaluation in Clinical Practice*.

Anya Plutynski (http://orcid.org/0000-0003-3791-7720) is Associate Professor of Philosophy at Washington University in St. Louis in the United States. Her areas of specialization are history and philosophy of biology and medicine. Her most recent book is *Explaining Cancer: Finding Order in Disorder* (Oxford University Press, 2018).

Federica Russo (https://orcid.org/0000-0002-1993-9697) is a philosopher of science and technology based in the Department of Philosophy and ILLC at the University of Amsterdam, the Netherlands. She has a long-standing interest in the methodology of the social sciences and biomedicine, and has written extensively about causal modeling, explanation, and evidence in the social and biomedical sciences and in public health. With Phyllis Illari, she has been Editor-in-Chief of the *European Journal for Philosophy of Science* since 2017. See russofederica.wordpress.com and @federicarusso.

Ritu Sadana (https://orcid.org/0000-0003-2989-3837) is a senior expert and unit head, and leads work on ageing and health and life course trajectories, at the World Health Organization's headquarters in Geneva, Switzerland. She coordinated the consultation and drafting of the *WHO Global Strategy on Ageing and Health (2016–2030),* and conceived of the Decade of Healthy Ageing, endorsed by WHO and UN member states for 2021–2030. She serves as an editorial advisor for the Bulletin of the World Health Organization.

Emily Sadecki (https://orcid.org/0000-0003-1631-5472) is an MD student at Mayo Clinic Alix School of Medicine and an MBE student at University of Pennsylvania, Philadelphia, in the United States. Her research interests include public health and vaccine ethics, and she plans on practicing medicine in a primary care specialty.

Harald Schmidt (https://orcid.org/0000-0003-4806-8816) is an Assistant Professor in the Department of Medical Ethics and Health Policy at the University of Pennsylvania's Perelman School of Medicine, in Philadelphia, in the United States. His work is centered on reducing disadvantage and improving opportunity in health promotion and priority setting.

Benjamin Smart (https://orcid.org/0000-0002-8364-4121) is an Associate Professor of Philosophy at the University of Johannesburg, South Africa, a member of the African Centre for Epistemology and Philosophy of Science, and director of the Future of Health Research Group at the Institute for the Future of Knowledge.

Maxwell J. Smith (https://orcid.org/0000-0001-5230-0548) is a public health ethicist and Assistant Professor of Bioethics and Health Policy in the Faculty of Health Sciences and Department of Philosophy at Western University in London, Ontario, Canada. His research and expertise are in infectious disease ethics and the ethical requirements of health equity and social justice in public health policy, practice, and research.

Tuhina Srivastava (https://orcid.org/0000-0002-9684-9759) is a doctoral candidate in Epidemiology in at the Perelman School of Medicine at the University of Pennsylvania, Philadelphia, in the United States. She has experience in infectious disease transmission and vaccine uptake research, both domestically and globally, and her current work focuses on health disparities in infectious disease risk and vaccination coverage in communities.

Daniel Steel (https://orcid.org/0000-0003-4448-3748) is Associate Professor at the W. Maurice Young Centre for Applied Ethics at School of Population and Public Health at the University of British Columbia, Vancouver, Canada. His research focuses on ethical issues that arise at the intersection of science and policy, especially with public health and the environment.

Jacqui Stevenson (https://orcid.org/0000-0002-1281-1607) is Gender Equality Consultant in the Department of Sexual and Reproductive Health and Research at the World Health Organization and is based in Geneva, Switzerland.

Ross E. G. Upshur (https://orcid.org/0000-0003-1128-0557) is a Professor in the Department of Family and Community Medicine and Dalla Lana School of Public Health in Toronto, Canada, where he also holds positions as Chair in Clinical Public Health and Head of the Division of Clinical Public Health. He is also an Affiliate Member, Institute for the History and Philosophy of Science and Technology, University of Toronto, the Associate Director, Lunenfeld-Tanenbaum Research Institute, and the Scientific Director, Bridgepoint Collaboratory for Research and Innovation, Sinai Health System.

Sridhar Venkatapuram (https://orcid.org/0000-0003-3076-0783) is Associate Professor of Global Health and Philosophy at King's College London in the United Kingdom. He is based at the Global Health Institute, where he is Deputy Director, and Director of Global Health Education. He publishes widely across various disciplines, has helped establish health justice philosophy, and has worked in various ethics advisory roles to public and global health institutions. He is the author of *Health Justice: An Argument from the Capabilities Approach* (2011) and co-editor of *Vulnerable: The Law, Policy and Ethics of Covid-19* (2020). He can be found at @sridhartweet.

Lavanya Vijayasingham (https://orcid.org/0000-0002-4424-4491) is a Research Fellow at London School of Hygiene and Tropical Medicine, UK. She was previously a Postdoctoral Fellow at the Gender and Health Hub, United Nations University International Institute for Global Health, in Kuala Lumpur, Malaysia.

Jeremy Youde (https://orcid.org/0000-0002-5449-1840) is the Dean of the College of Arts, Humanities, and Social Sciences at the University of Minnesota Duluth (United States). He previously held appointments at Australian National University, Grinnell College, and San Diego State University. His most recent book is *Globalization and Health* (2019).

INTRODUCTION
Philosophy and Public Health

Alex Broadbent and Sridhar Venkatapuram

"Public health" can refer to the field of professional practice that makes efforts to protect and improve health among certain groups of people, usually large in number, through means including but often outside of clinical medicine. The term can also refer to the property of health as it applies to "the public," whatever that might be. The relatively newer term "population health" is similarly used to refer to both a discipline and a property, with the additional stipulation by some authors that in its disciplinary sense, it refers to a specific kind of approach, one that foregrounds issues of justice, equity, and pays special attention to certain populations (Valles 2018). Beyond these two terms, the health disciplines in general are befogged by terminological variations even in technical aspects (Porta 2016; Rothman et al. 2008). We have not enforced any particular set of meanings on the authors contributing to this handbook, not least because doing so means adopting or aligning with one or another approach in these areas. So, without in any way judging the success of the arguments for or against one or another usage, our approach in this handbook is to be descriptive and permissive rather than normative and restrictive. However, as a rule of thumb, and certainly in this introduction, "public health" refers to the discipline (whether done in the way approved by advocates of "population health" approach; and whether done with optimally laudable goals in mind). And "population health" refers to the health of a population, that is, of a group of people however defined (and not only to identify particular populations who might be experiencing injustice). Both uses and their meanings, as can be seen, could benefit from further refinement.

This handbook is, therefore, a collection of original essays illuminating philosophical issues arising in the efforts made by diverse actors to improve the health of large numbers of people constituting various groups of interest. Which people and to whom they are of interest are among the philosophical questions at issue. These issues, and the long-standing need for a handbook such as this, may be loosely mapped as follows.

First, the nature of public health is an obvious point of contention, and one that cannot be solved or dissipated solely by empirical or practical activities. Disagreements and cross-talk arise partly because diverse disciplines contribute in various ways to public health, and partly because people may have different goals in mind while they try to improve the health of a population. People may also have different ideas about what a good health outcome would be, who the beneficiaries should be, how they should be distributed, and so forth.

DOI: 10.4324/9781315675411-1

Seven essays are included in Part 1 (Concepts and Distinctions) that parse the issue into distinct and manageable chunks. (The first part does not, however, focus on who should be the beneficiaries of public health efforts: the whole of Part 3 is devoted to that important question.) In Chapter 1, John Coggon considers what "public" in "public health" might mean: whether that term should be taken as referring to a coherent body of people, or whether a more individualistic conception of society (and perhaps one skeptical of the very notion of society) is better. Coggon digs deep into the various potential meanings of "public health" and in the process considers the role, actual and potential, of philosophy. Public health emerges as a diverse discipline in all respects, practical, conceptual, and ideological—a diversity that could be both a blessing and a curse.

In Chapter 2, Daniel Steel considers the relationship between public health and one of the diverse contributory disciplines: medicine. Starting from the obvious overlap in their respective concerns (namely, human health), Steel identifies the fundamental difference as being concerned primarily with individuals, in the case of medicine, and populations, in the case of public health. From this fundamental difference, several further differences flow: public health tends to be concerned with prevention as distinct from mitigating or curing illness; has stronger relationships than medicine with macro-level fields, including the social sciences; and faces distinct ethical issues. Steel's incisive analysis closes with an argument that these differences, while real, are ultimately of degree rather than kind.

If the relationship between public health and medicine depends on their respective concerns with group versus individuals, then we need an understanding of the relationship between groups and individuals, which Stephen John provides in Chapter 3. John distinguishes ethical tensions between perspectives of population and individual from the conceptual and epistemological challenges. He proceeds to reconcile these apparently different kinds of challenges with the novel proposal that public health is fundamentally concerned with supplying reasons, whether ethical or epistemic, that are suitable for deployment in the political realm.

Health and disease receive considerable attention in philosophy of medicine, and they are also important in philosophy of public health. In Chapter 4, Benjamin Smart guides us through the issues that arise in applying health-properties to populations. Smart sets out a number of analyses of the concepts of health and disease, and then tests their applicability at both organism and population levels. And he goes further, proposing a notion of health that can literally (not metaphorically) be applied to populations, as well as to individual organisms, namely, human beings.

In Chapter 5, the focus moves to the ethical foundations of public health. Sridhar Venkatapuram lays out the major frameworks of ethics and discusses how they might be applied to public health, as well as notes that their application to biomedical ethical problems is neither the same thing nor an adequate substitute for careful thinking about the ethics of public health. Venkatapuram also distinguishes political philosophy as another important domain of reflection that could usefully extend itself to consider questions raised by public health, which, since it recommends and informs policies, is inevitably political. Venkatapuram contemplates the appropriate methodology for ethical and political philosophical reasoning about public health, and offers some practical insights for engaging with ethics for non-philosophers.

Chapter 6 broaches one of the thorniest philosophical issues in any field: causation. Daniel Goldberg introduces fundamental cause theory, a framework from social epidemiology for thinking about the causes of health outcomes and, it is hoped, driving epidemiological research to grapple with causes that are in some important ways deeper and less superficial than others, especially the category of social determinants of health. Goldberg isolates the notion of causation currently in play, draws out some ethical implications, and provides a balanced review of criticisms, such as the persistent importance of understanding mechanisms even after acknowledging the importance of social determinants of health. Goldberg also points out the difficulty of explaining, with reference to a "fundamental cause," why health inequalities persist even when that cause is addressed (for example, by a generous welfare system).

The important theme of causation continues in Chapter 7, in which Federica Russo motivates pluralism as a reasonable stance for public health to take in response to the potentially bewildering range of philosophical efforts to promote a theory as capturing the one true meaning of "cause." Russo argues that this causal pluralism position is philosophically defensible, indeed superior to any given candidate, as well as practically useful for the public health context which, she argues, ought neither to be distracted by linguistic debates nor to be restricted by commitments to any given approach.

Public health is foremost a practical discipline and the six essays in Part 2 (Reasons and Actions) explore the intersection between conceptual issues and those that are practical. While the focus of this part is on evidential reasons, non-epistemic values intrude into nearly every chapter—an important observation in itself about the philosophy of public health. Chadwin Harris kicks off the part, tackling external validity in Chapter 8. External validity is often discussed as if it were obvious what it is, even if difficult to establish. Harris shows that some popular assumptions about external validity are hard to justify and in tension with each other, most notably between the trade-off view (that there is a trade-off between internal and external validities) and the prerequisite view (that internal validity is a prerequisite of external validity). Harris evaluates the complex literature and provides useful nuance to help avoid some of the more egregious methodological errors that this slippery concept can generate.

Moving from predictive concerns to the spaces of explanation in public health, in Chapter 9, Olaf Dammann summarizes the philosophical literature on why-questions, and doubts the utility of its outputs for public health practice. Instead, he offers a four-part classification of the *roles* explanations play in public health: scientific, justificatory, methodological, and prospective. He gives each of these a detailed explication in relation to the various processes of public health, then deals convincingly with the objection that only the scientific kind of explanation counts as a true explanation. For public health, this restrictive view hinders or is deficient in practice, and thus unacceptable in theory.

Evidence-based medicine (EBM) has dramatically influenced the practice of clinical medicine over the past few decades. In Chapter 10, Mathew Mercuri and Ross E. G. Upshur consider its younger cousin, evidence-based public health (EBPH). They usefully articulate the relationship between the two, partly by tracing their development, and go on to ask some tough questions of EBPH. Their approach is balanced, recognizing that the evidence movement has some roots in public health and has some strengths in that context. Yet, they argue that it is too restrictive for public health realities. They effectively illustrate their case with a study of mask-wearing and Covid-19.

Carrying on the link to data and evidence, profiling is the focus of Chapter 11. Winnie Ma contrasts the generally disparaging view of racial profiling by police with the uncertainty around acceptability of profiling in the public health and medical contexts. She responds in particular to recent work by Katherine Puddifoot, who argues that there are reasons both to stereotype and not to stereotype. Ma is broadly supportive of Puddifoot's stance (although differs on certain points), and Ma's contribution extends this "mixed bag" analysis to the medical and public health contexts. In these contexts, argues Ma, there are considerations both for and against profiling that differ from those that operate in the policing contexts. By identifying these, she provides a rigorous, sophisticated, and extremely useful analysis of the way that profiling can be fruitfully employed in medicine and public health, while avoiding its egregious uses.

Derek W. Braverman considers the opportunities and risk of using big data for public health in Chapter 12. He explains the big data methods of greatest significance for the field, and identifies four issues: the role of values; privacy; opacity; and health disparities. None of these issues is unique to big data at the general level, but each is relevant to the proper development and application of big data techniques in public health. Braverman takes us on a critical tour of the claims made for big data and the counter-claims that have been raised against it, concluding with a discussion of its application to omics research.

On a related theme, in Chapter 13, Thomas Grote and Alex Broadbent discuss the philosophical issues arising from potential and actual applications of machine learning (ML) to public health. The headline applications of ML have been to clinical medicine rather than public health, but Grote and Broadbent predict an upsurge of interest in the wake of Covid-19, which has prompted data scientists and major ML research groups to engage much more seriously with epidemiological and public health concerns. They provide a primer on ML and healthcare, then separate several problem bundles: ML for health monitoring and surveillance; fairness; privacy; and the changing nature of public health research itself, being driven not just by new techniques but by new actors—a process they call "Googlization." They conclude that philosophical consideration must encompass both the epistemological aspects of ML and the political economy of its development.

Political economy and ethics of the polity take center-stage in Part 3 (Distribution and Inequalities). Public health, from its roots in the nineteenth century, has been motivated by the health fate of the worst-off in society, and the contrast with the fate of the better-off. In the present day, access to clinical medicine is only one part of the explanation of this contrast. And, by taking an interest in what other changes in the circumstances of life might improve the health of the worst-off, public health inevitably strays into social, economic, and political territories, among others. The unfairness of avoidable and unequal health distributions ought, in theory, to be common ground shared by a wide range of political perspectives: a starting point of equal health is as much a precondition for unfettered liberties and competition as it is for a socialist utopia, just as hereditary wealth is anathema to both these diverse perspectives. Of course, the reality of politics does not reflect such theoretical common ground, and has many implications, as several of the chapters in this part show.

Chapter 14 includes the text of Michael Marmot's Amartya Sen Lecture delivered at the Human Development and Capability Association's 2016 conference, with an addendum reflection from late 2021. Marmot sets out his findings and stances on the social gradient of health over the course of his career: the fact that health tracks socioeconomic status at all levels, not merely below a "poverty line"; the difficulty of settling the direction of the causal arrow regarding socioeconomic position and health; the relationship between relative and absolute inequalities; the work of the World Health Organization's Commission on Social Determinants of Health and Health Equity; evidence-based policy; and whether there is a way to actually make a difference to health equity. The 2021 postscript reflects on the aftermath of the WHO commission and, of course, on the Covid-19 pandemic.

In Chapter 15, Mel Bartley presents a bold perspective on the concept of socioeconomic status, arguing that it is an outdated concept that should be abandoned. She provides a historical perspective on social class measurement in the United Kingdom and the role that eugenicist thinking plays in the genealogy of her target concept, socioeconomic status, via a functionalist understanding of that concept where an individual's function in society reflects their individual abilities and traits. She criticizes the conflation of social and economic properties and disaggregates them into social class, social status (prestige), income and wealth, and education. She then explores the relationship between inequality in each domain and public health, thus exemplifying the more nuanced approach she argues should replace vague gesturing at "socioeconomic status."

In Chapter 16, M. A. Diamond-Hunter discusses race and racism in public health. He starts at the foundations, discussing different ontological perspectives on race as they bear on the use of the concept in a public health context. He also elaborates the different senses of "racism," again with particular reference to their bearing on public health. He distinguishes different potential justifications for the use of race to support public health reasoning, including: it is at least in part related to some biological reality; and it is instrumentally valuable regardless of its ontological status. He also considers the position that it is not justifiable at all and should be abandoned. Also considered is the way that racism is understood as a public health issue—as a cause of ill-health. This careful discussion is completed with a useful forward-looking analysis of the options for proceeding in public health while carrying these difficult notions and their even more difficult underlying realities.

Sex and gender are the focus of Chapter 17, in which Avni Amin, Lavanya Vijaysingham, and Jacqui Stevens identify relevant blind spots and biases in health research. Neither biological sex nor sociological gender is systematically addressed in health research, they contend, despite the fact that both contribute to poor health outcomes. Tendencies to conflate sex and gender, and to think of male bodies as the norm, compounded by a lack of funding prioritization of research centered on sex and gender perpetuates great harms. They seek to identify those areas of health research where sex and gender need to be prioritized at the outset, and to identify means to bring this about. Guidelines are part of the answer, they argue. Another strategy is to improve uptake of existing capacity-building tools that have been developed.

The focus then turns to public health at the global level in Chapter 18, with Sara L. M. Davis considering the role of politics in shaping quantitative—and thus, perhaps, putatively objective—health indicators. Davis discusses how the definition of indicators becomes a means for global power imbalances to be exercised, creating global health inequalities, whether or not they were deliberately intentioned. Indeed, the intentions may be to reduce health inequalities. Those devising an indicator in Geneva, Switzerland or Seattle, USA may fail to appreciate how poorly it performs in Tanzania or Guyana. More conscious biases may also be at work in the creation of indices, for example, in those misrepresenting gender-based violence. Nonetheless, Davis asserts that global health indicators can be valuable in diverse ways, which is why health advocacy groups continue to insist on their improvement rather than for abandoning them.

In Chapter 19, Jeremy Youde explains how the securitization of health happens and is happening, and what it implies for public health. Securitization of a thing "X" is the process and practice of reframing X as a security threat. For health, this has potential benefits: focusing attention and resources on health, while recalibrating the concept of security to reflect the daily concerns of people (and not merely the concerns of leaders who may be more worried about securing international borders and economy than population welfare). However, securitization does not always lead to the best health policies (as has also been argued regarding securitization of environmentalism). It tends to assume that the enemy is external, especially regarding infectious diseases, which often leads to national isolationism. It can also provide a rationale for greater surveillance, promote militarization, and follow dubious priorities regarding whose security deserves protection. And, accountability is also threatened.

The upshot, Youde argues, is a mixed and complicated picture of a process and practice that ought to be handled with caution, despite seeming like health is being prioritized.

Chapter 20, by Samantha Fritz, Tuhina Srivastava, Emily Sadecki, and Harald Schmidt, reverts to a Global North focus to consider what the disproportionate impact of Covid-19 of racialized groups that are minorities in the US (but not globally) can tell us about distributive justice and health in the US. This deep dive into the American context lays out, in considerable detail, how national bodies sought to address inequalities between groups of different ethnicities and in different places, both in susceptibility to harmful Covid-19 outcomes and in vaccination uptake rates. A contrastingly general survey is offered of philosophical work on disadvantage. The lesson is that practical public health was advanced using the indicators described, and could potentially be applied in other areas of public health—a conclusion that must of course be carefully modulated by the various considerations raised by Davis in Chapter 18.

No discussion of public health would be complete without a discussion of rights and duties, and Part 4 (Rights and Duties) completes the volume with six essays covering both general and condition-specific issues.

It is often thought that public health is deeply committed to social justice as a normative or guiding framework. Maxwell J. Smith asks, in Chapter 21, whether this widespread assumption bears out under scrutiny. His plausible contention is that it does so only if the notion is sufficiently clear, and further that the commitment to social justice may cause disagreement, confusion, and even harm without such clarification. Smith begins with a lucid analysis of the concept of justice itself, explicating it as that which exists when individuals are rendered what is due to them—that to which they have a moral claim, in proportion to the strength and extent of that claim. He distinguishes distributive, relational, and procedural justice, and contrasts various conceptions of the object or currency of distributive justice (welfare, opportunities, capabilities, resources), as well as different target patterns of distribution (maximization, equality, priority, sufficiency). Against this background, Smith goes on to detail various conceptions of social justice in public health as relating to health equity, equality of opportunity, capability, well-being, structural fairness, and utilitarianism. He also considers the oft-neglected context of global health.

In Chapter 22, Michael Da Silva addresses the complex ways in which rights are related to health, public health, and healthcare. Rights are claimed in relation to health, and often imply—or are taken to imply—duties of states or other actors to do or provide something, and explanation when they do not fulfill the duties. What justifies such claims? Da Silva charts a careful course through the thicket of disagreements about what rights to health there are and what duties these imply upon which entities. He does so by means of a guiding question as to whether a philosophically (rather than merely rhetorically) useful formulation of an individual health-right can also recognize the moral priority of population health. He considers the grounds there are for a right to health, a right to healthcare, and a right to public health, before outlining his preferred approach: any satisfactory account of health-related rights must, he argues, include at least some consideration of the population perspective and must include both substantive rights and procedural stipulations, because no statement of substantive rights alone can avoid borderline cases.

Chapter 23 directs our attention to the fraught links between public health and disability. Agnès Berthelot-Raffard makes a case that public health has not been serving the full interests of disabled people because it recognizes the biomedical aspects of disability while ignoring the social and other relational aspects that make people disabled. If public health aims to mitigate or remove impairments, what is it to do about and with individuals who are disabled for the long term? This "public health versus disability rights" discussion is backgrounded by an argument that modern capitalism, ableism, and biostatistical theory of health have combined to marginalize the disabled. The view developed, in line with critical disability studies and activism, is that disability is in fact a form of social oppression. Berthelot-Raffard points toward a conception of disability justice that creates common ground between public health and the disabled community by first centering on the moral experience of being disabled, and extrapolating that knowledge to all people, as everyone will be disabled at one time or another in their lifetime.

In Chapter 24, Kebadu Mekonnen Gebremariam and Ritu Sadana address the way that justice concerns bear upon a growing concern across the world: population aging. There are increasing numbers of older people in countries, and many of the world's older people will live in low- and middle-income countries. Societies and global institutions are simply not ready to support larger number of older people. And one of the foremost issues is how to meet the needs of older people. They contrast perspectives that weigh the interests of distinct age groups with life-course perspectives, arguing that both can be linked to two mainstream conceptions of distributive justice: luck egalitarianism and sufficientarianism. They conclude with an analysis of the potential future scenarios regarding how the global society of nations will address the needs of older people.

Chapter 25 sets out the subtleties of cancer considered from a public health perspective. Anya Plutynski points out that the vast majority of research spending in recent decades has focused on basic science, clinical science, and pharmaceutical development. In the US, estimates for the proportion of health research spending on public health research are in the range of 1–5%. Plutynski homes in on the philosophical issues challenging public health research on cancer: the nature of causation, the best methods for discovering it, evidential underdetermination, and value trade-offs. Along the way, she highlights how health disparities arise, using race and cancer mortality as a case study.

Finally, in Chapter 26, Kristen Hessler contemplates the relationship between public health, human rights, and philosophy. She sees public health and philosophy as both undergoing transformations, and is optimistic about the prospects for a rights-based approach to public health. This will happen, provided that human rights and public health are understood non-traditionally, and thus evolve their conceptual frameworks appropriately. On the rights side, this means including social, economic, and cultural rights within the common understanding of human rights. And public health must see the preservation of rights not as a potential obstacle to effective interventions, but as a part of the mission of public health.

The volume thus ends in an optimistic mood, with the recognition of profound transformations within public health and philosophy. We hope that readers will find the handbook provocative on occasion and useful throughout.

References

Porta, M. 2016. *A dictionary of epidemiology.* 6th edition. Oxford University Press, Oxford.

Rothman, K. J., S. Greenland, and T. L. Lash. 2008. *Modern epidemiology.* 3rd edition. Philadelphia, PA: Lippincott Williams & Wilkins.

Valles, S. A. 2018. *Philosophy of population health science: Philosophy for a new public health era.* Routledge, Abingdon, Oxfordshire.

PART 1

Concepts and distinctions

1

THE PUBLIC IN PUBLIC HEALTH

John Coggon

Philosophy, public health, and the significance of context in framing the public in public health

The philosophy of public health, as evidenced in the chapters in this volume, embraces diverse points and sources of inquiry, analysis, and understanding. These include questions concerning our means of understanding what, why, and how the dynamics of public health are, by drawing, for example, from social ontology, theories of causality, and epistemology. The chapters also cover methods of explaining how things should be; engaging questions of health within the fields of social ethics and justice, and disciplines such as legal, moral, and political philosophies. And relatedly, they provide direction on how different actors, such as practitioners, researchers, government departments, or public officials, should behave or make decisions, here studying health through disciplines such as political science, behavioral economics, and psychology.

These broad bases and forms of analysis may stem from distinct areas of inquiry within the philosophy of public health, and from distinct structures of knowledge, understanding, and reasoning more widely (Venkatapuram and Bibby 2018). Nevertheless, they also have the clear potential to overlap and intersect. And the broad variety of "is" and "ought" questions they give rise to are endemic in public health research, policy, and practice. We may be designing an epidemiological study to advance our understanding of *the causes* of the incidence of cardiac disease. Or we may be engaging through social science methods with questions of how different communities, groups, or publics are *defined* and then *understood* to enjoy better or worse health. Or we may be considering what (if any) methods of regulation might *justifiably* be instituted to lower rates of unhealthy weight. In any such instance, or others that might be listed, public health activities are important because of three overlapping points. First, because health (whatever it is taken to mean) matters. Second, because it matters to look at health through a public (whatever that is taken to mean) lens. And third, because it matters to address health through public (again, whatever that is taken to mean) mechanisms. This chapter aims to elucidate some key issues in relation to these points by exploring what is distinctive in focusing on the public in public health.

To give a sense of the variety of ideas that may arise, I begin here with reference to my own earlier conceptual analysis in a book that explored the question "what makes health

DOI: 10.4324/9781315675411-3

public?" (Coggon 2012). That work looked at, among other things, the concepts of health, public, and public health. I argued that across different sources discussing or engaging with the idea of public health, we find it defined, characterized, or treated as holding a plurality of quite distinct meanings and functions. I represented these in summary as follows:

1   Public health as a political tool: in this sense, "public health" is used as an important end, denoting (supposedly) strong or compelling reasons for formulating policy. Here, the term may be seen to imply a social mission, a social theory, or a naturally good concept. [...]
2   Public health as government business: as a function of government, public health may be understood narrowly as relating to the competence or responsibility of specific health agencies, widely as any governmental power that affects health, or somewhere between these extremes.
3   Public health as the social infrastructure: in this sense, public health is taken to represent society's organisation [...] in respect to [...] non-State responsibility for health that nevertheless may described as public in character.
4   Public health as a professional enterprise: public health refers here to professional approaches [...] for example, to the scope of a professional's practical competence [...], to the nature of expertise that a professional has, or to his work's being health-related.
5   Public health as blind benefit/harm: public health may be used as a qualifier to represent probable benefits or harms within a population [...] to denote instances of certain harm where the specific identity of those harmed [or benefited] is unclear [..., or] instances where ex ante the ultimate beneficiaries are not known [...].
6   Public health as conjoined beneficiaries: here "the public" has moral, "solidaristic" connotations [...].
7   Public health as the population's health: this [...] refers to the health of a population, either in aggregate or by reference to distribution [...].

(Coggon 2012: 46–47)

This range of meanings and uses of public health indicates quite how broad-reaching an analysis of the public in public health might be. Public health means many things and is used to imply or provoke multiple ideas, even, at times, ideologies. For explanatory reasons, I will tease out in this chapter's analysis distinctions in more descriptive "is" questions and more normative "ought" questions when considering the public in public health. However, in practice, it is the very melding of descriptive and normative considerations that makes philosophical analysis so essential to understanding public health (Harper et al. 2010; Powers and Faden 2006; Venkatapuram 2011). Indeed, among public health communities, the links between ideas rooted in political theory and activism have a long and considerable legacy. And they necessarily have ongoing relevance to discussions of the philosophy and practice of public health (Mackenbach 2009). Of note too, within philosophical literatures more broadly, the idea of public health has long provided stock examples for critical discussion. These include analyses of the idea of public goods (see, for example, Geuss 2003), or questions concerning the justifiability (or otherwise) of state paternalism and policies such as the mandatory wearing of seatbelts in cars or helmets on motorcycles, placing prohibitions on substances such as narcotics, or moves to limit the use of—or ban—smoking tobacco (see, for example, Conly 2012; Feinberg 1989).

The culmination of these distinct factors and sources of normative concerns may be seen, in particular, in the scope and content of public health ethics. Public health ethics spans across professional values, social activist and governmental aims, and more "pure" or abstract points of philosophical inquiry (Jennings 2003). It has, over the past couple of decades, emerged as a discrete area of inquiry, an area of practical analysis that all of the contributors to this book have helped, and are helping, to develop. Nancy Kass explains how it formed as a field in its own right around the year 2000. Prior to that, Kass suggests, the majority of philosophical attention to public health was broadly contained in specific questions concerning health promotion agendas, HIV and AIDS, and rationales for different methods of resource allocation (Kass 2004). Significant and influential studies existed from within public health communities (broadly conceived), such as those embodied in works published in journals such as *Critical Public Health* and its previous manifestation *Radical Community Medicine* (Bunton and Wills 2004). However, the coming of age of the philosophy of public health *for and by philosophers* may be seen with the advent of journals such as *Public Health Ethics,* launched in 2008, and a broad surge around that time in academic attention through conferences, textbooks, monographs, and articles.

This book as a whole is motivated by a concern that better integration of philosophy within public health is needed: the philosophy of public health should not just be for and by philosophers. Yet, the formalization of fields such as public health ethics has as yet failed to gain the traction it promises to offer. As I hope to show in this chapter, it has also generated assumptions, norms, and understandings that may be measured against philosophical framings and ideological commitments that themselves are local to particular jurisdictions and cultures. These matters emphasize the need to invite better-engaged philosophical consideration of the work that might be done by the public in public health. Relatedly, they allow us to see how there is no neutral (in the sense of being unsituated) starting point for philosophical inquiry into public health as a phenomenon or cluster of phenomena. The philosophy of public health is unavoidably embedded in particular human societies and political communities.

In line with Kass' predictions on the direction of public health ethics, over the past twenty years, we have seen strong and rigorously argued positions on how to achieve global health with justice (see, for example, Gostin 2014; Gostin et al. 2019). Nevertheless, Sridhar Venkatapuram, one of the editors of this volume, has argued that progress in philosophy has not been matched by real-world improvements:

> The singular failure of philosophers and global health policy planners and practitioners has been our failure to create and engender moral motivation, a will—among those who are able—to prevent millions of human deaths and create conditions for good health within and across countries. The major global health actors, including funders, do not even share a minimal concept of commitment to equity.
>
> *(Venkatapuram 2021: 178)*

With those points made, it must bear stating that I write as a British, male, middle-aged, middle-class, white, legal scholar based in the United Kingdom (and more specifically still, in England). The greater part of my ideas is informed by the context and structural norms of the United Kingdom's political and legal systems, and their institutional and normative underpinnings, including being a parliamentary liberal democracy, with areas of political devolution (including for (public) health), a healthcare service that is free to access at the point of delivery, and a common law system. I engage in work with organizations that aim to serve and promote the public's health. And I recognize both the limitations, given my own positioning, and the broader structural limitations that Venkatapuram laments. At the same time, I am pleased to see how my work has been adapted to facilitate analysis in other jurisdictions and systems (see, for example, Kumar 2020a, 2020b). With due qualifications and caveats, I hope therefore that this indicates a utility in what follows beyond a United Kingdom-focused readership.

In approaching the idea of public health, I am particularly influenced by the seminal conceptual analysis by philosophers Marcel Verweij and Angus Dawson in their paper "The Meaning of 'Public' in 'Public Health'" (Verweij and Dawson 2007). Verweij and Dawson identify and review a series of influential definitions of public health and distill from them two particular concerns. Sometimes, they argue, the public in public health can denote the distinct points and insights learned or observed by considering or approaching health at a population level: whether from studying health effects of or between populations, by asking how and why different populations or sub-populations enjoy/suffer different levels of (ill) health, looking at the impacts of population-level interventions, and so forth. Alternatively, they argue, the public in public health can invite a focus on collective action or methods of social coordination: what "we as a society do," or how the "organized efforts of society" may operate, in order to protect and promote health. This may be about government responsibility for the public's health but could also be about the activities of nongovernmental actors. Although this second sense of public does not limit its focus to governmental public health activities, it implies a boundary between collective and shared responsibilities for health, on the one hand, and a private sphere where responsibilities for health remain personal or private matters, on the other. These distinct ideas around "public" both reflect and reflect back on the centrality of social, institutional, political, and scientific contexts.

I will flesh these ideas out more in the next part of this chapter. But anticipating the conceptual and normative challenges against which such analysis will take place, it is instructive to conclude this part of the discussion by presenting two dismissals of these respective ideas of the public in public health from critical, philosophical literatures. Both come from the liberal traditions associated with Anglo-American jurisdictions, and both preexisted the formalization of the field of public health ethics as described above. These are fundamental to how I frame my discussion: one concerns the ontology of the public and the other concerns the justification for acting on the public.

In relation to the idea of the public as a population and *its* health, the very first issue of the journal *Bioethics*, in 1987, contained a paper by Richard D. Mohr titled "Aids, Gays, and State Coercion" (Mohr 1987). Mohr argued that while there may be legitimate "metaphoric uses" of the term *public health:*

> No literal sense exists in which there could be such a thing as a public health. To say the public has a health is like saying the number seven has a color: such a thing cannot have such a property. You have health or you lack it and I have health or lack it, because we each have a body with organs that function or do not function. But the public, an aggregate of persons similarly disposed as persons, has no such body of organs with functions which work or fail.
>
> *(Mohr 1987: 96)*

Mohr's perspective raises questions of appropriate descriptive exercises: can we employ articulations such as "the health of the public" or "population health improvement" with more than (just) metaphorical meaning? And it gives rise to further questions of how policy approaches and justifications are framed: can health interventions be justified through population health framings?

Mohr's position may represent elements of liberal skepticism of the ontology of the social. These can be seen with much greater force in Petr Skrabanek's writings, which challenge the second sense of public in public health. Skrabanek aims to rebut the normative validity of governments and professional institutions engaging in public health promotion. Writing in the mid-1990s, in a characteristically scathing tone, Skrabanek presents and attacks the idea of "coercive healthism." Within Skrabanek's framing, what are generally presented as (public) health interventions are mere masks for practically-dangerous and philosophically-dubious political ideology. The roots of the dangerous and dubious ideas, according to Skrabanek, reside in the concept of health. For him, health is necessarily normative (value-laden), and is only properly defined by the individual, rather than the state or a professional elite (see also Illich 1995). Skrabanek argues:

> Health, like love, beauty or happiness, is a metaphysical concept, which eludes all attempts at objectivisation. Healthy people do not think of health, unless they are hypochondriacs, which, strictly speaking, is not a sign of health [...] It is the absence of health that gives rise to dreaming about health, just as the real meaning of freedom is only experienced in prison.
>
> *(Skrabanek 1994: 15)*

On Skrabanek's analysis, making health a matter of government policy or institutionalized professional activity is "a symptom of political sickness" (Skrabanek 1994: 15). Health, he argues, is an exclusively subjective phenomenon (contrast with Sen 2004). It follows that governments or professional hegemonies that fixate on and aim to protect a particular concept of health are actually alighting on and enforcing a particular, hidden ideology. This comes at the cost both of other, no less valid, conceptualizations of the good, and—crucially for Skrabanek—at the cost of a very broad understanding of individual freedom. In accordance with these ideas, what "we as a society" should do for the public's health is very little, beyond the aggregation of individually-led activities, which are functioning outside the direction of institutional actors such as governments and professional elites.

If the public in public health is to do philosophically coherent and legitimately productive work, we need to consider how we might respond to these sorts of challenges to the idea of thinking about the public's health or the place of government and other social actors in protecting and promoting health. The next part of the chapter, through three sections, accordingly addresses the conceptual and practical question of what, or who, is the public in public health.

What, or who, is the public in public health?

The first part of this chapter has shown that however we identify the public in public health, our understanding will depend on the practical context, as well as the critical or methodological approach we take to answering the question. Although this may seem a statement of the obvious, its implications for all of public health sciences, practice, and policy make it worth explaining, and underpin the importance of this book as a whole. As already indicated, context and approach directly influence what we may *do* with a public health framing—or how and why we may see resistance to framing something as a question of public health.

In the following three sections, I explain whether and how any philosophical coherence may be found in the idea of *public* health, and what normative or evaluative considerations come into play as we use that idea: what may be gained by focusing on the, or a, public, or something being public. Who or what is distinctively identified within a *public* health perspective? Without begging the questions of how, why, or in what ways health and health-affecting phenomena might be *shared* concerns (a point explored in what follows), we can stipulate up front that for the public in public health to mean something, it relates to points that underpin those questions. There are different ways that we might arrive at a positive answer to the conceptual coherence and practical good of looking at health through a "public" lens. Alex Mold and colleagues, for example, conceptualize the public in public health across three dimensions: "as a collection of people; as a space for action; and as a set of values" (Mold et al. 2019: 7). In what follows, I also look across three dimensions. These correspond with the three listed here, but do not overlap entirely. First, I look to what we might distinctively learn by observing health at population levels. I then consider conceptual questions about what a public is. And finally, I present a politico-legal framing about the idea of publicness. In each instance, I aim to explain some of the strengths and coherence that may be found, as well as challenges and problems.

The health of different publics

We saw above Mohr's claim that health is not something that can be possessed by a public. That position was rooted in the idea that health is a property of organic entities; and at most, a public is only metaphorically able to enjoy (or suffer ill) health. Bruce Jennings, a pioneer within the philosophy of public health, highlights similar problems in treating a public as a natural phenomenon in the sort of sense that Mohr guards against:

> This is a reified concept of the public; it conceives of the public as if it were a natural thing—an organic whole with its own interests, needs, and being—as opposed to a socially constructed, imaginary life-world. Reification—treating social reality as if it were material or natural reality—leads the theorist to predicate to the entity moral, legal, and other normative properties that are predicated to human persons. The public has rights, interests, obligations. It can be harmed or injured.
>
> *(Jennings 2007: 54)*

Does it follow from such views that it is outright mistaken to use articulations such as "the public's health"? One way to answer "no" to this question is to look at what is distinctively learned in population health sciences. That is, we might consider how lessons are learned by looking at the health of populations; of different publics.

At a basic and (apparently—contrast Harper et al. 2010) descriptive level, we might be interested in studying the health of publics because different health-related phenomena can be observed only by studying health dynamics among populations. These may include inferences regarding causation of disease, or observations about the different incidences of disease among different groups or communities. Such group- or population-level understandings, in turn, create avenues to alternative approaches to health protection and improvement: notably, but far from exclusively, some population-level interventions may not demonstrably benefit any specific individual but do provide demonstrable health benefits across a group of people. As reflected in Mohr's and Jennings' respective warnings, in liberal political philosophy and social ethics, there is long-standing disagreement about whether publics or "the social" exist as something that is meaningfully distinguishable from and applied against the individual people the public comprises. A seminal reference point to help elucidate how we achieve the distinct understandings found by looking at health at a population level is epidemiologist Geoffrey Rose's paper "Sick Individuals and Sick Populations" (Rose 1985).

Rose's analysis serves two purposes: an explanatory purpose regarding health status and its causes, and a critical and policy-oriented purpose, given his ideas' sociopolitical implications (on which more below). Regarding the first, explanatory goal, Rose discusses how looking at health dynamics between populations—engaging in epidemiological research across different populations—provides novel understandings. For example, it provides insights into the causation of disease that cannot be achieved when only looking at individuals within a single population, or with reference to individual risk factors that might be observed in clinical medicine. He illustrates this point with reference to our understandings of causation and the health harms of tobacco:

> If everyone smoked 20 cigarettes a day, then clinical, case-control, and cohort studies alike would lead us to conclude that lung cancer was a genetic disease; and in one sense that would be true, since if everyone is exposed to the necessary agent, then the distribution of cases is wholly determined by individual susceptibility.
>
> *(Rose 1985: 32)*

However, by looking at two populations, smokers and nonsmokers, we gain novel and distinct understandings. The higher-level disease among the smoking population would lead us to examine smoking as a causal factor. In developing the distinct insights from looking at different populations, Rose explains that these forms of understanding allow us then to draw inferences about how and why the frequency or incidence of disease differs across the different populations. Another example that Rose provides explains that the question of why men in Finland have higher average serum cholesterol levels becomes more readily answerable when they are compared to the men in Japan. It is because most Finnish men eat much more fat than Japanese men do.

So, looking at health (and disease) at a population level—at "a public's health"—allows inferences to be drawn about causal influences on people's health, and about disparities in levels of health across different populations. This supra-individual level of analysis provides insights that just could not be drawn by observing and comparing individuals as individuals. In so doing, and very importantly, it also allows us to identify *upstream* causes of ill health in the individual: to identify "causes of causes" of ill health in individuals. For example, we may see how our built environment, which is determined by social practices, may lead to higher rates of excess body fat in individuals. And we may see how this, in turn, may lead to higher incidence of diseases such as type-2 diabetes or cardiac disease in individuals within the population. Relatedly, population-level analysis allows us to observe factors—say, higher consumption of salt or use of statins—that do have influence on health where, at an individual level, the impact may be negligible or undiscernible among most lower-risk people (that is, people not showing clinical indications of susceptibility to disease).

In these senses, there is important meaning—and value—in looking at the health of publics, as opposed to just that of individuals. So far, this does not require the reification of publics. But it does lead to more than merely metaphorical value of talking about population health (or, in Mohr's words, "a public health"). It, in turn, also allows us to speak to the idea of healthier or less healthy causes, such as (public) spaces: interpreted here broadly to incorporate the natural, built, and social environments in which we live. Again, the suggestion is not literal—that a space itself can be "healthy"—but it is possible to show how environments impact on people's health opportunities and outcomes.

This brings us into the terrain of social epidemiology and the social determinants of health. The World Health Organization (WHO) defines these very broadly:

> The social determinants of health (SDH) are the non-medical factors that influence health outcomes. They are the conditions in which people are born, grow, work, live, and age, and the wider set of forces and systems shaping the conditions of daily life. These forces and systems include economic policies and systems, development agendas, social norms, social policies and political systems.
>
> The SDH have an important influence on health inequities—the unfair and avoidable differences in health status seen within and between countries. In countries at all levels of income, health and illness follow a social gradient: the lower the socioeconomic position, the worse the health.
>
> *(World Health Organization, n.d.)*

The social determinants of (ill) health have a broad reach, and within them public health scholars have focused on different aspects: for example, legal, commercial, and political determinants of health (see, for example, respectively, Gostin et al. 2019; McKee and Stuckler 2018; Ottersen et al. 2014).

Health sciences predominate the ideas discussed in this section. I therefore close with a qualified note of caution, in particular given the strong appeal of scientific neutrality or objectivity in the idea of evidence-based practice and policy. We can, and I would argue should, accept the distinct importance of population-level understandings. However, in doing so, we may still challenge the idea that observations in (social) epidemiology are purely descriptive. Normative ideas inevitably arise through the concept of health itself (Coggon 2012: Chapters 1 and 11). And as Sam Harper and colleagues have shown, the measurements selected to represent health data will rest on their own (often implicit) value judgments (Harper et al. 2010). Furthermore, the WHO brings normative terminology into its characterization of the social determinants of health, seeking identification of *inequities* and *unfair* differences. And when looking to implementing policy, Rose identifies another, ultimately normative, sociopolitical challenge, in the idea of the "prevention paradox": if our population-level, norm-shifting intervention also encompasses lower-risk individuals through policy measures, we are perhaps imposing a cost on these individuals through a regulatory burden, which may provide no (demonstrable), or only minimal, benefit in any given person's case. For example, a measure to change people's diet to lower the incidence of cardiac disease, targeted at lower-risk populations, may be demonstrably effective at a population level while individual beneficiaries of the policy prove impossible to identify. As such, while our analysis of the public in public health does well to look at the unique insights and understandings of population health research, we need as well to look further to the normative work of ideas of publics and things being public. These are addressed, respectively, in the following two sections.

The public, publics, community, and fragmentation

In the passage quoted above, Jennings argues against a reified understanding of "the public." However, this does not mean that he shuns *any* conceptual or practical rigor to entities being categorized as publics. In fact, he identifies a particularly strong concept of a population conceived as "a public" formed through the binds of *shared concerns* that generate what are recognized as political communities. He frames the ideas in these terms:

> Shared purposes or problems are not the same as individual purposes or problems that happen to overlap for large numbers of people. Of course, they do affect persons as individuals and as members of smaller groups, but they also affect the constitutions of a "people," a population of individuals as a structured social whole. An aggregation of individuals becomes a people, a public, a political community when it is capable of recognizing common purposes and problems in this way; and what allows it to have this kind of political understanding and imagination has largely to do with a dynamic interplay between what I shall call *action* and *structure* over time.
>
> *(Jennings 2007: 48)*

Jennings' arguments urge us toward a philosophy of public health rooted in ideas of civic republicanism. But his framing here is more generally applicable: it could also relate to a system of libertarianism such as that espoused by Skrabanek all the way through to highly collectivist political systems. What is important here is not the superiority of any given political system. Rather, it is the idea of the shared understanding and recognition, across time, of the identity of "a structured social whole." Such a group is bound together through shared recognition of political and legal systems of governance, with the special institutional status that those ideas imply. Jennings' work is directly informed by understandings from sociology and political sciences (Anderson 1991) and may be seen as mirrored in some ways in theories of legal positivism (Hart 1997). In relation to the public in public health of concern in this section, Jennings' ideas may be presented in more positive as well as more challenging terms.

More positively, the idea of shared political identity and common purposes promotes shared concerns for health: health is not—conceptually or practically—properly considered (without analysis) as just a matter for the individual. One person's health, or health-affecting activity, may well be the concern of another, and of the institutions of the society in which they live. The basis of such a position, and its practical extent, will necessarily rest on normative ideas about the very structure of political community (Coggon 2012: Chapters 7 and 8). But this means that even if we reject a reified concept of the public, we can recognize the public as something that exists, and within which shared responsibilities for health may function: for example, generating responsibilities to restructure social institutions, given evidence about social and institutional causes of disease from epidemiological research.

Against this idea, challenging questions may be seen to arise at two important levels. The first we may characterize as "internal." On the understanding of a public as a political community, we may consider, for example, "the British people," or the people who are within the jurisdiction of the United Kingdom. Among such a grouping, there will be complexities when and where there is inadequate sense of shared purposes or problems: this may be because, given structural conditions and institutional practices, particular groups or communities may be and/or feel marginalized or otherwise excluded or alienated. Or it may be because the politico-legal structures actively create an "othering" effect, as with the recent government efforts to create a "hostile environment" as part of the United Kingdom's immigration policy (Prabhat 2020).

From an "external" perspective, alternative problems arise in relation to *political* connectivity when we move beyond the conceptual and institutional boundaries of a nation-state or confederal structure and the ideas that these permit of "a structured social whole." This is most apparent when we consider questions of global interconnectedness and global health. Jennifer Prah Ruger, writing in 2011, presents the problem well in discussing ideas about governance and global health:

> Global health has experienced a record entry of private and public actors with unprecedented funding levels. This hyper-pluralism and fragmentation have received popular and academic attention, characterising them as anarchic and requiring coordination and control. [It is possible to illustrate the] congested, chaotic and complex nature of the activities of various global health actors. Public and private actors each pursue their own goals and preferences and not necessarily those of their "beneficiaries." Overlapping interests among donors can cause confusions and paralysis that dissipate or delay aid. Conflicts in donor priorities and requirements create competition and duplication of activities that overwhelm recipient countries' institutional capacities. By creating parallel facilities, systems and procedures, donors distort the design, implementation and sustainability of health programmes. So far, attempts to coordinate proliferating global health actors have fallen short.
>
> *(Prah Ruger 2012: 653; references omitted)*

As suggested by the quote from Venkatapuram in the first part of this chapter, almost a decade since Prah Ruger made these observations the landscape is not markedly different in how it might be characterized. In part, this may be due to the fragmentation that follows when conceiving of different publics in the sense of political communities: as Venkatapuram puts it, conceiving of "those people over there" (Venkatapuram 2021: 178).

In summary, this section has discussed how we may arrive at robust concepts of publics. These go beyond identification of groups by reference to particular individual characteristics, such as being a smoker, or a woman aged between 30 and 39. Concepts of publics can look to how *communities* and *institutions* are recognized and give rise to particular forms of normative orientation. Such ideas of publics may promote ideas of health as a shared and mutual concern, but as discussed, they may also alienate within and between publics, and in doing so, undermine efforts to act on health as a shared concern within and across societies.

Public versus private: liberal politico-legal framings of the "publicness" of health-affecting activities and spaces

As we focus on more political, normatively-loaded understandings, we may consider not just what is done by identifying someone as part of a public. We also do well to examine the idea of publicness: within a community, what makes a particular matter relating to health a public matter? Overall, I would argue, this is a question that will be inextricably linked to a basic political philosophy (Coggon 2012: Chapters 7 and 8, Coggon 2014). But a useful angle for framing ideas about approaching this issue comes from the contrasts that can be drawn between something being public and something being private (Coggon 2012: Chapter 2). Of different approaches that may be taken, it is instructive to consider the idea of privacy as it is presented in Article 8 of the European Convention on Human Rights (ECHR). Article 8 provides a qualified protection to a privacy right: that is, it stipulates a right to privacy, but also permits that government interference with the right will be permissible if it is lawful, necessary in pursuit of a legitimate aim, and proportionate.[1] The right itself is framed as follows: "Everyone has the right to respect for his private and family life, his home and his correspondence."

Within the United Kingdom, and in other jurisdictions where the ECHR applies, Article 8 is a significant reference point against which public health measures are evaluated. I do not refer to Article 8 jurisprudence because I think that it provides an authoritative source simply by virtue of its being law. Rather, judicial treatment of the right to private and family life allows a clear and well-formulated account of the potential for the intertwining of moral, personal, political, and legal considerations under the heading of privacy. That, in turn, gives an interesting philosophical framing for how and why we might consider something—for example, a health-affecting behavior such as smoking tobacco—to be a public as opposed to a private matter, a concern of others and of government, rather than just of the individual herself.

We may begin to drill into this with reference to an influential and clear framing from a decision of the House of Lords—the United Kingdom's then highest court, which has since been replaced by the Supreme Court—in which Baroness Hale formulated her ideas as follows:

> Article 8, it seems to me, reflects two separate but related fundamental values. One is the inviolability of the home and personal communications from official snooping, entry and interference without a very good reason. It protects a private space, whether in a building, or through the post, the telephone lines, the airwaves or the ether, within which people can both be themselves and communicate privately with one another. The other is the inviolability of a different kind of space, the personal and psychological space within which each individual develops his or her own sense of self and relationships with other people. This is fundamentally what families are for and why democracies value family life so highly. Families are subversive. They nurture individuality and difference. One of the first things a totalitarian regime tries to do is to distance the young from the individuality of their own families and indoctrinate them in the dominant view. Article 8 protects the private space, both physical and psychological, within which individuals can develop and relate to others around them. But that falls some way short of protecting everything that they might want to do even in that private space; and it certainly does not protect things that they can *only* do by leaving it and engaging in a very public gathering and activity.
>
> (R (Countryside Alliance) *2007: para. 116*)

The case in which Baroness Hale made this statement asked whether a legislative ban on fox hunting was compatible with the applicants' human rights. The reasoning allowed a private/public distinction to be drawn: first, in relation to the decisional motivation to undertake the activity and its personal significance—it was a matter of profound value to the individuals who were now banned from doing it—and, second, *where* the activity took place—it was very much a public activity in that sense. In the end, the balance between these led to the conclusion that the legislation was not an unlawful affront to the individuals' privacy rights.

To see how these ideas relate to a public health context, it is useful to read the Rampton smokers' case (R *(G and B)* 2008; R *(N)* 2009). This concerned a legal challenge to regulations made under the statute that provided for smoking bans in England and Wales: the Health Act 2006. The applicants were detained at Rampton, a secure psychiatric hospital. They argued that for people in their situation, an exemption should be provided against the general ban on smoking tobacco in enclosed and substantially-enclosed public and work spaces. This was on the basis that the law amounted, for people in their situation, to an outright ban on smoking: smoking indoors would be unlawful and smoking outdoors was not feasible. They accordingly claimed that it interfered with their right to respect for their private life and home.[2] The government and National Health Service Trust, against whom the challenge was brought, argued that Article 8 did not provide a "right to smoke." They also argued, in case that was not accepted, that if Article 8 were engaged, the interference with it would anyway be justifiable as a proportionate interference with the right in pursuit of a legitimate aim, namely, the protection of health.

In the Court of Appeal, the majority decision of Lord Clarke MR and Lord Justice Moses ruled in favor of upholding the ban. Of interest here is how the ideas of privateness/publicness within their reasoning were framed in line with Baroness Hale's ideas quoted above (and other rulings in that case). The judges' analysis of whether there could be justification for state interference with the decision to smoke rested on the following ideas:

- First, that we must consider two distinct sorts of questions of normative importance:
  - Questions about decisional importance: how significant·or fundamental a matter is to a person's physical or moral integrity, identity, or autonomy; and
  - Questions about place and space: how private or public is the space in which the activity is undertaken?
- Secondly, that we consider publicness as a graded concept: matters may be more or less private/public in each of the two senses, and the more private something might be in either sense, the higher the justification needed to demonstrate that it is legitimately treated as a public matter, a matter for law and policy (see *R (N)* 2009: paras. 30–52).

As indicated, I am not directly interested in whether the majority or minority were right in the decision in the case. Rather, I would argue that this framing is useful in considering how we might arrive at a conclusion on what makes health (or anything) "public" within a liberal system. The detainees' smoking—their health-affecting behavior—was made public because of its relative unimportance, in the majority judges' estimation, as a personal decision, combined with the relatively more public nature of their place of residence. In their words, "Rampton is not the same as a private home and the distinction is of significance" (*R (N)* 2009: para. 40). Thus, even after considering the significance of the liberal ideas of Isaiah Berlin (*R (N)* 2009: para. 42), and legal protections of "the right to act in a way that is or may be considered undesirable, foolish or irrational" (*R (N)* 2009: para. 47) they held:

> Since the nature of the place in which the appellants seek to smoke tells against any right protected by article 8, those seeking protection are compelled to rely to a greater extent on the importance of the activity they seek freedom to pursue. The less the appellant can rely upon the nature of the place in which the activity is pursued, the more he must rely upon the proximity of the activity to his personal identity or physical and moral integrity. Of course we accept that every activity a detained patient is free to pursue is all the more precious in a place where so many ordinary activities are precluded. But that does not mean that we must abandon the concept of private life which previous jurisprudence has sought to explain. Difficult as it is to judge the importance of smoking to the integrity of a person's identity, it is not, in our view sufficiently close to qualify as an activity meriting the protection of article 8.
>
> (R (N) *2009: para. 49*)

The way of approaching "publicness" here may work within a liberal state system. However, in closing this section, I would note, as in the previous section, challenges for international and global health that arise with these ideas of how health may be made public. These result from the contingent nature of some of their assumptions. The structure of the reasoning provides a basis in individual rights. But it also assumes an institutional architecture that relates to ideas of government. That works much more straightforwardly in the context of concepts of jurisdiction that are more recognizable at nation-state or federal levels than they are inter- and transnationally. The rigor of the sense of "publicness" that may gain purchase through the forms of reasoning identified in this section is not replicated to the same degree, given these points, at global institutional levels. That is, one could translate this idea of publicness in different societies with similar institutional and value contexts but could not apply it so simply as an idea across the world in the development and implementation of global policy.

Conclusions: challenges from and for the public in public health and motivating shared responsibility

When introducing the idea of public health in our 2017 textbook on public health law, Keith Syrett, A.M. Viens, and I wrote:

> Contemporary understandings of public health conceive a field whose breadth extends across political divides and transcends social and jurisdictional boundaries. Conceptually, public health is not limited to one sector or discipline. Rather it pervades governmental activities and social responsibilities [...]. It entails responding to and preventing disease, assuring a sound infrastructure to provide a sanitary environment, and understanding and addressing the social determinants of ill health.
>
> *(Coggon, Syrett, and Viens 2017: 3)*

The way these ideas may come to be unpacked—as a matter of practical or applied philosophy within Anglo-American liberal traditions—gives rise to what may be labeled "libertarian" and "jurisdictional" critiques (Coggon, Syrett, and Viens 2017: Chapter 1). The first of these concerns normative arguments about the legitimate business of government: challenges from those who would argue that health is properly treated (at least in the very greater part) as a private or personal matter, and thus a matter of individual rather than shared responsibility (for example, Skrabanek 1994). The second looks to the breadth and ambitions of public health when it reaches across sectors and into all policies: this position states, on essentially pragmatic grounds, that as a matter of government competence, public health should only be about the remit of a contained and designated department rather than something more pervasive (Rothstein 2002).

Within and through the philosophy of public health, it is possible that we may overcome conceptual challenges against the public in public health. However, these sorts of normative challenges, as explained in this chapter, represent how difficult it is, in theory and in practice, to overcome the principled difficulties in engaging the public in public health. This is in part because of the significance of political institutions and architecture. And it is also due to disagreement on fundamental ideas, such as justice, equity, rights, and indeed health itself. I have emphasized that my analysis is situated and partial; reflective of who I am, and where and when I write. Others within, as well as beyond, the United Kingdom will rightly disagree with some of the framings, emphases, and omissions in what I have written above.

If we consider, for example, the global coronavirus pandemic, the challenges become clear. A global policy, led by the WHO, might have arisen. However, we have seen fragmentation and difference rather than a meaningfully global public health response. This is explicable in part because of radical political as well as scientific disagreement; in part because of fragmentation and failures in cooperation; and, among further points too, in part because of unequal and competing interests among different "stakeholders." Similarly, at national levels, we have seen divisions within and across populations, and avoidable failures in government approaches.

In line with such points, this chapter has highlighted the importance of context in understanding the public in public health. I have approached the question of what it means to talk of the public in public health with reference to two liberal-skeptical challenges to the idea of public health. The first argues against the coherence of referring to population health, or the public's health. The second challenges the idea that health or health-affecting phenomena might be a shared concern within a public, the business of government. The analysis then explains how and why we might find both descriptively-oriented and normatively-oriented responses to the skeptical claims; and these have been framed with an analysis that is rooted in the sorts of liberal tradition from which the skepticism emanates.

At local, national, international, transnational, and global levels, key health challenges may be seen as hinging on the contests that exist within the public in public health. The recognition of social structures and political institutions, and ideas of community and solidarity present the firmer bases of shared responsibility for health. Yet, they also reinforce disjointedness and fragmentation, reaffirming "us and them" framings or fragmenting the institutional architectures that would otherwise orient and enact the bases of shared responsibilities for health. The paradigms of public and publicness that they represent themselves create and sustain challenges against efforts within and across national boundaries.

This chapter has not been about theories of justice, but it should have made clear how and why the study and practice of public health must be entrenched in understandings of ethics and equity, of the consolidations of power within and across society, and how these things are and may be mediated through social and political institutions (Coggon 2020). The public in public health does a great deal of work in the cause of promoting health and justice, but it may also do damage. If we are to make (health) equity a meaningful goal, we need prior understanding, and potentially reformulation, of the public in public health. Initiatives such as this volume, which invite critical engagement, development, and indeed rejection of ideas such as those explored in this chapter, are to be embraced if the real-world generation of better and fairer health opportunities and outcomes is to be found.

Notes

1 The full paragraph providing for lawful derogation from Article 8 says:

> There shall be no interference by a public authority with the exercise of this right except such as in accordance with the law and is necessary in a democratic society in the interests of national security, public safety or the economic well-being of the country, for the prevention of disorder or crime, for the protection of health or morals, or for the protection of the rights and freedoms of others.

2 The applicants also argued, under Article 14 ECHR, that the regulations unlawfully discriminated against them, as detained psychiatric patients, when contrasted with other groups for whom exemptions were provided, such as people in palliative care.

References

Anderson, B. 1991. *Imagined communities: Reflections on the origin and spread of nationalism (revised edition).* London: Verso.

Bunton, R. and J. Wills. 2004. Editorial: 25 years of *Critical Public Health*. *Critical Public Health* 14, no. 2: 79–80. https://doi.org/10.1080/09581590412331290576.

Coggon, J. 2012. *What makes health public? A critical evaluation of moral, legal, and political claims in public health.* Cambridge: Cambridge University Press.

Coggon, J. 2014. Global health, law, and ethics: Fragmented sovereignty and the limits of universal theory. In *Law and global health*, ed. M. Freeman, S. Hawkes, and B. Bennett, 369–385. Oxford: Oxford University Press.

Coggon, J. 2020. Legal, moral and political determinants within the social determinants of health: Approaching transdisciplinary challenges through intradisciplinary reflection. *Public Health Ethics* 13, no. 1: 41–47. https://doi.org/10.1093/phe/phaa009.

Coggon, J., Syrett, K., and Viens, A. M. 2017. *Public health law: Ethics, governance, and regulation.* London: Routledge.

Conly, S. 2012. *Against autonomy: Justifying coercive paternalism.* Cambridge: Cambridge University Press.

Feinberg, J. 1989. *The moral limits of the criminal law volume 3: Harm to self.* Oxford: Oxford University Press.

Geuss, R. 2003. *Public goods, private goods.* Princeton, NJ: Princeton University Press.

Gostin, L. O. 2014. *Global health law.* Cambridge, MA: Harvard University Press.

Gostin, L. O., J. T. Monahan, J. Kaldor et al. 2019. The legal determinants of health: Harnessing the power of law for global health and sustainable development. *The Lancet* 393, no. 10183: 1857–1910. https://doi.org/10.1016/s0140-6736(19)30233-8.

Harper, S., N. B. King, S. C. Meersman, M. E. Reichman, N. Breen, and J. Lynch. 2010. Implicit value judgments in the measurement of health inequalities. *The Milbank Quarterly* 88, no. 1: 4–29. https://doi.org/10.1111/j.1468-0009.2010.00587.x.

Hart, H. L. A. 1997. *The concept of law.* Oxford: Oxford University Press.

Illich, I. 1995 [originally published 1976]. *Limits to medicine—Medical nemesis: The expropriation of health.* London: Marion Boyars.

Jennings, B. 2003. Frameworks for ethics in public health. *Acta Bioethica* 9, no. 2: 165–176. http://dx.doi.org/10.4067/S1726-569X2003000200003.

Jennings, B. 2007. Public health and civic republicanism. In *Ethics, prevention, and public health*, ed. A. Dawson and M. Verweij, 30–58. Oxford: Oxford University Press.

Kass, N. E. 2004. Public health ethics: From foundations and frameworks to justice and global health. *Journal of Law, Medicine and Ethics* 32, no. 2: 232–242. https://doi.org/10.1111/j.1748-720x.2004.tb00470.x.

Kumar, A. 2020a. Caste and public health. *Frontline* (May): 47–53.

Kumar, A. 2020b. Reading Ambedkar in the time of Covid-19. *Economic and Political Weekly* 55, no. 16: 34–37.

Mackenbach, J. P. 2009. Politics is nothing but medicine at a larger scale: Reflections on public health's biggest idea. *Journal of Epidemiology and Community Health* 63, no. 3: 181–184. https://doi.org/10.1136/jech.2008.077032.

McKee, M. and D. Stuckler. 2018. Revisiting the corporate and commercial determinants of health. *American Journal of Public Health* 108, no. 9: 1167–1170. https://doi.org/10.2105/ajph.2018.304510.

Mohr, R. D. 1987. Aids, gays, and state coercion. *Bioethics* 1, no. 1: 35–50. https://doi.org/10.1111/j.1467-8519.1987.tb00003.x.

Mold, A., P. Clark, G. Millward, and D. Payling. 2019. *Placing the public in public health in post-war Britain, 1948–2012.* London: Palgrave MacMillan.

Ottersen, O. P., J. Dasgupta, C. Blouin et al. 2014. The political origins of health inequity: Prospects for change. *The Lancet* 383, no. 9917: 630–667. https://doi.org/10.1016/s0140-6736(13)62407-1.

Powers, M. and R. Faden. 2006. *Social justice: The moral foundations of public health and health policy.* Oxford: Oxford University Press.

Prabhat, D. 2020. Unequal citizenship and subjecthood: A rose by any other name…? *Northern Ireland Legal Quarterly* 71, no. 2: 175–191. https://doi.org/10.53386/nilq.v71i2.321.

Prah Ruger, J. 2012. Global health governance as shared health governance. *Journal of Epidemiology and Community Health* 66, no. 7: 653–661. https://doi.org/10.1136/jech.2009.101097.

R (Countryside Alliance and others) v *Her Majesty's Attorney General and another* [2007] UKHL 52.

R (G and B) v *Nottinghamshire NHS Trust; R (N)* v *Secretary of State for Health* [2008] EWHC 1096 (Admin).

R (N) v *Secretary of State for Health; R (E)* v *Nottingham Healthcare NHS Trust* [2009] EWCA Civ 795.

Rose, G. 1985. Sick individuals and sick populations. *International Journal of Epidemiology* 14: 32–38. https://doi.org/10.1093/ije/30.3.427.

Rothstein, M. 2002. Rethinking the meaning of public health. *Journal of Law, Medicine and Ethics* 30, no. 2: 144–149. https://doi.org/10.1111/j.1748-720x.2002.tb00381.x.

Sen, A. 2004. Health achievement and equity: External and internal perspectives. In *Public health, ethics, and equity*, ed. S. Anand, F. Peter, and A. Sen, 263–268. Oxford: Oxford University Press.

Skrabanek, P. 1994. *The death of humane medicine and the rise of coercive healthism*. Bury St Edmunds: St Edmundsbury.

Venkatapuram, S. 2011. *Health justice: An argument from the capabilities approach*. Cambridge: Polity Press.

Venkatapuram, S. 2021. Global health without justice or ethics. *Journal of Public Health* 43, no. 1: 178–179. https://doi.org/10.1093/pubmed/fdaa001.

Venkatapuram, S. and J. Bibby, eds. 2018. *A recipe for action: Using wider evidence for a healthier UK*. London: Health Foundation.

Verweij, M. and A. Dawson. 2007. The meaning of "Public" in "Public Health." In *Ethics, prevention, and public health*, ed. A. Dawson and M. Verweij, 13–29. Oxford: Oxford University Press.

World Health Organization. n.d. Social determinants of health. https://www.who.int/health-topics/social-determinants-of-health#tab=tab_1 (accessed November 11, 2021).

This work was made possible by the Tackling Root Causes Upstream of Unhealthy Urban Development consortium, award reference: MR/S037586/1, supported by the UK Prevention Research Partnership, which is funded by the British Heart Foundation, Cancer Research UK, Chief Scientist Office of the Scottish Government Health and Social Care Directorates, Engineering and Physical Sciences Research Council, Economic and Social Research Council, Health and Social Care Research and Development Division (Welsh Government), Medical Research Council, National Institute for Health Research, Natural Environment Research Council, Public Health Agency (Northern Ireland), The Health Foundation and the Wellcome Trust.

2

MEDICINE AND PUBLIC HEALTH

Daniel Steel

Introduction

Almost everyone has a basic familiarity with medicine, either through having received medical treatment or through portrayals of physicians and other healthcare workers in popular media. In contrast, public health is all around us but, except for times of crisis such as pandemics, usually out of sight and out of mind. As a result, when popular attention is drawn to public health, people may have a rather vague sense of what it involves and tend to assume that it is merely a branch of medicine. The purpose of this chapter, then, is to clarify the contrasting but overlapping relationship between medicine and public health.

The two fields share a common concern with health but differ in their primary targets. While medicine responds to the health needs of individual patients, public health interventions address the health of populations. This basic difference results in a number of other commonly noted differences between medicine and public health, three of which will be explored here. First, public health interventions usually focus on primary and secondary prevention (for example, vaccinations and smoking cessation, respectively), while medicine more commonly involves tertiary prevention (that is, treatment of illness).[1] Second, social science, geography, urban planning, environmental sciences, and other fields relevant to understanding the health of populations play a more prominent role in public health than medicine. Third, different ethical issues are paramount in medicine and public health. While biomedical ethics focuses on ethical conundrums arising from interactions among patients and healthcare workers in a clinical setting (for example, patient autonomy versus paternalism), public health ethics focuses on issues arising at the population level (for example, health of the population versus individual liberty, and unjust health inequalities).

Nevertheless, medicine and public health overlap in important ways. For example, implementation of public health interventions may involve the healthcare system, as in the case of vaccinations. Moreover, medicine can be viewed from a system-wide perspective, in which case populations rather than individual patients are the foci. Consequently, proposed reforms of healthcare systems, such as extending access to services, system-wide improvements of information sharing to reduce rates of medical errors, or reducing discrimination against minority groups, are examples of overlap between medicine and public health. A consequence

DOI: 10.4324/9781315675411-4

of such overlaps is that there may be research and interventions that lie in a gray area between these two fields.

The structure of this chapter is as follows. The first section discusses definitions of public health and medicine. Since public health is less familiar to most than medicine, the focus is primarily on definitions of public health. The next section, explores the contrasts between medicine and public health noted above in greater depth. The final section concludes.

What is public health?

The report, *The Future of Public Health*, published by the United States-based Institute of Medicine in 1988 famously characterized public health as "what we, as a society, do collectively to assure the conditions in which people can be healthy" (Committee for the Study of the Future of Public Health, Division of Health Care Services 1988: 1). The report notes the contributions of "private organizations and individuals" to public health but also emphasizes the special role of government at various levels (1998: 7). Other definitions of public health, including some proposed by philosophers, similarly emphasize joint action at a social level and a population focus as key aspects of public health. For example, according to Ross Upshur, "The focus of public health is directed to populations, communities and the broader social and environmental influences of health" (2002: 101). And according to James Childress and colleagues, "public health systems consist of all the people and actions, including laws, policies, practices, and activities, that have the primary purpose of protecting and improving the health of the public" (2002: 170). Childress and his colleagues note that the scope of public health is broader than medicine, since it is not only concerned with medical treatment but also with "fundamental social conditions" that shape health. They also distinguish between three relevant senses of "public": numerical (the population), political (the government), and communal (social organizations that are not part of the government, such as health advocacy groups or trade associations). But like the Institute of Medicine, Childress and his colleagues observe that government has a special position in public health, as it alone has the legal authority to institute necessary public health actions.

While many further definitions could be cited, those given so far are sufficient to highlight some of the central themes that would be found in almost any general description of public health. The most basic feature is that public health is concerned with the health needs of populations. A population can be the inhabitants of a country, province, state, or city, or the members of a community, and it might also be a collection of individuals identified by a demographic categorization, such as White males, or a shared condition, such as people living with HIV. The fact that populations are the targets of public health interventions has consequences for how those interventions are implemented and by whom. Plainly, public health interventions are not simply interactions between an individual patient and a physician in a clinic, although they may involve such interactions. Instead, public health interventions require the action of social organizations, which usually but not always or exclusively means government.

Consider vaccination, which is an example of a core public health action. Government health agencies or ministries commonly undertake measures such as monitoring infectious diseases and vaccination rates, producing a schedule of recommended or essential vaccinations, educating the public about vaccines, and facilitating access to vaccinations. Other branches of government might institute legal incentives or requirements intended to increase vaccination rates, such as making vaccination a prerequisite for enrollment in public schools. However, government is far from being the only player. The vaccines are likely to have been developed and manufactured by private pharmaceutical corporations. Private health providers may be involved in administering the vaccinations and private health insurers may cover the costs of vaccinations for some people. Organizations not affiliated with the government may advocate for or against vaccination, or for better access to vaccines for a specific subpopulation. Associations of medical professionals may weigh in on which vaccines should be deemed essential and which not, or on the appropriate schedules for administering them. Health researchers can contribute to the knowledge that influences vaccination policies even if they work autonomously from government health agencies (although often with government funding), and so on. All of this is to say that while vaccinations themselves often occur within the walls of medical clinics, vaccination as a public health intervention unfolds in a public forum where it is shaped by a variety of actors.

Vaccinations also illustrate some of the other features of public health noted above. Vaccines are a clear example of the important role of disease prevention in public health. Moreover, vaccinations illustrate the importance to public health of scientific research that takes a macro-level view of humans and their surroundings. While biomedical research is obviously relevant to the development of vaccines and their delivery to patients, epidemiology as well as a variety of social and environmental sciences are also very significant for the issue from a public health perspective. For instance, rates of infectious disease can depend on a number of social and environmental factors, such as housing arrangements and air or water quality (Croft et al. 2019). Infectious diseases with zoonotic origins also demonstrate the importance of interdisciplinary social and environmental sciences for public health. Vaccination is also a clear case of overlap between public health and medicine. Vaccinations are central concern for public health, but they are also a routine component of medical care, especially in pediatrics.

But it is important to bear in mind that there are many public health issues in which the overlap with medical and healthcare systems is much less prominent. For example, public health can include efforts to improve air or water quality, or to redesign urban areas to make them safer for pedestrians and bicyclists, or to improve access to green spaces. Moreover, there is a long tradition of public health research on the impacts of social and economic inequalities on population health (Ratcliff 2017). Such examples draw attention to the field of population health and its relation to public health. David Kindig identifies three ways of defining the term "population health": (1) as a framework for thinking about health disparities in populations, the causes of these disparities, and the policy responses these entail; (2) as the aggregate health outcomes in a population; and (3) as the empirical study of the social and environmental determinants of health and health disparities in populations (Kindig 2007: 145). Those interested in population health are typically concerned with all three of these elements (cf. Valles 2018). There is some discussion in the literature about the relationship between public and population health, and about whether the two are actually distinct or merely different names for the same thing (Kindig 2007; Raphael and Bryant 2002). And there is a closely related discussion about whether a broader or more narrow view of public health should be preferred (Verweij and Dawson 2007).

According to the narrow conception, public health is a matter of health-promoting interventions taken by government health agencies or ministries, such as vaccination drives or anti-smoking campaigns (Holland 2015; Kindig 2007: 139; Rothstein 2002). According to the broader conception, measures to address social determinants of health, especially social and economic inequalities, which are typically beyond the traditional purview of health ministries and which often involve nongovernment actors, also fall within the remit of public health. Thus, the broad conception of public health is very similar to the notion of population health described above. It is associated with the slogan "health in all policies," according to which health should be a concern for government actions and policies generally (for example, in transportation, taxation, urban planning, and education) and not merely for actions taken by government agencies specifically dedicated to health issues (Valles 2018: 14). Due to its emphasis on health disparities, population health is often associated with an explicit ethical commitment to promoting social equity (Valles 2018). Advocates of population health also tend to be critical of biomedical models of health and approaches to health promotion that emphasize biomedical solutions, such as creating new disease categories and prescription pharmaceuticals to treat them (Valles 2018: 9–10).

Defenders of the narrow conception raise several objections to the broad understanding of public health. For example, some argue that the broad concept makes the boundaries of public health overly vague, pushes the field into arenas in which its practitioners can claim no special expertise, and risks making public health overly politicized (Broadbent 2013; Gostin 2001; Rothstein 2002). In response to such concerns, one might argue that vague boundaries of a field are not necessarily a problem. After all, the world does not neatly divide up into discrete problems and phenomena, so it is natural that there will be a good deal of overlap between different fields of scientific research and public policy. And social determinants of health are in any case central rather than fringe concerns within the field of public health. For example, the accrediting body for schools of public health in the United States includes knowledge of population health and social determinants of health among its list of core competencies for masters and doctoral-level students (Valles 2018: 6–7). Moreover, since there is a long tradition of research on the topic of social determinants of health, it cannot be reasonably suggested that public health practitioners would be stepping outside the bounds of their expertise by addressing this topic. The third concern about the broad conception of public health—that an explicit commitment to health equity would make public health overly politicized—raises complex questions about value-neutrality of science that are beyond the scope of this chapter (Douglas 2009; Lacey 1999; Valles 2018). But whatever stance one takes on this philosophical debate, it is clear that health is a core value for both medicine and public health. Thus, since obesity, for example, is detrimental to the health of an individual person, medical doctors have reason to advise their patients to maintain a moderate weight. Similarly, since social inequalities exert adverse effects on population health, they are a concern for the field of public health. An interest in social equality, then, is a consequence of the population focus of public health together with research findings on social determinants of health (Ratcliff 2017).

In what follows, therefore, I will presume the broader conception of public health, in which public health is concerned with social and environmental determinants of health like economic inequality and air pollution, as well as with proximal causes of health in the population, such as rates of vaccination, obesity, and smoking. Public health, then, differs from medicine in its population focus, and this, in turn, entails a variety of other contrasts, which we will examine in greater detail in the subsequent section.

Contrasts

This section explores the three contrasts between public health and medicine noted in the introduction: (1) public health places greater emphasis on prevention than medicine; (2) fields that take macro-level views of humans and society are more deeply involved in public health than medicine; and (3) distinct ethical issues are salient in public health and medicine. The subsections that follow examine these three contrasts.

Prevention

Public health is generally thought to have a greater emphasis on prevention than medicine (Upshur 2002), and this fact may seem so obvious as to stand in no need of explanation. However, it is important to keep in mind that prevention is often a routine aspect of medicine, as illustrated by scheduled vaccinations as part of pediatric care, while inequities in access to medical treatments are a public health issue. So, it is worth considering the nature of public health's focus on prevention, and the reasons for it, more carefully.

There are several reasons why medicine would mostly focus on treatment. Since seeking medical care can be inconvenient and costly (for example, because it requires taking time away from work), people naturally avoid doing so unless they have some health problem that demands attention. Moreover, although treatments for many illnesses are fairly routine, medical treatment frequently requires tailoring interventions to suit the specific needs and circumstances of the patient. For instance, while a course of antibiotics would be routinely prescribed for pneumonia, which antibiotic is chosen can vary according to the history of adverse reactions of the patient or which bacterial strain the patient is infected with. And other aspects of the treatment could vary according to the severity of the case.[2] In sum, treatment of illness must often be individualized: two individuals may be diagnosed with the same disease but respond differently to treatment, or differ in their circumstances and preferences in ways that necessitate distinct treatment plans. It is unsurprising, then, that treatment primarily occurs at an individual, and therefore medical, level.

In contrast, interventions targeted at populations are typically limited in the extent to which they can be tailored to individual needs and preferences, although they may be designed or implemented in ways that favor the interests of some subpopulations over others. Preventive measures, therefore, are a natural fit for the population focus of public health. Prevention often applies similarly to a population, as examples such as potable water, air free of fine particulate matter, and immunization illustrate. And the case of vaccinations illustrates that, even when delivered via the medical system, public health interventions tend to be more standardized than medical care typically is. Of course, not every individual in a population will respond to a public health intervention in the same way, and a public health intervention, even when beneficial overall, may be harmful for some. The possibility that public health interventions may increase health disparities (for example, by primarily benefiting groups that are already healthier) will be discussed below in connection with the issue of health inequities. Nevertheless, similar conditions often prevent illness across a population, whereas treatments for already existing illnesses typically must be individualized to patient needs. As a result, the population focus of public health naturally leads to an emphasis on prevention rather than treatment. When public health does focus on medical treatment, it generally does so at a system-wide level appropriate for interventions targeted at populations. Examples include extending access medical services (for example, by broadening publicly funded health insurance) or reducing racial discrimination in medical practice (Ben et al. 2017).

Consider an extended example to illustrate the points made above. The efforts of the English physician John Snow to provide evidence for waterborne transmission of cholera in the nineteenth century constitute one of the most celebrated cases in the history of public health. Snow's treatise, *On the Mode of Communication of Cholera* (1855), traced cholera epidemics in England to contamination of drinking water by sewage. Snow is often remembered for his use of "shoe leather" epidemiology, such as collecting door-to-door data on people's sources of drinking water, and his use of maps to communicate the results of his investigations

(McLeod 2000). Famously, Snow's work in the Soho district of London linked a cholera outbreak to a pump on Broad Street that drew water from a well contaminated by a nearby cesspit, leading Snow to recommend that the handle on the pump be removed. Historians have critiqued the mythos surrounding Snow. For instance, Snow's recommendation to remove the handle from the Broad Street pump occurred after the cholera outbreak in that quarter of London was already subsiding, and Snow was not particularly successful in persuading his contemporaries of his ideas about the transmission of cholera or of his proposed solutions (Hempel 2006; Koch and Denike 2009; McLeod 2000). Nevertheless, Snow can be rightfully credited as a pioneer in recognizing the linkage between careful epidemiological research and government action in preventing the spread of infectious disease.

Snow's research suggested that digging cesspits for outhouses or disposing human waste in rivers, which might have previously seemed matters that could be left to the discretion of individuals, were in fact urgent public health concerns that should be regulated by the government. Moreover, prevention of waterborne transmission of infectious diseases, such as cholera, requires publicly funded water and sewerage systems that are carefully designed and maintained to keep the two streams separate. Naturally, such a system cannot be designed to suit the particular needs and preferences of every individual in the population. For instance, a single system might be chosen and built for a metropolitan area, and all inhabitants of that area would have to learn to live with it. However, the absence of sewage-derived pathogens from drinking water is generally beneficial to health. So, this is a clear case in which the health benefits of prevention, in contrast to the more individualized nature of medical treatment, can be enjoyed in a similar manner by an entire population.[3]

These observations also suggest something about the ways in which medicine and public health overlap. One type of overlap, illustrated by the case of vaccination, occurs when the healthcare system is unavoidably involved in the delivery of a public health intervention. Vaccinations may be delivered in a standardized manner to a large population, but medical and pharmaceutical expertise is nevertheless required to prepare the shots and to inject them into arms. A second type of overlap arises from the fact that access to needed medical care is generally beneficial to health. In other words, while patients vary enormously in the specific medical treatments they need, practically everyone will stand in need of some medical treatment at some points of their lives. Thus, obstacles to obtaining medical treatments, such as systematic racism in healthcare settings or gaps in publicly funded healthcare coverage, are also important public health concerns. Access to medical care, therefore, is similar to access to potable water insofar as both are conditions that are generally beneficial to health in a population notwithstanding individual differences and preferences. The difference in the latter case is that the relevant interventions (that is, well-designed and maintained public water and sewerage systems) are not implemented via the healthcare system.

The example of John Snow and cholera also illustrates the point made above that public health need not be limited to actions taken by government agencies specifically dedicated to health. Public health is also inherent in central government functions, such as building, maintaining, and regulating public utilities. Of course, this does not mean that public health dictates all of these functions. Rather, it simply means that it is one voice at the table among others.

Sciences at the macro-level

Due to its population focus, scientific fields that study humans and society at broader, macro-scale are more prominent in public health than medicine. While almost all medical practitioners are educated in human biology and physiology, public health researchers may be trained in epidemiology, sociology, economics, political science, urban planning, environmental sciences, social psychology, or other fields. A number of examples could be given to illustrate the prominence of such fields within public health. In this subsection, I describe public health research on urban green spaces, including the relationship of this issue to health disparities along economic and racial lines (Jennings, Browning, and Rigolon 2019).

The positive association between health and urban green spaces has become well established, but the reasons for it are complex (Jennings, Browning, and Rigolon 2019). Increased physical exercise does not appear to explain all of the association, and some studies find only weak associations between green spaces and exercise (Jennings, Browning, and Rigolon 2019; Maas et al. 2008; Richardson et al. 2013). A variety of biological, psychological, and social explanations of the relationship between green spaces and health have been proposed and investigated: green spaces may reduce stress, improve cognitive functioning, provide opportunities for socialization with neighbors, and provide exposure to a broader range of non-pathogenic bacteria that improve immune function (Jennings, Browning, and Rigolon 2019, 11–13). In addition, some research suggests that the health benefits of green spaces may not accrue to everyone equally. For instance, some studies suggest that the health benefits of green spaces appear to be more pronounced in men than women (Jiang, Chang, and Sullivan 2014; Richardson and Mitchell 2010), and the benefits appear to vary according to the lifespan (Astell-Burt, Mitchell, and Hartig 2014). Moreover, efforts to improve access to urban green spaces for lower-income communities sometimes yield paradoxical effects as a result of gentrification and relocation of lower-income residents (Wolch, Byrne, and Newell 2014).

In addition, public health work on urban green spaces is often linked to environmental justice and thereby to health equity. The 2019 book, *Urban Green Spaces*, by Jennings, Browning, and Rigolon, dedicates a chapter to this issue. Environmental justice movements were inspired by observations that noxious land uses are more likely to be located in or adjacent to predominantly racial minority and low-income communities (Bullard 2018). The health benefits of urban green spaces, therefore, suggest the possibility of a flipside disparity, wherein racial majority and higher-income neighborhoods have better access to well-maintained parks and green spaces. A 2016 systematic review of work on this topic concludes that "low socioeconomic and ethnic minority people have access to fewer acres of parks, fewer acres of parks per person, and to parks with lower quality, maintenance, and safety than more privileged people" (Rigolon 2016: 160). In addition to work focusing on this issue from a distributional perspective, some studies examine the processes, such as decisions about zoning or how to distribute funding for parks within a metropolitan area, that impact the citing and maintenance of urban green spaces (Jennings, Browning, and Rigolon 2019: 54–56).

This summary of research on health and urban green spaces serves to emphasize the important role of fields that take a macro-level view of society to public health. Public health research on green spaces runs the gamut from to epidemiological and geographical studies that examine associations between proximity to green spaces and various health outcomes (Richardson and Mitchell 2010), to research on the social and community impacts of green spaces (Jennings, Browning, and Rigolon 2019: 17–19), to studies that focus on public health and green spaces from the perspective of urban planning and health equity (Wolch, Byrne, and Newell 2014). But as before, it is important to keep in mind that contrasts between public health and medicine here is a matter of degree, and not absolutes. The field of health economics and the existence of a journal titled *Social Science & Medicine* indicate that the social sciences are relevant to medicine as well. So, while social and other sciences that adopt a macro-level perspective are clearly important to public health, one may wonder whether they are really more important to public health than to medicine. One argument that this is indeed the case is that social and other macro-level sciences are most relevant to medicine in contexts wherein medicine and public health overlap. For instance, studies of the economic efficiency of different approaches to providing health insurance take on a population-level issue concerning access to medical care, and hence fall squarely within the area of overlap between medicine and public health. Thus, when social sciences are relevant to medicine, they are typically also tied to public health. But the converse does not hold, as the discussion of urban green spaces illustrates. While poor access to urban green spaces may be a distal cause of medical conditions that ultimately require treatment, their role in medical interventions is mostly limited to a background condition that can facilitate following a physician's advice to reduce stress or exercise more regularly. Within public health, by contrast, the distribution of urban green spaces and processes by which these distributions are decided can be direct foci of interventions. For instance, researchers have generated guidelines for how to improve green space access and quality in lower-income neighborhoods without sparking a cycle of gentrification (Jennings, Browning, and Rigolon 2019: 23–24; Wolch, Byrne, and Newell 2014). Moreover, the case of urban green spaces is hardly unique in this regard. Similar points could be made for issues such as water and air quality, or for topics such as legal requirements to wear seatbelts. In all of these cases, research from a broad array of fields outside the bounds of biomedicine is directly relevant to deciding which interventions should be adopted and why.

Public health ethics and biomedical ethics

The final contrast has to do with which ethical issues are most salient in public health and medicine. Biomedical ethics tends to focus on ethical concerns arising in the context of interactions of healthcare workers and patients, such as informed consent, or issues raised by new biomedical technologies, such as medical applications of artificial intelligence (Beauchamp and Childress 2019). In contrast, public health ethics focuses on ethical issues that arise at the population level. These include health equity and the liberal challenge to public health, the latter of which refers to the potential for interventions that improve population health to conflict with the emphasis on individual freedom enshrined in liberalism. Given the influential status of principlism in biomedical ethics (Beauchamp and Childress 2019), it is not surprising that a variety of principles for public health ethics have been proposed (Childress et al. 2002; Coughlin 2008; Kass 2004; Kenny, Sherwin, and Baylis 2010; Swain, Burns, and Etkind 2008; Upshur 2002). Principlist approaches to public health ethics often focus on the liberal challenge to public health (Childress et al. 2002; Upshur 2002), and this focus is also shared by some textbooks on public health ethics (Holland 2015). However, the importance of equity is also a significant feature distinguishing public health and biomedical ethics. Unlike medicine, public health interventions usually cannot be tailored to suit individual needs, and hence may produce winners and losers within the affected population. Furthermore, disparities related to socioeconomic status, discrimination, gender, and other factors are commonplace in population health data. In short, once one takes a population focus, the existence of morally significant health inequalities becomes obvious. This subsection, then, explains how the population focus of public health brings a distinctive set of ethical concerns to the fore.

Biomedical ethics is often associated with Tom Beauchamp and James Childress' famous four principles: respect for autonomy, beneficence, non-maleficence, and justice. Several authors advise against directly transporting these principles to the domain of public health. For example, Stephen Holland (2015) explains that while the heavy emphasis on autonomy inherent in Beauchamp and Childress' principlism is reasonable in a medical context wherein patients have a right to decide and be informed about what interventions they will undergo, such an emphasis is question-begging in a public health context where trade-offs between individual freedoms and population health are core ethical concerns. Similarly, Upshur argues that because populations are composed of individuals and subpopulations with differing preferences and interests that often conflict, "the straightforward application of the principles of autonomy, beneficence, non-malfeasance and justice in public health practice is problematic" (2002: 101). One cannot assume a consistent set of values, preferences, or needs across a population as might be present for a single patient, and a public health intervention may not impact everyone in the population in the same way. In short, the fact that public health is concerned with the health of populations rather than individuals has significant ethical consequences.

So, what might principlism look like if adapted to public health? Consider the following list of public health ethics principles proposed by Upshur: the harm principle, least restrictive or coercive means, reciprocity, and transparency (2002: 102). The harm principle, borrowed from John Stuart Mill (1859), asserts that the state can restrict the freedom of an individual only to prevent harm to others. The second two principles concern cases in which such restrictions are enacted. The second principle requires that the measures should be no more restrictive or coercive than necessary, while the third, reciprocity, demands that the state facilitate individuals in following public health requirements. Finally, transparency states that public health officials have a responsibility to explain the rationale for public health interventions to the public. Legal requirements to be vaccinated against certain diseases can illustrate these principles. Given the harm principle, such requirements can only be justifiable on the grounds of preventing harm to others, and the measures put in place should be no more restrictive or coercive than needed to obtain vaccination rates sufficient for herd immunity. Moreover, reciprocity requires that governments make it easy for people to receive the required vaccinations, for instance, by making vaccines free and conveniently available, and transparency requires that the reasoning for all these decisions be clearly explained to the public.

Upshur's principles of public health ethics focus on the liberal challenge to public health. They are designed to guide judgments about when and how individual freedom can be justifiably restricted in the name of promoting the health of a population. Moreover, Upshur's inclusion of the harm principle gives his principles a strongly libertarian character. For instance, interventions that restrict freedom for the individual's own good, such as laws requiring that seatbelts be worn in automobiles, would be unjustifiable according to Upshur's principles. And the harm principle would also appear to prohibit interventions that restrict individual freedom for the benefit of others, such as imposing taxes to support programs that provide access to healthcare, public schools, and green spaces. Other principlist approaches to public health ethics are less libertarian than Upshur's. For instance, Childress and colleagues' proposal shares Upshur's focus on the liberal challenge to public health, but does not include the harm principle and instead insists that benefits of a public health intervention must outweigh any countervailing moral concerns (Childress et al. 2002: 173). Other authors who approach public health ethics from a principlist perspective suggest additional principles, such as the precautionary principle and a principle of solidarity or interdependence (Coughlin 2008; Swain, Burns, and Etkind 2008). Furthermore, some variants of principlism in public health emphasize justice as a central principle (Kenny, Sherwin, and Baylis 2010; Swain, Burns, and Etkind 2008). For example, Nuala Kenny and colleagues criticize what they view as the excessive individualist focus of much work in public health ethics, and emphasize relational approaches to autonomy and social justice as crucial (Kenny, Sherwin, and Baylis 2010).

The above discussion illustrates that principlism might be adapted to public health in a variety of ways that reflect differing theoretical orientations and foci problems. Despite their differences, however, all of these versions of principlism highlight that the salient ethical issues in public health are distinct from those in medicine. In the remainder of this subsection, I explore this point in greater depth by means of a closer look at the liberal challenge to public health and health equity.

The Covid-19 pandemic has brought public health to the forefront of public consciousness, and public health ethics has trailed along closely behind. While a number of ethical challenges arise in connection with Covid-19—triage of patients when medical resources are scarce, economic and racial disparities in Covid-19 mortality, global inequities in vaccine access, among others—this subsection homes in on the liberal challenge to public health. Prior to the widespread vaccination, slowing the spread of Covid-19, and ultimately reducing the prevalence and incidence of cases to a manageable level, required changes to behavior that became familiar to people around the globe: mask wearing in public places, social distancing, restriction of travel, self-isolation and quarantine for infected individuals, and cancellation of large gatherings. Such measures frequently constrain individual freedoms, and often do so in ways that carry significant psychological, economic, and health burdens. As a result, public health mandates aimed at curbing Covid-19 have generated opposition among some in the general public and among some political leaders. In short, Covid-19 has emerged as a dramatic example of the liberal challenge to public health. Not surprisingly, then, ethics discussions of this topic often highlight principles, such as those proposed by Upshur, that were developed to for situations in which public health interventions constrain liberty. For example, Lawrence Gostin, Eric Friedman, and Sarah Wetter (2020) emphasize that Covid-19 measures should be no more restrictive than necessary and that transparency is essential for maintaining public trust.

Consider how the liberal challenge to public health raises distinct ethical concerns from analogous conflicts between physician beneficence and patient autonomy in biomedical ethics. Both situations are similar insofar as involving a trade-off between doing what experts see as best for health and respecting the freedom of individuals to choose autonomously. However, the population focus of public health generates a number of distinctive ethical concerns. As illustrated by the case of Covid-19, public health interventions can target seemingly personal decisions that create risk of harms to others, such as the transmission of infectious disease. Moreover, the imposition of risks created by refusing to wear masks or social distance can also limit the freedom of others to carry on daily activities without fear of exposure, so the trade-off is not simply a matter of liberty against health but also one person's freedom against another's. In addition, it is typically not possible to consult and obtain consent from all individuals impacted by a public health intervention. And indeed, in many cases, intransigent differences of values within the population would preclude universal acceptance of any policy. Furthermore, public health measures in Covid-19 are administered by the government and therefore may be backed up by police powers, creating potential issues of civil liberties that are typically absent in discussions of patient autonomy in bioethics. And public health interventions, such as restrictions on travel from the source of an infectious disease outbreak, can risk stigmatizing some subpopulations and promoting ethnic violence. Finally, since the target of the intervention is a population rather than an individual, disparities in difficulty of abiding by restrictions can create inequities along lines of class or race. And at a global scale, Covid-19 lockdowns may have more severely adverse impacts on welfare in less-wealthy nations (Broadbent et al. 2020).

The above discussion also illustrates the crucial role of equity and justice concerns for public health ethics. A long-standing finding of population health research is that social and economic inequalities generate health disparities that are not erased by universal access to healthcare (Ratcliff 2017). For example, the long running Whitehall study of British civil servants found that every level of the civil service hierarchy enjoyed a lower rate of mortality than the level below, even though none were poor in an absolute sense and all had access to healthcare (Abell et al. 2018; Marmot 2006; Marmot et al. 1991; Marmot and Shipley 1996). In addition, there is an emerging body of research documenting the role of racism in generating health disparities within populations (Cave et al. 2020). A number of different theoretical approaches to health equity can be found within literature public health ethics. These include approaches that frame the issue in terms of a trade-off between maximizing the aggregate health of a population and preventing health inequalities (Anand 2006), neo-Rawlsian approaches to health equity (Daniels 2008; Peters 2006), capabilities approaches (Sen 2006; Venkatapuram 2011), a relational justice approach (Kenny, Sherwin, and Baylis 2010), and approaches to justice and the health of Indigenous peoples in settler colonial states (Matthews 2019). However, for the present purposes, the theoretical differences between these several approaches are less important than the broader contrast between public health and medicine when it comes to equity.

It is important to keep in mind that equity is also a concern in medicine, as illustrated by examples such as universal access to healthcare and the distribution of scare medical resources. As discussed above, such examples are areas of overlap between public health and medicine because they concern features of healthcare systems that impact populations. But as explained in the previous paragraph, concern with equity in public health ethics extends beyond access to healthcare to encompass broader social inequalities and injustices that produce disparities in health outcomes along the lines of socioeconomic status and race. As a consequence, issues of equity in public health are much more deeply entangled with broader social concerns, such as economic inequality, social class, racism, and colonialism. Critics of a broad conception of public health warn that it is risky to engage with such politically controversial topics (Rothstein 2002). However, the fact remains that public health research and policy *does* currently address these subjects (Valles 2018), and that they raise a plethora of thorny philosophical challenges regarding equity and justice.

Conclusions

Public health and medicine are both concerned with the human health and well-being but differ in that the latter focuses on the needs of individual patients, while the former is concerned with populations. This basic difference leads to other contrasts: (1) a greater emphasis on prevention in public health; (2) a greater role of research in public health that studies humans and their surroundings from a macro-perspective; and (3) different salient ethical issues in public health and medicine. However, it is important not to oversimplify these differences. The contrasts are matters of degree, not absolute, and there are large areas of overlap between public health and medicine. Public health and medicine, therefore, should be seen as complementary and mutually supporting enterprises.

Notes

1 In common parlance, tertiary prevention might not seem like prevention at all. However, medical treatment can be viewed as aiming to prevent harmful effects of a health condition.
2 Similar observations could be made for other diseases, such as malaria.
3 However, this is not to disregard the fact that decisions could be made to not cover certain areas under a public utility system or to maintain better systems in some areas than others, decisions which might reflect long-standing social inequalities.

References

Abell, J., M. Kivimäki, A. Dugravot et al. 2018. Association between systolic blood pressure and dementia in the Whitehall II cohort study: Role of age, duration, and threshold used to define hypertension. *European Heart Journal* 39, no. 33: 3119–3125. https://doi.org/10.1093/eurheartj/ehy288.

Anand, S. 2006. The concern for equity in health. In *Public health, ethics, and equity*, ed. S. Anand, F. Peter, and A. Sen, 15–20. Oxford: Oxford University Press.

Astell-Burt, R., R. Mitchell, and T. Hartig. 2014. The association between green space and mental health varies across the lifecourse: A longitudinal study. *Journal of Epidemiology and Community Health* 68, no. 6: 578–583. https://doi.org/10.1136/jech-2013-203767.

Beauchamp, T., and J. Childress. 2019. *Principles of biomedical ethics.* 8th edition. Oxford: Oxford University Press.

Ben, J., D. Cormack, R. Harris, and Y. Paradies. 2017. Racism and health service utilisation: A systematic review and meta-analysis. *PLoS One* 2, no. 12 (December): e0189900. https://doi.org/10.1371/journal.pone.0189900.

Broadbent, A. 2013. *Philosophy of epidemiology.* London: Palgrave MacMillan.

Broadbent, A., D. Walker, K. Chalkidou, R. Sullivan, and A. Glassman. 2020. Lockdown is not egalitarian: The costs fall on the global poor. *The Lancet* 396, no. 10243: 21–22. https://doi.org/10.1016/s0140-6736(20)31422-7.

Bullard, R. 2018. *Dumping in Dixie: Race, class, and environmental quality.* 3rd edition. New York: Routledge.

Cave, L., M. Cooper, S. Zubrick, and C. Shepherd. 2020. Racial discrimination and child and adolescent health in longitudinal studies: A systematic review. *Social Science & Medicine* 250: 112864. https://doi.org/10.1016/j.socscimed.2020.112864.

Childress, J., R. Faden, L. Gaare et al. 2002. Public health ethics: Mapping the terrain. *Journal of Law, Medicine & Ethics* 30, no. 2: 170–178. https://doi.org/10.1111/j.1748-720x.2002.tb00384.x.

Committee for the Study of the Future of Public Health, Division of Health Care Services, Institute of Medicine. 1988. *The future of public health.* Washington, DC: National Academy Press.

Coughlin, S. 2008. How many principles for public health ethics? *Open Public Health Journal* 1, no. 1: 8–16. https://dx.doi.org/10.2174%2F1874944500801010008.

Croft, D., W. Zhang, S. Lin et al. 2019. The association between respiratory infection and air pollution in the setting of air quality policy and economic change. *Annals of the American Thoracic Society* 16, no. 3: 321–330. https://dx.doi.org/10.1513%2FAnnalsATS.201810-691OC.

Daniels, N. 2008. *Just health: Meeting health needs fairly.* Cambridge: Cambridge University Press.

Douglas, H. 2009. *Science and the value-free ideal.* Pittsburgh, PA: University of Pittsburgh Press.

Gostin, L. 2001. Public health, ethics, and human rights: A tribute to the late Jonathan Mann. *Journal of Law, Medicine & Ethics* 29, no. 2: 121–130. https://doi.org/10.1111/j.1748-720x.2001.tb00330.x.

Gostin, L., E. Friedman, and S. Wetter. 2020. Responding to Covid-19: How to navigate a public health emergency legally and ethically. *Hastings Center Report* 50, no. 2: 8–12. https://doi.org/10.1002/hast.1090.

Hempel, S. 2006. *The medical detective: John Snow and the mystery of cholera.* London: Granta.

Holland, S. 2015. *Public health ethics.* 2nd edition. Cambridge: Polity Press.

Jennings, V., M. Browning, and A. Rigolon. 2019. *Urban green spaces: Public health and sustainability in the United States.* Cham: Springer.

Jiang, B., C. Chang, W. Sullivan. 2014. A dose of nature: Tree cover, stress reduction, and gender differences. *Landscape and Urban Planning* 132: 26–36. https://doi.org/10.1016/j.landurbplan.2014.08.005.

Kass, N. 2004. Public health ethics: From foundations and frameworks to justice and global public health. *Journal of Law, Medicine & Ethics* 32, no. 2: 232–242. https://doi.org/10.1111/j.1748-720x.2004.tb00470.x.

Kenny, N., S. Sherwin, and F. Baylis. 2010. Re-visioning public health ethics: A relational perspective. *Canadian Journal of Public Health* 101, no. 1: 9–11. https://dx.doi.org/10.1007%2FBF03405552.

Kindig, D. 2007. Understanding population health terminology. *Milbank Quarterly* 85, no. 1: 139–161. https://dx.doi.org/10.1111%2Fj.1468-0009.2007.00479.x.

Koch, T. and K. Denike. 2009. Crediting his critics' concerns: Remaking John Snow's map of Broad Street cholera, 1854. *Social Science & Medicine* 69, no. 8: 1246–1251. https://doi.org/10.1016/j.socscimed.2009.07.046.

Lacey, H. 1999. *Is science value free? Values and scientific understanding.* London: Routledge.

Maas, J., R. Verheij, P. Spreeuwenberg, and P. Groenewegen. 2008. Physical activity as a possible mechanism behind the relationship between green space and health: A multilevel analysis. *BMC Public Health* 8, no. 206: 1–13. https://doi.org/10.1186/1471-2458-8-206.

Marmot, M. 2006. Social causes of inequalities in health. In *Public health, ethics, and equity*, ed. S. Anand, F. Peter, and A. Sen, 37–61. Oxford: Oxford University Press.

Marmot, M., G. Davey Smith, S. Stansfeld et al. 1991. Health inequalities among British civil servants: The Whitehall II study. *The Lancet* 337, no. 8754: 1387–1393. https://doi.org/10.1016/0140-6736(91)93068-K.

Marmot, M., and M. Shipley. 1996. Do socioeconomic differences in mortality persist after retirement? 25 year follow up of civil servants from the first Whitehall study. *British Medical Journal* 313, no. 7066: 1177–1180. https://doi.org/10.1136/bmj.313.7066.1177.

Matthews, R. 2019. Health ethics and indigenous ethnocide. *Bioethics* 33, no. 7: 827–834. https://doi.org/10.1111/bioe.12610.

McLeod, K. 2000. Our sense of Snow: The myth of John Snow in medical geography. *Social Science & Medicine* 50, no. 7–8: 923–935. https://doi.org/10.1016/s0277-9536(99)00345-7.

Mill, J. 1859. *On liberty*. London: John W. Parker & Son.

Peters, F. 2006. Health equity and social justice. In *Public health, ethics, and equity*, ed. S. Anand, F. Peter, and A. Sen, 93–106. Oxford: Oxford University Press.

Raphael, D. and T. Bryant. 2002. The limitations of population health as a model for a new public health. *Health Promotion International* 17, no. 2: 189–199. https://doi.org/10.1093/heapro/17.2.189.

Ratcliff, K. 2017. *The social determinants of health: Looking upstream*. Cambridge: Polity Press.

Richardson, E., and R. Mitchell. 2010. Gender differences in relationships between urban green space and health in the United Kingdom. *Social Science & Medicine* 71, no. 3: 568–575. https://doi.org/10.1016/j.socscimed.2010.04.015.

Richardson, E., J. Pearce, R. Mitchell, and S. Kingham. 2013. Role of physical activity in the relationship between urban green space and health. *Public Health* 127, no. 4: 318–324. https://doi.org/10.1016/j.puhe.2013.01.004.

Rigolon, A. 2016. A complex landscape of inequity in access to urban parks: A literature review. *Landscape and Urban Planning* 153: 160–169. http://dx.doi.org/10.1016/j.landurbplan.2016.05.017.

Rothstein, M. 2002. Rethinking the meaning of public health. *Journal of Law, Medicine & Ethics* 30, no. 2: 144–149. https://doi.org/10.1111/j.1748-720x.2002.tb00381.x.

Sen, A. 2006. Why health equity? In *Public health, ethics, and equity*, ed. S. Anand, F. Peter, and A. Sen, 21–33. Oxford: Oxford University Press.

Snow, J. 1855. *On the mode of communication of cholera*. 2nd edition. London: John Churchill.

Swain, G., K. Burns, and P. Etkind. 2008. Preparedness: Medical ethics versus public health ethics. *Journal of Public Health Management Practice* 14, no. 4: 354–357. https://doi.org/10.1097/01.phh.0000324563.87780.67.

Upshur, R. 2002. Principles for the justification of public health intervention. *Canadian Journal of Public Health* 93, no. 2: 101–103. https://doi.org/10.1007/bf03404547.

Valles, S. 2018. *Philosophy of population health: Philosophy for a new public health era*. New York: Routledge.

Venkatapuram, S. 2011. *Health justice: An argument for the capabilities approach*. Hoboken, NJ: Wiley & Sons.

Verweij, M., and A. Dawson. 2007. The meaning of "public" in "public health." In *Ethics, prevention, and public health*, ed. Angus Dawson and Marcel Verweij, 13–29. Oxford: Oxford University Press.

Wolch, J., J. Byrne, and J. Newell. 2014. Urban green space, public health, and environmental justice: The challenge of making cities "just green enough." *Landscape and Urban Planning* 125: 234–244. https://doi.org/10.1016/j.landurbplan.2014.01.017.

3

GROUPS AND INDIVIDUALS

Stephen John

Introduction

Epidemiology and public health policy generate and use population-level knowledge to secure population-level goods, such as reductions in health inequalities. However, it is individuals who are sick or well, who live or die. This gap gives rise to a fundamental conceptual question in public health: *How should we reconcile the population- and individual-level perspectives?*

On the face of it, this question has an *ethical* aspect and an *epistemological* aspect. Under the first heading, we have questions like whether we can restrict individuals' liberties—for example, their freedom to buy cigarettes—for the sake of a population-level goal, like reducing lung cancer rates. Under the second heading, we have questions such as how we can move from population-level patterns—on average, smokers are more likely to develop lung cancer—to claims about individual-level outcomes—say, that smoking will probably be bad for this person. This chapter complicates this distinction: we should not think of the ethical and epistemological questions as distinct, because resolving the epistemological puzzles about the population- and individual-level perspectives affects the ethical questions, and vice versa. We need an *integrated philosophy of public health*.

In Sections "Introduction" and "Motivating the individual perspective," I use case studies of paradigmatic public health problems, screening and mass vaccination, to outline some ethical tensions between individual- and population-level perspectives. In Section "Prevention paradoxes," I discuss three of the concepts which frame these problems: chance, categorization, and causation. Each of these three concepts raises tricky puzzles, which require both epistemic and ethical analyses. The concluding section, "The epistemic aspect," sketches ways of combining the ethical and epistemological issues to create an integrated philosophy of public health.

Motivating the individual perspective

Consider two paradigm cases of public health policy:

> Breast cancer screening: In the U.K., every woman between 50 and 71 is invited to breast cancer screening triennially. It is estimated that the U.K.'s program "saves" 1,300

DOI: 10.4324/9781315675411-5

lives *per annum* (Marmot et al. 2013). Unfortunately, screening also has costs: most notably, through "overdiagnosis," where women will be treated for cancer when the cancer would not have gone on to cause symptoms or early death; but also through anxiety caused by false positives, and, arguably, through medicalizing everyday life.

(Plutynski 2012)

Vaccination policy: Cervical cancer is typically associated with contraction of the human papillomavirus virus (HPV). Many countries have introduced programs which vaccinate against HPV. The most effective strategies for reducing cervical cancer rates involve vaccinating not just young women but also young men, because, although men are very unlikely to fall ill from contracting HPV, they can act as carriers of the virus.

(Lowy 2011)

In both cases, securing the best population-level outcome requires us to do things which we know will harm at least some individuals: reducing breast cancer rates involves some women having unnecessary mastectomies; reducing cervical cancer rates involves some men suffering side effects from a vaccination which brings them no protective benefit.

In medical ethics, there is a strong norm of non-maleficence—more colloquially, "do no harm" (Beauchamp and Childress 2001). Interpreting this norm is tricky; for example, it is clear that it is permissible for a surgeon to cut the patient with a scalpel, "harming" her, as part of the operation of removing the tumor. However, one thing the principle does seem to imply is a strong default norm against harming some patients for the sake of helping *other* patients (John and Wu, 2022). Consider a standard case in introductions to medical ethics, where we could kill one person and redistribute her organs to save five lives. Even if cutting up friendless loners who wander too close to hospitals would do more "good" than "harm" overall, doing so would be wrong. Cancer screening or mass vaccination seems structurally similar to the organ redistribution case, as they involve knowingly harming some to help others, apparently violating this non-maleficence concern. How, then, might they be justified?

One possible response is that there is a disjunction between public health ethics and clinical ethics, such that, in public health policy, *all* that matters are population-level consequences. To use terms from moral philosophy, even if clinical practice should be governed by "deontological" norms, we should be "consequentialists" in public health (see Goodin 1995). There is a lot to be said for this approach, because public health policy clearly differs from clinical practice in its focus on securing and promoting population-level outcomes. While a doctor saves an individual patient from disease, a public health policy-maker aims to improve outcomes across populations, where it may be impossible to identify individual "winners" or "losers" (Verweij 2015). Unsurprisingly, then, many familiar debates in public health ethics concern which population-level consequences we should pursue: for example, lives saved or life-years saved; aggregate health outcomes or also health inequalities (Anand, Peter, and Sen 2004; Hausman 2015).

However, even leaving aside worries that public health programs are often administered by physicians, it seems odd to think that public health policy should *only* be concerned with the population perspective. There are interesting debates over the metaphysical relationships between individuals and populations; ultimately, however, populations are composed of individuals, and any moral concern we have about population-level outcomes is based on a concern about individual-level outcomes. It seems implausible that we can just sacrifice individuals for collective health. A full ethical accounting of public health policy needs to find some place for the individual- as well as population-level perspectives.

A second way to reconcile the population and individual perspectives is to turn to notions of consent and choice. We might hold that programs are justifiable only when individuals do or can make *informed choices* about participation. For example, we might say that screening programs are permissible only when individuals can choose whether to attend. This move captures intuitions that respect for autonomy is a foundational value (Beauchamp and Childress 2001). It also provides a response to "non-maleficence" concerns on the basis of the *volenti non fit injuria* principle—according to which those who consent to some course of action in full knowledge of its consequences have no moral complaint when they are harmed as a result.

Unfortunately, this consent strategy for reconciling the population- and individual- level perspectives is problematic. First, it is unclear that it can be generalized to all public health interventions. For example, it is odd to say that a policy mandating clean air or a tax on sugar in soft drinks is permissible only if each and every affected individual gives her consent to the relevant legislation (O'Neill 2002). (And in some cases, such as vaccination, each could opt out, but there would not be any point pursuing the program if they did.) Second, the approach seems to assume that the programs *are* worth pursuing and the question is how to ensure that no one can complain about being harmed; our initial question, however, is whether, given their foreseeable effects, it is permissible to pursue the policies *at all*. If you consent to being punched, then, plausibly, you cannot complain if I punch you; it would be odd, though, for a professional cage-fighter to boast about her commitment to "do no harm" despite making a living from fighting (John and Wu, 2022)!

Appeals to consent can, though, be understood as attempts to articulate a more plausible way of understanding how public health programs could be ethically justifiable: when they seem to be a "good deal" of the kind a rational agent would accept—more formally, when they are in each affected individual's *ex-ante* interests. Consider a simple example: paying £1 for a lottery ticket where you have a 99% chance of winning £100 does not *guarantee* that you will be better off (you might get the one-in-a-hundred unlucky ticket). Nonetheless, prior to the lottery draw—from the *ex-ante* perspective—you are better off holding the ticket than not. Using this concept of *ex-ante* interests, we can understand how a screening policy might be permissible, even when we know that some will lose out. For some individual entering screening, although there is some chance that she will "lose," through overdiagnosis, there is also a chance that she will "gain," through a life-saving operation. Being screened might be in her *ex-ante* interests, as long as the chance of gain is higher than the chance of loss. Plausibly, we can ensure that some screening programs are in the *ex-ante* interests of each affected individual. As long as we think about harm and benefit in terms of changes to *ex-ante* interests, the screening program does not violate "non-maleficence," even if some do "lose out" as a result of participation. (The general principle that policies which are in the *ex-ante* interests of each are permissible is sometimes called "*ex-ante* Pareto": see Fleurabey and Voorhoeve 2013.)

In support of this approach, a concern for individuals' *ex-ante* interests is baked into the ways in which we assess screening policies. For example, consider James Wilson and Gunnar Jungner's early account of the ethics of screening (1968), since widely adopted, according to which, "the risks [of being screened], both physical and psychological, should be less than the benefits" (Brindle and Fahey 2002: 56). This principle looks a lot like the approach articulated above, because it holds that a good screening program does not just improve population-level outcomes but benefits each screenee.

The notion of *ex-ante* interests seems to provide a neat way of bridging the gap between the population- and individual-level perspectives. Unfortunately, although this problem is often hidden in discussions of screening (John and Wu, 2022), the reconciliation is not complete: because it is easy to confuse the claims that a program does more good than harm overall, so is in the *ex-ante* interests of the *average* attendee, with the claim that it is in the *ex-ante* interests of *each* attendee. I return to related concerns in Section "Prevention paradoxes" below. Before doing so, however, it is important to note further problems in reconciling individuals' *ex-ante* interests with the population perspective: the prevention paradoxes.

Prevention paradoxes

The key problem in these cases stems from what the British epidemiologist Geoffrey Rose called the "fundamental axiom of preventive medicine": "a large number of people exposed to a small risk may generate many more cases [of disease] than a small number of people exposed to a high risk" (Rose 2008: 53). For example, the most effective strategy to tackle alcohol-related morbidity and mortality may not be to influence the behavior of "high-risk" heavy drinkers, but to change the habits of the large number of "moderate" drinkers. Although each individual's risk reduction is far less in the second intervention than the first, the aggregate gains are far higher, because the second population is so much larger (John 2018). Rose's principle is counter-intuitive, or at least non-obvious, but why think is there any reason to think that it is deeply troubling?

Indeed, there are some reasons to worry about Rose's prevention principle, which Rose himself termed "paradoxes of prevention." First, there are "relative prevention paradoxes," concerning how heavily we should weigh individuals' *ex-ante* interests in deciding which public health policies to pursue (John 2014; Thompson 2018). For example, compare a policy of screening every woman between 50 and 70 with a policy of screening all and only women with the BRCA1 and BRCA2 variants for breast cancer. Given the extremely high elevated risk associated with these two variants, the second policy would do far more to improve each affected individual's *ex-ante* interests. One might think that the most vulnerable have a special claim on social help (Wolff and De-Shalit 2007). Therefore, focusing on the individual perspective, one might take public health policy to have most reasons to help the BRCA1/BRCA2 women. Nonetheless, given that there are very many more women between 50 and 70 than women with BRCA1/2, the first program would foreseeably do much more population-level good. If, then, we have limited resources and cannot follow both policies, we must choose whether to help those at greatest risk or to save the greater number of lives.

This is a difficult choice, made more difficult by its intersection with debates over the "identified victims" bias (Cohen, Daniels, and Eyal 2015). There is a well-documented psychological tendency to prefer helping "identified" rather than "statistical" victims, even when helping "statistical" victims would do more aggregate "good." For example, we are far more likely to be willing to donate £10 when told that doing so will save the life of a specific, named individual, rather than when we are told that the sum will reduce a 1-in-10,000 risk of death suffered by 20,000 people, even though the latter course of action will foreseeably save more lives. A preference for saving the most-at-risk may seem related to this general tendency, insofar as it tends to be far easier to identify high-risk individuals than the many more people at moderate risk. On the one hand, we might use this link to debunk the "save the most at risk" principle as irrational; for example, we might say that the principle simply reflects the fact that we find it hard to think about probabilities and big numbers. On the other hand, however, some have argued that we can (at least partially) vindicate the apparent "bias" as reflecting a deep and important moral concern (Daniels 2012; Frick 2015).

Second, it seems possible to generate "absolute prevention paradoxes," where the very same policy seems to be both *worse* for each affected individual in terms of her *ex-ante* interest and yet *improve* population-level outcomes (John 2014). Assume that, for each individual woman between 50 and 70, the expected health benefits of screening ever so slightly outweigh the expected health harms. However, each woman also dislikes the discomfort associated with a mammography, such that, from her individual perspective, going to screening is not in her *ex-ante* interests. When, however, we calculate the population-level benefits of screening, we tend to focus only on aggregate *health-related* costs and benefits, not including "feelings of discomfort" in the "costs" column. This may be because they are hard to measure (Alexandrova 2017), but there are also arguments why we should *not* measure such harms or consider them relevant, stemming from more general philosophical concerns (Kelleher 2013). Either way, when assessing the policy from a population-level perspective, we might judge that its overall population-level effects are positive. So, the very same policy seems to make each individual *worse off*—and yet to improve aggregate health outcomes!

Either we focus on assessing and justifying policies solely in terms of their expected population-level effects or (at least in part) in terms of individuals' *ex-ante* interests. In Section "Introduction," I suggested that just adopting the first perspective risks sacrificing individuals for the sake of a "population-level" good. However, if we adopt the second perspective, taking *ex-ante* interests seriously might lead us to policies which seem clearly sub-optimal from a population perspective. This is not a minor concern. Think again about the debate over identified and statistical victims. On the face of it, if we can choose a measure which helps more people or fewer people, it seems better to help more people: that the people we help are not identifiable does not mean that they are not real people!

Furthermore, these dilemmas and problems in the screening case only become more complicated in other cases, such as vaccination. As Section "Introduction" explained, some vaccination policies involve vaccinating some individuals because they can act as disease vectors, even though vaccination is not in their own interests. (Note that this tension does not just arise in HPV; for example, vaccinating children against chickenpox is best understood as protecting fetal health (Malm and Navin 2020).) Again, this problem can be framed as a concern about the relationship between the population perspective and a concern for *ex-ante* interests. The best "population-level" outcomes seem to require policies that improve the *ex-ante* interests of some—young women—but worsen the *ex-ante* interests of others—young men. So, we face a question of whether and how a policy's effect on the *distribution* of *ex-ante* interests is ethically relevant.

In turn, this is a difficult question. Consider the distribution of scarce vaccines during a pandemic. One obvious principle is to distribute the vaccine which maximizes (expected) impact on overall population-level mortality and morbidity. However, some philosophers argue that this efficiency principle is *unfair*, and that it would be preferable to distribute doses using a fair lottery, ensuring that each has an *equal chance* of benefit (Peterson 2008). Resolving this debate requires, then, that we have some sense of how to balance concerns about the *distribution* of *ex-ante* chances and concerns about population-level outcomes. And, to add an extra twist, even if we adopt the individual *ex-ante* perspective, you might think that our focus should not be on ensuring equal chances, but on helping the most vulnerable. For example, the initial UK government guidelines for distributing the Covid-19 vaccine seem to have focused on helping those most vulnerable to disease, rather than helping the greatest number or equalizing chances (Joint Committee on Vaccination and Immunisation 2020); of course, it is possible that helping the most vulnerable coincides with helping the greatest number, but Rose's work reminds us that this cannot be guaranteed. We are back, then, to the "relative prevention paradox"!

The vaccination case is further complicated, because, unlike the screening case, it involves risk imposition. If an individual woman chooses not to get screened for breast cancer, this choice does not affect anyone else's risks of suffering ill-health. By contrast, unvaccinated men who choose to have unprotected sex with women impose a risk of HPV on their partners. In turn, then, we might argue that, regardless of *their own* prospects, young men have an obligation to get vaccinated (Giublini 2019). Indeed, Jessica Flanigan (2014) has argued that people who choose not to vaccinate are ethically equivalent to people who sit on their doorsteps casually firing guns at their neighbors! This kind of consideration is, though, extremely hard to spell out. Plausibly, every time I ride my bicycle, I impose a tiny risk of harm on pedestrians compared to the alternative of staying at home, but it would be odd to say that every cycle ride harms other people; however, choosing to drive to the shops in my giant SUV, when I could as easily have cycled, seems more likely to be problematic. Even if we can solve these puzzles, we face a further mystery, of how concerns about individual obligations and rights fit into the "consequentialist" calculations typically used in public health policy (Hausman 2006).

So far in this chapter, I have distinguished the population-level and individual-level perspectives in public health policy and explored ethical principles we might use to think through each of perspective. In the face of this kind of complex ethical situation, we have two options: *monism*, one perspective, and one principle within that perspective, is the *only* correct approach (so, for example, *all* we should care about is maximizing aggregate population health or ensuring equal chances); or *pluralism*, that both perspectives, and various principles within each, are valid, and ethical reasoning involves balancing considerations. The first option seems implausible, given our complex intuitions. The second is appealing in some cases—where it helps us identify policies which look good according to *every* principle—but, whenever we have a tension, it risks being ad hoc. So, public health ethics requires difficult choices. Unfortunately, rather than making those choices here, I will now suggest an even more fundamental set of concerns about reconciling the population- and individual-level perspectives.

The epistemic aspect

In this section, I explore three concepts which mediate the population- and individual-level perspectives: chance, causation, and categorization. Before going on, it is important to note the limits to my discussion. There is a huge literature on how we establish various claims at the population level; for example, how we might establish that some intervention, like screening, actually *does* lead to a decrease in cancer mortality (Saquib, Saquib, and Ioannidis 2015). In this section, I place these questions to one side to focus, instead, on the question of how and when we can move *from* claims about population-level relationships to claims *about* individuals. Following Jonathan Fuller and Luis Flores (2015), I am less interested in questions about how we can "generalize" claims from epidemiological studies to target populations—for example, how and when we can move from "the intervention was effective in the study population" to "the intervention will be effective in the general population"—and more interested in how we "particularize" from population-level to individual-level claims; for example, from "it works for most people in the population" to "it will work for this individual."

First, consider, again, the case of screening. Why invite women over 50 to routine screening, but not women under 50? The standard answer is that breast cancer risk increases with age, and it is only when women are over 50, when their ten-year breast cancer risk is 2.85%

that screening starts to become effective (Pashayan et al. 2018). We can use standard epidemiological tools to calculate the proportion of cases of breast cancer in the under-50s and the over-50s, generating the 2.85% figure. Even if we have well-established population-level data, it does not obviously follow, however, that each woman under 50 is at a lower risk of breast cancer than each woman over 50. It seems, for example, that a 35-year-old with BRCA1 and BRCA2 is at a higher breast cancer risk than a 52-year-old without them. Again, though, we should be careful here. For example, plausibly, even if they don't have the BRCA1/2 variants, 52-year-old women with a family history of breast cancer are at a higher risk than women without such a family history, so we should be careful not to treat the 52-year-olds without BRCA1/2 as homogenous (Pashayan et al. 2018). Indeed, identifying different ways of identifying at-risk individuals is a mini-industry, with one paper comparing 49 common models for calculating breast cancer risk (Cintalo-Gonzalez et al. 2017).

We often talk of an individual's risk of disease as akin to something like her blood pressure, a measurable quantity which can directly be affected by various interventions, for example, when we distinguish between "controllable" and "uncontrollable" risk factors for disease. However, plausibly, there is no quantity of *this individual's risk*. Rather, claims about risk—at least as employed in public health policy and epidemiology—are best understood as claims about some individual considered as a member of some population (Fuller 2020). So, for example, the claim that Jane is at a higher risk of breast cancer than Priya *and* the claim that Priya is at a higher risk of breast cancer than Jane can *both* be true, as long as we specify that, in the first case, we are comparing the two women in terms of BRCA status, and, in the second, in terms of age. Unfortunately, there are no further facts, Jane and Priya's *true* risks—similar to their true blood pressure—relative to which we can resolve the apparent disagreement over whose risk is *actually* higher. This may seem too strong, because you might think that there is a clear sense in which gaining more information about an individual gets us to a better estimate of her risk; say, we are better off calculating Jane's risk relative to her age and family history than just her age. There are difficult conceptual issues here. All I want to suggest is that there is a difference: when two blood pressure monitors give different readings, at most one can be correct, but two apparently contradictory risk scores can *both* be correct.

(You might respond that all of the concerns above are premised on denying that there are things such as "objective" chances. This is a topic which takes us into tricky metaphysical issues. All I note here is that even if there are objective, individual chances—"my risk of cancer" akin to "my blood pressure"—it is deeply unclear that we can interpret epidemiologically based claims about individual risks as attempts to measure those "things.")

Why think this feature of risk estimates is so problematic? Consider vaccination. As we saw in Section "Motivating the individual perspective," during the recent Covid-19 pandemic, the UK's vaccination programs were aimed at helping the most vulnerable (Joint Committee on Vaccination and Immunisation 2020). Who counts as the "most vulnerable"? The UK government's answer to this question was the oldest members of society. This is reasonable, because Covid-19 risk increases with age. However, we also know that Covid risk varies with sex and with ethnicity (Spiegelhalter 2020). It may well be true that the average 75-year-old is more vulnerable than the average 65-year-old, but it is not at all obvious that a white, female 75-year-old is more vulnerable than a Black, male 65-year-old. Should we have subdivided the population differently? Any decent answer to this question has to take account of our knowledge of the world, what statistics we can compile, and our causal knowledge of the effects of inequality. However, ultimately, we cannot answer that question without also engaging with distinctively ethical concerns. For example, consider the claim that the epidemiology of Covid-19 stems in part from background structural inequalities

(Horton 2020). One might argue that this claim implies that, even if age and ethnicity are both risk factors for Covid-19 risk, we *should* identify the "most vulnerable" using ethnicity, rather than age, because doing so responds to a background *injustice*. Any such claim, however, involves contentious ethical claims, about the nature of (in)justice and how justice should be balanced against other social goods. In turn, these differences are not merely "theoretical" or "semantic": they might make an important difference not only to who lives or dies, but to how many people live or die. When justice considerations demand that we save fewer lives than we could otherwise, we face a fundamental ethical problem about balancing competing ethical norms.

These remarks on *chance* lead to my second concept, *categorization*. A core concern in public health ethics is the nature of health inequality (Hausman 2007). For example, one worry about breast cancer screening is that if there is differential uptake across social classes, then the programs will increase inequalities between different socioeconomic groups, even as they improve population health. Consider, now, a feature of concerns about inequality: typically, measures of health inequity or inequality focus on differences between members of different groups (Eyal 2018). (These might be differences in *access* or in *outcomes*, reflecting, again, a distinction between *ex-ante* and *ex-post*, but nothing here turns on that issue.) For example, we might measure inequalities in screening access between members of different socioeconomic classes or different ethnicities. Therefore, claims about the extent of inequality within a population turn on how we divide that population into sub-populations: there might be high levels of health inequality between socioeconomic groups, but low inequality between ethnic groups.

Many agencies are committed to tackling health inequalities; for example, reducing health inequalities is one of the six key goals of the UK's National Health Service (NHS). However, there are, of course, multiple inequalities the NHS could tackle: for example, in the UK, there is life-expectancy inequality between White men and Afro-Caribbean men, and life-expectancy inequality between men and women. If we focus on the first inequality, Jack, a White man, will not have any special entitlement to help; if we focus on the latter, he might have some claim to help. Which inequality should we focus on, then? One way of addressing this question is to ask whether the relevant categories—of ethnicity, of sex—are really scientifically respectable, in the sense that they can usefully serve as the basis for purposes of explanation and prediction (Franklin-Hall 2015). Ultimately, however, there may be more than one scientifically respectable way of carving up the natural and social worlds (Dupré 1995); plausibly, categories of ethnicity and of sex are *one* way of carving up the world, but not the only way—classification by social class, say, might *also* be a "respectable" ground for explanation and prediction. In choosing which inequality to care about, then, we seek explanations for the inequalities in the thought that certain sorts of explanations might render the relevant inequalities more or less ethically worrying. For example, you might think that if ethnic differences reflect social discrimination, whereas sex differences stem from biological differences, then we should care about the former rather than the latter. Such choices, which might have a large impact on specific individuals like Jack, are, of course, shot through with ethical assumptions about topics such as the nature and harm of discrimination.

Finally, consider causation. Clearly, one reason we care about—and one way in which we use—epidemiological data is to identify interventions on individual behavior; for example, we move from claims about the average effects of statin consumption in a population to claims about the benefits to individuals of consuming statins. This blurring of the population and individual perspectives has been intensified by the ways in which the influential "Evidence-Based Medicine" movement has suggested that the tools used to identify causation in (some areas of) epidemiology have an important role in establishing causal claims in the clinic, blurring the lines between public health and clinical care (Howick 2011; see also Mercuri and Upshur, this volume). Furthermore, as the examples above suggest, claims about causation are central to ethical and political theorizing; we want to know the causes of ill-health not only as a way of identifying effective interventions, but also for understanding the grounds of where we should intervene, or, indeed, whether we have ethical reasons to intervene at all. Plausibly, if ethnic inequalities are "our" fault, we have a particularly strong reason to act, but notions of fault clearly piggyback on notions of cause.

However, causation is another contested notion. Two concerns are worth noting. First, plausibly, any outcome has numerous causes: cancer is the result of mutations, but the rate of mutation may be affected by diet, but diet may be affected by food availability, which is affected by policy. When we talk of *the* cause of an outcome, we choose which of these causes to prioritize. Some epidemiological approaches insist that we should only treat "controllable" causes as causes of disease (Broadbent 2015). However, while there might be methodological reasons to define causal hypotheses carefully, such claims are multiply problematic: judgments about what can be changed or controlled may be heavily biased and, even when correct, what *can* be controlled or changed may not be what *ought* to be controllable or changeable. We need to recognize, then, that claims about which causes are "most important" or "relevant" need to be shaped and assessed through explicitly ethical argument.

Second, a familiar claim in theories of causation is that causal explanation is contrastive: an answer to "why did X happen?" is best understood as having an implicit "foil"—"why did X happen, rather than Y?" Therefore, an answer to the question of why X happened might differ depending on the (implicit) foil. For example, if our question is "why did Jack contract the disease rather than stay healthy?" a good answer might be "because he contracted the virus," given that this is a key difference between the *actual* world, where Jack falls ill, and a counterfactual scenario where he does not. However, if our question is "why did Jack fall ill when Jill did not?" the best answer will have to point to some difference between Jack and Jill. If Jill was also exposed to the virus, then the best answer will have to be something like "Jack had a pre-existing susceptibility to the infection" (Lipton 2003). This contrast-sensitivity gives us a further difficulty in moving from population-level claims, which typically compare differences between outcomes in groups, to claims about individuals, because we cannot assume that the contrasts used to address population-level questions will be the most relevant for addressing individual-level concerns. It may well be correct to say, at the population level, that the best explanation for the different health outcomes in different groups is relative socioeconomic deprivation. It does not thereby follow that the best explanation of why some individual member of some lower socioeconomic group fell ill is that she was (relatively) deprived. Using population-level claims at an individual level requires us to think about which kinds of contrasts are relevant. In turn, again, such judgments go well beyond the purely epistemic, to include concerns about which comparisons are ethically or politically important.

In this section, I have investigated three concepts—chance, categorization, and causation—which mediate between the "population" and the "individual" perspectives. Being able to "particularize" our population-level knowledge—to talk about the risks individuals face, or to make predictions based on their membership of sub-populations, or to talk about individual-level causes—is useful for clinical care and prediction. It is also ethically important. In each of my cases, however, there seem to be *too many* ways in which we could move from population- to individual-level claims. For any individual, given the very same population-level data, there are multiple ways of describing *her* risk of harm, of categorizing *her*, and of talking about *the* causes of *her* ill-health.

Sometimes, realizing that individual-level claims are underdetermined by population-level data is liberating. For example, rather than worrying about whether, in using age rather than race to calculate individual risk we have identified the *really* at-risk people, we can, instead, just accept that both approaches *could* be valid, depending on ethical interests. At other points, however, this abundance is destabilizing, because it seems hard to take any *particular* claim seriously—help *me* because I am at a high risk or a member of such a community or my health is caused by this unjust situation—when some other claims would be equally valid. So, we need ways of deciding which risks or categories or causes matter.

An integrated philosophy of public health

At this point, you might feel worried: to resolve the clash of ethical principles which we discussed in Sections "Introduction" and "Motivating the individual perspective," we need to know that cases are properly described, but to describe those cases we need to know how to balance principles. Should we give up any hope of reconciling the population- and individual-level perspectives?

I suggest not. Rather, I think that the real lesson to be taken here is that we need to focus attention on the kinds of reasons, both epistemic and ethical, we can give for framing a case a particular way. How might we do that? There is not space here to address that challenge fully. However, an obvious suggestion is to think about inference from population to individual as something which should be open to broadly political forms of debate and discussion. For example, Norman Daniels and James Sabin have argued that we should assess decisions about healthcare allocation in terms of how well they match norms of deliberative democracy (Daniels and Sabin 2002). Plausibly, we might think about the move from population- to individual-level claims along similar lines, asking if they pass norms of procedural justice; for example, rather than treat the cut-off point for inviting women to breast cancer screening as if it were purely a technical matter, we might seek to create forums where these decisions are discussed and debated through proper democratic means.

These approaches from political philosophy mesh neatly with recent arguments in philosophy of science, which have stressed the importance of deliberation and debate for uncovering and refining non-epistemic values which structure scientific research. For example, Helen Longino has argued that scientific inference must always rest on some sets of untestable non-epistemic assumptions and has suggested broadly democratic procedures for ensuring that these assumptions are not ethically, socially, or politically problematic (Longino 1990). So, too, we might argue that we need critical scrutiny of the values which implicitly structure our move from population to individual. Again, the example of cancer screening is helpful here: rather than decide eligibility by a procedure which assumes a particular utilitarian end, we might, instead, seek to prompt public debate and discussion, which would allow us to uncover potential biases in how we frame our decision.

The notion that how we infer from population to individual is not only "scientific" but also "political" may seem worrying or utopian or some mixture of the two. However, the general approach sketched here dovetails with real-life debates. One way of thinking about the ethics of screening is to assume that various official estimates of the "costs" and "benefits" are correct, then to ask how we should balance or compare them; this is the kind of approach I adopted in Section "Introduction." However, a key part of the real-world debate over screening concerns what we should count as a cost in the first place. For example, many critical commentators point out that standard approaches to screening fail to take account of the psychosocial effects of medicalization (Klawiter 2008). In raising these concerns, critics are not arguing over how best to balance the costs and benefits of screening, but over how to frame the problem in the very first place. So, we can see how many real debates over public health policy do not fit neatly into an "ethical" or "epistemic" camp. In this case, we have ethical arguments about what we should try to count (and how it should be counted). It should be no surprise, then, that something similar might be true about the cases of chance, categorization, and causation.

In turn, thinking about how we want to represent the world will also uncover options for improving it. In both screening and vaccination cases, ethical problems arise because it seems that the claims of different groups are in tension: in the screening case, there is an apparent tension between the interests of women between 50 and 70 and women in the BRCA1/2 groups; in the case of HPV vaccination, there is an apparent tension between the interests of men and women. However, we should not be so quick to assume that these apparent tensions are genuine. Rather, we should first ask ourselves whether we think that categorizing people by, say, age, or genetic profile, or sex, is something we should be doing in public health policy in the first place: who has objections to doing this? How strong are those objections? What are our alternatives? In turn, working through these questions might, plausibly, help us find different ways of framing our decisions which at least alleviate or remove problems. Of course, there will always remain tensions between the population- and individual-level perspectives. However, we will not understand what those tensions *are*, or how they might be avoided, without thinking about the ethical dimensions of population to individual inference. To reconcile the population- and individual-level perspectives, we need an integrated philosophy of public health policy.

References

Alexandrova, A. 2017 *A philosophy for the science of well-being.* Oxford: Oxford University Press.

Anand, S., F. Peters, and A. Sen, eds. 2004 *Public health, ethics and equity.* Oxford: Oxford University Press.

Beauchamp, T. L. and J. F. Childress. 2001. *Principles of biomedical ethics.* New York: Oxford University Press.

Brindle, P. and T. Fahey. 2002. Primary prevention of coronary heart disease. *British Medical Journal* 325, no. 7355: 56–57. https://dx.doi.org/10.1136%2Fbmj.325.7355.56.

Broadbent, A. 2015. Causation and prediction in epidemiology: A guide to the "methodological revolution." *Studies in History and Philosophy of Biological and Biomedical Sciences* 54: 72–80. https://doi.org/10.1016/j.shpsc.2015.06.004.

Cintolo-Gonzalez, J. A., D. Braun, A. L. Blackford et al. 2017. Breast cancer risk models: A comprehensive overview of existing models, validation, and clinical applications. *Breast Cancer Research and Treatment* 164, no. 2: 263–284. https://doi.org/10.1007/s10549-017-4247-z.

Cohen, I., N. Daniels, and N. Eyal, eds. 2015. *Identified versus statistical lives: An interdisciplinary perspective.* Oxford: Oxford University Press.

Daniels, N. 2012. Reasonable disagreement about identified vs. statistical victims. *Hastings Center Report* 42, no. 1: 35–45. https://doi.org/10.1002/hast.13.

Daniels, N. and J. Sabin. 2002. *Setting limits fairly: Can we learn to share medical resources?* Oxford: Oxford University Press.

Dupré, J. 1995. *The disorder of things: Metaphysical foundations of the disunity of science.* Cambridge, MA: Harvard University Press.

Eyal, N. 2018. Inequality in political philosophy and in epidemiology: A remarriage. *Journal of Applied Philosophy* 35, no. 1: 149–167. https://doi.org/10.1111/japp.12150.

Flanigan, J. 2014. A defense of compulsory vaccination. *HEC Forum* 26, no. 1: 5–25. https://doi.org/10.1007/s10730-013-9221-5.

Fleurbaey, M. and A. Voorhoeve. 2013. Decide as you would with full information. In *Inequalities in health: Concepts, measures, and ethics,* ed. N. Eyal, S. A. Hurst, O. F. Norheim, and D. Wikler, 113–128. Oxford: Oxford University Press.

Franklin-Hall, L. 2015. Natural kinds as categorical bottlenecks. *Philosophical Studies* 172, no. 4: 925–948. https://doi.org/10.1007/s11098-014-0326-8.

Frick, J. 2015. Contractualism and social risk. *Philosophy & Public Affairs* 43, no. 3: 175–223. https://doi.org/10.1111/papa.12058.

Fuller, J. 2020. Epidemiological evidence: Use at your "Own Risk?" *Philosophy of Science* 87, no. 5: 1119–1129. https://doi.org/10.1086/710540.

Fuller, J. and L. J. Flores. 2015. The risk GP model: The standard model of prediction in medicine. *Studies in History and Philosophy of Biological and Biomedical Sciences* 54: 49–61. https://doi.org/10.1016/j.shpsc.2015.06.006.

Giubilini, A. 2019. *The ethics of vaccination.* Cham: Springer Nature.

Goodin, R. E. 1995. *Utilitarianism as a public philosophy.* Cambridge: Cambridge University Press.

Hausman, D. M. 2006. Valuing health. *Philosophy & Public Affairs* 34, no. 3: 246–274. https://doi.org/10.1111/j.1088-4963.2006.00067.x.

Hausman, D. M. 2007. What's wrong with health inequalities? *Journal of Political Philosophy* 15, no. 1: 46–66. https://doi.org/10.1111/j.1467-9760.2007.00270.x.

Hausman, D. M. 2015. *Valuing health: Well-being, freedom, and suffering.* Oxford: Oxford University Press.

Horton R. 2020. Offline: COVID-19 is not a pandemic. *The Lancet* 396, no. 10255: 874. https://doi.org/10.1016/S0140-6736(20)32000-6.

Howick, J. H. 2011. *The philosophy of evidence-based medicine.* London: John Wiley & Sons.

John, S. D. 2014. Risk, contractualism, and Rose's "prevention paradox." *Social Theory and Practice* 40, no. 1: 28–50. https://doi.org/10.5840/soctheorpract20144012.

John, S. 2018. Should we punish responsible drinkers? Prevention, paternalism and categorization in public health. *Public Health Ethics* 11, no. 1: 35–44. https://doi.org/10.1093/phe/phx017.

John, S. and J. Wu. 2022. First, do no harm? Non-maleficence, population health and the ethics of risk. *Social Theory and Practice.* online-first https://doi.org/10.5840/soctheorpract2022218152

Joint Committee on Vaccination and Immunisation. 2020. Advice on priority groups for COVID-19 vaccination, 30 December. https://www.gov.uk/government/publications/priority-groups-for-coronavirus-covid-19-vaccination-advice-from-the-jcvi-30-december-2020/joint-committee-on-vaccination-and-immunisation-advice-on-priority-groups-for-covid-19-vaccination-30-december-2020 (accessed December 13, 2021).

Kelleher, J. P. 2013. Prevention, rescue, and tiny risks. *Public Health Ethics* 6, no. 3: 252–261. https://doi.org/10.1093/phe/pht032.

Klawiter, M. 2008. *The biopolitics of breast cancer: Changing cultures of disease and activism.* Minneapolis: University of Minnesota Press.

Lipton, P. 2003. *Inference to the best explanation.* London: Routledge.

Longino, H. E. 1990. *Science as social knowledge: Values and objectivity in scientific inquiry.* Princeton, NJ: Princeton University Press.

Lowy, I. 2011. *A woman's disease: The history of cervical cancer.* Oxford: Oxford University Press.

Malm, H. and M. C. Navin. 2020. Pox parties for grannies? Chickenpox, exogenous boosting, and harmful injustices. *American Journal of Bioethics* 20, no. 9: 45–57. https://doi.org/10.1080/15265161.2020.1795528.

Marmot, M. G., D. G. Altman, D. A. Cameron et al. 2013. The benefits and harms of breast cancer screening: An independent review. *British Journal of Cancer* 108, no. 11: 2205–2240. http://doi.org/10.1038/bjc.2013.177.

O'Neill, O. 2002. *Autonomy and trust in bioethics.* Cambridge: Cambridge University Press.

Pashayan, N., S. Morris, F. J. Gilbert, and P. D. Pharoah. 2018. Cost-effectiveness and benefit-to-harm ratio of risk-stratified screening for breast cancer: A life-table model. *JAMA Oncology* 4, no. 11: 1504–1510. https://doi.org/10.1001/jamaoncol.2018.1901.

Peterson, M. 2008. The moral importance of selecting people randomly. *Bioethics* 22, no. 6: 321–327. https://doi.org/10.1111/j.1467-8519.2008.00636.x.

Plutynski, A. 2012. Ethical issues in cancer screening and prevention. *Journal of Medicine and Philosophy* 37, no. 3: 310–323. https://doi.org/10.1093/jmp/jhs017.

Rose, G. 2008 *The strategy of preventive medicine.* Oxford: Oxford University Press.

Saquib, N., J. Saquib and J. P. Ioannidis. 2015. Does screening for disease save lives in asymptomatic adults? Systematic review of meta-analyses and randomized trials. *International Journal of Epidemiology* 44, no. 1: 264–277. https://doi.org/10.1093/ije/dyu140.

Spiegelhalter, D. 2020. What are the risks of COVID? And what is meant by "the risks of COVID?" *Medium,* May 13. https://medium.com/wintoncentre/what-are-the-risks-of-covid-and-what-is-meant-by-the-risks-of-covid-c828695aea69 (accessed May 14, 2020).

Thompson, C. 2018. Rose's prevention paradox. *Journal of Applied Philosophy* 35, no. 2: 242–256. https://doi.org/10.1111/japp.12177.

Verweij, M. 2015. How (not) to argue for the rule of rescue. In *Identified versus statistical victims: An interdisciplinary perspective,* ed. G. Cohen, N. Daniels and N. Eyal, 137–149. Oxford: Oxford University Press.

Wilson, J. and G. Jungner. 1968. *Principles and practice of screening for disease.* Geneva: World Health Organization.

Wolff, J. and A. De-Shalit. 2007. *Disadvantage.* Oxford: Oxford University Press.

4

CONCEPTS OF HEALTH AND DISEASE IN PUBLIC HEALTH

Benjamin Smart

Introduction

Given that notions of health and disease ground the practices of all medical sciences, it is unsurprising that analyzing these concepts has always been a core component of philosophy of medicine. Christopher Boorse (1975, 1977, 1997, 2014), Rachel Cooper (2002), Jerome Wakefield (1992), and many others have written papers discussing the nature of disease, but all of these focus on the domains of clinical medicine and pathology. Some work on the philosophy of public health has been published (Nijhuis and Van der Maesen 1994, 2000; Valles 2018; Weed 1999), but little in the way of detailed analysis of the concepts of health and disease within this context of public health has been presented.

Harry Nijhuis and Laurent van der Maesen identify two ontological categories characterizing the nature of "public" in public health. The first emphasizes the individual over the collective, and the second the collective over the individual. In this chapter, I will discuss the nature of disease in the context of both the individuals that make up a population, and in Section "Conclusions," consider how the "health" predicate can meaningfully be applied to the collective.

Let us use the term "public health" broadly as "the science of protecting and improving the health of people and their communities [...] by promoting healthy lifestyles, researching disease and injury prevention, and detecting, preventing and responding to infectious diseases" (CDC Foundation 2021).

Nijhuis and Van der Maesen, in a 1994 editorial on the philosophical foundations of public health, suggest four "categories of ontological interpretations of public health," two pertaining to "public" and two to "health."

> [Public] Category [PC1] emphasises the individual. In this view, the public is primarily comprised of the actions and motives of discrete individuals. "Public" category [PC2], on the other hand, emphasises the collective over the individual. "Health" category [HC1] is a mechanistic view that emphasises the traditional medical distinction between disease and non-disease in the individual, whereas [Health] category [HC2] views health as the degree to which an individual reaches an equilibrium state with somatic, psychological, and social influences.
>
> *(Weed 1999: 99)*

DOI: 10.4324/9781315675411-6

Nijhuis and Van der Maesen claim that "The great majority of scientific and other public health work, including epidemiological research and preventive programmes … is based on the concepts in categories [PC1 and HC1]. Most of the policy statements of 'health promotion' seem to be founded on perspectives [PC1 or PC2 and HC2]" (1994: 2).

Drawing on work published in the *Journal of Evaluation in Clinical Practice* (Smart, Stevens, and Verbakel 2018), I show in this chapter how these four categories can be applied to existing analyses of disease in the context of clinical medicine and pathology, and then apply these analyses to public health. I conclude with a plausible, comparative account of health that can be applied to populations as a collective (as opposed to the individuals comprising the collective).

The context-dependency of the disease concept

The literature on "what is health/disease?" is rapidly growing, broadly speaking covering two related but distinct philosophical projects. The first concerns disease as an ontological category, where the goal is to determine what types of particulars and/or processes and/or properties constitute diseases (for example, Whitbeck 1977; Fuller 2018). The second is a project in conceptual analysis. This second project comprises an attempt to discover the meaning of the term "disease," in other words, to work out the necessary and sufficient conditions for an individual to be diseased (assume diseases pertain only to individuals for now), without recourse to "not healthy."[1] If one interprets this as "what do 'we' mean when we use the term 'disease'"—and this is a dangerous interpretation—then one finds oneself in a quandary. "We," as a proxy for a definite description of a particular group of persons, is not, without qualification, particularly useful. Does "we" refer to all (alive) persons? Does it refer to all (alive) persons in academia? Does it refer to all (alive) persons working in the medical sciences? And so on. If one takes "we" to refer to the class of all (alive) persons, then there is the further question of "does the term 'disease' always mean the same thing, or can it change its meaning when used in different contexts or at different times?" This chapter is concerned primarily with the second category of conceptual analysis, although as we (all readers of this chapter) shall see, reference to the ontological category is inevitable.

It will become clear during the course of this chapter that "disease" is a fluid concept—its meaning changes depending on who is uttering the term, and under what circumstances. The search for necessary and sufficient conditions for *the* concept of disease will therefore always be fruitless, since those conditions are subject to change. One should thus adopt a pluralist approach. That is not to say that attempts to cash out notions of health and disease are necessarily fruitless, only that one must specify the context prior to presenting one's analysis. Boorse does exactly this. He states that his analysis is one of disease qua "pathological condition" (Boorse, 1977: 542)—the theoretical concept of disease employed by the pathologist. Others are guilty of being less explicit in this regard. Cooper (2002) criticizes Boorse on the ground that disease cannot be a value-free concept, but Cooper's analysis is, at least on the face of it, entirely inappropriate for the pathologist with no direct access to the patient (it is often impossible for the pathologist to determine whether the patient considers the condition to be a "bad thing to have," so how *could* the value assessments of the patient play any role?). In this chapter, I consider three contexts in which the concept of disease is employed within the medical sciences: pathology, clinical medicine, and the health of a human population as a collective.

PC1 considers the "public" in terms of a collection of individuals. This, the individual organism, is where the majority of literature on concepts of health and disease has focused.

PC2 considers the collective over the individual, and in the final section, I outline what "healthy populations," in this sense, might look like. In the following sections, I provide an overview of a number of analyses of health and disease from the PC1 perspective, since public health draws on concepts of health applied to both PC1 and PC2.

The pathologist

Pathology is the branch of medical science that describes the study of physiological subsystems (fluids, cells, tissues, organs) for the purpose of diagnosing and establishing the cause(s) of disease. The job of pathologists is thus, at least in part, to examine surgically removed tissue and/or fluids (or perhaps an entire body, in the case of an autopsy) and identify the abnormalities typical of specific diseases. It is this focus on discovering abnormalities that motivates the biostatistical theory (BST). Over the course of these debates, Boorse has set out BST in a number of different ways. I will assume, however, the most recent schema at the time of writing. It runs as follows:

1   The *reference class* is a natural class of organisms of uniform functional design, specifically, an age group of a sex of a species.
2   A *normal function* of a part or process within members of the reference class is a statistically typical contribution by it to their individual survival [or] reproduction.
3   *Health* in a member of the reference class is a normal functional ability: the readiness of each internal part to perform all its normal functions on typical occasions with at least typical efficiency.
4   A *disease* [later, pathological condition] is a type of internal state which impairs health, i.e. reduces one or more functional abilities below typical efficiency (Boorse 2014: 684).

Boorse takes a physiological subsystem to be diseased if and only if it performs its function subnormally, relative to the reference class to which the organism in question belongs. This is often illustrated by a graph such as in Figure 4.1.

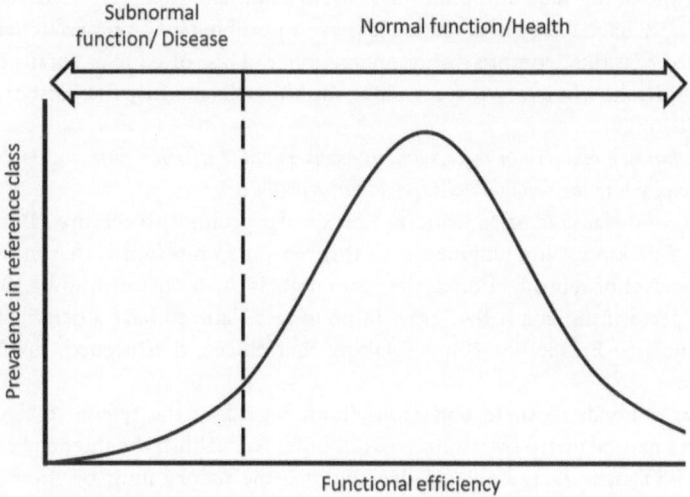

Figure 4.1   The biostatistical theory

Most physiological subsystems have a "natural function"—subsystems *do* something specific that positively contributes to the health of the organism.[2] Let us take Figure 4.1 to represent the functional efficiency of lungs for some reference class *R*. Some members of *R* have incredibly healthy lungs that perform their function (of absorbing oxygen into the bloodstream) extremely efficiently, whereas other members of *R* have lungs that barely absorb sufficient oxygen to keep those members alive. These individuals fit into the far right and far left hand sides of Figure 4.1. The area to the left of the dotted line represents those lungs performing their function "subnormally," that is, those members of *R* with diseased lungs. More generally, the areas to the right of the dotted line represent organs operating with normal (or, to the far right, supernomal) functional efficiency (for *R*). For a member of *R* to be diseased with respect to some trait *T* is just to fit into the area to the left of the dotted line the chart representing *T* for *R*.

BST is a mechanistic account of health in individuals. It falls into Nijhuis and Van der Maesens' "health" category HC1. However, individual health states are grounded by the health (qua functional efficiency of the physiological subsystems of members) of populations. Health and disease are not states wholly determined by the physiological state of the individual, but those states relative to the average physiological states of the population, estimated through epidemiological studies. It is worth examining the core claims in the schema, since most have been criticized in one way or another (although, in my opinion, for the most part not all that successfully).

1   *The reference class is a natural class of organisms of uniform functional design, specifically, an age group of a sex of a species.*

   The first clause has been criticized on at least two grounds: first, that contrary to Boorse's claim, BST is not a naturalist conception of disease. In selecting age, sex, and species type, Boorse is making value judgments regarding the saliency of particular properties to determine the members of each reference class and, *ipso facto,* the biostatistical norms and functional limits for disease states. Second, that age, sex, and species type are the *only* qualities relevant to selecting the members of reference classes is questionable. Cooper (2002) claims that many more than three qualities are relevant, including race and a number of environmental factors—cyclists, for example, typically have lower heart rates. It is even possible that some reference classes are so detailed that they comprise only one member. This, of course, entails that the one member is healthy in every respect, since she alone determines the biostatistical norms (Smart 2016: 28).

2   *A normal function of a part or process within members of the reference class is a statistically typical contribution by it to their individual survival [or] reproduction.*

   The second clause is often criticized on similar grounds to the first: Boorse is again accused of making value judgments. In this case, the objection is that in *choosing* individual survival or reproduction as the natural goals of an organism, over, say, writing a novel or performing in a ballet, one can no longer claim to have a genuinely naturalist conception (see Ereshefsky 2009). Making that choice, it is argued, involves a value judgment.

   Boorse responds to these objections (both regarding the reference classes and the organism's natural goals) by arguing that in order to establish the intended conclusion—that the BST is, in fact, a value-laden theory—the theory must be shown to include value-laden concepts. "A correct definition of concept H in terms of concepts C1, C2, … Cn is value-laden precisely if one of the Ci is value-laden: that is, if a judgement of the form 'x is Ci' is a value judgement" (Boorse 2014: 12). How the various concepts are chosen is irrelevant, and since none of the concepts involved in BST (statistical normality, survival, reproduction, organism, part, process, species, sex, age, and causation) are value-laden concepts, the theory remains value-free.

Boorse acknowledges that the nature of the reference class can have a profound effect on what counts as pathological. However, he claims that the BST reference classes simply draw from how biologists deal with taxonomy. "When biologists describe and classify organisms, they sort them into species, subspecies, separate them by sex in sexual species, and distinguish immature from adult forms" (Boorse 2014: 15). The alternatives offered by Cooper (2002) (with the exception of race, which Boorse has always said may need to be added (1977: 558; 1987: 370)), simply do not feature in how biologists classify organisms, and thus should not feature in an analysis of disease that is designed to encompass all species.

3   *Health in a member of the reference class is a normal functional ability: the readiness of each internal part to perform all its normal functions on typical occasions with at least typical efficiency.*

Boorse's conception links health states to biostatistical norms, but what is biostatistically normal changes over time—this causes at least two problems for BST:

i   Most would agree that, given the progression of modern medicine, improvements in diet and hygiene, and indeed the vast increase in life expectancy, population health has improved significantly since the Middle Ages, but if biostatistical normality is the mark of health, then the same percentage of the population is diseased now as were diseased in the sixteenth century. Surely, any conception of disease with this implication should be discarded (Guerrero 2010).

ii A sudden infectious disease epidemic (tuberculosis, for example) could, at least in principle, considerably lower the average functional efficiency of the lungs across a population/reference class. The implication for BST is that the functional efficiency necessary for healthy lungs drops significantly over a very short period of time.

Suppose my lungs are currently diseased due to cancer; for BST, this is just to say that my lungs perform their function subnormally. But I would surely maintain that my lungs are diseased, no matter how poor the species-typical functional efficiency becomes during a tuberculosis epidemic. Health status should not be subject to Cambridge changes (see Geach 1969) in this way, since changes in health status should, at least on the face of it, pertain only to changes in the intrinsic properties of the organism.

Boorse provides a threefold response to David Guerrero's Cambridge change objection:

(1) The theoretical possibility of a Cambridge change in someone's health status seems to be entailed by any view of health as normality, an idea basic to scientific medicine. But (2) it is far more difficult than Guerrero thinks for such a change to occur, and (3) the only realistic ways in which one could occur are of no importance to medical practice.

(Boorse 2014: 35)

Boorse bases normal functional efficiency on what he terms "a reasonable time-slice of the species" (1997: 66). The exact duration of this time-slice will vary from species to species, since some species have a life expectancy of only a few days, whereas others can reasonably hope to live for more than 100 years. However, given that statistical normality is not only calculated based on the properties of those animals currently living, an epidemic of the sort described above will not affect the species-typical functional efficiency of physiological subsystems as dramatically as it first appears. The time-slice, in human populations, would extend into the past, long before the tuberculosis epidemic began. An individual's health status is thus not relative only to the existing population, but to those who existed prior to the onset of the epidemic within the time-slice.

4   *A disease [later, pathological condition] is a type of internal state which impairs health, i.e. reduces one or more functional abilities below typical efficiency.*

Perhaps the most pressing concern regarding tenet 4 of BST is the "Line-Drawing Problem" (Schwartz 2007). If BST required the same percentage of physiological subsystems to be classified as functioning subnormally in all reference classes, then the same percentage would necessarily be classified as diseased, no matter how healthy or sick the reference class. This would be highly problematic, since some diseases affect a large proportion of a reference class, and others are very rare. Similarly, some diseases affect a much larger proportion of some reference classes than others.

Boorse does not, however, impose this condition. The BST, he states, "is consistent with disease prevalence of 35%, 20%, 5%, 1% or, I suppose, even 0%, and with prevalence varying from disease to disease" (Boorse 2014: 34). It is not consistent, as Boorse acknowledges, with disease prevalence of >50%, and this might prove problematic in the very elderly.

There is no particular place in which "the line" demarcating the normal and subnormal is drawn—rather, the location of the line is chosen by "medicine."

Boorse's concept of disease qua pathological condition has, as I have demonstrated here, received much criticism since its first publication in the mid-1970s. However, despite these objections, it remains perhaps the most discussed naturalist analysis of disease in the literature. Its target is explicitly what Nijhuis and Van der Maesen refer to as HC1; that is, the "mechanistic view that emphasises the traditional medical distinction between disease and non-disease in the individual" (Weed 1999: 99) with its remit is firmly within PC1, where the individual is emphasized over the collective. Its prominence in the literature is testament to how well it has stood up to these critiques.

Public health is interested in more than just the biological function of physiological subsystems, but there are certainly aspects of public health where this is the primary concern. The development and testing of pharmaceutical treatments, determining "the normal range" of biological markers in the blood (and elsewhere), and so on, seem to fit this model very well. Boorse's model helps us distinguish between the pathological and the normal, but it does not help determine where public health resources should be directed. Values may not be fundamental to (or even play any role in) pathology, but public health policymakers need a richer concept of disease than that of the pathologist. Policymakers need to know what interventions and treatments should be implemented and when in order to improve public health, and this inevitably requires value judgments.

Value-laden accounts of disease

In this section, I consider three value-laden accounts of disease. The first, which I refer to as Cooper's "tripartite account," has no criteria concerning population health, and no criteria concerning the "functional efficiency" of physiological subsystems whatsoever. The second and third accounts, those of Wakefield (the Harmful Dysfunction Account (HDA)) and myself (the Harmful Function Account (HFA)), take the concept of disease to have both a value-laden and a value-free component. In neither case does the value-free component directly refer to biostatistically average functional efficiencies; rather, the degree of functional efficiency to be expected is determined by evolutionary considerations. In this way, both HDA and HFA are tied to mechanistic concepts of health, and thus to Nijhuis and Van der Maesen's "health" category no. 3. As we shall see, although Cooper's account focuses on the "traditional medical distinction between disease and non-disease in the individual" (category no. 3), there is no mention of physiological mechanisms.

Cooper's tripartite account

Cooper begins her account of disease with a disclaimer: "that a neat account of disease cannot be achieved" (2002: 271). Perhaps the two most reliable ways of rejecting a conceptual analysis A of a concept C are (i) to provide examples that satisfy all the criteria set out in A, but are not cases of C; or (ii) to provide examples of C that do not satisfy all the criteria set out in A. On the face of it, one cannot reject Cooper's analysis on either ground since the disclaimer allows for cases of both (i) and (ii). Cooper is right. The concept of disease is messy. It is certainly the case that the meaning of "disease" is context-dependent, and perhaps even within specific contexts no one set of necessary and sufficient conditions is going to be a perfect fit for all our intuitions. That being said, below I present Cooper's view, and criticize it in exactly the same way as I would those analyses whose defenders do not assert this prior disclaimer (after all, what else can one do?).

Cooper's tripartite account (2002: 271) states that "we" (note the unqualified "we") take a physiological condition to be a disease if and only if:

1   the condition is "a bad thing to have" for the individual patient;
2   one would consider "the afflicted person to have been unlucky"; and
3   the condition "can potentially be medically treated."

Cooper is of course speaking of diseases in individuals rather than in populations, so once again this is an analysis of health in PC1. But this is not a biostatistical account—it does not rely on the statistically normal functional efficiencies of the collective, but is based only on the intrinsic properties of the individual patient, and society's attitudes toward those properties.

Condition 1 of Cooper's view jumps straight into the value-laden quality of the disease concept. That diseases are bad naturally comes to mind when thinking about health and disease. In other words, the value component seems to form a part of the lay concept of disease. It most likely forms a part of the clinician's concept, too. For Cooper, the primary reason for including the "bad thing to have" criterion is that biological abnormality without a normative component is simply not enough to draw conclusions about health states. Having ginger hair, she points out, is a biological abnormality, but it is not a disease (2002: 272). Perhaps the most intriguing benefit of Cooper's account, at least as an account of health and disease within a clinical context, is that it allows for physiological conditions to be diseases for some people and not others. A daisy, she says, "can be a weed in one garden but a flower in another, depending on whether or not it is a good thing in a particular garden" (274). A gardener will not remove the daisy, nor will she consider it a weed, when she likes it in her garden. Similarly, a patient will not treat some physiological condition, nor consider it a disease, when she takes it to be a good thing to have. For myself, male pattern baldness (MPB) might well come out as a disease under Cooper's definition. However, for some, baldness is a valued part of their identity (think of actor Patrick Stewart, for example).

Condition 2 (that the patient must be considered to be unlucky) eliminates some of the obvious counterexamples. By unlucky, Cooper does not mean unpredictable by medical science, but rather "'unlucky as judged by the uninformed layman', that is, roughly, worse off than the majority of humans of the same sex and age" (Cooper 2002: 276). Cooper (strangely enough, considering my own example above) uses MPB as an example of a condition that is clearly not a disease to warrant the "unlucky" criterion. For her, MPB is obviously not a disease, precisely because men cannot be considered unlucky if they have it.

Cooper uses a second example of a 90-year-old man who cannot walk as far as he could when he was younger. Since that is to be expected of any man, it is not unlucky, and thus not a disease. I would urge Cooper to apply similar reasoning to MPB. It is true that 70-year-olds can expect hair loss, but only 16% of 18–29-year-olds have MPB (Rhodes et al. 1998). At the very least, it is arguable whether or not MPB can be a disease in young men, whereas it is certainly not arguable that 90-year-olds who cannot walk as far as when they were younger are diseased. Why? If Cooper is right, it is precisely because the former are unlucky, and the latter are not. The argument about whether MPB in a young man (who does not want to be bald) is a disease, then, is really just an argument about whether that man is unlucky to have the condition.

Cooper's "unlucky" condition is questionable, even if cashing out only the lay concept of disease. We saw that Cooper uses the example of a 90-year-old who struggles to walk as a case of poor, but biologically normal functional efficiency. This is not a disease for Cooper, since it does not count as unlucky. This coheres nicely with our intuitions, but there are at least some potential counterexamples—cases where a patient is not unlucky by Cooper's definition (since she is not worse off than the majority of people her age and sex) but is nonetheless diseased. It is not particularly unlucky (at least not in Cooper's sense) for a very elderly man to suffer from severe arthritis. It is a very common condition in the elderly. The same is true of hearing loss, and even mild dementia in very elderly patients. These states are (surely) all pathological, and typically require intervention(s) no matter how old the patient. It seems that condition 2 is not a necessary condition after all.

Further, I have argued elsewhere that all three of Cooper's conditions can be satisfied, without the afflicted individual being diseased:

> Suppose Sam decides to get a tattoo reading "peace and love" on her arm, and, as is the fashion, decides to have it written in Chinese characters … The tattoo artist gets confused, and instead of "peace and love", Sam finds herself with "I hate China" decorating her arm [in Chinese symbols she does not understand]. Given that Sam is about to go to China, this is definitely bad and unlucky, but fortunately for her, this is also medically treatable. Nonetheless, it is not a disease.
>
> *(Smart 2016: 8)*

Cooper's view looks to satisfy the concept of health for PC1, but not using the solely mechanistic approach typical of the naturalist accounts. Rather, it includes aspects of Nijhuis and Van der Maesen's HC2—the somatic, psychological, and social aspects of disease. On the face of it, it is a good contender for an appropriate concept of disease in the clinical context— that which determines not only whether some condition counts as pathological, but whether it should be treated and how.

Nonetheless, we have seen that Cooper's conception of disease is problematic in two ways. First, not all of the supposed necessary conditions are necessary. Second, they are not always together sufficient for disease status. Cooper recognizes that her analysis (along with all others) is likely to fail in some instances, however, and her view exposes some important features of the lay concept of disease.

The introduction of the value criterion is also important for clinical medicine, in a way that it is not for the theoretical/pathological account provided by naturalists such as Boorse. Following Wakefield, however, I believe that a more plausible account of disease can be constructed by combining a value criterion with a value-free criterion—one that is more suitable in the context of public health.

Mixed accounts: disease as harmful function/harmful dysfunction

The value-laden accounts of Wakefield (the HDA) and myself (HFA) take the concept of disease to have both a value-laden and a value-free component. In neither case does the value-free component directly refer to biostatistically average functional efficiencies; rather, the degree of functional efficiency to be expected is determined by evolutionary considerations. In this way, both HDA and HFA are tied to mechanistic concepts of health, and thus to Nijhuis and Van der Maesen's HC1.

Wakefield provides the second of the three value-laden accounts of disease presented in this chapter. He suggests that:

> A condition is a disorder in and only if (a) the condition causes some harm or depriva-tion of benefit to the person as judged by the standards of the person's culture (the value criterion), and (b) the condition results from the inability of some internal mechanism to perform its natural function, wherein a natural function is an effect that is part of the evolutionary explanation of the existence and structure of the mechanism (the explan-atory criterion).
>
> *(Wakefield 1992: 384)*

For Wakefield, the harm of the condition is judged by the standards of the person's culture, rather than (only) by the patient himself/herself. It is an account of what it is to be diseased *within a particular cultural context/population*. Wakefield's view, then, implies that those who are not sterile as a matter of choice (i.e. did not voluntarily, and without coercion, have a vasectomy/tubal occlusion) are diseased since this would be deemed harmful by the stan-dards of the person's culture. Further, Wakefield's view is not subject to the Cambridge change objection, since disease status does not hinge on the health of others within the population.

For Nijhuis and Van der Maesen, in the context of public health policy, "public" is "pri-marily conceived of as populations within social, economic, and political systems" (PC2), and "health" as "the degree to which an individual reaches an equilibrium state with so-matic, psychological, and social influences" (HC2) (Weed 1999: 99). Wakefield's account of health implicitly incorporates both.

I take there to be a sizeable problem with Wakefield's account, however. Wakefield states that for a condition to be a disease, the harm caused by it must be a result of the *failure* of some physiological subsystem to perform its natural function. It is certainly true that in the case of some pathological conditions, an organ, tissue, or cell might be to perform its natural function. During myocardial infarction, the heart ceases to pump blood around the body effectively, for example. But in many (if not most) cases of disease, those biological parts continue to perform their natural function; that is, they continue to perform the process which explains its continued existence through the evolutionary process—they just perform that function at a poor level of efficiency.

Disease as harmful function

I propose an adjustment to Wakefield's account that eliminates the part-dysfunction criterion. My account of disease in clinical medicine, as an amended version of Wakefield's above, runs as follows:

a   The condition causes some harm or deprivation of benefit to the person as judged by the standards of the person's culture (Wakefield's value criterion).
b   The condition results from an internal mechanism either (i) failing to perform its natural function, or (ii) performing its natural function at a harm-causing level of efficiency, "wherein a natural function is an effect that is part of the evolutionary explanation of the existence and structure of the mechanism" (the explanatory criterion) (Smart 2016).

This account of disease as harmful function deals with the counterexamples to Cooper in much the same way as Wakefield's account of disease as harmful *dysfunction*. Further, it functions well as a concept of disease in the public health concept since it draws on both health categories HC1 and HC2 of Nijhuis and Van der Maesen's model—HC1 insofar as the condition results from an internal mechanism of the individual, and HC2 insofar as disease status is also partially dependent on somatic, psychological, and social determinants. However, it better accounts for diseases whereby physiological subsystems continue to function, but do so inefficiently, than Wakefield's position. Elsewhere (Smart, Stevens, and Verbakel 2018), I have looked to chronic kidney disease (CKD) of a good example of where this applies.

Kidneys clean waste products from the blood, regulate the production of red blood cells, control the body's fluids, and release hormones that regulate blood pressure. There are various ways of measuring the functional efficiency of the kidneys, but most measures relevant to defining CKD at least refer to the "glomerular filtration rate" (GFR), which estimates how much blood passes through the glomeruli (filters in the kidney that cleans the blood of waste products) each minute. The evolutionary explanation for the kidney's existence is thus the need to filter blood of waste products, with the normal/healthy range being 90–120 mL/min/1.73 m^2.

One can see that at CKD stage 5, as the GFR dips below 15, the kidneys malfunction to the extent that dialysis is (typically) required to keep the patient alive. However, even though functional efficiency (as measured by GFR) is below the normal/healthy level, CKD stages 2–4 do not involve "dysfunction." The kidneys of a 20-year-old patient with CKD stage 3 *are* performing that function which explains their continued existence through the evolutionary process—they are filtering the blood of waste products—but they are doing so rather poorly for someone of that age. If one grants that stage 3 CKD is a disease, then, one must do so on the basis of *how* efficiently the kidneys are performing their natural function, rather than *whether* they are performing that function. HFA thus takes disease to poor efficiency of natural function, as opposed to failure to perform a natural function.

Table 4.1 US National Kidney Foundation (NKF) Kidney Disease Outcomes Quality Initiative (KDOQI) definition and classification of stages of chronic kidney disease (columns 1–3), and remarks on symptomatic status (column 4)

KDOQI Definition and classification of stages of chronic kidney disease[a]			Remarks
CKD stage	Description	GFR (mL/ min/1.73 m²)	
1	Kidney damage with normal or elevated GFR	>=90	Asymptomatic except: Increased risk of cardiovascular disease Increased risk of stage 2 CKD and beyond
2	Kidney damage with mild decreased GFR	60–89	Asymptomatic except: Associated with a greater risk of cardiovascular disease than stage 1, but less than stage 3 CKD Increased risk of stage 3 CKD and beyond
3	Moderate decreased GFR	30–59	Asymptomatic except: Associated with a greater risk of cardiovascular disease than stage 2, but less than stage 4 CKD Increased risk of stage 4 CKD and beyond
4	Severe decreased GFR	15–29	Asymptomatic except: Associated with a greater risk of cardiovascular disease than stage 3, but less than stage 5 CKD
5	Kidney failure	<15 (or dialysis)	End stage CKD Associated with a greater risk of cardiovascular disease than stage 4 CKD Kidneys malfunctioning such that dialysis of transplant is needed to stay alive.

a   2002 Guidelines; from http://kidneyfoundation.cachefly.net/professionals/KDOQI/guidelines_ckd/index.htm.

Healthy populations

PC2 emphasizes the collective over the individual. Corresponding concepts of health and disease must therefore reflect this, and not focus on the pathophysiological mechanisms of the individual. Rather, they should reflect the functions of society as a whole.

The properties of health and disease in medicine are more often viewed as properties of individual organisms, but talk of "healthy populations" is not entirely foreign. Indeed, arguably the primary concern of public health is the health of the collective/population (Kindig 2007). What, then, should one take this to mean? In this section, I consider the possibility of attributing the property of health to populations as a collective, as opposed to the individuals that make up that collective.

In their follow-up paper to the 1994 editorial, Nijhuis and Van der Maeson write: "Our proposition is that health is primarily an attribute of individual subjects. Notions such as healthy communities or healthy populations evoke confusion. A healthy population metaphorically refers to a population that is doing well, culturally and economically" (2000: 135).

While I agree that the primary concern of medicine is health and disease in individuals, it is not clear to me that health and disease can only be viewed as applying to groups in a metaphorical sense. When Boorse sets out his BST, he does so with a view to it being applicable across all species. Let us, for now, consider a species where the idea of a healthy (or diseased) population is more easily construed as a literal property ascription.

Bee colony health indicators

Honeybees, which play an important role in human health through plant pollination, honey production, and its associated economic impact, are facing a crisis. There is a growing concern that the drastic global rise in colony collapse disorder (CCD) will result in severely depleted bee populations, which could have devastating consequences not only for beekeepers (and their bees), but for the environment more generally. As the name suggests, CCD is not a disorder of an individual bee. It is a disorder of the colony, whereby the majority of worker bees in a colony leave the hive and do not return. They abandon the queen bee, the honey they have produced, and the juvenile bees. This quickly results in a collapse of the colony.

Fabrice Requier, in his 2019 paper "Bee Colony Health Indicators, Synthesis and Future Directions," writes that: "Honey bee colonies can be assimilated to a complex system for which survival depends on its individual quality, its adaptive capacity and its threshold of resilience to pressures" (Requier 2019: 1).

Beekeepers, when they speak of the health of their colony, are not speaking metaphorically. CCD is a real disorder, and one that applies to the colony (the collective), not to individual bees, which, despite abandoning the hive, may themselves suffer from no pathological conditions as individuals. One might question whether the "health" property, as attributed to a colony, is the very same property as that one attributes to the individual bee. Arguably not, but simply because an analysis of "colony health" will differ substantially to that of "individual bee health" does not imply that the term is being used metaphorically. After all, as we have seen above, the content of the disease concept in individuals differs substantially from one context to another. Health/disease as concepts at the population/group/colony level is just another context in which these meaningful concepts can be usefully deployed.

The health of human "colonies"

Requier defines a healthy hive as a "colony that does not show any symptomatic diseases and includes adequate population sizes of adult bees and brood and an adequate production of honey in relation to the annual life cycle of the colony and the geographical location" (2019: 2). While this same definition would be inappropriate for modern human populations (perhaps, in the past, low population sizes might have been an issue for some human populations), it shows that *contra* Nijhuis and Van der Maesen, the literal use of "health" as a predicate applying to "Public Category 2" (the collective) need not evoke confusion. Of course, one might simply object that "humans are not bees,"[3] but I contend that the literal use of health as a property applicable to human populations is very plausible. It merely needs careful exposition. In this section, I provide a tentative analysis of healthy human populations, based on the statistical model of Boorse and key markers of flourishing healthy human populations.

First, let us consider what it is about bee colonies that enable one to speak of their health status. One cannot meaningfully talk of the health of any random collection of bees from multiple hives. One does not even speak of the health of the dyad of two adjacent hives. The health/disease property is ascribed only to individual bee colonies, with a single queen and all the worker bees servicing the honey production and the development of that colony's juvenile bees. Each bee plays a particular role or function within its community, contributing in some way to the continued survival of the colony. It is this quality, I argue, that makes a bee colony a suitable collective/population for the disease predicate. The colony has, to use Boorse's terminology, certain "natural goals." The individual bees have certain functional roles that contribute to the attainment of these goals, and sometimes those bees fail to perform those functions. When those functions are no longer adequately performed, the colony can accurately be described as diseased.

Human societies are not unlike bee colonies, in this way. One cannot arbitrarily pick out a group of unconnected humans, call them a population, and ascribe a health status. Some classes of humans are suitable candidates for health/disease predicates, and others are not. The key principle that distinguishes the two is an interconnectedness, with each member contributing (or potentially contributing) toward the collective flourishing of the group. Individual countries, for example, often comprise millions of taxpayers, some of whom work in the health sector, others in the financial sector, others in farming, and so on. The success of, for example, a country's economy affects each and every one of its citizens in innumerable ways, including their individual health and well-being. When unemployment rates are high, or a country is poorly administered by a corrupt government, the functional efficiency of important sectors within society begins to fail. Currencies collapse, access to basic commodities such as food, water, and electricity become restricted, healthcare services start to deteriorate, and so on. It is the interconnectedness of the bees that qualifies the bee colony for a health status, and the same interconnectedness demarcates those classes of humans that qualify for a health status, from those that do not.

Nicolae Morar and Joshua August Skorburg (2018) have argued along similar lines for their "hypothesis of extended health." They claim that the bearer of health need not be an individual organism, but that "certain features of our biological and social environment can be so tightly integrated as to constitute a unit of care extending beyond the intuitive boundaries of skin and skull" (Morar and Skorburg 2018: 341). Borrowing from S. Orestis Palermos (2014), and using the example of the relationship between the gut microbiome and the human organism, Morar and Skorburg identify "ongoing feedback loops" as the key feature in identifying those interconnected organisms that qualify for a combined health status. This, they claim, can meaningfully be extended to the parent-child dyad, partly because interventions such as obesity treatments "targeting only the parent might also turn out to be effective at producing weight loss in the untreated child" (Morar and Skorburg 2018: 363). At least for the purposes of healthcare interventions, then, Morar and Skorburg take the parent-child dyad to be a suitable bearer of the health property. Of course, when one talks of healthy populations, we are not referring to dyads (although the term is vague, a "population" comprises more than two members). But nevertheless, the same "ongoing feedback loop" principle can be applied. There is an ongoing feedback loop between members of those populations that qualify as bearers of the health predicate—the actions of those working in the financial sector, as many found out during the 2007/2008 financial crisis, have a profound impact on everyone, and even the actions of those who do not substantially contribute to the economy affect others through their consumption of water, goods, and services. Where no ongoing feedback loop exists, for example, random humans from distinct societies, that "population" cannot qualify as a bearer of the health property.

Markers of healthy populations

Like bees, human populations are prone to diseases, and require an adequate food supply. They also need housing, access to good medical care, and access to education and jobs. Mental health and economic productivity are also important factors in a healthy human population. In addition to the individual HC1 healthy needs of the individuals making up the population, these are the somatic, psychological, and social aspects of Nijhuis and Van der Maeson's HC2. Key markers for the health of a population will thus include measures to this effect. I do not set out to provide a comprehensive list here, but healthy populations will be characterized by:

- low extreme poverty rates (Lotter 2011: 27–32);
- access to sanitation facilities;
- access to education;
- low child mortality rates;
- high life expectancy;
- low levels of inequality;
- low levels of mental-health disorders; and
- low rates of unemployment.

It may sound odd to classify a human population as health with respect to, for example, levels of poverty, but such an approach to targeting public health problems need not be viewed as problematic. Public health aims not only to promote individual health and well-being, but the overall flourishing of a society.

I remain agnostic as to whether one should label "the absence of health" as "disease" in human populations. One could just as easily label high inequality or high unemployment as a "public health problem," without loss of meaning. If labeling an unhealthy (in the context of public health) human population as "diseased" evokes confusion, this move can be side-stepped, as I demonstrate in the next section.

What counts as collective health? A tentative solution

Boorse's BST focuses on part-function; that is, he does not provide a definition of what it means for the organism as a whole to be diseased; rather, he considers the health state of the physiological subsystems in terms of their contribution to the natural goals of the organism. I propose a similar system for health and disease at the PC2 level; that is, when analyzing the health of a human population as a collective, one can consider the performance of each of these key indicators independently (although they are, undoubtedly, interconnected—as indeed the health of our physiological subsystems often are). I further suggest that rather than distinguishing between diseased and healthy populations, public health is better suited to a "comparativist theory of health" (Schroeder 2013).

Comparative theories of health avoid trying to define a particular state (health or disease) in favor of the relational concept "healthier than," which holds between two or more organisms—or in the case of PC2, two or more populations, or two or more possible states in the same population. Andrew Schroeder argues that this comparative model should be adopted at the PC1 level for HC1 (mechanistic) health measures. This, he argues, resolves a number of problems associated with attempting to identify an absolute distinction between the healthy and diseased (as per the BST model), including those arising from increasingly healthy populations. This debate is beyond the scope of this chapter, but on the face of it, Schroeder's proposed solution eradicates concerns regarding distinguishing diseased from healthy populations when applied at the PC2 level.

Consider "multidimensional poverty" as a health measure. The Multidimensional Poverty Index (MPI) does not focus only on meeting the income requirements determined by the international poverty line (i.e. earning more than a fixed amount). It acknowledges that poverty is not just about low income, but also (among other things) access to education, toilet facilities, electricity, and clean running water. The MPI also includes health measures, such as nutrition and child mortality (Alkire et al. 2020). It thus serves as a good measure of multiple aspects of public health.

Countries with a high level of multidimensional poverty are less healthy in these respects than those countries with low levels of multidimensional poverty, and a single country can improve its population's PC2 health by lowering its multidimensional poverty levels. Of course, each component of the MPI could be assessed individually, and the health of the population with respect to its absolute poverty level, for example, or access to education, or access to adequate nutrition could be individually compared with that of another population. However, as an overall assessment of relative population health, the MPI is a good contender since it encompasses many of the key indicators mentioned above.

Conclusions

Philosophical literature on public health remains fairly sparse, but Nijhuis and Van der Maesen's (1994, 2000) papers and the response by D.L. Weed have made some inroads toward a philosophy of public health. The earlier article advances four ontological categories: PC1, PC2, HC1, and HC2, which form the basis of public health. To separate the metaphysical understanding of the population/public into PC1 (which emphasizes the individual over the population) and PC2 (the collective over the individual), and health into HC1 (medicine's traditional mechanistic understanding of health) and HC2 (the somatic, psychological, and social aspects of public health), lays good groundwork for further analysis.

In assessing the health of a bee colony, one must first identify whether the individual bees are suffering from any diseases (a PC1 and HC1 concept). Public health is concerned not only with the pathological conditions of individuals, however, but also the somatic, psychological, and social qualities of health. Analysis of health at the colony/population level thus requires including aspects of both HC1 and HC2. Boorse's HC1 analysis provides a useful analysis of what it is to be a pathological condition, but this is insufficient for public health purposes, since it provides no guidance for public health policy, which is an inherently value-laden process. A more appropriate HC1 analysis can thus be found by including a value criterion. While Cooper includes a value criterion, I have shown her analysis to be problematic in a number of ways. Wakefield's account, which includes both an explanatory criterion and a value criterion, seems much closer to the mark, but I recommend a slight adjustment to Wakefield, proposing an account of disease as a "harmful function." This novel account of disease is, I maintain, suitable to play the HC1 role within the context of public health. The value criterion focuses on the patient's reaction to somatic, psychological, and social influences, and the explanatory criterion on the biological functions that distinguish disease states from other harmful states.

Where Nijhuis and Van der Maesen have argued that the literal use of "health" at the PC2 ontological category can evoke confusion, I have shown that its use is already commonplace in the scientific discussion of the health states of other species, highlighting the example of the honeybee. Although I concede that demarcating diseased from healthy populations is difficult, this does not, I contend, hinder the correct and literal use of the health concept for human populations at the PC2 level. Instead, I propose that we follow Schroeder's lead (in the PC1 context) and implement a comparative theory of health at the level of the collective. In this way, we can compare the health of populations by appeal to key markers of population health, such as those included in the MPI. Individual assessment of those factors included in the MPI can guide public health policymakers on how best to improve the overall health of populations.

Notes

1 Suggesting "not healthy" as a definition of disease is not useful unless one already has a solid analysis of the concept of health. In short, one must pick one concept to focus on—which one does not matter if they are deemed negation of one another (but whether health is equivalent to "not diseased" is also up for debate).
2 There are vestigial physiological subsystem, such as goosebumps and possibly the appendix, but those shall be ignored, for now.
3 My thanks to Alex Broadbent for raising this objection.

References

Alkire, S., P. Conceição, C. Calderón et al. 2020. Multidimensional Poverty Index (MPI): Charting pathways out of multidimensional poverty—Achieving the SDGs. United Nations Development Programme, Human Development Reports. http://hdr.undp.org/sites/default/files/2020_mpi_report_en.pdf (accessed December 13, 2021).

Boorse, C. 1975. On the distinction between disease and illness. *Philosophy and Public Affairs* 5, no. 1: 49–68. http://www.jstor.org/stable/2265020.

Boorse, C. 1977. Health as a theoretical concept. *Philosophy of Science* 44, no. 4: 542–573. https://doi.org/10.1086/288768.

Boorse, C. 1997. A rebuttal on health. In *What is disease? Biomedical ethics reviews,* ed. J. M. Humber and R. F. Almeder, 1–134. Totowa, NJ: Humana Press.

Boorse, C. 2014. A second rebuttal on health. *Journal of Medicine and Philosophy* 39, no. 6: 683–724. https://doi.org/10.1093/jmp/jhu035.

CDC Foundation. 2021. What is public health? https://www.cdcfoundation.org/what-public-health (accessed August 10, 2021).

Cooper, R. 2002. Disease. *Studies in History and Philosophy of Science* 33, no. 2: 263–282. http://dx.doi.org/10.1016/S0039-3681(02)00018-3.

Ereshefsky, M. 2009. Defining "health" and "disease." *Studies in History and Philosophy of Biological and Biomedical Sciences* 40, no. 3: 221–227. https://doi.org/10.1016/j.shpsc.2009.06.005.

Fuller, J. 2018. What are chronic diseases? *Synthese* 195, no. 7: 3197–3220. https://doi.org/10.1007/s11229-017-1368-1.

Geach, P.T. 1969. *God and the soul.* London: Routledge.

Guerrero, D. 2010. On a naturalist theory of health: A critique. *Studies in History of Philosophy of Biological and Biomedical Sciences* 41, no. 3: 272–278. https://doi.org/10.1016/j.shpsc.2009.12.008.

Kindig, D. A. 2007. Understanding population health terminology. *The Milbank Quarterly* 85, no. 1: 139–161. https://dx.doi.org/10.1111%2Fj.1468-0009.2007.00479.x.

Kingma, E. 2007. What is it to be healthy? *Analysis* 67, no. 294: 128–133. https://doi.org/10.1093/analys/67.2.128.

Lotter, H. P. P. 2011. *Poverty, ethics and justice.* Cardiff: University of Wales Press.

Morar, N. and J. Skorburg. 2018. Bioethics and the hypothesis of extended health. *Kennedy Institute of Ethics Journal* 28, no. 3: 341–376. https://doi.org/10.1353/ken.2018.0020.

Nijhuis, H. and L. J. van der Maesen. 1994. The philosophical foundations of public health: An invitation to debate. *Journal of Epidemiology and Community Health* 48, no. 1: 1–3. https://dx.doi.org/10.1136%2Fjech.48.1.1-a.

Nijhuis, H. and L. J. van der Maesen. 2000. Continuing the debate on the philosophy of modern public health: Social quality as a point of reference. *Journal of Epidemiology and Community Health* 54, no. 2: 134–142. https://dx.doi.org/10.1136%2Fjech.54.2.134.

Palermos, S. 2014. Loops, constitution, and cognitive extension. *Cognitive Systems Research* 27, no. 1: 25–41. http://dx.doi.org/10.1016/j.cogsys.2013.04.002.

Requier, F. 2019. Bee colony health indicators: Synthesis and future directions. *CAB Reviews* 14, no. 56: 1–13. http://dx.doi.org/10.1079/PAVSNNR201914056.

Rhodes, T., C. J. Girman, R. C. Savin et al. 1998. Prevalence of male pattern hair loss in 18–49 year old men. *Dermatologic Surgery* 24, no. 12: 1330–1332. https://doi.org/10.1111/j.1524-4725.1998.tb00009.x.

Schroeder, S. A. 2013. Rethinking health: Healthy or healthier than? *British Journal for the Philosophy of Science* 64, no. 1: 131–159. https://doi.org/10.1093/bjps/axs006.

Schwartz, P. H. 2007. Natural selection, design, and drawing a line. *Philosophy of Science* 74, no. 3: 364–385. https://doi.org/10.1086/521970.

Smart, B. T. H. 2016. *Concepts and causes in the philosophy of disease*. London: Palgrave Macmillan.

Smart, B. T., R. J. Stevens, and J. Y. Verbakel. 2018. Is "chronic kidney disease" a disease? *Journal of Evaluation in Clinical Practice* 24, no. 5: 1033–1040. https://doi.org/10.1111/jep.13018.

US National Kidney Foundation. 2002. NKF KDOQI guidelines. http://www2.kidney.org/professionals/KDOQI/guidelines_ckd/p4_class_g1.htm (accessed December 13, 2021).

Valles, S. 2018. *Philosophy of population health: Philosophy for a new public health era*. New York: Routledge.

Wakefield, J. 1992. The concept of mental disorder: On the boundary between biological facts and social values. *American Psychologist* 47, no. 3: 373–388. https://doi.org/10.1037//0003-066x.47.3.373.

Weed, D. 1999. Towards a philosophy of public health. *Journal of Epidemiology and Community Health* 53, no. 2: 99–104. https://dx.doi.org/10.1136%2Fjech.53.2.99.

Whitbeck, C. 1977. Causation in medicine: The disease entity model. *Philosophy of Science* 44, no. 4: 619–637. https://doi.org/10.1086/288771.

5

PUBLIC HEALTH AND ETHICS

Sridhar Venkatapuram

Introduction

Ethical reasoning within and about public health is something that everyone should be familiar with—whether they are public health researchers and practitioners, educators, industry leaders, policymakers, or citizens affected by public health; and that means everyone. The Covid-19 pandemic has made it clear that a health threat to populations, and the social and policy responses to that threat can have profound impacts on each of our daily lives. The causes of the spread of the virus between and within societies, prevalence levels of disease and deaths, social distribution patterns of disease and deaths, social responses, including lockdowns and vaccine development and procurement, and other dimensions are right or wrong, good or bad, fair or unfair, as well as who is responsible to do what, when, where, and so forth are all matters with an ethical dimension. Yet, such ethical dimensions of public health are not unique to this pandemic but have always been there and will be in the future. Nevertheless, there are several reasons why even public health policymakers, researchers, and doctoral students are not familiar with public health ethics or it being something distinct from medical or research ethics.

First, public health training in most graduate schools in North America and Europe, and most wealthy countries, is largely organized as training in scientific and technical skills. This is because public health is thought to be an applied or instrumental science. While there may be some attention given to ethics of doing research on human subjects, broader ethical concerns and philosophical aspects of public health are not recognized or given much time. Indeed, that is why an aim of this handbook is to help make the space for more philosophy in public health training and practice, even if it is currently envisioned as largely scientific and technical training.

Second, public health ethics as a distinct academic field of inquiry and practice emerged recently in the mid-1980s and 1990s in response to the novel and difficult issues raised by the spread of HIV/AIDS in rich counties (Bayer 1988; Bayer and Fairchild 2004; Mann 1997). Bioethics (that is, medical ethics and research ethics) had limited capacity to offer ethical guidance for policies addressing the spread of a fatal infectious disease among people—a health issue with ethical implications that included but went much beyond the scope of an ethical rubric centered on an individual patient in a healthcare/research setting. And, while

DOI: 10.4324/9781315675411-7

academic public health ethics has moved beyond HIV/AIDS and infectious diseases, public health educators and practitioners more broadly have been diffident about engaging robustly with ethics.

While the unfamiliarity and neglect of public health ethics may be explainable, public health without ethics can become quite a gruesome endeavor. Public health has just as much potential as biomedical science has for generating morally controversial if not unjust and repugnant consequences. Moreover, public health without coherent and transparent ethical reasoning risks being (and frequently is) rejected by the "public" it seeks to serve, whether in free and democratic societies or otherwise. The debates related to the Covid-19 pandemic about the moral legitimacy of lockdowns and mask or vaccine mandates illustrate this. A more ethically engaged and sophisticated (global) public health community might have anticipated the libertarian, egalitarian, communitarian and other ethical concerns earlier and responded more effectively. They might even have settled on different pandemic policies for different contexts, especially in low- and middle-income countries (LMICs) where the social lockdown polices have been catastrophic. In any case, public health education and practice are overwhelmingly focused on framing health problems, analyses, research, and responses largely in terms of scientific and increasingly economic concepts, as if (social and political) ethics is a minor or marginal aspect.

Notwithstanding the importance of doing excellent science, the consequences of the neglect and proactive diminution of ethics to the margins of public health have enormous negative consequences. Again, there is no better example than the response to the Covid-19 pandemic, particularly at the global level. Immense rhetoric such as "follow the science" and "science is the only exit strategy" reflected a view that the public health crisis was being caused by a natural organism that requires global (natural and medical) science to find a solution. Such a view, in addition to billions of dollars invested into pharmacological research, did indeed produce a number of effective vaccines. At the same time, the view also produced a situation where only the few richest countries in the world had first access to the vaccines and are hoarding billions of more doses than the amounts needed for their own populations. Large stocks are regularly being destroyed due to expiry dates, and other stocks will likely be distributed to poorer countries slowly over time, according to the donor country's national interests. All this is happening while millions of people in LMICs are dying preventable deaths directly from Covid-19 or indirectly from other causes resulting from social shocks. Then, there is the possibility of harmful new variants arising from parts of the world where there is low vaccine uptake due to limited supply or mistrust. The United Nations (UN) Secretary-General Antonio Guterres best summed up the situation in September 2021. Speaking to world leaders at the UN General Assembly, he stated, "This is a moral indictment of the state of our world. It is an obscenity. We passed the science test. But we are getting an F in Ethics" (United Nations Regional Information Centre for Western Europe 2021).

The pandemic has clearly brought to the forefront the fact that public health without robust ethical reasoning can result in huge moral failures as well as being self-defeating. This chapter presents a discussion that sits in between the extant and largely implicit ethics in some parts of public health and the absolute lack of ethical reasoning in other parts. On the one hand, it seeks to motivate making the implicit ethics more explicit and into "living things"—up for scrutiny, and open to further iterations and development. On the other hand, it seeks to motivate the integration and development of ethical reasoning in other parts of public health, as well as in addressing novel public health issues and areas of research and policy. The chapter seeks to achieve these aims by presenting how to think about public health and ethics, or public health ethics, by providing an introduction to ethics for non-philosophers; identifying some salient differences between bioethics and public health ethics; and reviewing some prominent kinds of philosophical methods used in doing public health ethics. This is attempted in a fair manner, but inevitably there will be some authorial perspective. Importantly, the chapter is not a survey of public health ethics issues. There are a growing number of books and journals available for that purpose, including many chapters in this handbook (Bayer and Beauchamp 2007; Dawson 2011; Dawson and Verweij 2007; Freeman 2010; Gostin and Wiley 2018; Holland 2015; Mastroianni, Kahn, and Kass 2019).

Before the main discussion, it may be helpful to make a few points directed especially to readers who may be coming to this subject from backgrounds outside of philosophy or academia. The first point has to do with the use of the term "ethics." Many professional associations and organizations ask individuals to abide by certain ethical codes of behavior. While these ethics codes are important, they can raise confusion in public health organizations. That is because there is a difference between the ethical conduct of an individual (in a professional role and setting), and the ethical assessment of a policy, such as the ethical evaluation of both its means and its ends. Such policy assessment cannot be guided by any professional code of conduct. Further confusion may arise when medical professionals work in public health organizations and their medical professional code of conduct includes how to ethically provide medical treatment to patients (that is, the four bioethics principles). Consequently, they and others may assume the bioethics principles jointly with other professional and organizational ethics standards, including those related to theft and corruption, sexual harassment, discrimination, and so forth, are relevant and sufficient ethical resources for ensuring that a public health policy or program is ethical. Needless to say, such diverse ethics resources may be relevant, but they are not sufficient.

Just as a public health policymaker may see value in requesting a health economist to produce cost-effective analyses of various public health interventions to help decision-making, the growth of public health ethics signals the importance and value in assessing ethical dimensions of public health policies and programs based on a distinct and evolving set of public health ethics resources. Furthermore, aside from being an additional input into the development and evaluation of a candidate policy or program, public health ethics can stand independently and produce ethical demands for or motivate designing and implementing public health interventions. For example, illuminating how the persistent ill-health of African Americans in the United States, or of indigenous populations in Brazil as being unjust, should then motivate initiating particular public health interventions to ameliorate the injustices. So, the reach of public health ethics, if understood properly, can be in an assistive role to policymakers and planners as well as going far beyond to clarifying and asserting foundational principles of public health and its organizations, as well as all social institutions that impact health more broadly. In light of all the above, confusion arises in health agencies and public health organizations when the term "ethics" could be referring to professional ethics, organizational standards, clinical ethics, research ethics, public health ethics, or something else. The confusion, miscommunication, poor policies, and other consequences directly result from ethics, despite its great diversity and broad reach, being relegated to the margins of public health.

The final point is about how academic philosophers work. In their teaching and research, philosophers tend to put aside arguments with blatantly poor reasoning, that are clearly self-interested, and other kinds of politics and contextual issues in order to identify and examine the "core" philosophical issues or puzzles. While this helps push forward philosophical knowledge, it also paves the way for poor reasoning, self-interest, and partisan politics to influence policy unchallenged in various domains. Those individuals seeking to apply ethics in public health practice do not have the luxury of refusing to acknowledge or engage with these realities. For example, the Covid-19 pandemic has made it abundantly clear that politicians and other national leaders are the ultimate decision-makers of public health policy. A public health policy that is rigorously reasoned regarding its ethical foundations and principles may be stillborn in certain contexts or get badly transformed as it goes through the political channels. This brings to the forefront a long-standing open question about the right role of philosophers in real-world health and public policymaking (Brock 1987; Kamm 1990; Nussbaum 2000; Van der Vossen 2015; Swift 2008). Divergent as the views may be, it is hard to imagine public health engaging more robustly with ethics or the related concept of equity without the involvement of trained philosophers willing and able to engage with the contextual realities of policymaking.

Ethics 101

This section presents a synopsis of ethics as it is usually categorized and taught in introductory courses in many Anglo-American and European universities. According to common contemporary views, ethics is about guiding action toward what is right or good. These action guides are only rarely and often partially codified in law or professional regulations. They are usually articulated as principles, rules, frameworks, imperatives, and so forth. Some thinkers have sought to make a distinction between ethics and morals/morality (Williams and Moore 2011). However, such internecine niceties are not helpful for our purposes here and will be set aside. In this discussion, ethics and morals mean exactly the same thing. And usually, introductory ethics is divided into five different areas (Shafer-Landau 2020). Three areas are distinct kinds or "schools" of ethics and grouped together under the heading of normative ethics. These three schools of ethics are consequentialism, deontology, and virtue ethics.

Consequentialism

In the consequentialist approach to ethics, the right thing to do is reflected in the final outcome or end result (Darwall 2003). Or, to put it another way, the outcome is what matters—and the only thing that matters—in assessing the rightness or goodness of an action, or prospectively determining what we ought to do. One prominent example of this type of ethics is utilitarianism. It posits that the right thing to do is to act in a way that creates the greatest amount of a valued good (originally happiness) (Mill and Sher 1979; Sen and Williams 1982; Smart and Williams 1973). Because this good, and only this good, is what is morally valuable, we ought to act to produce as much of that good as possible (maximize). To give a public health example, imagine Policy A that would save 100 lives and Policy B that would save 1,000 lives. All things considered, utilitarian ethics would guide you to choosing Policy B as it produces more lives/happiness. Choosing B is not just a nice thing to do; it is morally required.

It is important to note that utilitarianism is a prominent but only one form of consequentialism. Other forms can result from replacing the valued good of happiness with some other good or even complex outcomes (for example, freedoms, procedures, and so on). Furthermore, there could also be alternative ways to aggregate the good aside from maximizing (for example, one could instead seek to ensure that the worst-off individual is better off than in any alternatives; add a condition that everyone has enough according to a defined standard, and so on). What matters in consequentialist reasoning is the coherence and justification of the end result. Again, to take a public health example, an argument could be made that the right action is one that leads to everyone having a sufficient amount of healthcare. This example also shows how one could argue for consequentialism without being a utilitarian. The policy resulting in sufficient healthcare for all might produce less total overall health in the group compared to a utilitarian-maximizer who provides more healthcare to those individuals who could produce the most health overall. Consequentialism and utilitarianism are discussed further in the methodologies section because they are so prevalent in public health.

Deontology

In contrast to a singular focus on outcomes, deontological ethics assert that the right thing to do is to act according to certain rules or principles, irrespective of the outcomes. Take, for example, principles such as "you shall not kill another human being," or "you shall not lie." Such principles demand that we should or should not act in a certain way and not consider the consequences of doing so, nor act according to principles because of their consequences. Many religions provide such principles or edicts and justify them as being handed down by God. We must act according to certain ethical principles because God has told us to do so. And trying to take into account the consequences is often said to be beyond our human capacities and understanding. In contrast, the foremost source of the contemporary secular deontological tradition is Immanuel Kant (Rohlf 2020). He argued (non-equivalently) that (i) we should act in accordance with rules that could hold for everyone (the principle of universalizability), and (ii) that people should be treated as ends and never as a means, even if we are pursuing the greater good (the categorical imperative). The most well-known among deontological principles is the respect for the autonomy of every human being.

Deontological ethics differs from consequentialist ethics in its specific moral verdicts, and most obviously in cases where following a categorical imperative results in less overall utility/valued good. For example, deontology would require telling a would-be murderer where to find their intended victim, if a person with that knowledge is asked, on the basis of the principle, "it is absolutely wrong to lie to someone." Another difference is that deontologists often (though not always) hold that acts and omissions (for example, doing harm and allowing harm to happen) are morally different. This is because the target of assessment in deontology is the act, and where there is no act (an omission), there is nothing to assess. In contrast, the scope of consequentialism usually includes acts and omissions because the target of assessment in both is their consequences. Furthermore, while consequentialism is strictly focused on the outcomes, deontological ethics circumscribe the means of action. There are some things that must never be done, or some things that must always be done. The concept of moral rights—claims that individuals have by virtue of their status as a human being—is a particular species of deontological ethics. For example, it is argued, following Kant, we should never violate a person's right to autonomy because autonomy reflects something valuable about their humanity, their status as a human being.

Virtue ethics

The third type of normative ethics, called virtue ethics, focuses on personal moral character (Crisp and Slote 1997; Hursthouse and Pettigrove 2018). In contrast to focusing on consequences or the act itself, virtue ethics approaches locate the target of moral assessment inside the person taking action (although acts or consequences will feature in determining whether a person is virtuous or not). The focus on moral character shifts from external rules and principles, including the rights-claims that others may have on us, to our internal dispositions. Certain virtues are seen to be worthy of developing for the sake of the virtues themselves and not for other reasons, such as the valued consequences that may result, or for being the kind of character that follows rules. Moreover, virtues are not superficial traits or habits, but reflect a certain complex mindset. Many professional codes of conduct seek to elevate certain virtues, but usually often fall short in many ways because the code itself does not produce the underlying complex mindset in the target professionals. Things become even more confounding when such codes of conduct, while initially addressing moral dispositions, then also include decision-making principles that constrain the application of exactly the highlighted dispositions by drawing directly upon consequentialist or deontological considerations. Virtues that have often been considered exemplary include a sense of justice, wisdom, honesty, and beneficence, among others.

Metaethics

In addition to the above three types of normative ethics, a fourth area of ethics is metaethics (McPherson and Plunkett 2017; Sayre-McCord 2014). Reflecting the prefix *meta*, this area of study and reasoning focuses directly on the nature of ethical principles themselves (whether those be utility, deontological principles, or virtues). For example, what is the nature of the moral "ought?" Is ought a fact like the existence of a pen or atom, or does it exist in a different way, or not at all? Are our ethical beliefs really beliefs, or are they emotional or other non-cognitive attitudes masquerading as beliefs, and actually lacking propositional content? Metaethics can entail highly abstract philosophical reasoning involving metaphysics where we aim to distinguish between what exists in the world versus what we are able to perceive of it, and our different valuations of what we perceive as well as the reality being perceived. However, it can connect directly to practical concerns because metaethical considerations may influence the way in which decisions are justified (the epistemology of ethical claims) and how ethical disagreements are resolved. Such influence is rarely made explicit at present but could usefully clarify persistent disputes, for instance, where religious and secular factions are opposed on an issue. And public health policies and programs often produce such conflicts.

Applied ethics

The fifth area is that of applied ethics, where the three kinds of normative ethics as well as arguments from metaethics are applied to (and sometimes modified or rejected in response to) real-world issues (Chadwick 1998). These discussions can range from how we as individuals should act regarding a particular issue as well as how our communities, societies, and the human species should act regarding specific issues. The reasoning and research in applied ethics can range from the highly abstract, such as addressing the methodology of applying ethical principles, rules, and frameworks to generic cases across to highly specific and contextual consideration of an issue (for example, the allocation of ventilators in mass emergencies; the prioritization of vaccinations in short supply; the implementation of a sugar tax; and so on).

While public health ethics can, indeed, be understood as the application of ethics to public health issues, there is ever-increasing breadth and depth to what is currently underway.

That is to say, there is a growing amount of philosophical literature and practical ethical guidance that starts with a pressing public health issue and applies certain ethical approaches to produce a recommendation about how to act. Such applied ethics is recognizable starting from literature on population growth and famines in the 1970s, HIV/AIDS in the 1980s and 1990s, up to the Covid-19 pandemic in the 2020s. At the same time, rapid developments in public health sciences, particularly social epidemiology and health economics, have motivated reexamination and modifications to established abstract principles and theorizing in ethics. As examples, the reality of an infectious disease spreading through social interactions and inequalities, within and across national borders, motivates rethinking of the individual as fully autonomous, being treated only as an end in themselves, as well as reconsidering the theoretical assumptions regarding benefits and burdens of social cooperation that are at the foundation of social contract theories.

Religious ethics

While the discussion so far has followed how ethics is often presented in courses and textbooks, at least two points are worth noting about such a presentation. First, it may have been noticed that there has been little mention of religion or religious ethics. Life, death, birth, pain, suffering, and other aspects of health are often central concerns of religions. And religions typically provide followers with guides on what to value and how to act. And the three types of normative ethics presented above come out of the European Enlightenment tradition, though their original sources can be traced to thinkers from centuries before. One of the hallmarks of the Enlightenment tradition is that thinkers sought to use reason to argue and justify rather than rely on faith and received instructions from religious sources. Contemporary philosophical training, particularly in nonreligious institutions, largely follows the Enlightenment tradition. This, however, does produce gaps or disconnects between academic discussions and literature on ethics, various religious traditions also producing ethical guidance, as well as the ethical practices of people who give place to religion in their lives. Such disconnects often come to the fore when individuals and groups seek religious exemptions from public health and medical interventions, or in advocating for or against certain public policies. While this chapter does not afford the space to delve into diverse religious ethics, it is necessary to acknowledge their existence and significance as well as their wide influence in the daily lives of individuals, including and especially policymakers, implementers, and political leaders.

Non-dominant ethical traditions

Another point about what has been presented above as basic knowledge about ethics is that it has been derived largely from European and North American traditions and developed by mostly men. Regarding the first point, neither philosophy nor ethics is found only in European and American traditions, nor did they begin in Ancient Greece. There are important texts on ethics, both religious and secular, from ancient India, China, and the Middle East. There are also many other ethical principles and practices all over the world, including many that are not written (for example, the *ubuntu* tradition widespread in sub-Saharan Africa long predates literacy in that region) as well as in social groups not geographically defined (for example, the stereotypical "honor among thieves"). Regarding the latter point about men, starting in the 1980s, there has emerged a strong body of work that shows that the great men of philosophy have commonly ignored issues predominantly affecting females, and also failed to consider whether girls and women might prioritize different values, or even have different epistemological attitudes or ways of knowing. A strong feminist ethics literature seeks to correct this, focusing on ethical reasoning by and for girls and women, and more recently, other genders (Hall and Ásta 2021; Jaggar 2018; Norlock 2019). And care ethics has emerged as a distinct category of normative ethics that particularly reflects feminist concerns (Held 2018; Robinson 2018).

The reasons for acknowledging other types of ethics and reasoning are manifold. First, it makes us recognize that categories, reasoning, and applications that may initially appear universal or generalizable are, in fact, coming from certain places and sources. The normative guidance also may not have much salience if and where other ethical reasoning is functioning and dominant. Second, reasoning about ethics often proceeds by confronting a chosen approach with various kinds of moral intuitions and real-world cases while also showing how competing ethical approaches would have less coherent solutions. The acknowledgment of non-secular, non-Euro-American, and non-male developed traditions motivates extending such dialectical reasoning to engage with these other approaches. This is especially necessary, if indeed, the arguments and guidance being put forward are meant to be relevant and applied to these "other" kinds of people and places. With some important exceptions (for example, recent work situating *ubuntu* in the global discourse, including both Western and Eastern traditions), we are currently only at the stage of seeking out or presenting (in English) coherent representations of some non-dominant ethical traditions or schools functioning in the world (Boyle and Novak 2008; Metz 2010). We (exceptions aside) are not yet at a stage where ethicists are routinely engaging with different ethical traditions outside of the dominant ones, even where the ethicists in question are based outside the Euro-American geographies (Tsai 2005). Keeping all this in mind, anyone anywhere in the world interested in public health ethics should understand the dominant discourse of ethics as presented above. It is a necessary foundation to engage with, further evolve, expand, or fundamentally challenge.

Bioethics versus public health ethics

Public health ethics emerged as a distinct area of research and practice in the 1980s in response to difficult practical issues being raised by the spread of HIV/AIDS and the limitations of bioethics, the usual go-to resource for health-related ethical guidance. The inadequacy or limits of bioethics can be located in various places. First, the focus of bioethics was and still largely remains the individual patient or human research subject. The HIV/AIDS pandemic brought into focus the fact that not all ethical concerns about populations could be solved by ethical considerations at the individual level, such as when the health problems concern an entire "key population" at a high risk of a fatal infection. In fact, given the specific epidemiology of HIV/AIDS, there could be a whole range of vulnerable subpopulations, including pregnant women, children, injection-drug users, undocumented migrants, sex workers, gay men, and so forth. The group concerns could not be fully addressed one individual at a time. Second, a "principlist" approach, discussed further below, had become dominant where most health-related ethical concerns were analyzed using four ethical principles: respect for persons (autonomy), beneficence, non-maleficence, and justice. While these four principles are also applicable in public health, they are not particularly illuminating with regard to some classic public health problems, such as resource allocation, health inequalities within a population, access to medicines, and so forth. Bioethics principles, and perhaps principlism more generally, may be useful where individuals are making decisions about themselves or regarding other individuals. But they are not adequate guides where polities and institutions are making policy decisions affecting populations. These decisions are simply more complex, and the populations and institutions themselves bear more complex moral properties than individuals.

Furthermore, in the HIV/AIDS case, and in many other ways, the bioethics principles actually constrain established public health strategies to contain and control infectious diseases, and other interventions (Selgelid 2005). For example, the respect for autonomy constrains interventions such as isolation, contact-tracing, and compulsory medical management of highly transmissible infections. Moreover, the bioethics principles were silent on various pressing HIV/AIDS issues, such as access to information and healthcare, community mobilization, and discrimination in non-healthcare settings. So rather than centering on individuals in clinical or research settings, public health ethics starts elsewhere. Namely, it is a population, and specifically the population's health, that is the primary target of moral concern. And second, public health ethics requires ethical resources that can guide the actions of governments, social organizations, and other actors that impact publics, whether small or large. As has been helpfully described, bioethics draws on moral philosophy, while public health ethics draws on political philosophy—theories and conceptions of what makes up a good society, a good government, the rights and responsibilities of citizens, distributive justice, and so forth (Wikler and Brock 2008).

To someone external to academic philosophy and ethics, this distinction between moral and political philosophies may seem small. Could this not just require those working in bioethics to shift slightly in order to work in public health ethics? Indeed, this is a plausible view and reflects some work in public health ethics. As will be discussed more below (and notwithstanding the remarks above), some bioethicists have put forward ethical principles for public health akin to the four bioethics principles for healthcare and research. The idea is that public health is similar to medical care but about population health(care); therefore, principlism is a plausible method to develop public health ethics. At the same time, there has been a growing body of literature grounded in political philosophy, and particularly in debates of theories of social justice ("health justice") and metaethics. All these diverse kinds of engagements with public health ethics should be welcomed as there is clearly a recognizable need for ethical reasoning and guidance for public health beyond bioethics.

Methodologies

The differences between bioethics and public health ethics as presented above are not only about scope and sources, but also about methodology. Bioethics is dominated by a principlist methodology, while the growth of public health ethics is from ethical reasoning using diverse methods. While discussions on philosophical methods can be expansive, the focus here is on the methods and structure of arguments and guidance. Methodology and the particular methods used in public health ethics are important to explicitly recognize and assess because they can limit the scope of which issues can be addressed—through what kind of ethical reasoning is possible—and illustrate how certain issues require certain kinds of ethical reasoning rather than others. For example, surveying a sample population about what they believe is the right thing to do about an issue X versus an individual reasoning through argumentation about the right response to the issue X are very different methods than can be used to produce guidance on how to act. The following sections discuss the most visible methods of doing ethics in public health, including consequentialism (which is often implicit), principlism, and theories of social and global justice, and a note on doing ethics research.

Consequentialism as a method

Normative ethics, by definition, guide actions through identifying what is to be valued (the target of moral concern) as well as how to pursue or relate to the valued good. But consequentialism in its most basic form could be understood as not asserting any substantive values aside from telling us to value and assess only the consequences. So we could argue for an absurd consequentialist position that an act is morally right if it increases rabbit numbers in Oslo. What this shows is that only a subset of consequentialist ethical precepts that have justifiable outcomes is plausible. Utilitarianism, the paradigm case of consequentialism, clearly asserts that what is valuable is happiness, though the term "well-being" is also often used. Utilitarianism also tells us that it is morally required to act so as to maximize total happiness. Public health, policies, and programs usually do not focus on happiness or well-being, but on a related notion of health (often implicit), on disease (thought of as absence of health), a narrowly construed conception such as life-years lost, or even some other non-standardized concepts. All of these kinds of things are accepted implicitly or otherwise, as valued outcomes. And the aim of interventions is often to maximize the outcome. Take, for example, two different vaccines approved for use, and each will produce different numbers of averted cases of disease. All things being equal, because disease is dis-valued, we choose the vaccine that will result in the largest number of averted disease cases. This may seem not only morally right but also the *logical or rational* choice. This illustrates the extent to which consequentialist reasoning, and almost classic utilitarianism are pervasive in much of public health. This occurs across epidemiological research, health technology assessment, policy planning, implementation, and monitoring and evaluation. And yet, there are numerous potential challenges to deploying such consequential and utilitarian reasoning.

One important challenge comes from deontological ethics. Showing respect for every person's unique status as human being, their humanity or dignity, entails not violating their autonomy, bodily integrity, choices, and so forth. So maximizing averted deaths cannot be carried out if it violates respect for some or all persons. This conflict comes to the fore in cases when maximizing health in a group involves redistributing health burdens. Think of a vaccination program that produces rare but fatal reactions; those few who die serve as the means to others' survival. They die earlier than they would have because of the vaccinations, and they contribute to reducing circulating viruses and transmissions in the group, maximizing health. On a Kantian view, this is never permissible no matter how many others' lives are at stake. Within and across countries, there are different settlements of this sort of confrontation between utilitarian and deontological approaches in relation to diverse public health issues. Part of the diffidence in public health education and practice to engaging robustly with ethics may be explained by the strong hold that consequentialist and utilitarian reasoning has in public health. To some within public health, non-consequentialist/ non-maximizing ethical approaches to issues can seem irrational, illogical, unscientific, and even unethical for not maximizing health outcomes.

Principlism

In contrast to consequentialism and utilitarianism that are deeply embedded in diverse areas of public health, a second prominent kind of method being used explicitly to develop ethical precepts is principlism. Following on from the enormous success of bioethics principles in clinical medicine and health research, various principles to guide public health are being put forward. One form of principlism is to take a "bioethics-plus" approach whereby new principles are added to the four bioethics principles. And, the proposed principles include ensuring respect for community, realizing solidarity, social justice, reciprocity, health maximization, efficiency, and proportionality (Schroder-Back et al. 2014). A second method unlinks from bioethics principles, perhaps because of the clear tensions between the focus on the individual in healthcare versus groups in public health, to produce stand-alone principles (Bernheim, Nieburg, and Bonnie 2007; Kass 2001). Of the few examples available, they visibly move away from asserting the principles as strong ethical imperatives. Rather, they are meant to serve as a guide or framework to think through ethical implications of a public health issue.

There are various benefits of using the principlism method in developing public health ethics. Foremost is that it is possible to construct a list of ethical principles fairly quickly and with modest effort. For example, during the early months of the Covid-19 pandemic in the United Kingdom, many lists of ethics principles for the allocation of limited intensive care beds and ventilators were rapidly produced by diverse professional organizations, government entities, hospitals, and even individuals. What made this public health ethics was that the principles were clearly in response to a sudden and large increase in numbers of people requiring care and aimed to guide decisions about how to allocate resources across groups, and large numbers of people presenting at the hospital as well as those predicted to arrive in the near future.

While the principlism method can enable quick and easy development of ethical guidance, such as in an emergency, there are many shortcomings of such an approach whether during a crisis or normal times. Such shortcomings can be avoided if ethical concerns are given more forethought. Ease of devising ethics checklists under time pressure or otherwise should not be confused with ease of using them to achieve optimal ethical outcomes. A bad ethics framework or checklist will produce unethical outcomes in a crisis or otherwise.

Principlism in bioethics has received great scrutiny and criticism, too extensive to be repeated here (Clouser and Gert 1990; Petrini 2010). What is germane here are some of the particular limits of principlism when used to develop public health ethics. One big indicator of its limits is found in the framing of proposed principles as a framework, analytical tool, checklists, worksheet, and so forth. It indicates that proposed principles are not strong ethical prescriptions for what things to value or how to act. Instead, they are considerations and discussion points. This can render them ineffectual or overly malleable and limit their capacity to offer a meaningful direction for decisions arising in practice. Conversely, because checklists are inevitably devised in rarefied settings away from the heat of the action, they may fail to anticipate important features. Or they may undermine or fail to credit a front-line practitioners' ability to weigh moral issues as they arise, with all their real-life complexities.

A second problematic aspect of such lists is that they make "ethical assessment" perform an *assistance* function to public health policymaking, which is inconsistent with the fact that public health is *fundamentally* a normative discipline, aimed at furthering a presumed *moral* good (that is, a public's health). In clinical care, the primary objective is to address disease in an individual presenting in the clinical setting, and bioethics principles help pursue that goal without violating any important ethical principles or virtues. Similarly, the current examples of public health ethics principles are meant to assist a public health policy planner or implementer achieve their goal without violating any important moral principles while upholding some new ones. However, there is a profound difference in assistance functions to clinical care versus public health. Bioethics principles do not motivate or compel doctors to go out in search of patients to treat (with ethics). And, similarly, by taking on an assistive perspective, these extant public health principles also do not motivate public health practitioners and policymakers to seek out and address public health problems. If public health ethics do not motivate seeking out and addressing public health problems, rather than helping after a particular policy has been tabled, then there is something inadequate about such ethics.

A third, and perhaps, most significant challenge to principlism in public health ethics is that the principles can be incoherent and inconsistent in a variety of ways. One type of incoherence is that they can have disparate levels of abstraction and operation. Unlike bioethics principles, which are all functioning between the doctor and patient or researcher and subject, proposed public health ethics principles can range from respecting individuals and involving populations in decision-making to ensuring social justice or that social solidarity is realized. Another type of incoherence occurs when the lists of principles are contradictory or incommensurable. Remember that above, consequentialist ethics can be contradictory to some types of deontological ethics. And yet, the lists of public health ethics principles contain consequentialist, utilitarian, deontological, and virtue ethics, and more. In the bioethics-plus approach example and others, the advocates list as imperatives both health maximization of a population and justice, understood as fair distribution of health outcomes in society (Schroder-Back et al. 2014). Maximization and fair distribution are usually incommensurable. And a further type of incoherence can be that some principles may be misrepresenting ethical concepts, ideas, and theories. On the one hand, some of the principles may refer to things such as community, reciprocity, solidarity, and so forth without a grounding in a conceptual theory, debates, or literature to produce a thick conception. On the other hand, principles such as social justice or solidarity caricature large bodies of philosophical literature and profound disagreements. Indeed, putting social justice, in particular, as one among other principles misunderstands what a conception of social justice is and does. Stated simply, it puts the mother (social justice) inside a child (framework) while describing a well-ordered family. Moreover, presenting the social justice principle as referring to the take-aways from one preferred conception or theory of social justice among contested and diverse options is disingenuous.

Theories of health justice

Given the drawbacks of consequentialism and principlism, are there methods for producing public health ethics that are substantively grounded, coherent, and have a methodological approach? Such aspects are what philosophical theories of social justice seek to have. Indeed, there may also be other methods to derive a coherent set of ethical principles for social action, including public health. But theories or approaches to social justice are compelling resources to draw upon. Many theories of social justice seek to answer a set of overlapping questions, including how should we live together in a community, what do we owe each other in light of our humanity, and what does the respect for the equal moral worth of every human being entail in terms of how we treat each other. Keeping in mind the different kinds of normative ethics, different philosophers have sought to construct conceptions of a good society that are coherent and produce various principles for social organization and functioning. In recent times, the period between 1970 and 2000 saw enormous activity in this area where various theories of social justice were put forward, described as social contractarian, libertarian, communitarian, capabilitarian, luck egalitarian, feminist, and others (Clayton and Williams 2004; Kymlicka 2002; Reisch 2014). Some of these theories take health and public health as being central to social justice; others do not. And "health justice" literature considers how each of these and other types of theories of justice would address health, public health, health inequalities, social determinants of health, and so forth (Asada and Schokkaert 2019). One upshot of this is that while each theoretical school might produce robust ethical principles for guiding public health institutions, it is unlikely that there will be great overlap across the approaches as each is internally consistent to one kind of normative ethics. Despite the incommensurability of different approaches, public health ethics would be well served with more coherence, clarity, internal consistency, and other such aspects the theories can offer. Moreover, there has been much work on how to proceed in public policy decision-making where there are diverse and incommensurable social values, and conceptions of social and health justice (Sen 2018; Sunstein 1995).

Systematic reviews

A final and prosaic comment about methodology may be useful to readers. In health sciences, as in social and natural sciences, the number of times a piece of research is cited is often thought to indicate the significance of the publication; it made a significant contribution to the understanding of the subject. In social sciences, a literature review is also often used to identify the contour or terrain of a subject. How frequently certain topics or themes repeatedly appear indicates the dominant topics under the broader subject of interest. Public health practitioners and researchers may seek to apply these same methods to identify what is the right way to address a pressing ethical concern. However, using the same science research methodology to gather ethics knowledge can yield misleading results because it does not account for valence. Frequency of citations in ethics literature can mean that the work is a significant contribution and/or that it has been repeatedly challenged and shown to be lacking in diverse ways. An analogy would be that the attacks on the Twin Towers may be repeatedly discussed, but overwhelmingly with negative rather than positive valence.

Philosophical reasoning is largely dialectical, and positions that are widely considered false attract attention because they are widespread but false on reflection (for example, when an equivalence is presumed between concepts that are actually non-trivial to reconcile, such as liberty and equality), or because they are intuitively false but hard to refute (for example, anti-natalism—bringing a person into existence is necessarily to harm them and is, therefore, wrong). Other work may be cited simply because it is sloppy or represents egregious error that requires refuting—a task that is often presumed to be completed by the peer-review process in the sciences but falls to other philosophers in philosophy. Thus, ethics literature requires much closer scrutiny of the cited references and related literature to recognize the proper significance and quality of a publication, and the rightness of the argument presented. The same too can be said for the frequency of certain topics appearing repeatedly. Perhaps, more than in the sciences, one philosophy publication can show how an entire line of debate was misplaced. Conducting a systematic review of a particular ethics topic can lead to a dead end when that one single publication is missed, or when it is weighed the same as the many it decisively refutes. The significance of a certain ethical argument or ethical topics has to be determined through engagement with the topics, and some familiarity with evolutions of debates, and not primarily through citation or other metrics.

Conclusion

The aim of this chapter has been to situate public health ethics in between the implicit ethics already present in many parts of ethics and the lack of ethical reasoning in others, where it is clearly needed. The discussion began with describing some standard categories of ethics and then proceeded to discuss how bioethics differs from public health ethics, and finished with a discussion on some prominent methods currently being used to develop public health ethics. As stated in the introduction, public health ethics is a relatively new area of research and application. The discussion hopefully motivates the reader to engage and contribute to its further development. It is much needed.

References

Asada, Yukiko and Erik Schokkaert. 2019. Introduction to the special issue on justice and health: Different perspectives in different disciplines. *Social Justice Research* 32, no. 2: 1–12. https://doi.org/10.1007/s11211-019-00334-8.

Bayer, R. 1988. AIDS and the ethics of public health: Challenges posed by a maturing epidemic. *AIDS* 2, suppl. 1: S217–S221. https://doi.org/10.1097/00002030-198800001-00033.

Bayer, R. and A. L. Fairchild. 2004. The genesis of public health ethics. *Bioethics* 18, no. 6: 473–492. https://doi.org/10.1111/j.1467-8519.2004.00412.x.

Bayer, Ronald and Dan E. Beauchamp. 2007. *Public health ethics: Theory, policy, and practice.* New York: Oxford University Press.

Bernheim, Ruth Gaare, Phillip Nieburg, and Richard J. Bonnie. 2007. Ethics and the practice of public health. In *Law in public health practice,* ed. Richard A. Goodman, Richard E. Hoffman, Wilfredo Lopez, Gene W. Matthews, Mark Rothstein, and Karen Foster, 110–135. New York: Oxford University Press.

Boyle, Joseph M. and David Novak. 2008. Religious and cultural perspectives in bioethics. In *The Cambridge textbook of bioethics,* ed. A. M. Viens and Peter A. Singer, 377–378. Cambridge: Cambridge University Press.

Brock, Dan W. 1987. Truth or consequences: The role of philosophers in policy-making. *Ethics* 97, no. 4: 786–791. https://doi.org/10.1086/292891.

Chadwick, Ruth F. 1998. *Encyclopedia of applied ethics.* 4 vols. San Diego, CA: Academic Press.

Clayton, Matthew and Andrew Williams. 2004. *Social justice.* Malden, MA: Blackwell.

Clouser, K. Danner and Bernard Gert. 1990. A critique of principlism. *Journal of Medicine and Philosophy* 15, no. 2: 219–236. https://doi.org/10.1093/jmp/15.2.219.

Crisp, Roger and Michael Slote. 1997. *Virtue ethics.* Oxford: Oxford University Press.

Darwall, Stephen L. 2003. *Consequentialism: Blackwell readings in philosophy* 7. Malden, MA: Blackwell.

Dawson, Angus. 2011. *Public health ethics: Key concepts and issues in policy and practice.* Cambridge: Cambridge University Press.

Dawson, Angus and M. F. Verweij. 2007. *Ethics, prevention, and public health.* Oxford: Clarendon.

Freeman, Michael D. A. 2010. *The ethics of public health.* Farnham, Surrey: Ashgate.

Gostin, Lawrence O. and Lindsay F. Wiley. 2018. *Public health law and ethics: A reader.* 3rd ed. Oakland: University of California Press.

Hall, Kim Q. and Ásta. 2021. *The Oxford handbook of feminist philosophy.* Oxford: Oxford University Press.

Held, Virginia, ed. 2018. *Justice and care: Essential readings in feminist ethics.* New York: Routledge.

Holland, Stephen. 2015. *Public health ethics.* 2nd edition. Cambridge: Polity.

Hursthouse, Rosalind and Glen Pettigrove. 2018. Virtue ethics. In *The Stanford encyclopedia of philosophy,* ed. Edward N. Zalta. https://plato.stanford.edu/archives/win2018/entries/ethics-virtue/ (accessed December 14, 2021).

Jaggar, Alison M. 2018. *Living with contradictions: Controversies in feminist social ethics.* New York: Routledge, Taylor & Francis Group.

Kamm, Frances M. 1990. The philosopher as insider and outsider. *Journal of Medicine and Philosophy* 15, no. 4: 347–374. https://doi.org/10.1093/jmp/15.4.347.

Kass, N. E. 2001. An ethics framework for public health. *American Journal of Public Health* 91, no. 11: 1776–1782. https://dx.doi.org/10.2105%2Fajph.91.11.1776.

Kymlicka, Will. 2002. *Contemporary political philosophy: An introduction.* 2nd edition. Oxford: Oxford University Press.

Mann, Jonathan M. 1997. Medicine and public health, ethics and human rights. *Hastings Center Report* 27, no. 3: 6–13. https://doi.org/10.2307/3528660.

Mastroianni, Anna C., Jeffrey P. Kahn, and Nancy E. Kass. 2019. *The Oxford handbook of public health ethics.* New York: Oxford University Press.

McPherson, Tristram Colin and David Plunkett. 2017. *The Routledge handbook of metaethics*. London: Routledge.

Metz, T. 2010. African and Western moral theories in a bioethical context. *Developing World Bioethics* 10, no 1: 49–58. https://doi.org/10.1111/j.1471-8847.2009.00273.x.

Mill, John Stuart and George Sher. 1979. *Utilitarianism*. Indianapolis: Hackett.

Norlock, Kathryn. 2019. Feminist ethics. In *The Stanford encyclopedia of philosophy*, ed. Edward N. Zalta. https://plato.stanford.edu/entries/feminism-ethics/ (accessed December 14, 2021).

Nussbaum, Martha C. 2000. Four paradigms of philosophical politics. *The Monist* 83, no. 4: 465–490. http://dx.doi.org/10.2307/27903701.

Petrini, C. 2010. Theoretical models and operational frameworks in public health ethics. *International Journal of Environmental Research and Public Health* 7, no. 1: 189–202. https://doi.org/10.3390/ijerph70101899.

Reisch, Michael. 2014. *Routledge international handbook of social justice*. New York: Routledge.

Robinson, Fiona. 2018. *Globalizing care: Ethics, feminist theory, and international relations*. New York: Routledge.

Rohlf, Michael. 2020. Immanuel Kant. In *The Stanford encyclopedia of philosophy*, ed. Edward N. Zalta. https://plato.stanford.edu/entries/kant/ (accessed December 14, 2021).

Sayre-McCord, Geoff. 2014. Metaethics. In *The Stanford encyclopedia of philosophy*, ed. Edward N. Zalta. https://plato.stanford.edu/archives/sum2014/entries/metaethics/ (accessed December 14, 2021).

Schroder-Back, P., P. Duncan, W. Sherlaw, C. Brall, and K. Czabanowska. 2014. Teaching seven principles for public health ethics: Towards a curriculum for a short course on ethics in public health programmes. *BMC Medical Ethics* 15: 73. https://doi.org/10.1186/1472-6939-15-73.

Selgelid, M. J. 2005. Ethics and infectious disease. *Bioethics* 19, no. 3: 272–289. https://doi.org/10.1111/j.1467-8519.2005.00441.x.

Sen, A. 2018. The importance of incompleteness. *International Journal of Economic Theory* 14, no. 1: 9–20. https://doi.org/10.1111/ijet.12145.

Sen, Amartya and Bernard Arthur Owen Williams, eds. 1982. *Utilitarianism and beyond*. Cambridge: Cambridge University Press.

Shafer-Landau, Russ. 2020. *The fundamentals of ethics*. 5th edition. New York: Oxford University Press.

Smart, J. J. C. and Bernard Williams. 1973. *Utilitarianism: For and against*. London: Cambridge University Press.

Sunstein, Cass R. 1995. Incompletely theorized agreements. *Harvard Law Review* 108, no. 7: 1733–1772. https://doi.org/10.2307/1341816.

Swift, Adam. 2008. The value of philosophy in nonideal circumstances. *Social Theory and Practice* 34, no. 3: 363–387. http://dx.doi.org/10.5840/soctheorpract200834322.

Tsai, D. F. 2005. The bioethical principles and Confucius' moral philosophy. *Journal of Medical Ethics* 31, no. 3: 159–163. https://dx.doi.org/10.1136%2Fjme.2002.002113.

United Nations Regional Information Centre for Western Europe. Covid-19: UN Secretary-General says the world has failed an ethics test. https://unric.org/en/covid-19-un-secretary-general-says-the-world-has-failed-an-ethics-test/ (accessed December 14, 2021).

Van der Vossen, B. 2015. In defense of the ivory tower: Why philosophers should stay out of politics. *Philosophical Psychology* 28, no. 7: 1045–1063. https://doi.org/10.1080/09515089.2014.972353.

Wikler, Daniel and Dan W. Brock. 2008. Population-level bioethics: Mapping a new agenda. In *Global bioethics: Issues of conscience for the twenty-first century,* ed. Ronald Michael Green, Aine Donovan, and Steven A. Jauss, 15–35. Oxford: Clarendon Press; New York: Oxford University Press.

Williams, Bernard and A. W. Moore. 2011. *Ethics and the limits of philosophy*. London: Routledge.

6

THE PHILOSOPHICAL IMPLICATIONS OF FUNDAMENTAL CAUSE THEORY

Daniel Goldberg

Introduction

This chapter aims to (1) describe "fundamental cause theory"; (2) analyze the idea of causation at work in "fundamental cause theory"; (3) analyze two significant ethical implications that arise from "fundamental cause theory"; and (4) explain several significant criticisms of "fundamental cause theory." The chapter represents an attempt to analyze both epistemological and ethical components of "fundamental cause theory." Although, as will be noted, "fundamental cause theory" (FCT) is well regarded as a conceptual and practical framework, relatively few exponents have delved deeply into either the philosophical foundations of the schema or relevant ethical concerns that attend it. This chapter aims to help fill the gap.

Description of FCT

Bruce G. Link and Jo C. Phelan, sociologists working at Columbia University's Mailman School of Public Health, are the creators and principal architects of FCT. Its first published exposition appeared in a special issue of the *Journal of Health & Social Behavior* in 1995, titled simply "Social Conditions as Fundamental Causes of Disease" (Link and Phelan 1995). In it, Link and Phelan articulate the notion that, while many variables and factors play a role in the causal chain to disease and population health outcomes, only some of them qualify as a "fundamental cause." Link and Phelan submit three criteria a putative cause must satisfy in order to qualify as a fundamental one: "First, fundamental causes tend to cause multiple diseases. Second, fundamental causes determine multiple risk factors. Third, fundamental causes tend to persist" (Goldberg 2014: 1839). These criteria are most easily perceived via example, as in the case

> of an individual forced into prostitution as a subsistence strategy; such a person may be entirely unable to avoid known risks. But the sex acts themselves are intervening mechanisms rather than upstream causes, which in this case would likely be some combination of material deprivation, inadequate income, oppressive power structures, etc.
>
> *(Goldberg 2014: 1839)*

DOI: 10.4324/9781315675411-8

Link and Phelan offer a more detailed example, one also intimately connected to the history of public health: that of sewerage. In the mid-to-late nineteenth-century United States, access to sewerage was a significant risk factor for waterborne disease, but it was one that was distributed unequally largely along class lines. Subsequently, gradients in such access began to flatten, followed predictably by flattening of the curves in waterborne disease prevalence and incidence. Yet, as Link and Phelan point out, overall population health inequalities did not contract. People of lower socioeconomic status (SES) remained significantly less healthy than people of higher SES—even as access to sewerage ceased to stratify outcomes for waterborne disease in terms of class. Link and Phelan argue that new mechanisms arose to mediate the relationship between socioeconomic position (SEP)[1] and disease, such as widespread tobacco consumption and poor nutrition.

According to Link and Phelan, SEP therefore qualifies as a fundamental cause of disease. It is strongly correlated with a wide variety of diseases, both infectious and noncommunicable. It also predicts the distribution of a number of important risk factors for disease. That is, it is not simply the case that important outcome measures such as prevalence, incidence, and mortality are correlated with SEP (although they are). In addition, important risk factors for these outcomes such as tobacco consumption, substance abuse, and social isolation also track a social gradient. Although this point might seem to follow *a fortiori* from the first point, it has important normative and policy implications, which will be discussed below. Finally, the robust links between SEP and important metrics of population health persist even when the intervening mechanisms shift or disappear completely, as the sewerage example demonstrates. Access to sewerage became much less significant within affluent populations as a mechanism linking SEP to health; yet, the SEP–health connection remained strong as new mechanisms arose to mediate the causal pathways between SEP and health outcomes.

Although these are merely the rudiments of FCT, they suffice to explain the basic parameters of the approach. As the following sections excavate more deeply the philosophical foundations and implications of FCT, further specification of FCT will be provided as needed.

Concepts of causation and FCT

Obviously, FCT is about causation—it says as much in the title of the theory! But the claims about causation at the core of FCT are hugely important. At its most basic level, the novelty and epistemological significance of the theory rest on its capacity to promote ideas of disease causation that advance the field itself and that translate into important directions for policy and practice. Link and Phelan expressly endorse the latter objective in their original 1995 piece. But the background context of causation in epidemiology renders the point even more important. Causation is a continually contested topic in epidemiology. There are multiple reasons for this.

First, disease causation in general is problematic from an epistemological perspective. Multiple factors and variables often converge to cause disease in a single person. Compounding such variables across large populations increases the complexity exponentially. Thus, in the US contexts, plaintiffs alleging injury from medical negligence or defective medical products often have enormous difficulty demonstrating that a specific exposure (that is, ingestion of a drug, implantation of a medical device, and so on) caused a particular injury or harm because there are so many potential causes for the conditions claimed for, even if the statistical probability that any one of these causes the outcome is remote (Brennan 1987; Callahan 1991). Similarly, in November 2020, a court in South Korea rejected a compensation request by the National Health Insurance Service against a major Korean tobacco manufacturer in part because it could not rule out the possibility that lung and laryngeal cancers are "caused by other factors, such as individual lifestyle, genetics and job-related characteristics" (Yonhap 2020).

Second, proving causation in epidemiologic research is exceptionally difficult both because of time/money considerations and because of ethical limitations on research. Especially as to the kinds of chronic, noncommunicable diseases that constitute an increasingly larger share of the global burden of disease in both the developed and the developing world, running large-scale randomized controlled trials (RCTs) that might permit causal inferences between exposure and outcome would take decades, because outcomes are not proximate to exposure. For example, outcomes in coronary artery disease or type 2 diabetes can take decades to develop, and running a large, sophisticated research study with rigorous adherence to study protocols for such a time period is difficult and sometimes not feasible.

Perhaps more important than these obstacles are the ethical limitations to such research. While there is widespread agreement that RCTs provide the most robust justification for exposure-outcome causal inferences, such RCTs are uncommon in epidemiology—partly for the time/cost reasons noted above. But such RCTs are often also ethically dubious. Frequently, known risks to particular exposures often appear well in advance of the point at which the relative effects of *levels* of those exposures are known. This means, for example, that while it may be of significant value to understand the precise levels of benzene toxicity in children, it would be obviously unethical to intentionally expose children to benzene in order to identify the point or specify the range at which it causes an adverse health impact (Goldberg 2014). Even if the specific level at which benzene causes illness is unknown, the risks are sufficient to justify intervention.

In other words, evaluating whether a given exposure causes illness may require exposing subjects to risks of harm widely viewed as unacceptable in human participants' research. As such, even where RCTs are feasible, they may be ethically intolerable. This means that much epidemiologic research depends on retrospective cohort studies. Methodologically, such studies can provide strong evidence that given exposure-health correlations are unlikely to be spurious. But by design they are unable to control for confounding variables in the ways that some RCTs can.

The problem of causation is a thorny one, and this has not escaped the attention of epidemiologists. One of the most popular tools for addressing this within the practice are the Bradford Hill "criteria," a set of nine "aspects of association," which can be used to justify causal inferences within epidemiology. They are as follows:

1   strength of association;
2   consistency;
3   specificity;
4   temporality;
5   biological gradient;
6   plausibility;
7   coherence;
8   experiment; and
9   analogy.

Explicating these in detail is beyond the scope of this analysis (Fedak et al. 2015). However, at a broad level, the dimensions are interesting insofar as each of them, if sufficiently "strong" enough, increases the probability that a given association justifies causal inference. Taken together, a correlation that features sufficient levels of most or all of these "aspects" counts as evidence strong enough to justify causal inference. Alex Broadbent, a leading philosopher of epidemiology, notes that this account is actually an instance of "inference to the best explanation" (IBE):

> The core idea of IBE is that, in some circumstances, we can infer the truth of an explanation on the basis that it is good. For example, if you hear a roaring noise outside the window, you can reasonably infer that a bus or car is revving its engine. The noise could be coming from a recording, or from a helicopter, but these are probably less good explanations of the sound because they are more complex or raise further questions (e.g., why would someone play a recording of an engine outside the window?).
>
> *(Broadbent 2017: 252)*

Essentially, IBE is a qualitative judgment, a kind of "triangulation," in Broadbent's words. The idea is to "tak[e] into account as much evidence as possible, from as many sources as possible—and, crucially, [to consider] the question of whether there is a *better* possible explanation" (2017: 252).

Broadbent notes that despite the long tradition of an IBE approach to causation in epidemiology, a newer framework, which he terms the "potential outcomes approach" (POA), has grown in popularity. According to a POA,

> in order to make a meaningful causal claim, one must clearly specify the intervention one has in mind to bring about the difference between the exposed group and the unexposed group. It is not enough, according to this approach, merely to seek to investigate the effects of obesity on mortality, for example. There are many ways to intervene so as to reduce (or increase) body mass index (BMI), and these may have different effects on mortality.
>
> *(Broadbent 2017: 253)*

In other words, the POA "insists that investigators clearly specify the counterfactuals whose truth they are investigating" (Broadbent 2017: 253). This has methodological implications as well—experimental studies are regarded as epistemically superior to observational studies "because in such studies the investigator actually makes an intervention to create the exposed and control groups."

The IBE and POA approaches of course do not exhaust theories of disease and epidemiologic causation. Nevertheless, they arguably account for the bulk of explicitly causal claims made in epidemiology.[2] Do either of these fairly characterize FCT? And, if so, what are the implications?

It seems fairly obvious that the causal claims at the heart of FCT reflect an IBE approach. Link and Phelan are hardly the first investigators to note the existence of robust correlations between a variety of indices of social and economic status and health outcomes. However, consistent with the problem of causation in epidemiology in general, the crucial question is whether these consistent correlations justify causal inference. Is it the case that adverse social conditions cause poor health? The problem of reverse causality is also significant, since in a variety of times and places, poor health can be utterly ruinous to key social factors such as family structure, income, wealth, and work. It is, of course, possible that confounding variables might render the strong correlations between social conditions and health outcomes spurious. But Link and Phelan want to suggest that there are no better explanations for these strong and persistent links than the operation of the factors they identify as fundamental causes.

Although I consider criticisms of FCT in more detail in Section "Conclusion," the issue for this IBE is whether there are plausible competing explanations for the links between social conditions and health outcomes that might justifiably undermine the qualitative judgment of causation. One way of evaluating this question is to subject FCT to empirical tests. Several attempts have been made. One of the questions Link and Phelan seek to answer in their extended work on FCT is how exactly social conditions create differential health outcomes. Why is it, for example, that social gradients in health persist even as intervening mechanisms change?

The primary reason Link and Phelan offer is the idea that social conditions enable access to "flexible" resources that can be used to protect health, either by preventing disease or by minimizing its impact once it occurs (Link et al. 2008; Link and Phelan 1995; Phelan et al. 2004). This aspect of FCT facilitates empirical evaluation of the theory. If the core mechanism that drives the causal influence on disease outcomes is the access to resources that enable more advantaged groups to prevent, mitigate, or buffer the health impact of adverse risk factors, it follows that social gradients *should* be stronger for preventable diseases and health conditions. Specifically, Link and Phelan suggest that this prediction is particularly applicable where we possess good knowledge regarding how to prevent certain diseases—if the resources needed to act on that knowledge are unequally distributed, we would predict that the ensuing prevalence/incidence and outcomes should also track the social gradient.

Mackenbach et al. (2015) conducted a specific test of FCT and published the results in 2015. Tracking Link and Phelan's preferred methodology for such evaluation, Mackenbach et al. reasoned that inequalities in mortality in nineteen European populations should be larger for conditions that can be prevented with an infusion of the resources. Link and Phelan posit that marginalized groups tend to lack. Consistent with the theory's prediction, Mackenbach et al. found larger inequalities among conditions more amenable to "behavior change, medical intervention, and injury prevention" (Mackenbach et al. 2015: 59). This provides support for FCT. However, Mackenbach et al. also noted considerable variance in the strength of the association, as well as multiple exceptions to the general trend, in some regions and for some populations, in gender (Mackenbach et al. 2015).

Earlier, in 2009, Virginia Chang and Diane Lauderdale used statins as the key variable for evaluating the solidity of FCT. Analyzing income gradients for cholesterol and statin use in the United States between 1976 and 2004, they found that "income gradients for cholesterol were initially positive, but then reversed and became negative in the era of statin use. While the advantaged were previously more likely to have high levels of cholesterol, they are now less likely" (Chang and Lauderdale 2009: 245). This finding supports the prediction of FCT inasmuch "as an expensive new technology that treats an asymptomatic condition, statins may have been disproportionately adopted by those with greater resources, promoting disparities in cholesterol that favor the wealthy" (Chang and Lauderdale 2009: 246).

Here, it is worth noting that most of the evaluations of FCT in which either Link or Phelan have been involved posit the use of technological innovation as a key driver in widening socioeconomic mortality gradients. There is something peculiar about the postulation of this specific mechanism as the key proof for the validity of the IBE apparatus at the core of FCT because there is excellent evidence that access to healthcare technologies are *not* prime determinants of health and its distribution in human populations. Although a great deal depends on what exactly is defined to constitute "technological innovations," there is ample historical and contemporary evidence that social structures located distal to the onset of disease are much more powerful determinants of health outcomes than access to healthcare and medical services—including healthcare technologies.

For example, the well-known McKeown Thesis charts the rapid and substantial decline in English mortality in the nineteenth and early twentieth centuries that had mostly finished well before the advent of the first effective antibiotic drugs (the sulfa drugs of the 1930s) (Colgrove 2002). As a historian of public health Simon Szreter (2005: 99) concludes:

> [The McKeown Thesis] effectively demonstrated that those advances in the science of medicine forming the basis of today's conventional clinical and hospital teaching and practice, in particular the immuno- and chemo-therapies, played only a very minor role in accounting for the historic decline in mortality levels. McKeown simply and conclusively showed that many of the most important diseases involved had already all but disappeared in England and Wales before the earliest date at which the relevant scientific medical innovations occurred.

Or consider the Whitehall Studies, which documented a sharp social gradient of health even where all study participants had access to basic healthcare services and technologies (Marmot et al. 1991). Of course, Link and Phelan might counter that improvements in public health interventions qualify as the kind of intervention they document. At a deeper level, they might note that their analysis of health innovations simply examines a mediator of the SEP-outcome connection. The effects of this mediator are evidence of the causal pathway linking SEP to disease outcomes just insofar as social gradients are sharper as to more preventable diseases. Nevertheless, directionality and effect size, which are consistent difficulties for causal inference in epidemiology, seem confusing in these assessments. Which variable is causally most significant? SEP? Knowledge (that is, health literacy, which often is a robust predictor of outcomes)? Access to healthcare technologies?

The causal pathways become even more confusing upon consideration of the internecine debate within social epidemiology regarding the connections between unequal social conditions and unequal health outcomes. As Simon Szreter and Michael Woolcock (2004: 650) put it, the contest

> has centred on the persistence of health inequalities in affluent societies, and the extent to which more effective research and policies should prioritize the psychological experience of individuals and their relationships to others in their community and society, or the material deprivations due to overall economic structures and national political choices.

Richard Wilkinson and colleagues argue for the former, suggesting as primary the "psycho-social effects of widening levels of socioeconomic inequality" (Szreter and Woolcock 2004: 652). Wilkinson argues that these increasing gaps in post-epidemiologic-transition societies "are characterized by individuals with increased anxiety and declining social support institutions, and by rising levels of violence and disrespect between citizens" (Szreter and Woolcock 2004: 652). Note that if this argument is correct, that poses a problem for the mechanism proponents of FCT what have generally deployed to evaluate the validity of theory. The causal links between social conditions and outcomes would of course remain, but under the Wilkinson account, they do not exist because of access to material resources so much as are mediated by declining levels of what has been termed "social capital."[3]

Critics of the Wilkinson account, categorized by Woolcock and Szreter as the "neo-materialists," "have argued that inequalities in health are always fundamentally rooted in differences of access to material resources (including housing and relevant neighbourhood amenities), which are, in turn, ultimately the product of political and ideological decisions" (Lynch et al. 2000; Szreter and Woolcock 2004: 652). The neomaterial account seems much friendlier to FCT, or at least to the methodology Link, Phelan, and other proponents have recommended and used as a means of evaluating the theory.

Although time and space preclude a deeper analysis of the debate itself and the implications for FCT, the issues involved have significant normative and policy ramifications. Specifically, at what points and at which levels should policymakers intervene? Should proportionally larger efforts be expended on increasing access to healthcare technologies, or on increasing health literacy, or on radical income redistribution? The latter approach would most likely be favored by Wilkinson and colleagues, at least as a means of building the social capital they deem the most powerful cause of unequal health outcomes. Yet, if unequal social conditions cause unequal health outcomes primarily because of unequally distributed access to material resources, relieving such deprivation and "giving people more things" would seem to be the highest priority. But even in the latter case, questions abound. Which things are most significant? Access to pharmaceutical products, like the statins studied in the Chang-Lauderdale study? Or access to early childhood education, as favored by many social epidemiologists?

Note of course that there is no false choice here. All of these interventions can be favored, but stakeholders cannot devote equal resources to all of them. The fact of scarcity alone demands efforts be made to prioritize possible interventions. Thus, one of the key normative issues that follows from FCT is the implications for priority-setting in public and population health. Which interventions ought to be prioritized, and why?

Ethical implications of FCT

Virtually, all commentators agree that FCT presents a novel and interesting way of conceptualizing the (causal) connections between social conditions and health outcomes. However, few scholars have explicitly analyzed the normative implications thereof. One of the pressing questions that immediately jumps out is whether FCT actually contributes anything substantial to axiological commitments that are widely shared among public health leaders across the globe. That is, aside from FCT, an immense body of evidence demonstrates the robust correlations between social conditions and health outcomes. Indeed, an entire subfield of epidemiology (social epidemiology) is devoted to documenting the link and providing a rigorous empirical basis on which to base policy and practice. Much of this evidence antedates the existence of FCT.

Public health leaders across the globe—by their public statements—are generally committed to collective action on the social determinants of health and seem at least somewhat invested in compressing health inequalities. In any event, to the extent such commitments are not shared, there is little evidence that FCT in and of itself is likely to generate them. Although FCT may provide supplemental reasons for believing that the highest moral priority is intervening on adverse and unequally distributed social risk factors that impede access to resources, it is less clear that, given the extensive epidemiologic evidence on social determinants of health, FCT is either necessary or sufficient to generate the normative conclusion.

Nevertheless, in prior work, I have argued that FCT, when applied to an ethical framework that has particular relevance and suitability for population health, can assist with difficult problems of priority-setting in public health (Goldberg 2014). Madison Powers and Ruth Faden's health sufficiency model of social justice (2006) is attractive because it is closely tethered to the same social epidemiologic evidence base that animates FCT. One aspect of this base is of particular importance for clear thinking about priority-setting: compound disadvantage. This natural concept refers to the tendency for disadvantage to cluster in the aggregate around social groups (Powers and Faden 2006). That is, if a person is a member of a group that experiences one form of social disadvantage, they are more likely, as a member of that group, to experience multiple additional social disadvantages. So, a person who is a member of a group that experiences low SEP is much more likely to also experience low educational attainment, exposures to violence, stigma, discrimination, poor housing, and so on. This is obviously not applicable for all members of the group, but at the aggregate level, it holds often enough to constitute a distinct empirical phenomenon.

Powers and Faden argue that these "densely-woven patterns of disadvantage" are morally significant because they help order priorities: those factors that drive these patterns, that contribute to the accumulation of social disadvantage, are of most significance because it is these factors that most drastically undermine health sufficiency (Powers and Faden 2006). Moreover, Powers and Faden expressly label their model a "twin aims" theory because it aims to maximize two goals: improvements in overall population health and compression in health inequalities.

It is easier than most think for public health interventions to advance one at the expense of the other (Benach et al. 2013). For example, in the United States, a variety of interventions aimed at reducing the prevalence and incidence of tobacco consumption have proved effective over the last few decades. Predictably, as prevalence and incidence have decreased, metrics of overall population health have improved. However, at the same time, the inverse gradient of tobacco consumption—more affluent people tended to be more likely to consume tobacco products—began to flatten and reverse slope. Over time, poorer and more disadvantaged groups in the United States became more likely to consume tobacco. As a result, while overall population health improved, inequalities in smoking and tobacco-related diseases increased. Although this is not necessarily morally unjustifiable, it is obvious that this is not ethically optimal public health policy. Optimally, overall population health increases at the same time that health inequalities between the least well-off and the most well-off contract. And note that what matters is not simply absolute values—whether the sum total of inequality expands or contracts—but also the relative value of the change in inequality. Thus, other things being equal, interventions that make the most well-off slightly healthier but dramatically contract health inequalities seem preferable to those that make the most well-off slightly healthier but marginally contract SEP-related health inequalities.

How does this relate to FCT and Powers and Faden's health sufficiency model of social justice? Understanding the complexity and the potential trade-off between absolute and relative population health values is crucial for priority-setting in public health policy. Applying FCT to Powers and Faden's model suggests that those variables that satisfy the criteria for fundamental causation are extremely likely to belong to the set of factors that drive densely woven patterns of disadvantage. In other words, FCT does not simply replicate the results of decades of epidemiologic studies documenting the effects of social conditions on health but provides a pathway to identifying those social conditions that are of paramount importance in producing health and its distribution in population. Consider Link and Phelan's example of sanitation:

> Presuming an equitable distribution of sanitation, the whole population's health will improve. At the same time, because the least well-off bear disproportionate burdens of

waterborne disease, sanitation-induced health gains will be greater for the poor than for the affluent. Sanitation both improves absolute health and compresses health inequities and is therefore ethically optimal.

(Goldberg 2014: 1840)

Tracking Geoffrey Rose's work (2001) on the preferability of whole-population-based interventions, Simon Capewell and Hilary Graham (2010) point out that many of the public health interventions that seem most likely to expand health inequalities are those they term "agentic." Agentic interventions depend for their efficacy on the particular level of resources that an individual agent can bring to bear. Such interventions therefore tend to benefit disproportionately the most well-off, which means that insofar as they are effective, they will expand health inequalities. Rose points out that, paradoxically, even approaches targeting the least well-off might expand inequalities to the extent that more affluent groups are more able to realize the gains enabled by such interventions. Rose documents that such focused approaches can increase health inequalities. Instead, he argues that interventions targeted at whole populations would be more likely to satisfy the twin aims.

Integrating Rose's whole population approach with the capacity to distinguish mediate variables from true fundamental causes enabled by FCT arguably informs debates over priority-setting in public health policy in novel ways. Of course, a normative framework is required to cash out the ethical implications of Rose's approach and FCT, but Powers and Faden's health sufficiency model seems reasonably well suited to the task.

To take one example of the way this process might work, consider the issue of stigma. The harms of stigma in health contexts are well known, but typically clinical literature focuses on the ways in which health and illness stigma can impede access to care. In the case of communicable diseases, such impediments can have profound population health concerns beyond the individual patient. However, proponents of FCT, including Link and Phelan (who are also leading stigma scholars), have recently (Hatzenbuehler, Link, and Phelan 2013) issued a more dramatic claim: stigma is best understood as a fundamental cause of disease. It seems to satisfy the three criteria; stigma is linked with multiple diseases, is linked with multiple risk factors, and persists over time. Stigma is a particularly powerful form of social disadvantage because of the way, to paraphrase Erving Goffman (2009), it spoils identity. A stigmatized person carries the taint of that stigma as they move through their social worlds, and the devastating social consequences of that taint are not limited to the particular context or paradigm in which the stigma occurs. Thus, where a person experiences weight stigma in a healthcare encounter, they may decide to avoid applying for a job they were considering, or otherwise carry the psychosocial impact of the stigma experience well beyond the confines of the clinical setting.

Applying Powers and Faden's model to FCT in this case justifies a moral argument that stigma is of significant priority. Stigma is corrosive to overall health and is disproportionately likely to be experienced by already-disadvantaged groups. Moreover, because stigma is such a powerful form of disadvantage, it is a perfect example of a social force that intensifies existing inequalities and perpetuates densely woven patterns of disadvantage. Intervening with specific anti-stigma mechanisms is therefore justified as a critical public health intervention—efficacy in such interventions promises both to improve overall population health and to have disproportionate impact on the least well-off, thereby satisfying the twin aims.

In spite of the above analysis, some commentators continue to question the extent to which FCT has important practical and ethical implications beyond that already justified based on the epidemiologic evidence base regarding the social determinants of health.

Emphasis on upstream versus downstream causes is not original to FCT, and Rose's emphasis on the significance of whole population approaches and his warnings against prioritizing action on proximal causes directed at high-risk groups was novel when he first proposed it in 1985. Stigma may well merit higher priority in public health action, but it is unclear that, even absent designation as a fundamental cause, the existing epidemiologic evidence is insufficient to justify such a priority designation.

Further objections to FCT

Challenges about novelty are of course hardly the only objections to FCT. First, critics can marshal some of the same concerns regarding the broad scope of FCT-based public health action as they can with any policy action targeted at root social determinants of health. Even if it is the case that such interventions are important, it does not follow that public health organizations and actors should be charged with their implementation. Rothstein (2002), perhaps the most vigorous critic of a broad model of public health, argues that social engineering in the name of public health risks damaging credibility and eroding support for essential public health services. Moreover, such concerns dovetail with the well-known boundary objection. If it is the case that upstream social conditions are the prime determinants of health and its distribution, then the legitimate scope of public health action is boundless. Literally, every public policy can be health policy.

I have considered and rejected these criticisms in prior work. The boundary objection is actually a category error:

> If the ethical justification for prioritizing attention to fundamental causes is valid, the fact that doing so might erode boundaries between traditional policy domains is a non sequitur. Even if true, the organizational problems that animate the boundary objection do not undermine the ethical justification for emphasizing attention to fundamental causes. Perhaps, if ought implies can, boundary problems sufficient to render impossible intervention on fundamental causes undermine the ethical case for the latter. But there is little indication that such is actually the case, and it is a high bar to show that action on fundamental causes is literally impossible where there is no shortage of examples of policies and programs across the globe that do so.
>
> *(Goldberg 2014: 1841)*

Moreover, the fact that virtually every public policy has population health implications is a feature, not a bug. Social policy literally is health policy, and policy approaches such as "Health in All Policies (HiAP)" make this point the keystone of the scheme.

A second set of criticisms addresses the explanatory power of FCT. Deriving principally from Mackenbach (2012), one of the major inequality researchers in the world, the critique begins by questioning "the persistence of health inequalities in modern welfare states." Mackenbach and colleagues pose an important question: if welfare policy is the key to ameliorating the adverse and unequal impact of social conditions on health, why do significant health inequalities persist in countries with the most generous welfare regimes in the world (principally located in Northern and Western Europe)? Moreover, "this paradoxical situation is made even more puzzling by the lack of association between the extent or intensity of welfare policies in a country on the one hand, and the magnitude of its health inequalities on the other hand" (Mackenbach 2012: 762). In a 2012 paper, Mackenbach considered nine different theories that might serve to explain the paradox, including FCT. Consistent with the analysis above, he summarized the novelty of FCT in terms of its focus on root social causes: "[According to FCT,] it is the social forces underlying social stratification that ultimately cause health inequalities, and not exposure to the proximal risk factors, which are usually studied by social epidemiologists (like smoking, psychosocial stress, working conditions etc.)" (2012: 762). Mackenbach labels FCT as "elegant," and suggests that "the paradox may actually be seen as an example of the workings of this theory" (2012: 764). Nevertheless, he judges that FCT is dangerously nonspecific; it fails to "provide a specific explanation of the paradox" (2012: 764). It is unclear what intervening mechanisms replace those "eliminated or attenuated by the welfare state," or whether the persistence of health inequalities can be explained solely by the fact that more affluent groups "make better use of these welfare resources" (2012: 764). The latter point seems to resemble the concern raised by Rose and others regarding the extent to which social policies aimed at helping the least well-off are in many cases likely to benefit the affluent disproportionately.

In a 2017 follow-up paper, Mackenbach again takes up the persistence of health inequalities in modern welfare states. He considers various sociological theories, but argues that all of them, including FCT, leave unanswered "the even more fundamental question of why these resources are unequally distributed, and why this unequal distribution is so persistent" (Mackenbach 2017: 114). This seems something of an odd criticism, since sociology as a field can hardly be accused of ignoring the pathways by which social structures produce (health) inequalities. While it is true that FCT does not contain within its domain a full tracing of these pathways and histories, it is unclear why it should be tasked with doing so. And in any event, even a rudimentary understanding of the historical flows of power, money, and capital across the globe suggests no independent reason for doubting the explanatory capacity of FCT.

To summarize, then, the most obvious objection to FCT is that while it may be an elegant formulation, it has no further implications for public health policy beyond those already suggested by decades of research in social epidemiology. It is not entirely clear why interventions targeting upstream social determinants of health were not justified based on the weight of the evidence prior to the development of FCT. As noted above, there are responses to this objection, centering largely on the ways in which FCT can, when paired with a robust normative framework, guide difficult processes of priority-setting in public health.

Other possible criticisms of FCT are not necessarily FCT-specific (such as the family of concerns often labeled the "boundary objection") but may well impact the validity of FCT to the extent that they are adjudged persuasive. Finally, Mackenbach's critique, while gentle, suggests that FCT does not illuminate the specific mechanisms through which health inequalities persist even in the face of relatively generous social welfare regimes. Mackenbach also contends that the available evidence does not demonstrate conclusively that health inequalities can be explained simply by virtue of the fact that more affluent groups have better access to needed resources. This point may cohere with the concern raised in Section "Ethical implications of FCT" regarding the peculiarity of using evidence of access to pharmaceutical products as a proof of the validity of FCT.

Conclusion

It is important to recall that FCT is a relatively young theory, with the seminal and introductory paper on the subject appearing in 1995. It has generated a lively body of scholarship and discussion since, and there are multiple published papers attempting to evaluate the theory's explanatory capacity. Given the increasing attention given to problems of causal inference from within the field of epidemiology, and the urgency of setting normative priorities in public health policy and practice, it is reasonable to suggest that further scholarly and practical attention to FCT is warranted.

Notes

1 In 1995, when Link & Phelan introduced FCT, the chief variable used to link measures of income, class, and wealth was SES. Although SES remains widely used as a key variable, methodological challenges have led some to argue that SEP is a better proxy for that which public health scientists seek to account for in connection with health outcomes.

2 Admittedly, there is a distinction to be drawn here between the structure of causal claims made within the field of epidemiology and the sociological fact of what epidemiologists claim to be doing when making explicitly causal claims. It is theoretically possible, for example, that epidemiologists could claim to be drawing causal inferences based on the Bradford Hill framework when in fact a close analysis of the reasoning at play demonstrates that the claims are in fact based on a POA approach. Birds, as Broadbent (2017) notes, are not ornithologists, and there are obvious potential differences between how professionals in any field claim to be reasoning and sociological facts about the structure of their reasoning. Nevertheless, there seems to be a little question both that epidemiologists frequently draw on the Bradford Hill framework in making causal claims and that in so doing they are utilizing an IBE approach to causal attribution.

3 Social capital is both a controversial and a well-studied topic. Szreter and Woolcock (2004) liken it to the energy flowing through electrical wires; the extent of the connections between different "wires" is correlated with population health outcomes.

References

Benach, J., D. Malmusi, Y. Yasui, and J. M. Martínez. 2013. A new typology of policies to tackle health inequalities and scenarios of impact based on Rose's population approach. *Journal of Epidemiology and Community Health* 67, no. 3: 286–291. https://doi.org/10.1136/jech-2011-200363.

Brennan, T. A. 1987. Causal chains and statistical links: The role of scientific uncertainty in hazardous–substance litigation. *Cornell Law Review* 73, no. 3: 469–533. https://scholarship.law.cornell.edu/cgi/viewcontent.cgi?article=3362&context=clr (accessed December 14, 2021).

Broadbent, A. 2017. Philosophy of epidemiology. In *The Routledge companion to philosophy of medicine,* ed. Miriam Solomon, Jeremy R. Simon, and Harold Kincaid, 248–256. London: Routledge.

Callahan, C. L. 1991. Establishment of causation in toxic tort litigation. *Arizona State Law Journal* 23: 605.

Capewell, S. and H. Graham. 2010. Will cardiovascular disease prevention widen health inequalities? *PLoS Medicine* 7, no. 8: e1000320. https://doi.org/10.1371/journal.pmed.1000320.

Chang, V. W. and D. S. Lauderdale. 2009. Fundamental cause theory, technological innovation, and health disparities: The case of cholesterol in the era of statins. *Journal of Health and Social Behavior* 50, no. 3: 245–260. https://doi.org/10.1177/002214650905000301.

Colgrove, J. 2002. The McKeown thesis: A historical controversy and its enduring influence. *American Journal of Public Health* 92, no. 5: 725–729. https://dx.doi.org/10.2105%2Fajph.92.5.725.

Fedak, K. M., A. Bernal, Z. A. Capshaw, and S. Gross. 2015. Applying the Bradford Hill criteria in the 21st century: How data integration has changed causal inference in molecular epidemiology. *Emerging Themes in Epidemiology* 12, no. 1: 1–9. https://doi.org/10.1186/s12982-015-0037-4.

Goffman, E. 2009. *Stigma: Notes on the management of spoiled identity.* New York: Simon and Schuster.

Goldberg, D. S. 2014. The implications of fundamental cause theory for priority setting. *American Journal of Public Health* 104, no. 10: 1839–1843. https://dx.doi.org/10.2105%2FAJPH.2014.302058.

Hatzenbuehler, M. L., J. C. Phelan, and B. G. Link. 2013. Stigma as a fundamental cause of population health inequalities. *American Journal of Public Health* 103, no. 5: 813–821. https://dx.doi.org/10.2105%2FAJPH.2012.301069.

Link, B. G. and J. Phelan. 1995. Social conditions as fundamental causes of disease. *Journal of Health and Social Behavior* (extra issue): 80–94. https://doi.org/10.2307/2626958.

Link, B. G., J. C. Phelan, R. Miech, and E. L. Westin. 2008. The resources that matter: Fundamental social causes of health disparities and the challenge of intelligence. *Journal of Health and Social Behavior* 49, no. 1: 72–91. https://doi.org/10.1177/002214650804900106.

Muntaner, C., Lynch, J. and G.D. Smith. 2000. Social capital and the third way in public health. *Critical Public Health* 10, no. 2: 107-124. https://doi.org/10.1080/713658240

Mackenbach, J. P. 2012. The persistence of health inequalities in modern welfare states: The explanation of a paradox. *Social Science & Medicine* 75, no. 4: 761–769. https://doi.org/10.1016/j.socscimed.2012.02.031.

Mackenbach, J. P. 2017. Persistence of social inequalities in modern welfare states: Explanation of a paradox. *Scandinavian Journal of Public Health* 45, no. 2: 113–120. https://doi.org/10.1177/1403494816683878.

Mackenbach, J. P., I. Kulhánová, M. Bopp et al. 2015. Variations in the relation between education and cause-specific mortality in 19 European populations: A test of the "fundamental causes" theory of social inequalities in health. *Social Science & Medicine* 127: 51–62. https://doi.org/10.1016/j.socscimed.2014.05.021.

Marmot, M. G., Stansfeld, S., Patel, C., North, F., Head, J., White, I., Brunner, E., Feeney, A. and G. D., Smith. 1991. Health inequalities among British civil servants: the Whitehall II study. *The Lancet*, 337, no. 8754: 1387–1393. https://doi.org/10.1016/0140-6736(91)93068-K

Phelan, J. C., B. G. Link, A. Diez-Roux, I. Kawachi, and B. Levin. 2004. "Fundamental causes" of social inequalities in mortality: A test of the theory. *Journal of Health and Social Behavior* 45, no. 3: 265–285. https://doi.org/10.1177/002214650404500303.

Powers, M. and R. R. Faden. 2006. *Social justice: The moral foundations of public health and health policy.* New York: Oxford University Press.

Rose, G. 2001. Sick individuals and sick populations. *International Journal of Epidemiology* 30, no. 3: 427–432. https://doi.org/10.1093/ije/30.3.427.

Rothstein, M. A. 2002. Rethinking the meaning of public health. *Journal of Law, Medicine & Ethics* 30, no. 2: 144–149. https://doi.org/10.1111/j.1748-720X.2002.tb00381.x.

Szreter, S. 2005. *Health and wealth: Studies in history and policy.* Rochester: University of Rochester Press.

Szreter, S. and M. Woolcock. 2004. Health by association? Social capital, social theory, and the political economy of public health. *International Journal of Epidemiology* 33, no. 4: 650–667. https://doi.org/10.1093/ije/dyh013.

Yonhap. 2020. Court rules against state health insurer in damages suit against major tobacco firms. *Korea Herald*, November 20. http://www.koreaherald.com/view.php?ud=20201120000256 (accessed December 14, 2021).

7

CAUSAL PLURALISM AND PUBLIC HEALTH

Federica Russo

Introduction

Public health (PH) is a diverse field in which a number of disciplines and approaches contribute to establishing a knowledge base for the design and implementation of PH interventions (Beaglehole and Bonita 2004; Brownson 2003; Guest 2013; Killoran and Kelly 2009; Tannahill 1985; WHO 2021; Winslow 1920). While epidemiology is arguably the main generator of evidence to feed the knowledge base, many other disciplines from the health and social sciences are part of this joint enterprise to a lesser extent: from bio-chemistry to sociology of health (Haveman-Nies and Jansen 2017; Mackenbach 1995; Pearce 1996). The diversity of PH is not just in terms of its "composing disciplines," but also in terms of the "people that make PH." PH scholars are academics from different fields, as well as officers in various non-academic organizations. I mention this kind of diversity too, as it may sociologically explain the difficulty in transferring academic knowledge outside the walls of academia, including using jargon and highly specialized vocabulary. The notion of causality, with its conceptually and historically loaded baggage, is a case in point.

Despite its inter- and multidisciplinary approach, PH appears to be dominated by one narrative about health and disease, one that owes its origin to the success of the biomedical approach, and that traces the causes of health and diseased down to the (alleged) measurable biological realm (Engel 1980; Kelly and Russo 2017; Meloni et al. 2018). Thus, while few in PH will question nowadays the importance of social factors, and the strong and steady correlation between health (inequalities) and social factors, the vast majority of interventions still tackle biological factors, rather than social ones. This may be due to the fact that it is easier to conceptualize causality between biological factors and biological outcomes, rather than across factors and outcomes of different natures.

I will return to this point later in the chapter, but for now it is important to note that causality *is* central, albeit not always explicit, in the generation of the knowledge base as well as in the design of PH interventions. The centrality of causality should be obvious to see from the fact that PH interventions aim to *bring about change:* in individuals' behavior, in populations' health, in risk exposures, in the burden of disease, and so on.

But given the multidisciplinary nature of PH, it is also easy to imagine what creates a barrier to thinking productively about causality: each and every domain works with different

DOI: 10.4324/9781315675411-9

concepts of causality and holds different epistemic norms or methodological standards to establish causal relations. However, just as PH is diverse in its knowledge base, goals, and implementation, so is the philosophy of causality. As I shall argue in the remainder of the chapter, causal pluralism can be of help, in order to keep diversity and plurality of methods, and to understand what concepts can help advance the field and design good interventions.

The chapter is organized as follows. In Section "Causal challenges in PH," I introduce six causal challenges in PH. These six causal challenges are meant to motivate the need for a pluralistic approach to causality. In Section "Conceptualizing causality and the prospects of causal pluralism," I explain why monistic approaches to causality are bound to fail and present causal pluralism, and in particular the causal mosaic approach. This approach has the peculiar feature of distinguishing philosophical and scientific questions of causality, for which specific concepts are needed, also depending on the scientific or policy context under investigation. In Section "What is causal pluralism good for?" I return to the six causal challenges and explain how the causal mosaic approach can help at both the stage of establishing the knowledge base and the stage of design and implementation of PH interventions.

Causal challenges in PH

In this section, I present six causal challenges that PH faces in the process of establishing a knowledge base and then designing interventions.

The first challenge [Challenge 1] is a most general issue in PH: choose the most effective causal narrative to explain disease and then intervene (direct paths versus very indirect paths). This is distinctively a causal problem because, arguably, narratives of aetiology, of intervention, and of prevention are different, because they identify different factors as the relevant ones (Kelly and Russo 2017). Any PH intervention is subject to this challenge. But Covid-19 will serve as a handy example. While it did not take very long to isolate the virus and understand (some of) the bio-chemical aspects of infection (aetiology), these are not the immediate "actionable" factors to contain the spread of the virus (prevention and intervention) (Greenhalgh 2020; Khalatbari-Soltani et al. 2020; Marmot et al. 2020). In other words, they provide only some clues, but insufficient to design effective strategies to control infection control.

The next two challenges I call "vertical" and "horizontal." The vertical challenge [Challenge 2] is about the level of aggregation of individuals into groups and population. The issue at stake is to pitch the right or best level of intervention: individual versus population, different types of social aggregation (family versus school versus peers …). This is distinctively a causal problem because causal relations may work differently at different levels of aggregation, and also because levels interact and interfere with each other. This "unit of analysis" problem is well-known in social science, as instantiated in the debates about methodological individualism versus holism (Zahle and Collin 2014). Smoking prevention programs are a good example of Challenge 2, because such programs need tailoring to different groups, for example, targeting teenagers in schools, or certain types of workers (Santiago, Talbert, and Benoza 2019; Strickland et al. 2015). It is well-known that what works for one group may not work for another, and this is true for individuals as well.

The horizontal challenge [Challenge 3] is about choosing the right or best factor(s) to intervene upon. In part, such choice will depend on one's metaphysical views about disease causation. Simply put, one can reduce disease causation to bio-chemistry or hold the view that socioeconomic factors (broadly construed) are also real causes. This is distinctively a causal problem, and for multiple reasons. To begin with, it has been (and still is) a struggle of some strands of social epidemiology and of medical sociology to establish the "social" as a legitimate, real causal factor, as opposed to a useful and informative classificatory device with respect to health and disease (Kelly, Kelly, and Russo 2014; Kelly and Russo 2017). Moreover, and relatedly, it is not obvious that the best factor to target is always biological even when we hold thorough knowledge about the bio-chemistry of health and disease. In part, this traces back to Challenge 1, about distinct causal narratives in place, but in part this is a distinct metaphysical question about disease causation. A good example of this challenge is the MEND (Mind, Exercise, Nutrition…Do It!) program against child obesity.[1] Part of these interventions, in fact, target parents rather than children directly, exploiting "remote", behavioral, and social (rather than "proximate", biological) factors, and on a quite indirect (rather than direct) path.

The next two challenges concern methodological issues in establishing the knowledge base. Challenge 4 is about understanding the complex conceptual relation between cause and risk. This is clearly a causal problem because the conceptual borders between "risk" and "cause" are not so clear-cut, but the problem also pertains to the actionability of risks and causes, and to the communication to general public (Covello, Von Winterfeldt, and Slovic 1987; Gigerenzer et al. 2007; Giroux 2011; Schooling and Jones 2018). The debate around the classification of red and processed meat as carcinogenic to humans (Group 1) by the International Agency for Research on Cancer (IARC) illustrates well the subtle difference between cause and risk, and the potential for misunderstandings, from the perspective of the general public (IARC 2018).

Challenge 5 concerns the assessment of evidence and the choice of methods to form the knowledge base and to design interventions. More specifically, one question is to assess how much evidence of correlation and/or of mechanisms is needed to have a solid enough knowledge base. Another issue, related to the previous one, concerns the use of quantitative and/or qualitative approaches to generate evidence of correlation and mechanisms. These are distinctively causal problems because, on the one hand, it is contested that we always have enough of these types of evidence. On the other hand, qualitative and quantitative methods (and of different kinds) come with specific assumptions, and especially about which causes are the "right" ones. Some methodological debates in epidemiology and PH illustrate this challenge. For instance, the use of statistical methods such as the potential outcome model has been considered by some as a gold standard method because of their rigor and for their requirement to work with "well-defined" interventions (Hernán and Robins 2020; VanderWeele 2018). However, some scholars have been critical of the approach precisely because of the impossibility of defining interventions "well enough" and for the assumption that causes be manipulable factors, thus excluding gender, ethnicity, or other key social factors (Vandenbroucke, Broadbent, and Pearce 2016). Similarly, the recent rise of qualitative methods in epidemiology testifies to the need for a plurality of methodological approaches that nonetheless come with very different epistemic assumptions (Bannister-Tyrrell and Meiqari 2020).

The final challenge [Challenge 6] is that concepts of health and disease are not "causally neutral." The problem here is really about the way health and disease are to be conceptualized. And this is distinctively a question about causation, because depending on how we conceptualize them, this will impact what causes we look for and what actions could/should follow (Russo 2021). Concepts of health and disease that reduce them to their biology are not just conceptually different from bio-social ones. They are accompanied by different *epistemologies* about how we can find out about health and disease, and they are also accompanied by a different *normative framework* about which interventions should (not) follow from said conceptualization. Differently put, in the context of PH, the concepts of health and disease that are part of the knowledge base are not just value-laden, but they are also *value-promoting*. A good example of this challenge are the European Union (EU) directives to fight obesity, which explicitly mention that social and behavioral factors are a key target, but in fact only regulate food labeling (Erixon 2017; European Commission 2007; WHO 2014). Arguably, these directives do not target the social aspects of obesity in a structural and systematic way (as stated in the documents), but instead implicitly appeal to the biology and chemistry supporting certain food labeling recommendation rather than others. Additionally, they leave the burden of choice to individuals, without introducing any structural changes, for instance, at the level of food industry.

In sum, establishing a solid knowledge base goes well beyond establishing the alleged biological, "hard" facts of disease causation. Instead, establishing the knowledge base should be done trying to make the complexity of the phenomena of health and disease intelligible and tractable. There is a sheer diversity in the type of causal challenges that PH faces. For this reason, it is a wrong move to assume any monistic or monolithic view about causation. In the next section, I will explain why monistic approaches to causality are bound to fail, and why we should seriously look into pluralistic options to advance the production of the knowledge base or the design process of interventions.

Conceptualizing causality and the prospects of causal pluralism

The search for the-one-theory of causality

The philosophy of causality has a long history in Western and non-Western traditions. It is clearly beyond the scope of this chapter to retrace these histories, and the reader may want to refer to the work of others (see, for example, Beebee, Hitchcock, and Menzies 2009; Illari and Russo 2014; Rabins 2015) to understand the development of causality across time and disciplines.

I instead focus on the debate on causality in the past 50 or 60 years, and particularly the one that mostly happened in English-speaking circles. In the reconstruction of this recent history of the philosophy of causality, a main strategy has been to analyze the concept of causality, as it occurs in natural language, and as is used by competent (English) speakers (Illari and Russo 2014). Such a strategy is rooted in the analytic tradition of philosophy of language. The goal was to reach *The-One-Definition* of causality, capable of resisting all kind of counterexamples. A main limitation of this approach was to appeal to competent speakers' intuition, and also to tie the concept to its linguistic formulation. Another limitation was that ordinary language analysis may be quite unilluminating when it comes to the specific meaning a concept like causality acquires in, say, physics, biology, and in PH.

A first important way to liberalize the philosophy of causality was to relocate the analysis within proper scientific domains. Philosophers of science thus investigated causality in specific contexts such as physics, and over the years, in biology, social science, and very recently also in medicine. Nevertheless, these investigations remained very "discipline-oriented," while trying to reach *The-One-Definition*. The philosophy of causality managed to produce an impressive variety of accounts that cashed out causality in terms of processes, mechanisms, capacities or dispositions, inferential practices, etc. It is not difficult to understand that the challenge of making *one concept* fit *all* scientific domains is real and bound to fail. For this reason, some philosophers of causality turned their attention to causal pluralism. When the community started investigating causal pluralism, philosophers of science had not yet paid attention to PH as a legitimate scientific domain worth of philosophical investigation. The situation has now changed, and the six causal challenges presented in Section "Causal challenges in PH" offer further ground for exploring causal pluralism, which I present next.

Pluralistic approaches to causality

Simply put, causal pluralism is the view that causality cannot or should not be reduced to one notion or kind of thing only. In the philosophy of causality, this is a strategy that has already been explored, partly as a reaction to the difficulty of finding *one* notion or concept that fits any domain, context, or problem. Phyllis Illari and Federica Russo (2014) also note that there are different variants of causal pluralisms. I lack the space here to undertake a comprehensive and exhaustive discussion of all the approaches that adopt a pluralist strategy. I will therefore offer a simple roadmap through this literature and motivate for the approach I favor, namely, "causal mosaic."

It should be noted that while pluralism is becoming an increasingly popular option in philosophy of causality, the Aristotelian theory of four causes (formal, material, efficient, and final) was already pluralistic about *types of causing.* Also about types of causing, but more related to the analysis of ordinary language, is Elizabeth Anscombe's idea that causality is (linguistically) couched into transitive verbs such as pulling, pushing, or binding, that all express ways in which causes act (Anscombe 1975), an approach that has been further developed by e.g. Nancy Cartwright (2004).

More recently, philosophers of causality tried pluralistic strategies, for instance, with regard to *concepts* of causation. Ned Hall (2004), for instance, famously held the view that we have two concepts, one to be cashed out in terms of "dependence" and one in terms of "production," which are applicable in different contexts. The proposal of Erik Weber (2007), instead, is to use different concepts of cause/causation, depending on the scientific context (for example, natural science versus social science). Other accounts centered on the idea that *causal inference* can be of different types; thus, for instance, Julian Reiss (2012) thinks that it is important to distinguish inferences about the model and the target. Another strategy is pluralism about *evidence* for causal relations. This was initiated by Federica Russo and Jon Williamson (Russo and Williamson 2007), who argued that to establish causal claims in medicine, one typically needs evidence of difference-making and evidence of mechanism. The original paper sparked a lively debate and a research program, to which I will return later in this section.

All these pluralistic strategies capture something true about causality and causal methods, as they are used and developed in different (scientific and philosophical) contexts and settings. But it is the approach of the "causal mosaic" developed by Illari and Russo that, I submit, can be of help in the case of PH. The approach of causal mosaic also starts from the observation that, until now, no single concept of causality fits all domains and contexts. This approach is maximally liberal: it allows for different kinds of causing as well as a variety of causal methods and concepts. But this approach goes a step further in motivating the project philosophically: no single concept of notion or causality can simultaneously answer the following different philosophical questions about causality:

1 Metaphysics (or ontology): What is causality? What are causal relata?
2 Epistemology: What concepts guide causal reasoning or govern causal knowledge?
3 Methodology: What methods to use to discover/explore/confirm causal relations?
4 Semantics: What is the meaning of "cause"/"causality" in natural or scientific language?
5 Use: What can we do (or not do) in the presence/absence of causal knowledge?

The approach of causal mosaic is also motivated *scientifically:* causality is not "one thing," or "one problem," as the sciences deal with different types of causal problems, notably:

1   Inference: Does C cause E? To what extent?
2   Explanation: How or why does C cause or prevent E?
3   Prediction: What can we expect if C does (not) occur?
4   Control: What factors should we hold fix to understand the relation between C and E? Or to modify C so that E accordingly change?
5   Reasoning: What considerations enter into establishing whether/how/to what extent C causes E?

Causal reasoning is arguably the broadest of the scientific problems, as it concerns all the ways we think about causality in science, whether explicitly and implicitly, and it lies at the intersection of science and philosophy.

To remain within the metaphor of the "mosaic," causal theories, notions, or concepts developed in the literature thus far constitute the "tiles" to juxtapose to one another in order to form an image. We choose the tiles as they help us address philosophical questions and scientific problems. For instance, the concept of (causal) mechanism may help with explanatory practices in e.g. biology (epistemology, methodology), while concepts of capacities or dispositions may instead help address ontological questions about biological phenomena. Or, the concept of (causal) process may help with tracing "world-line" trajectories in physics contexts or in social science (metaphysics), while some explanatory practices in the social domain may need a concept of "function" rather than mechanism. The image generated by choosing the tiles and by selecting which philosophical questions and scientific problems are at stake can be different for different problems in different fields, and even within a same field it may change substantially over time. It is worth clarifying that, in the mosaic approach, once the appropriate "tiles" are chosen and placed next to each other, an image will appear. The approach to causality thus produced is not static, rigid, or immutable. In many ways, it is a pragmatic approach to causality, rather than a substantive one that seeks to nail down "The One Concept" of causality. However, causal mosaic is not an "anything goes" strategy, but instead it is about selecting and choosing appropriate notions for appropriate contexts, keeping in mind that while we can ideally distinguish elements within the philosophical questions and scientific problems above, they are in practice intertwined. What makes a concept more or less appropriate is its fitness to a given goal. For instance, probabilistic theories of causality fare pretty badly with explanation, but they were never intended to be explanatory in character, but are rather about inferences of different kinds. Thus, the ultimate goal of the causal mosaic approach is to select and use "compatible" notions across philosophical questions and scientific problems. The approach of causal mosaic can offer a pretty sophisticated way of synergistically using many of the existing accounts, always specifying the philosophical question(s) and scientific problem it intends to address at any given time. It is part of the philosophical and scientific debates to establish which tiles best satisfy the intended function—i.e. whether and to what extent they address the selected philosophical questions and/or scientific problem—and to keep the search open for always better suited accounts in case none of the available ones works.

In an applied context such as PH, philosophical questions about causality are clearly phrased mainly in terms of use, namely, using causal knowledge for the purpose of designing an intervention. Yet, questions of use are not independent of other philosophical issues. For instance, Challenge 6, which is about defining health and disease, is clearly an ontological or metaphysical problem, but one that has important links with causal epistemology/

methodology, and with use. As for the other scientific challenges, PH may be concerned with any of the scientific problems of causality mentioned above, but possibly at different moments or stages of the process. Consider the different scientific problems first. Most of the time, we will need *some* level of explanation of a phenomenon of interest in order to make decisions about intervention and control. But in some cases, descriptive and correlational claims will have to serve as a basis for intervention and control, even in the absence of firm and sound explanations, according to the knowledge base established at any given time. Consider now the different philosophical questions. While defining health and disease (a question of metaphysics or ontology) are likely to remain, implicitly or explicitly, central through the whole process, from forming the knowledge base to the design of intervention proper, other questions, such about epistemology, methodology, or semantics, can be of variable relevance.

Causal mosaic has been developed as a general pluralistic approach to causality. In the next section, I use PH as a "stress test" for causal mosaic: how does causal mosaic really help PH with its tasks and challenges?

What is causal pluralism good for?

In this section, I seek to explain how causal mosaic can help to address the general task of PH (how to pass *from* conceptualizing/understanding a causal relation *to* acting on the causal relation), and the different causal challenges in PH.

The two stages of PH and causal pluralism

I begin with the general task of PH. The inference from conceptualization/understanding of causes to action/intervention is clearly not an easy one. For the sake of clarity, I cash out this inference as corresponding to the (conceptual) distinction of two following stages: (i) establishing the knowledge base and (ii) designing and implementing interventions. Though highly intertwined in practice, this conceptual distinction is directly related to Challenge 1: choosing the most effective causal narrative to explain disease, or to intervene, or to prevent, and this has to do with the identification of direct or indirect causal paths. Causal mosaic helps with Challenge 1 because it distinguishes between different scientific problems of causality, each having their proper formulation of the question, and appropriate methods. Explanation, intervention/control, or prevention are different, and their difference is conceptually and methodologically acknowledged in causal mosaic. With the causal mosaic approach, we can nuance these different scientific tasks, their import toward forming the knowledge base, and consequently their import toward the design and implementation of interventions.

A problem that cuts across the two stages is Challenge 6: the conceptualization of health and disease will influence a great deal how we form our knowledge base or how we design interventions. Causal mosaic helps with this challenge because it takes the most liberal stance about the metaphysics of causation, and for that matter about disease causation. This means that disease causation can be as inclusive as possible, to incorporate social and biological factors (I return to this later), and to open a space for the direct inclusions of values (epistemic, moral, political), into the formation of concepts such as health and disease (Russo 2021; Schramme 2017; Valles 2019). Let me elaborate further. The conceptualization of health and disease as primarily or solely biological phenomena, or as bio-*social* ones has very important consequences at the methodological and ethico-political levels. To begin with, a reduction to health and disease to "the biological" sphere restricts causal methods to the ones used in bio-medicine, in some sub-fields of epidemiology, and in evidence-based medicine. But it largely excludes direct contributions of sociology and anthropology of medicine or of narrative medicine. Such choices are underpinned by different epistemic values and norms in selecting methods and concepts. But all this also has profound consequences at the ethico-political level. Again, reducing health and disease to the biological sphere excludes socioeconomic, sociocultural, and sociopolitical factors not just from the *explanation* of health and disease, but also from the basket of *intervenable* factors in a PH intervention. For instance, if obesity is a bio-social (rather than just biological) phenomenon, intervening on the socioeconomic, structural factors that favor the obesity epidemic is *also* a clear normative standpoint—for instance, about the role of governments with respect to individuals or to the food industry, and these stances are de facto ethico-political in character.

In the rest of the section, I provide further explanation of how causal mosaic helps thinking about causality in these two moments and through the six challenges of PH, and how it may help with communication outside specialist circles, for example, from PH scholars to PH officers, and from PH officers to the general public.

Establishing the knowledge base

As mentioned earlier in this chapter, establishing the knowledge base may need different disciplinary and methodological approaches. This is captured by Challenge 5: assessing evidence and choosing methods to form the knowledge base and to design interventions. Specifically, we are interested in assessing how much evidence of correlation and/or of mechanisms is needed, and in choosing between and from quantitative versus qualitative approaches. In conceptual (philosophical) terms, the most general way of expressing this is that we need to admit, generate, and evaluate a whole variety of evidence. This is precisely the point of *evidential pluralism*, which is one of the tiles of causal mosaic, and a distinct pluralistic strategy.

Evidential pluralism is the epistemological and methodological view according to which, in order to establish a causal claim, we need different sources of evidence, and notably evidence of correlation and of mechanisms (Clarke et al. 2014; Illari 2011; Parkkinen et al. 2018; Russo and Williamson 2007). The thesis has been developed in the philosophy of causality and of medicine, partly as a reaction to evidence-based medicine and the use of evidence hierarchies, which put too much emphasis on evidence of correlation (especially in the form of randomized controlled trials (RCTs) and meta-analyses), at the expenses of any other form of evidence, from the ones generated by observational studies, or by experimental studies (for example, lab studies about mechanisms), or expert opinion. Evidential pluralism, it is important to note, is not about what causation is, but about what is needed in order to deem a relation causal—it is in this sense that the thesis is epistemological and methodological. Slightly different forms of pluralism about evidence and methods have been in recent times supported by, for example, Alex Broadbent, Jan Vandenbroucke, and Neil Pearce (2016); Vandenbroucke, Broadbent, and Pearce (2016), and Susan Haack (2009), and are certainly part of the history of epidemiology (Hill 1965).

Evidential pluralism holds that we need to establish *some* correlation and *some* mechanism in order to have *some* level of explanation of the phenomenon to address. The big problem is that none of these "some" can be fixed, as we cannot provide exact thresholds for when we have enough (or not) of these correlations and mechanisms. But the whole process of reasoning (one of the scientific causal problems of the causal mosaic) about the "quality" and "quantity" of mechanisms and correlations available *is* valuable to return a balanced report on what is the available knowledge base. For instance, the EBM+ group designed a number of tools for evaluating knowledge bases (Parkkinen et al. 2018, chapter 4).[2] Using these tools, we can clarify how much evidence of correlation is available, and assess its quality, and how much evidence of mechanisms is available, and assess its quality. In a similar vein, the CauseHealth group has explored the philosophical underpinnings (for example, causal complexity or individual variation) of several aspects of the medical profession evidence of mechanisms (Anjum, Copeland, and Rocca 2020), and the role of evidence of mechanisms in clinical practice, notably in establishing claims about safety or about efficacy (Pérez-González and Rocca 2022).[3] These important contributions notwithstanding, a question that deserves further discussion is how quantitative and qualitative methods can contribute to generating evidence. In evidence-based medicine, it is an established view that RCTs and meta-analyses are the gold standard for the generation of evidence of difference-making, but other methodologies—from lab research to observational methods to qualitative-oriented research—likewise contribute to generating evidence of both difference-making and mechanisms.

The principles of evidential pluralism, as developed by the EBM+ group, have been in part implemented in the United Kingdom's National Institute for Health and Care Excellence (NICE) and IARC methodologies (IARC 2019; NICE 2014; Samet et al. 2020),[4] and further work should tailor evidential pluralism to the specific needs of PH. Evidential pluralism, when properly understood, is likely to help with communication from academia to the policy world. In fact, the conceptual separation between evidence of difference-making and evidence of mechanism can be cashed out in terms of "knowing that" versus "knowing how," which is possibly easier to grasp than the categories of evidential pluralism. For instance, we have long established *that* smoking causes lung cancer, but understanding *how* smoking causes cancer required more time and resources. Additionally, the "how" part of smoking is not reducible to the bio-chemistry of the inhalation of substances such as tar, but also involves a whole variety of social practices, from imitation to stress release to "social smoking." "That" and "how" would, in *ideal* situations, license different inferences and interventions. Increasing smoking taxation targets the "that" part. But targeted interventions may instead focus on specific parts of the "how," for instance, prevention programs in schools.

Yet, we all know that the design and implementation of intervention are done in far from ideal situations or conditions. Very often, we need to intervene on the basis of some established "that" part, and without much understanding of the "how" part. This is exactly what happened with general lockdown strategies in 2020, at the beginning of the Covid-19 pandemic. But now that we have gathered more information about the mode of transmission, and also data about the exposure, morbidity, and mortality in different socioeconomic and age groups, arguably we are in a position of better exploiting the "how" part for targeted interventions (for example, in designing specific protocols for schools).

So, at the very least, we can design interventions with more awareness about what is solidly grounded in the "how" and what is instead solely grounded in the "that." Again, in ideal situations, it would be best to have as much of "that" and of "how" in our knowledge base, but in practice we need to be able to say why "that" can be enough to act, and this may be justified with arguments that do not necessarily appeal to the knowledge strictly speaking, but to arguments of precaution, urgency, or other values.

Designing and implementing an intervention

Ideally, in order to design and implement effective PH interventions, one should base them on the best available knowledge base. We have just seen that, even if we are typically far from being in ideal conditions, evidential pluralism offers tools to assess what evidence is (not) available. From a causal perspective, in the process of designing an intervention, we may need to distinguish two questions, which also maps onto specific causal problems:

1 How much do we really need to know about the target population to properly intervene? (Explanation, control)
2 How likely it is that implementing X we'll get the sought result Y? (Inference, prediction)

The two questions are not independent, but they are nonetheless distinct. Arguably, the first question is really about explanation, while the second is about inference, and notably about prediction. Being clear about these two questions will be of great help in the design of an intervention, because the link between the two may or may not be essential. The "Semmelweis case" provides a useful illustration. The case is debated in the literature, and in no way I will be able to do justice to the wealth of its historical and philosophical scholarship (Broadbent 2011; Gillies 2005; Kadar and Croft 2020; Tulodziecki 2013) in this chapter. Briefly put, the case is about Ignaz Semmelweis, a doctor active in Vienna in the first half of the nineteenth century. He was hypothesizing that puerperal fever was caused by some kind of infection; he proposed hand disinfection with chlorinated lime solutions for doctors in wards of the obstetrical clinic. As the story goes, Semmelweis's recommendations encountered lots of resistance from the medical community of the time, and in part because there was no scientific theory to support the proposed intervention, as the germ theory of disease was yet to be developed. The exact historical reconstruction of this case does not matter here, and its basic facts are not disputed, but the philosophical lessons to draw from the case are. It is contentious, in philosophical circles, whether the community at that time was right in rejecting Semmelweis's proposed intervention. Yet, it is to be hoped that one lesson to learn from this story is that, at least in some cases, we can accept to carry out an intervention, even in the absence of a good enough explanation of its underlying mechanism. Making masks mandatory during the Covid-19 pandemic is another good example of the difference between the two questions above, and would be supported by arguments from precaution, rather than from a fully established knowledge base in terms of both difference-making and mechanisms (Greenhalgh et al. 2020).

The approach of causal mosaic is pluralistic about metaphysics or ontology too, and for this reason it helps address Challenge 2, that is, picking the right/best level of intervention, depending on the types of social aggregation, and Challenge 3, that is, targeting the right/best factor to intervene upon, social or biological. Let me explain further. Causal mosaic does not take the biological level as prior or foundational to the social level: health and disease can be caused by bio-chemical *and* by socioeconomic factors. Much of medicine (broadly construed) since the second half of the nineteenth century has been about opening the opaque box of health and disease, down to the molecular level. But this has been at the expense of socioeconomic factors, which gradually lost their status as causes proper. The development of epigenetics and of the life-course approach in epidemiology requires a non-reductionist ontology for disease causation (Blane et al. 2013; Castagné et al. 2018; Kelly-Irving, Tophoven, and Blane 2015; Lock 2015; Sacker et al. 2016). It is in this sense that causal mosaic opens the doors for exploring the (causal) relations between the biological and the social spheres in health and disease, and for an ontology of disease that is not reductive in character. Likewise, causal mosaic does not fix that causation is primarily a token or type thing, or that it has a privileged level of aggregation at which it happens. With causal mosaic, we can legitimately talk about causal relations happening "inside the body," at the bio-chemical level, or at the level of the individual, or at some level of aggregation—for instance, social or working environment—and across any of these levels. These different levels may call for very different types of interventions, from the individual, clinical one, to a PH level proper, for instance, in occupational health. These are *all* legitimate levels at which *real* causal relations operate, but levels that arguably need different methods of analysis and likely different types of interventions.

Let me give an example of different levels of PH interventions, using different types of interventions in the case of Covid-19. A general lockdown, for the whole country, some would argue, does not need much "local" knowledge of different groups, environments, or other. The likelihood of reducing infection rates solely depends on reducing to a maximum any contact as a vehicle of infection. Partial lockdowns, for instance, targeting specific professions, or schools, or other targets, need a lot of local knowledge about the target populations or groups. This argument has something going for it, but also masks some important reasons why, after all, general lockdowns have been less effective than hoped for. In fact, general lockdowns target the whole population, without making distinctions about living conditions of specific areas or households, or which socioeconomic groups actually benefit, to a greater or lesser extent (Broadbent and Smart 2020). Similarly, consider banning smoking in public places versus designing prevention programs in schools. The same reasoning applies here, and actually traces back to the two key elements of evidential pluralism: "how" versus "that." In any of these situations, socioeconomic and sociocultural factors loom large, in terms of explaining exposure, identifying more or less direct pathways to disease outcomes, and for prevention. If it is true that even very general interventions, such as the ones just mentioned, do require "local" knowledge, the right question to ask is not in absolute terms about their efficacy, but in terms of their usefulness, for some specific purposes. A general lockdown may still be helpful, in the state of emergency, to gain time to develop strategies that are more tailor-made. The evaluation of generic interventions such as taxation of tobacco, sugar, or alcohol is different, and should weigh in also the simultaneous implementation of several other "local" programs.

The approach of causal mosaic can help with formulating clearer expectations and more transparent reasoning in the design process, which may, in turn, help with the communication from PH officers to politicians and general public. This is because, within this approach, we are prompted to specify which scientific problem we want to tackle, whether it is inference and prediction, explanation, or control. Moreover, assuming that the whole process is carried out with the least vexed interests and with the highest level of intellectual honesty, making clear what the expectations are and being transparent about the evidence base should lend support to the choices made, and find a middle ground between two equally deleterious attitudes: scientism and skepticism toward science. In fact, while not having "The Truth" all the time or for everything, science still has *some* base to act. Also, decisions are not the simple product issued from the knowledge base, but incorporate other dimensions too, including values, economic priorities, cultural aspects, or other elements. There must be a way in which we can succeed in communicating these subtleties about the scientific and policy process beyond the ivory towers of our specialisms.

Another pressing issue in PH is captured by Challenge 4: the complex conceptual relation between cause and risk. Causal mosaic helps with addressing Challenge 4 because it allows for a conceptual distinction and use of "cause" versus "risk," and also of "probabilistic cause" versus "deterministic cause." Grasping the difference between a "cause" and a "risk" is a well-known problem, and not just for the general public, but also for doctors (Gigerenzer et al. 2007). Thus, if causal mosaic can return a useful semantics of these concepts, together with fine-grained analyses of the concepts that will be of immense help to PH (Giroux 2011,

2013). It is important to acknowledge that these notions are complex from a philosophical and scientific perspective and their meaning is not univocally fixed (yet) in the sciences (of health and disease). At the same time, these terms *are* part of the technical jargon and their precise meaning ought to be better conveyed to the general public. Thus, any quick slip from the language of correlation and association into the language of *deterministic* cause should be avoided. It should be noted that, in epidemiological circles, causal talk is not always well received. Arguments to drop the term "causality" are regularly made (Hernán and Robins 2020; Lipton and Odegaard 2005). Adopting an explicit causal perspective does not imply that we have to always find causes, or that these causes are deterministic, but that we *can* distinguish between causes and risks, without reducing everything to the nebulous and dubious claim that, ultimately, we can never establish causes. In this sense, concepts of probabilistic causality, and the distinction between generic and single-case causality can be of much help to PH in recovering a "healthy" causal talk.

An effort can and should be made to better communicate the difference between causes and risks, notably by making clear what kind of studies have been conducted on problem X, whether there is experimental evidence, whether meta-analyses exist, whether similar interventions have already been done, and so on. It is not just a matter of degree. Partly, it is a matter of conceptually distinguishing (again) the "that" and "how" of causal relations, and partly it is a matter of distinguishing other dimensions of causality, notably between individual- and group-levels. In this way, we can hopefully better explain the difference between risk and cause to the public, disclosing, whenever possible, elements of the knowledge base and of the rationale behind interventions. It goes without saying that nothing can replace good literacy in general, but the idea is that causal pluralism can help the quality of science communication.

Concluding remarks

PH interventions face a number of challenges. In this chapter, I have identified six of them, all inherently causal, and I have introduced a pluralistic approach to causality to address them. Specifically, the form of pluralism I advocate is "causal mosaic" because of its distinction between philosophical and scientific questions of causality, and for its explicit stance that we need to select concepts of cause/causation that suit specific problems, questions, or domains. Causal mosaic can help to establish a more solid knowledge base, to better specify the rationale behind PH interventions, and also to improve on the communication between different actors and stakeholders involved in the process (scholars, officers, the public).

Acknowledgments

I would like to thank Alex Broadbent for his helpful review comments on this chapter, as well as Sridhar Venkatapuram, Alison Lockhart, and the participants of the workshops for this book. My thanks also to Mike Kelly for insightful comments on an earlier version of the chapter.

Notes

1 See, for example, https://healthyweightpartnership.org (accessed December 14, 2021).
2 http://ebmplus.org (accessed December 14, 2021).
3 https://causehealthblog.org (accessed December 14, 2021).

4   The 2019 version of the IARC Preamble explicitly references Parkkinen et al. (2018), and changes to the methods are also described in Samet et al. (2020). These changes resulted from a collaboration during the AHRC-funded project Evaluating Evidence in Medicine (https://blogs.kent. ac.uk/jonw/projects/evaluating-evidence-in-medicine/, accessed December 14, 2021). Update in the NICE manual since 2018 includes, inter alia, a more explicit recognition of the importance of evidence of mechanisms in identifying sub-populations, using the terminology of "mechanisms of action" rather the more generic "pathophysiological basis."

References

Anjum, Rani Lill, Samantha Copeland, and Elena Rocca. 2020. Medical scientists and philosophers worldwide appeal to *EBM* to expand the notion of "evidence." *BMJ Evidence-Based Medicine* 25, no. 1: 6–8. https://doi.org/10.1136/bmjebm-2018-111092.

Anscombe, G. E. M. 1975. Causality and determination. In *Causation and conditionals*, ed. E. Sosa, 63–81. Oxford: Oxford University Press.

Bannister-Tyrrell, Melanie and Lana Meiqari. 2020. Qualitative research in epidemiology: Theoretical and methodological perspectives. *Annals of Epidemiology* 49 (September): 27–35. https://doi. org/10.1016/j.annepidem.2020.07.008.

Beaglehole, R. and R. Bonita. 2004. *Public health at the crossroads: Achievements and prospects.* 2nd edition. Cambridge: Cambridge University Press.

Beebee, Helen, Christopher Hitchcock, and Peter Charles Menzies, eds. 2009. *The Oxford handbook of causation.* Oxford: Oxford University Press.

Blane, David, Michelle Kelly-Irving, Angelo d'Errico, Melanie Bartley, and Scott Montgomery. 2013. Social-biological transitions: How does the social become biological? *Longitudinal and Life Course Studies* 4, no. 2: 136–146. http://dx.doi.org/10.14301/llcs.v4i2.236.

Broadbent, Alex. 2011. Inferring causation in epidemiology: Mechanisms, black boxes, and contrasts. In *Causality in the sciences*, ed. Phyllis McKay Illari, Federica Russo, and Jon Williamson, 45–69. Oxford: Oxford University Press.

Broadbent, Alex and Benjamin Smart. 2020. Why a one-size-fits-all approach to Covid-19 could have lethal consequences. *Africa at LSE* (blog), March 27. https://blogs.lse.ac.uk/africaatlse/2020/03/27/ coronavirus-social-distancing-covid-19-lethal-consequences/ (accessed December 14, 2021).

Broadbent, Alex, Jan P. Vandenbroucke, and Neil Pearce. 2016. Response: Formalism or pluralism? A reply to commentaries on "Causality and causal inference in epidemiology." *International Journal of Epidemiology* 45, no. 6: 1841–1851. https://doi.org/10.1093/ije/dyw298.

Brownson, Ross C. 2003. *Evidence-based public health.* Oxford: Oxford University Press. http://site. ebrary.com/id/10375108.

Cartwright, Nancy. 2004. Causation: One word, many things. *Philosophy of Science* 71, no. 5: 805–819. http://dx.doi.org/10.1086/426771.

Castagné, Raphaële, Valérie Garès, Maryam Karimi et al. 2018. Allostatic load and subsequent all-cause mortality: Which biological markers drive the relationship? Findings from a UK birth cohort. *European Journal of Epidemiology* 33, no. 5: 441–458. https://doi.org/10.1007/s10654-018-0364-1.

Clarke, Brendan, Donald Gillies, Phyllis Illari, Federica Russo, and Jon Williamson. 2014. Mechanisms and the evidence hierarchy. *Topoi* 33, no. 2: 339–360. https://doi.org/10.1007/s11245-013-9220-9.

Covello, Vincent T., Detlof von Winterfeldt, and Paul Slovic. 1987. Communicating scientific information about health and environmental risks: Problems and opportunities from a social and behavioral perspective. In *Uncertainty in risk assessment, risk management, and decision making*, ed. Vincent T. Covello, Lester B. Lave, Alan Moghissi, and V. R. R. Uppuluri, 221–239. Boston, MA: Springer US. https://doi.org/10.1007/978-1-4684-5317-1_19.

Engel, G. L. 1980. The clinical application of the biopsychosocial model. *American Journal of Psychiatry* 137, no. 5: 535–544. https://doi.org/10.1176/ajp.137.5.535.

Erixon, F. 2017. Europe's obesity challenge. ECIPE Policy Briefs. https://ecipe.org/publications/ europes-obesity-challenge/?chapter=all (accessed December 14, 2021).

European Commission. 2007. A strategy for Europe on nutrition, overweight and obesity related health issues. White Paper. https://ec.europa.eu/health/archive/ph_determinants/life_style/nutrition/documents/nutrition_wp_en.pdf (accessed December 14, 2021).

Gigerenzer, Gerd, Wolfgang Gaissmaier, Elke Kurz-Milcke, Lisa M. Schwartz, and Steven Woloshin. 2007. Helping doctors and patients make sense of health statistics. *Psychological Science in the Public Interest* 8, no. 2: 53–96. https://doi.org/10.1111/j.1539-6053.2008.00033.x.

Gillies, Donald. 2005. Hempelian and Kuhnian approaches in the philosophy of medicine: The Semmelweis case. *Studies in History and Philosophy of Biological and Biomedical Sciences* 36, no. 1: 159–181. https://doi.org/10.1016/j.shpsc.2004.12.003.

Giroux, Élodie. 2011. Contribution à l'histoire de l'épidémiologie des facteurs de risque. *Revue d'histoire des sciences* 64, no. 2: 219. https://doi.org/10.3917/rhs.642.0219.

Giroux, Élodie. 2013. The Framingham Study and the constitution of a restrictive concept of risk factor. *Social History of Medicine* 26, no. 1: 94–112. https://doi.org/10.1093/shm/hks051.

Greenhalgh, Trisha. 2020. Will COVID-19 be evidence-based medicine's nemesis? *PLOS Medicine* 17, no 6: e1003266. https://doi.org/10.1371/journal.pmed.1003266.

Greenhalgh, Trisha, Manuel B. Schmid, Thomas Czypionka, Dirk Bassler, and Laurence Gruer. 2020. Face masks for the public during the Covid-19 crisis. *BMJ* 369, April, m1435. https://doi.org/10.1136/bmj.m1435.

Guest, Charles, ed. 2013. *Oxford handbook of public health practice*. 3rd edition. Oxford: Oxford University Press.

Haack, Susan. 2009. *Evidence and inquiry: A pragmatist reconstruction of epistemology*. 2nd edition. Amherst, NY: Prometheus Books.

Hall, Ned. 2004. Two concepts of causation. In *Causation and counterfactuals*, ed. L. A. Paul, E. J. Hall, and J. Collins, 225–226. Cambridge, MA: MIT Press.

Haveman-Nies, Annemien and Maria Jansen. 2017. *Epidemiology in public health practice*. Wageningen: Wageningen Academic Publishers.

Hernán, M. A. and J. M. Robins. 2020. *Causal inference: What if.* Boca Raton, FL: Chapman & Hall/CRC. https://www.hsph.harvard.edu/miguel-hernan/causal-inference-book/.

Hill, A. B. 1965. The environment and disease: Association or causation? *Proceedings of the Royal Society of Medicine* 58, no. 5: 295–300. https://doi.org/10.1177%2F003591576505800503.

IARC (International Agency for Research on Cancer). 2018. *Red meat and processed meat.* https://publications.iarc.fr/Book-And-Report-Series/Iarc-Monographs-On-The-Identification-Of-Carcinogenic-Hazards-To-Humans/Red-Meat-And-Processed-Meat-2018 (accessed December 14, 2021).

IARC (International Agency for Research on Cancer). 2019. *Preamble to the IARC monographs.* Lyon: IARC. https://monographs.iarc.who.int/wp-content/uploads/2019/07/Preamble-2019.pdf (accessed December 14, 2021).

Illari, Phyllis McKay. 2011. Mechanistic evidence: Disambiguating the Russo–Williamson thesis. *International Studies in the Philosophy of Science* 25, no. 2: 139–157. https://doi.org/10.1080/02698595.2011.574856.

Illari, Phyllis McKay and Federica Russo. 2014. *Causality: Philosophical theory meets scientific practice.* Oxford: Oxford University Press.

Kadar, Nicholas and Russell D. Croft. 2020. Why Semmelweis's doctrine was rejected: Evidence from the first publication of his results by Friedrich Wieger, and an editorial commenting on the results. *British Journal for the History of Science* 53, no. 3: 389–395. https://doi.org/10.1017/S0007087420000229.

Kelly, Michael P., Rachel S. Kelly, and Federica Russo. 2014. The integration of social, behavioral, and biological mechanisms in models of pathogenesis. *Perspectives in Biology and Medicine* 57, no. 3: 308–328. https://doi.org/10.1353/pbm.2014.0026.

Kelly, Michael P. and Federica Russo. 2017. Causal narratives in public health: The difference between mechanisms of aetiology and mechanisms of prevention in non-communicable diseases. *Sociology of Health & Illness* 40, no. 1: 82–99. https://doi.org/10.1111/1467-9566.12621.

Kelly-Irving, Michelle, Silke Tophoven, and David Blane. 2015. Life course research: New opportunities for establishing social and biological plausibility. *International Journal of Public Health* 60, no. 6: 629–630. https://doi.org/10.1007/s00038-015-0688-5.

Khalatbari-Soltani, Saman, Robert G. Cumming, Cyrille Delpierre, and Michelle Kelly-Irving. 2020. Importance of collecting data on socioeconomic determinants from the early stage of the COVID-19 outbreak onwards. *Journal of Epidemiology and Community Health* 74, no. 8: 620–623. https://doi.org/10.1136/jech-2020-214297.

Killoran, Amanda and Mike P. Kelly. 2009. *Evidence-based public health.* Oxford: Oxford University Press. https://doi.org/10.1093/acprof:oso/9780199563623.001.0001.

Lipton, Robert and Terje Odegaard. 2005. Causal thinking and causal language in epidemiology. *Epidemiological Perspectives and Innovations* 2: 8. https://dx.doi.org/10.1186%2F1742-5573-2-8.

Lock, Margaret. 2015. Comprehending the body in the era of the epigenome. *Current Anthropology* 56, no. 2: 151–177. https://doi.org/10.1086/680350.

Mackenbach, J P. 1995. Public health epidemiology. *Journal of Epidemiology & Community Health* 49, no. 4: 333–334. https://doi.org/10.1136/jech.49.4.333.

Marmot, M. G., J. Allen, P. Goldblatt, E. Herd, and J. Morrison. 2020. *Build back fairer: The COVID-19 Marmot review—The pandemic, socioeconomic and health inequalities in England.* London: Institute of Health Equity. http://www.instituteofhealthequity.org/resources-reports/build-back-fairer-the-covid-19-marmot-review/build-back-fairer-the-covid-19-marmot-review-full-report.pdf (accessed December 14, 2021).

Meloni, Maurizio, John Cromby, Des Fitzgerald, and Stephanie Lloyd, eds. 2018. *The Palgrave handbook of biology and society.* London: Palgrave Macmillan.

NICE (National Institute for Health and Care Excellence). 2014. *Developing NICE Guidelines: The Manual.* Updated 2020. https://www.nice.org.uk/process/pmg20/chapter/introduction (accessed December 14, 2021).

Parkkinen, Veli-Pekka, Brendan Clarke, Phyllis Illari et al. 2018. *Evaluating evidence of mechanisms in medicine: Principles and procedures.* Cham: Springer International Publishing. https://doi.org/10.1007/978-3-319-94610-8.

Pearce, N. 1996. Traditional epidemiology, modern epidemiology, and public health. *American Journal of Public Health* 86, no. 5: 678–683. https://doi.org/10.2105/AJPH.86.5.678.

Pérez-González S, Rocca E. Evidence of Biological Mechanisms and Health Predictions: An Insight into Clinical Reasoning. Perspect Biol Med. 2022;65(1):89-105. doi: 10.1353/pbm.2022.0005. PMID: 35307703.

Rabins, Peter V. 2015. *The why of things: Causality in science, medicine, and life.* New York: Columbia University Press.

Reiss, Julian. 2012. Causation in the sciences: An inferentialist account. *Studies in History and Philosophy of Biological and Biomedical Sciences* 43, no. 4: 769–777. https://doi.org/10.1016/j.shpsc.2012.05.005.

Russo, Federica. 2021. Value-promoting concepts in the health sciences and public health. Preprint. PhilSci Archive. http://philsci-archive.pitt.edu/id/eprint/19287.

Russo, Federica and Jon Williamson. 2007. Interpreting causality in the health sciences. *International Studies in the Philosophy of Science* 21, no. 2: 157–170. https://doi.org/10.1080/02698590701498084.

Sacker, Amanda, Mel Bartley, London University College, Department of Epidemiology and Public Health, Economic and Social Research Council (Great Britain), and International Centre for Life-course Studies in Society and Health. 2016. *Never too early, never too late: Social and biological influences on health and disease over the lifecourse.* https://www.ucl.ac.uk/icls/publications/booklets/N2EN2L.pdf (accessed December 14, 2021).

Samet, Jonathan M., Weihsueh A. Chiu, Vincent Cogliano et al. 2020. The IARC monographs: Updated procedures for modern and transparent evidence synthesis in cancer hazard identification. *Journal of the National Cancer Institute* 112, no. 1: 30–37. https://doi.org/10.1093/jnci/djz169.

Santiago, Suzanne, Emily C. Talbert, and Gem Benoza. 2019. Finding Pete and Nikki: Defining the target audience for "The Real Cost" campaign. *Fifth Anniversary Retrospective of "The Real Cost," the Food and Drug Administration's Historic Youth Smoking Prevention Media Campaign* 56 (2, Supplement 1): S9–S15. https://doi.org/10.1016/j.amepre.2018.07.040.

Schooling, C. Mary and Heidi E. Jones. 2018. Clarifying questions about "risk factors": Predictors versus explanation. *Emerging Themes in Epidemiology* 15, no. 1: 10. https://doi.org/10.1186/s12982-018-0080-z.

Schramme, Thomas. 2017. Classic concepts of disease. In *International encyclopedia of public health*, 44–50. https://doi.org/10.1016/B978-0-12-803678-5.00075-8.

Strickland, J. R., N. Smock, C. Casey, T. Poor, M. W. Kreuter, and B. A. Evanoff. 2015. Development of targeted messages to promote smoking cessation among construction trade workers. *Health Education Research* 30, no. 1: 107–120. https://doi.org/10.1093/her/cyu050.

Tannahill, Andrew. 1985. What is health promotion? *Health Education Journal* 44, no. 4: 167–168. https://doi.org/10.1177/001789698504400402.

Tulodziecki, Dana. 2013. Shattering the myth of Semmelweis. *Philosophy of Science* 80, no. 5: 1065–1075. https://doi.org/10.1086/673935.

Valles, Sean A. 2019. *Philosophy of population health science: Philosophy for a new public health era*. New York: Routledge.

Vandenbroucke, Jan P., Alex Broadbent, and Neil Pearce. 2016. Causality and causal inference in epidemiology: The need for a pluralistic approach. *International Journal of Epidemiology* 45, no. 6: 1776–1786. https://doi.org/10.1093/ije/dyv341.

VanderWeele, Tyler J. 2018. On well-defined hypothetical interventions in the potential outcomes framework. *Epidemiology* 29, no 4: e24–e25. https://doi.org/10.1097/EDE.0000000000000823.

Weber, Erik. 2007. Conceptual tools for causal analysis in the social sciences. In *Causality and probability in the sciences*, ed. Federica Russo and Jon Williamson, 197–213. Rickmansworth: College Publications.

WHO (World Health Organization). 2014. European food and nutrition action plan 2015–2020. EUR/RC64/14. https://www.euro.who.int/__data/assets/pdf_file/0008/253727/64wd14e_FoodNutAP_140426.pdf (accessed December 14, 2021).

WHO (World Health Organization). 2021. WHO definition of public health. https://www.publichealth.com.ng/who-definition-of-public-health/ (accessed December 14, 2021).

Winslow, C. E. A. 1920. The untilled fields of public health. *Science* 51, no. 1306: 23–33. https://doi.org/10.1126/science.51.1306.23.

Zahle, Julie and Finn Collin, eds. 2014. *Rethinking the individualism-holism debate: Essays in the philosophy of social science*. Cham: Springer International Publishing. https://doi.org/10.1007/978-3-319-05344-8.

PART 2

Reasons and actions

8

EXTERNAL VALIDITY AND PUBLIC HEALTH

Chad Harris

Introduction

External validity, the problem of inferring from the discovery of a causal relationship in one context to the existence of the same causal relationship in a different environment, is steadily evolving from being a sterile and esoteric methodological concern into a contentious and lively topic in public health discourse. One indication of its increasing prominence is the feedback emerging from studies into Covid vaccine hesitancy. The most popular reasons offered as justifications for refusing vaccination include concerns about the safety of the vaccines as well as the speed at which Covid vaccines were developed and administered (Machingaidze and Wiysonge 2021: 1338). What this suggests is a growing awareness that there is more to the decision to adopt a treatment than just the narrow consideration of whether it has been deemed effective in trials. At the same time, there is an emerging acknowledgment that external validity is a neglected concern in public health research in comparison to its counterpart, internal validity (Rothwell 2005: 82), which received significant scrutiny by the evidence-based medicine movement. In this chapter, I discuss the way the problem of external validity has been theorized in the context of public health. I evaluate the predominant approach to dealing with external validity in public health, which I describe as a "compliance" approach and suggest an alternative framework for guiding inferences about external validity. To prepare the ground for this discussion, I start with some background relating to the distinction between internal and external validities and clarify the important role these terms play in our understanding of experimental method.

Understanding external validity

The genesis of the debate around external validity can be traced to a distinction pertaining to experimental validity drawn by psychologist Donald Campbell:

> Validity will be evaluated in terms of two major criteria. First, and as a basic minimum, is what can be called *internal validity*: did in fact the experimental stimulus make some significant difference in this specific instance? The second criterion is that of *external validity, representativeness*, or *generalizability*: to what populations, settings, and variables can this effect be generalized.
>
> *(Campbell 1957: 297)*

DOI: 10.4324/9781315675411-11

This distinction yields two separate imperatives that researchers need to keep in mind when designing experiments or establishing experimental claims. Establishing internal validity involves trying to warrant the conclusion that there is a causal relationship between the variables or constructs of interest in the sample population. Establishing external validity is about considering whether the same causal relationship will hold in another target population outside of the sample or can be generalized throughout the entire population from which the sample was drawn.

Campbell's distinction, although framed for use in psychology and the social sciences, also influenced other disciplines requiring frameworks for guiding the way experiments are envisioned and designed. This includes public health research where the distinction between internal and external validities mirrors a distinction in drug trials between efficacy and effectiveness testing. The efficacy stage of testing, corresponding to the internal validity stage in experimental validity, is the stage consisting of "highly controlled studies that answered the question of whether a proposed intervention would have the desired effect under ideal circumstances" (Steckler and McLeroy 2008: 10). The effectiveness stage of testing, corresponding to external validity, is concerned with "studies that carried out the proposed intervention in less controlled and more real-life situations."

Over time, certain problematic assumptions about the relationship between internal and external validities have become entrenched in the discourse around these topics. It is important to clear these up because they threaten to muddy the waters when we get to the discussion on approaches to external validity in public health. The first problematic assumption is that there is some kind of trade-off between the two types of validity, even though internal validity is supposed to be a prerequisite for external validity. The seed for this is Campbell's comment that the criteria (internal and external validities) are both "important although [...] to some extent incompatible, in that the controls required for internal validity often tend to jeopardize representativeness" (Campbell 1957: 297). This sentiment is echoed and deepened in the work of those, such as Francesco Guala (2005), who adopt Campbell's definition. Guala goes further than Campbell in his belief in a trade-off because he says that validity can be threatened in both directions: "The stronger an experimental design is with respect to one validity issue, the weaker it is likely to be with respect to the other. The more artificial the environment, the better for internal validity; the less artificial, the better for external purposes" (Guala 2005: 144). This rationale for accepting the trade-off view is also considered in the debates about evidence hierarchies where it is argued that different types of studies are stronger or weaker in internal or external validity. An example in public health research is the debate about the relative importance of randomized controlled trials (RCTs) in medical research (Rothwell 2005). The crux of this debate is the question whether RCTs are the gold standard when it comes to identifying and measuring treatment effects. There is also the related question of whether the characteristics that work in favor of RCTs in the pursuit of one sort of experimental validity are counterproductive when it comes to the other.

The trade-off view is motivated by worries about the artificiality of experimental settings as well as the types of idealizations required for experiments. According to Maria Jimenez-Buedo and Luis M. Miller, the concern is that

> the more we ensure that the treatment is isolated from potential confounds in order to ensure that the observed effect is attributable to the treatment, the more unlikely it is that the experimental results can be eloquent of phenomena of the outside world, since typically, in the outside world, many factors interact in the production of events that we are interested in.
> *(Jimenez-Buedo and Miller 2010: 302)*

Part of the intuitive appeal of this view, and something that Jimenez-Buedo and Miller give reasons for rejecting, is a general skepticism about the status of knowledge arising from experiments. It is argued that because the experimental setting is purposefully set up to ensure internal validity, there is always going to be the risk that the causal mechanisms found in the experiment will not hold outside the laboratory. Guala (2003), for example, argues that the concern with establishing external validity stems from what he terms "radical localism," or the worry that we are always burdened with the onus of explaining why conditions in one experimental setting will not result in a different outcome if the experiment is performed in another setting. Arthur Schram also expresses this concern when he argues that the artificiality of the experimental environment is a significant threat to external validity because if "the laboratory institutions and incentives do not sufficiently mirror those of the outside-the-laboratory situation they intend to study, the loss of external validity may be significant" (Schram 2005: 226).

However, when we look closely at exactly how the trade-off is meant to work, we start noticing problems in the idea. On the one hand, accepting the existence of a trade-off could mean accepting that, for any given experiment, we can change the design so that we improve internal validity at the expense of external validity (Jimenez-Buedo and Miller 2010: 304). Alternatively, it could mean that, for any given experiment, we can manipulate the design so as to improve external validity, but at the expense of the experiment's internal validity (2010: 304).

Of course, there may well be circumstances where researchers are primarily interested in the applicability of a causal claim across populations and hence do not focus their investigation on establishing internal validity. Presumably, these experimenters would base their hunch about the ubiquity of the causal relationship on evidence other than the establishment of the causal claim in experimentally accessible populations. But just because internal validity is not the focus of these investigations, it does not mean that these are circumstances where internal validity is traded off in the interests of external validity. In other words, in these scenarios, internal validity is simply not a concern for the experimenters, and hence the idea that they are after some sort of trade-off between internal and external validities does not make sense.

This leaves us with the first interpretation, which yields the claim that "in a given experimental setting, the design can be altered in order for the inferences from the experiment to have more internal validity at the expense of external validity" (Jimenez-Buedo and Miller 2010: 304). Jimenez-Buedo and Miller are skeptical of the existence of even this limited interpretation of the purported trade-off. The first reason they question it is because it is inconsistent with the other commonly held view of the relationship; namely, that internal validity is a prerequisite for external validity. "If we accept that an experiment cannot have external validity if it does not have internal validity, how then, can one tamper with the experimental setting in order to gain internal validity by trading it for external validity?" (2010: 305).

The other reason they give for doubting the trade-off is because the notion of the "artificiality" of experimental settings, used to justify its existence, is vague and ambiguous (Jimenez-Buedo and Miller 2010: 307). The difficulty in blaming the artificiality of experimental environments for external validity failure is that none of the proponents of this view explain in exactly which respects the environments are meant to differ. In any case, it is clear that there is a lot more to the external validity problem than just a concern about the artificiality of experimental settings. This can be seen by considering the case of so-called field experiments or observational studies, where causes and effects are observed in real-world settings. In these studies, there is nothing artificial about the experimental context; yet, the external validity question is still a legitimate concern. This is because we can have cases where a field experiment exposes a clear causal relation evident in one context, but this causal relation does not hold in a new context because of different confounding factors, for example.

The most compelling consideration against holding the trade-off view is the fact that considered normatively, both internal and external validities are goals that experimenters aspire to if they are after experimental success. As Floris Heukelom explains:

> Although Campbell noted that internal and external validity might sometimes be incompatible when controls for internal validity would jeopardize external validity, they were not presented as opposites. A bad experiment could be inferior in both the internal and external validity domain, and a good test or experiment would score high on both internal and external validity.
>
> *(Heukelom 2011: 16)*

If the trade-off view is true, this best-case scenario of high internal and external validities is not possible. This is why, as Jimenez-Buedo and Miller point out, the types of prescriptions given in the literature for how to solve the external validity problem, namely, things such as replication of the study across contexts, improve both the internal and external validities of the result. This means that we have to give up either the belief in the trade-off relationship, or the possibility of an experiment successful in terms of both internal and external validities. Given that there is no reason to doubt the possibility of experiments that are both internally and externally valid, it stands to reason that the belief which should be dropped is the purported trade-off.

The other questionable assumption about the relationship between internal and external validities is that internal validity is supposed to be a necessary condition for, or prerequisite of, external validity. This view starts from the premise that it makes no sense to want to transfer or generalize a causal relationship unless you know there is a causal relationship to begin with, and that "unless we ensure internal validity of an experiment, little, or rather nothing, can be said of the outside world" (Jimenez-Buedo and Miller 2010: 302). The prerequisite view is motivated by practical concerns related to the way experimental knowledge is typically achieved. The idea is that when aiming for knowledge through the experimental method, you have to start with the local, and then, once you have a result, see whether that result applies elsewhere.

However, the plausibility of this belief is undermined when you consider the nature of the causal relationships that are supposedly the result of an internally valid experiment. If the causal principles that experiments discover are expressed by "past tense, local statements concerning highly artificial experimental contexts" (Persson and Wallin 2012: 11), then it is unclear what sense there would be in wanting to know whether these specific cases of causal interaction can be generalized. In simple terms, if research is only about questioning why, for example, this specific match strike caused this specific flame, then there does not seem to be any role for external validity concerns. There also does not seem to be much point in learning about these causal relationships. It is more plausible to hold that we study cases like these to expand our knowledge about and guide our responses to future cases of causal relationships between event types. We want to know that this match strike caused this flame because it is informative about other scenarios where other matches will cause other flames. But as Johannes Persson and Annika Wallin point out, this implies that the prerequisite view is false:

The only way this kind of trivial causal statements could prove useful is if they connect with more substantial ones. In other words, internal validity of this kind could have a value in relation to external validity as providing one of the instances externally valid claims have to be true about. Now, internal validity is not prior to external validity in any interesting sense. If anything, it seems secondary.

(Persson and Wallin 2012: 11)

A related assumption is that external validity is, in some ways, superfluous to the requirements of experimental validity because once internal validity is properly established, the external validity problem should not even arise. This position is evident in the following argument:

Campbell seems to believe that it is possible to identify causal relationships between treatment and outcome within an experiment independently of both (a) whether treatment and outcome are effective indicators of the variables they are intended to represent and (b) the question of whether the relationship will be found elsewhere. To the extent that the terms "treatment" and "outcome" refer to particular events in the experiment, these two issues collapse into one and Campbell's distinction is undermined, since by its very nature a covariance between particular events cannot occur elsewhere. If, on the other hand, these terms refer to lower level variables that have been investigated because they are assumed to correlate with the theoretical variables, then the issues are separate. But even here the judgement that the lower level variables are causally related necessarily implies that the relationship will be found in other contexts.

(Hammersley 1991: 383)

The key criticism here is that given the way we are meant to understand internal validity, once an experimental result is internally valid, we should already have good grounds for believing that the experimental result will be generalizable, or externally valid. If the experiment is conducted properly, we end up with a result that says, for example, A causes B, and this says more than that at those specific occasions the individual denoted by "A" in the study caused the thing denoted by "B." This is not to deny that experimenters might be interested in having an experiment studying a once-off causal interaction between two objects. Obviously, in such a case, the external validity question never arises.

However, in most cases, experimenters are after knowledge about causal relationships between types of things, not individual instantiations of these causal relationships. The causal relata in the experimental result, A and B, should ideally be representative tokens of the A-type and B-type, respectively. Martyn Hammersley's point is that when an internally valid experiment yields the conclusion that A-types cause B-types, we immediately have grounds for believing that other A-types not studied in the experiment will cause B-types, other things being equal. If this is the case, it is not clear what would constitute an interrogation of the external validity of the experiment.

Another way Hammersley expresses his argument against the importance of external validity is through considering the reasons typically given for the failure of an experimental result to be replicated. Considered from this viewpoint, external validity "refers to whether the same experimental plan would produce the same conclusion about the validity of the hypothesis under test if performed on another occasion, with different subjects, in a different setting etc." (Hammersley 1991: 384). A common explanation in social science research for external validity failure is a phenomenon called interaction effects, which is basically when an experimental subject's knowledge that she is being experimented on changes her behavior or her answers to the study questions. Hammersley uses one such example of interactive factors from a United Nations (UN) study where, after the first set of interviews, the participants became more aware of the UN and their work. This, in turn, made the participants responsive to the campaign and changed the way they responded. Those who accept external validity see this as a case of an experiment with internal validity but poor external validity. Hammersley suggests other interpretations of why the failure occurred:

a   the covariance observed in the first experiment was a result of chance or of another systematic relationship and does not indicate a causal relationship between the variables measured.
b   one or more of the assumptions about the relationship between variables and indicators in the first and/or the second experiment were false. In other words, the problem is measurement error.
c   The causal relationship between the variables holds, but not under the conditions realized in the second experiment (Hammersley 1991: 384).

He argues that these interpretations of the failure, which are as convincing as the original explanation of the failure, imply that there were problems with the way the original experiment was designed, and so the failure can still be traced back to lack of internal validity. If we interpret the experiment's failure in this way, then there seems to be no work left for external validity to do once an experiment is internally valid.

What this is supposed to show is that external validity is superfluous to requirements if you take internal validity as your starting point. However, even Hammersley's examples demonstrate why we should not ignore external validity. Hammersley is correct that if the experiment was designed properly and if the studied populations were truly representative, and so on, then the flaws in the experiment would have been detected. But the fact that the reasons for rejecting the experimental result cannot always be picked up during the phase of the experiment governed by internal validity demonstrates why retaining external validity is important. Even if we accept Hammersley's alternative explanations for the failure of replication, we are still left with the problem that certain problems, certain reasons to reject the causal relationship of interest, can only be detected after the internal validity phase of testing is completed.

Another way of understanding my reservation about Hammersley's argument is to distinguish between the metaphysical and the epistemological aspect of external validity. Considered as a metaphysical category, the experimental result is either internally valid or invalid, and this is what the experimental controls are meant to detect. However, if testing goes awry, and we are led to the mistaken belief that a conclusion is valid when, in fact, it is invalid, what should we blame? Hammersley's point is that in cases like these the conclusion has been invalid all along, and so the blame should be placed on the original experiment.

This metaphysical, or what we could equally describe as "factive," notion of validity implies a very close connection between experimental validity (of either variety) and truth. If an experiment is valid, in either sense, then the connection between all the referents of both the variables, wherever they are, is in fact causal. Naturally, on this view, there is little sense in suggesting that the relationship is causal in one setting but not causal in another. The original experiment failed to detect the causal relationship of interest, which either holds or does not hold in both experimental and target environments.

However, if we interpret validity as having mostly epistemological, as opposed to metaphysical, import, then our assessment changes. If one holds the view that being internally valid means being justified, in some epistemic sense, in believing there is a causal relationship in the experimental environment, then one can still make sense of an important distinction between internal and external validities. In simple terms, internal validity involves being justified in accepting that there is a causal relationship in the experimental environment. This justification is a normative notion separate from considerations about the ultimate truth of the experimenter's belief. It implies that the epistemic agent has ticked all the appropriate boxes in the way she has conducted the experiment. On this epistemological conception, external validity becomes necessary simply because evidence for rejecting the existence of the causal relationship in the target environment is sometimes only accessible after the experimental stage. We can say that the experimenters were internally justified in asserting causality in the original experiment because there was good evidence for a causal relationship. However, they did not have the type of justification needed to render their conclusion externally valid.

Even Campbell, who was the progenitor of both assumptions about the relationship between internal and external validities, endorsed a far more nuanced position about the priority of internal validity in his later work. In his (2002) statement, he and his collaborators have the following to say on the matter: "*Internal validity is not the sine qua non of all research. It does have a special (but not inviolate) place in cause-probing research, and especially in experimental research, by encouraging critical thinking about descriptive causal claims*" (Shadish, Cook, and Campbell 2002: 98; italics in the original).

This is a clear indication that Campbell and his coauthors do not consider the attainment of internal validity as the most significant plateau for researchers to clear. Instead, they imply that not all the intellectual work has been done, in terms of understanding causes, once we have an internally valid result.

An approach that avoids these issues is understanding the external validity problem as a problem pertaining to a specific variety of inference. This should not be taken to mean that factors such as experimental design are irrelevant to our understanding of external validity. All it means is inferences are a crucial component of the problem of external validity; and, in my opinion, the reason it is a topic of concern is because it represents a real and significant problem for anyone in the position of having to make decisions about implementing a treatment or intervention based on studies showing their past efficacy.

In other words, those who are truly burdened by the external validity problem are those who have the task of making an inference from the fact that the experimental result was established (or that the causal relationship holds) in one specific context to the conclusion that it will hold in another target population outside of the sample or can be generalized throughout the entire population from which the sample was drawn. I call such inferences "EV inferences." The issue at hand pertains to scenarios where the first type of validity, internal validity, has been satisfactorily resolved but where the latter, external validity, is at stake. In other words, my concern here is with cases where we have confirmed the existence of a causal relationship in one context, but where we have to make an *extrapolation* about the existence of that relationship in a new environment where it has not been tested for. Accordingly, we can follow Daniel Steel's definition of extrapolation as "using a causal relationship found in one context as a basis for an inference about causal relationships in another that may differ in a number of relevant respects" (Steel 2013: 186).

This focus on EV inferences is consistent with the way experimental validity was initially defined. Even Campbell, the originator of the experimental validity distinction between internal and external validities, endorsed an interpretation of the external validity problem that stresses the importance of the inferences involved in the external validity context, as illustrated in the following definition: "External validity concerns inferences about the extent to which a causal relationship holds over variations in persons, settings, treatments, and outcomes" (Shadish, Cook, and Campbell 2002: 83). My position is that deepening our understanding of such EV inferences is crucial if we want to make progress in understanding the concept of external validity. If making EV inferences is an issue at the heart of the problem of external validity, then it stands to reason that a fundamental element of solving the problem is to give some sort of account of these inferences.

The compliance approach to external validity in public health

Now that the nature of the problem has been clarified, I move on to evaluating some of the advice proffered for dealing with external validity in public health. The first clear trend is the prominence of the idea that the most effective way of solving the external validity problem is to identify threats or limitations to external validity. This approach is not unique to the discussion of external validity in public health and medicine, but it is clearly a dominant approach in the field and is premised on the hope that the identification of these threats will allow researchers to avoid, or at least mitigate some of these factors, and hence improve the external validity of studies.

This approach is clearly demonstrated by Peter Rothwell's two influential papers (2005, 2006) arguing for increased attention to the external validity problem in clinical research. His aim is to provide advice to doctors and patients grappling with the task of making decisions about the applicability of clinical studies. In answering the question "To whom do the results of this trial apply?" Rothwell compiles a list of factors that are known to adversely affect the external validity of RCTs and systematic reviews. While there is no doubt that these checklists can be useful, the main shortcoming is that there is no clear and explicit criterion given for inclusion in the list of threats. One can infer that the list was compiled through a combination of judgment and empirical findings about factors that were blamed for a study result failing to hold in a new environment. The problem with this approach is that it is not systematic, and results in an ad hoc proliferation of factors to consider when making an EV inference. The result is that more and more items become included for consideration without regard for the relative importance of the newly added factors. This has meant that healthcare research has become inundated with these checklists (Dyrvig et al. 2014: 863) and it is becoming increasingly difficult to know exactly what is relevant and what is not. It is preferable to aim for the outcomes Laura Leviton calls for in the context of generalizing public health interventions:

> Public health should develop a program of research on external validity that focuses on frequent and important context features, because these are the features that have the most consequences for population health. Such a program should draw on the entire body of evidence, including descriptive and qualitative information, practitioner experience, correlational and regression studies, and tests of effectiveness. Doing so has several advantages. (a) A systematic approach explicates the undifferentiated bundle otherwise lumped as "context." (b) One can go beyond surface similarity to more powerful generalizations on the basis of program theory. (c) One can utilize practitioner knowledge in meaningful ways. (d) With the accrual of information, one can be increasingly specific about situations where a causal inference is likely to hold. (e) One can also be more selective about where to focus additional attention and resources, whether the focus is on causal inference or causal generalization.
>
> *(Leviton 2017: 387)*

A slight improvement to the approach premised on checklists of threats is to rather identify broad types or varieties of factors that could possibly threaten the external validity of study results. One of the earliest such attempts at such categorization is the work of Glenn H. Bracht and Gene V. Glass (1968) on population validity and ecological validity. On the one hand, external validity can be threatened because of differences between the people or things studied in the experiment and their counterparts outside of the experiment. This first type of threat, which they describe as threat of "population validity," concerns "generalizations to populations of persons (What population of subjects can be expected to behave in the same way as did the sample experimental subjects?)" (Bracht and Glass 1968: 438).

Concerns with population validity are also evident in the factors O. M. Dekkers et al. (2010) identify as the main threats to external validity in the medical literature. They point to the eligibility criteria for a medical study as a key reason for why it might fail to achieve external validity (2010: 92). The basic worry is that getting this wrong would mean that the population studied in the sample is not representative of the population of interest for the treatment. It is this concern with population validity that has led to increasingly advanced methods for ensuring representative sampling in experimental studies.

The second type of threat to external validity are those pertaining to "ecological validity" and these threats deal with "the 'environment' of the experiment (Under what conditions, i.e., settings, treatments, experimenters, dependent variables, etc., can the same results be expected?)" (Bracht and Glass 1968: 438). Another way of describing these ecological threats is in terms of interactive factors as is the case with William R. Shadish, Thomas D. Cook, and Donald T. Campbell, who see the answer to threats to external validity as "the search for ways in which a causal relationship might or might not change over persons, settings, treatments, and outcomes" (2002: 86).

While the separation of external validity failures into those due to population and ecological factors is useful as a way of envisioning potential threats, this neat division glosses over the interrelatedness of the two types of factors, as illustrated in the work of John G. Lynch (1982), who lists the following as the factors that influence our ability to generalize a conclusion:

1   The *true state of nature* – i.e. whether a particular background factor normally interacts or combines additively with the manipulated variables.
2   The researcher's intentional or inadvertent *sampling* of that background factor in designing the experiment – is it held constant, allowed to vary with marginal distribution similar to its counterpart in the target population, or allowed to vary with a marginal distribution that is dissimilar to its counterpart in the target population?
3   The researcher's *awareness* of the possible influence of the background factor in analyzing the data – i.e. if it has a main effect on the dependent variable and/or interactions with the treatments, does the experimenter have the insight to formally estimate those effects in analyzing the data, or does s/he simply average over all levels of the background variables to derive estimates of the treatment effects of primary interest? (Lynch 1982: 234–235).

What this illustrates is that environmental factors, which form part of the "true state of nature," are often responsible for the causally relevant differences between populations studied in experiments and the populations of interest. If environmental factors are responsible for differences in populations, it is difficult to argue for the total separation of the two types of factors. Nevertheless, envisioning potential threats to external validity in terms of factors related either to the studied population or to the wider environment can be a useful heuristic tool.

Even though this categorization framework is an improvement on approaches that simply list all known threats to external validity, it is still based on a problematic underlying assumption. This assumption is that the best way of thinking about the problem is to consider, when making an EV inference, whether the target population is sufficiently similar to the studied population. This emphasis on the idea of similarity of environment is questioned by Nancy Cartwright and Jeremy Hardie (2012) in their criticism of established methods for dealing with external validity:

> In the orthodoxy, a study has external validity when the "same treatment" has the "same result" in a specific target as it did in the study. The orthodox advice is that external validity can be expected if the target population is "sufficiently similar" to the study population. For us, the key question is how good a job this advice does in getting you from "it worked there" to "it will work here." The answer: you are lucky if it gets you anywhere.
>
> *(Cartwright and Hardie 2012: 46)*

They have the following major criticisms of the advice to policy implementers generated by the concept of external validity. First, the advice about studying similarities between the experimental and target environments is too vague because it is not always clear what exactly the "same effect" would be in the environments of interest. Sometimes, experimenters want to know if the same effect size can be expected, but at other times it is good enough for the effect direction to be the same. In most cases, argue Cartwright and Hardie, the most experimenters can hope for is that the factors that played a causal role in the experimental sample will play a similar role in the target populations (2012: 46). However, this does not mean that we should expect the causal relationship to be evident in the new context because the support factors that allow the causal principle to function in the original context might be missing.

They also argue that the advice about seeking similarities between the environments is too demanding because it is rarely the case that the environment where the policy needs to be implemented is similar to the experimental environment (Cartwright and Hardie 2012: 47) in all the relevant respects. It is possible that the treatments of interest play the same causal roles in very different environments, or that environments that seem very similar contain factors that will confound the studied causal relationship. For these reasons, the idea of similarity between studied and target population should not be relied upon as the ultimate determinant of external validity success or failure.

Toward an inferentialist approach

To advance the approach to external validity in public health, it is important to move beyond seeing the problem as merely one of compliance, or as the purely preventative mission of avoiding threats to the attainment of externally valid results. A workable solution to external validity must also include the positive element of constructing warrant for inferences that the causal relationship identified in the experiment will be present in the target. In constructing these inferences, and in lieu of threats, we should be guided by two considerations identified by Steel's (2008) account of the problems that beset extrapolation in the sciences:

> One challenge, which I call *extrapolator's circle*, arises from the fact that extrapolation is worthwhile only when there are important limitations on what one can learn about

the target by studying it directly. The challenge, then, is to explain how the suitability of the model as a basis for extrapolation can be established given only limited, partial information about the target.

(Steel 2008: 4)

Steel's second challenge arises from the fact that there are invariably differences between studied and targeted populations: "The second challenge arises from the inevitable presence [...] of causally relevant differences between the model and the target. Thus, any adequate account of extrapolation in heterogenous populations must explain how extrapolation can be possible even when such differences are present" (2008: 78–79).

With these considerations acting as guiding principles, we need recourse to a framework that allows us to build an argument about exactly what we should pay attention to in the target. An example of the type of constructive framework that would be suitable is the effectiveness argument outlined by Cartwright and Hardie in the context of evidence-based policy:

1 *x* works there (i.e. *x* genuinely appears in the causal principle that governs the production of *y* there post-implementation).
2 Here and there share that causal principle post-implementation.
3 The support factors necessary for *x* to contribute under that principle are present for at least some individuals here post-implementation. Conclusion. *x* works here (i.e. *x* genuinely appears in the causal principle that governs the production of *y* here post-implementation and the support factors necessary for it to contribute to *y* are present for at least some individuals here post-implementation) (Cartwright and Hardie 2012: 42).

This approach seemingly satisfies Steel's challenges because it explains what one would need to establish about the target, short of running another internally valid experiment there. Specifically, it exhorts the EV inference-maker to think about, first, whether the causal principle responsible for the causal relationship in the studied population would play a similar role in the target. By a "causal principle," Cartwright and Hardie are referring to a reliable and systematic connection between the cause and effect (2012: 22). The second crucial component to the inference would be some consideration of the support factors that played a role in the manifestation and strength of the causal principle, and whether the same configuration of support factors is present in the target.

Another framework that ostensibly satisfies Steel's challenges is his own comparative process tracing (Steel 2008, 2013). This approach is premised on identifying the mechanisms responsible for the causal relationship of interest. Doing so successfully yields the following method for making EV inferences: "First, learn the mechanism in the model organism [...] Second, compare stages of the mechanism in the model organism with that of the target organism in which the two are most likely to differ significantly" (Steel 2008: 89).

A similar mechanism-underpinned approach is suggested by the Russo and Williamson thesis (RWT) about causal inference in medicine (Williamson 2019). According to RWT, a strong EV inference can be made to the extent that one can establish that similar mechanisms are responsible for the correlation between cause and effect in the studied and target population. This means that EV inferences should be guided by the following considerations:

If the corresponding causal claim is established in the source population and it is also established that the mechanisms in the target population are sufficiently similar to those which underpin causation in the source population then this combination of evidence may be enough to establish correlation in the target population. If so, since mechanism in the target is also established, causality can be inferred.

(Williamson 2019: 53)

These methods give us a way of dealing with Steel's challenges of extrapolation because they specify exactly which aspects of the experimental and target populations need to be compared, namely, specific stages of the relevant mechanisms responsible for the causal relationship. As with the Cartwright-Hardie framework, mechanism-based approaches are thus appropriate frameworks for making good EV inferences.

Conclusion

The increased scrutiny being given to the problem of external validity challenges us to accelerate our efforts in understanding and exploiting frameworks that guide EV inferences. With these general frameworks in place, investigators are now able to leverage domain-specific knowledge related to public health to support EV inferences with information about the causal principles, interactive factors, and mechanisms responsible for the causal relationships studied in public health. This combination of a sturdy inferential framework and reliable subject knowledge promises to deliver EV inferences that are well warranted.

References

Bracht, G. H. and G. Glass. 1968. The external validity of experiments. *American Education Research Journal* 5, no. 4: 437–474. https://doi.org/10.2307/1161993.

Campbell, D. 1957. Factors relevant to the validity of experiments in social settings. *Psychological Bulletin* 54, no. 4: 297–312. https://doi.org/10.1037/h0040950.

Cartwright, Nancy and Jeremy Hardie. 2012. *Evidence-based policy: A practical guide to doing it better.* New York: Oxford University Press.

Dekkers, O. M., E. von Elm, A. Algra, J. A. Romijn, and J. P. Vandenbroucke. 2010. How to assess the external validity of therapeutic trials: A conceptual approach. *International Journal of Epidemiology* 39, no. 1: 89–94. https://doi.org/10.1093/ije/dyp174.

Dyrvig, A. K., K. Kidholm, O. Gerke, and H. Vondeling. 2014. Checklists for external validity: A systematic review. *Journal of Evaluation in Clinical Practice* 20, no. 6: 857–864. https://doi.org/10.1111/jep.12166.

Guala, F. 2003. Experimental localism and external validity. *Philosophy of Science* 70, no. 5: 1195–1205. https://doi.org/10.1086/377400.

Guala, F. 2005. *The methodology of experimental economics.* New York: Cambridge University Press.

Hammersley, M. 1991. A note on Campbell's distinction between internal and external validity. *Quality and Quantity* 25, no. 4: 381–387. https://doi.org/10.1007/BF02484586.

Heukelom, F. 2011. How validity travelled to economic experimenting. *Journal of Economic Methodology* 18, no. 1: 13–28. https://doi.org/10.1080/1350178X.2011.556435.

Jimenez-Buedo, Maria and Luis M. Miller. 2010. Why a trade-off? The relationship between the external and internal validity of experiments. *Theoria* 25, no. 3: 301–321. https://doi.org/10.1387/theoria.779.

Leviton L. C. 2017. Generalizing about public health interventions: A mixed-methods approach to external validity. *Annual Review of Public Health* 38: 371–391. https://doi.org/10.1146/annurev-publhealth-031816-044509.

Lynch, J. 1982. On the external validity of experiments in consumer research. *Journal of Consumer Research* 9, no. 3: 225–239. https://doi.org/10.1086/208919.

Machingaidze, S. and C. S. Wiysonge. 2021. Understanding COVID-19 vaccine hesitancy. *Nature Medicine* 27, no. 8: 1338–1339. https://doi.org/10.1038/s41591-021-01459-7.

Persson, J. and A. Wallin. 2012. Why internal validity is not prior to external validity. In *Philosophy of Science Assoc. 23rd biennial meeting (San Diego, CA) PSA 2012 contributed papers*. Phil Sci Archives. http://philsci-archive.pitt.edu/9171/ (accessed December 15, 2021).

Rothwell P. M. 2005. External validity of randomised controlled trials: "To whom do the results of this trial apply?" *The Lancet* 365, no. 9453: 82–93. https://doi.org/10.1016/S0140-6736(04)17670-8.

Rothwell, P. M. 2006. Factors that can affect the external validity of randomised controlled trials. *PLoS Clinical Trials* 3, no. 5: 1–5. https://doi.org/10.1371/journal.pctr.0010009.

Schram, A. 2005. Artificiality: The tension between internal and external validity in economic experiments. *Journal of Economic Methodology* 12, no. 2: 225–237. https://doi.org/10.1080/13501780500086081.

Shadish, W. R., T. D. Cook, and D. T. Campbell. 2002. *Experimental and quasi-experimental designs for generalized causal inference*. Belmont, CA: Wadsworth Cengage Learning.

Steckler, A. and K. R. McLeroy. 2008. The importance of external validity. *American Journal of Public Health* 98, no. 1: 9–10. https://doi.org/10.2105/AJPH.2007.126847.

Steel, D. 2008. *Across the boundaries: Extrapolation in biology and social science*. Oxford: Oxford University Press.

Steel, D. 2013. Mechanisms and extrapolation in the abortion-crime controversy. In *Mechanism and causality in biology and economics, history, philosophy and theory of the life sciences 3*, ed. Hsiang-Ke Chao, Szu-Ting Chen, and Roberta L. Millstein. Dordrecht: Springer Science+Business Media. https://doi.org/10.1007/978-94-007-2454-9_10.

Williamson, J. 2019. Establishing causal claims in medicine. *International Studies in the Philosophy of Science* 32, no. 1: 33–61. https://doi.org/10.1080/02698595.2019.1630927.

9

EXPLANATION IN PUBLIC HEALTH

Olaf Dammann

Introduction

What are the things that call for an explanation in public health? What types of explanation are used to do the explaining and what are their functions in public health practice?

Let me begin with a brief note on *explanation*. There are of course many definitions of the term, both in general dictionaries and in the philosophical literature. For example, the Merriam-Webster Thesaurus states that explanation is "a statement that makes something clear" and the Encyclopedia Britannica defines the philosophical concept of explanation as a "set of statements that makes intelligible the existence or occurrence of an object, event, or state of affairs."[1] In the philosophical literature, however, the meaning of the term is frequently restricted to *scientific explanation* (Skow 2015). While there is no consensus on how *scientific explanation* should be defined, there seems to be agreement that many scientific explanations can be characterized as answers to *why*-questions which explain *why* facts come about and events occur. On this view, an explanation is sometimes seen as an outline of the *etiology* of a fact or event by reference to its causal history (Lewis 1986; Lipton 1991; Salmon 1984). More recently, non-causal explanation has received increased attention by philosophers (Lange 2017; Reutlinger and Saatsi 2018).

I will not delve any further into models of explanation in this chapter. Instead, my survey of explanations used in public health includes but is not restricted to "*why*-question-response" explanations. Activities like data interpretation, decision-making, planning, and policy development also involve explanations that are nonscientific. Most of these activities are *based* on scientific evidence, but they also require types of explanation that are not answers to why-questions. The main reason not to restrict myself to the usual pattern of how explanation is generally discussed in the philosophical literature is that my topic is explanation in public health *practice* in which other types of explanation play important roles.

The types of explanation given in public health vary according to what is being explained (explanandum), what kinds of data are used to do the explaining (explanans), and for what purpose the explanation is given. I propose to distinguish four types of explanation that are used for the purpose of knowledge generation (scientific explanation), justification of

DOI: 10.4324/9781315675411-12

Table 9.1 Characteristics of types and subtypes of explanation in public health

Type	Subtype	Explanandum	Explanans	# in Figure 9.2
Scientific	Etiological	Occurrence of phenomenon	Causal-mechanical origin of phenomenon	1a
	Meta-epistemological	Knowledge gain	Description of knowledge generated	4a
Justificatory	Open	Reason for	Justification of action (scientific, economic, moral, etc.)	1b
	Moral	Obligation to act	Moral justification	2a
Methodological	Procedural	Intervention method	Means of intervention	2b
	Analytical	Success measurement	Means of measurement	3b
Prospective	Anticipatory	Anticipated	Clarify the expected intervention outcome	3a
	Destinatory	What's next?	Description of plan	4b

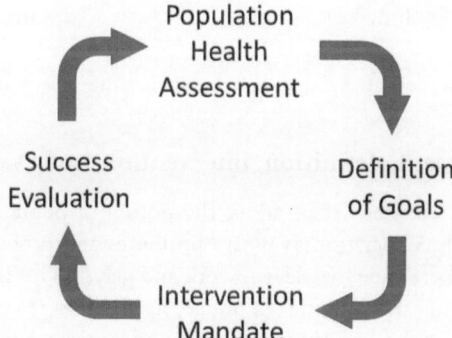

Figure 9.1 Four main activities in the cyclical public health research and practice workflow

action (justificatory explanation), data design (methodological explanation), and planning (prospective explanation) (Table 9.1). I do not suggest that this list exhausts all possible types of explanation.

Of note, I will be flexible regarding the distinction between *public health* and *population health* but will attempt to be mindful of potential differences when it comes to issues of explanation. In broad terms, I suggest thinking of *public health* as the institutionalized effort to protect the public's health and of *population health* as the health of populations, pragmatically defined by some as groups with >1 member (Keyes and Galea 2016).

In what follows, I will first introduce a simple four-step schema (Figure 9.1) that illustrates the sequential relationship among the abovementioned tasks in public health, then turn to the types of explanation (Table 9.1) that play a role in connecting them (Figure 9.2) into a continuous workflow and finally offer some comments in the last section.

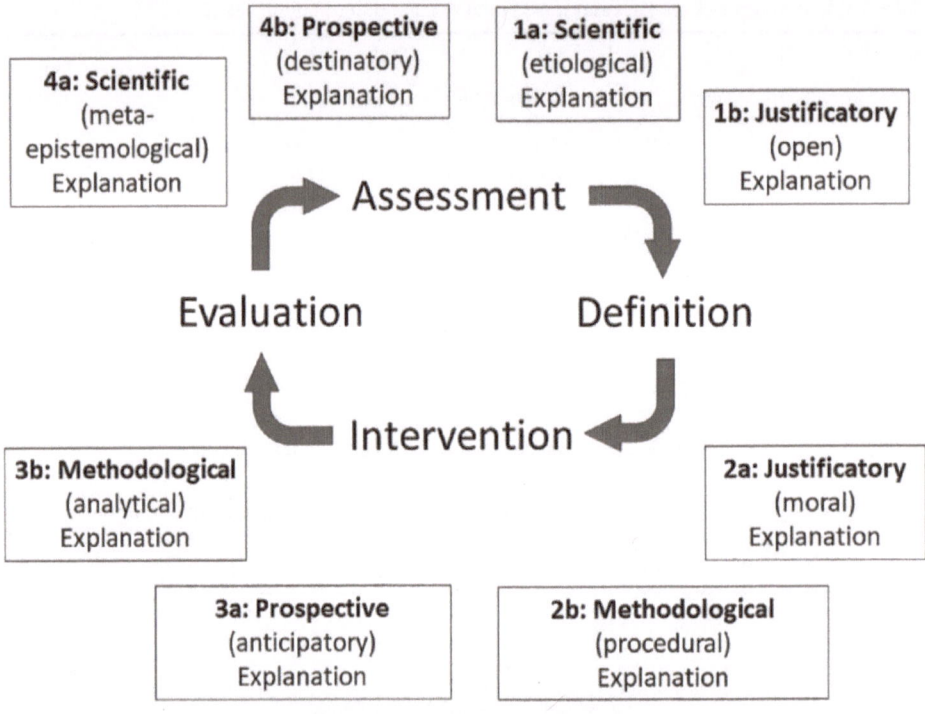

Figure 9.2   Types (and subtypes) of explanation in public health research and practice

Assessment, definition, intervention, and evaluation

For the purpose of this chapter, let us adopt the notion of public health proposed by the American Public Health Association as what "promotes and protects the health of people and the communities where they live, learn, work and play."[2] This is obviously an extremely broad definition, including the activities of police, firefighters, teachers, and so forth. I propose the following list of main activities in order to outline how public health workers (researchers and practitioners) accomplish that mission (Figure 9.1): population health *assessment*; *definition* of goals; an appropriate *intervention*; and *evaluation* of success.

The following sections briefly touch on the four types of explanation, each one with two subtypes as specified in Table 9.1 and depicted in Figure 9.2, that are part of the transition from each one of these activities to the next. They will be discussed in more detail later in this chapter.

From assessment to definition

As a first step in the development of a public health program, public health workers must be able to *assess* the state of the health of their target population accurately. Usually, those in charge of public health activities work in municipal or regional (in the United States: county or state) departments of public health. They are charged with overseeing public health activities to support the population residing in their catchment area. In order for their work to be evidence-based, the department has to collect evidence, that is, valid information about the state of health in this population, which is a research activity guided by scientific principles.

How is the occurrence of disease explained? A *scientific/etiological* explanation needs to be provided that tells decision-makers *why* and *how* a certain assessment result occurs (Figure 9.2, #1a). In the evidence-based public health framework (Brownson, Fielding, and Maylahn 2009), this explanation is based on type 1 scientific evidence, that is, data on the "size and strength of preventable risk—disease relationship (measures of burden, etiologic research)" (Brownson, Fielding, and Maylahn 2009: 179).

Before data from surveillance and epidemiological studies can be turned into a definition of public health action, an explanation needs to be given that specifies *why* the collected data justify a certain public health action (Figure 9.2, #1b). This *justificatory/open* explanation is called "open" because it needs to employ all kinds of justification (scientific, moral, economic, and so on). In the context of dangerous infectious diseases, this seems trivial and is, obviously, done a long time in advance and not just when the need arises. With other health indicators, however, such as a novel clustering of cancer cases in a certain community, the justificatory explanation will be made only after the new data have become available.

From definition to intervention

Public health agencies like the Centers for Disease Control and Prevention (CDC) in the United States are mainly concerned with the definition of surveillance measures. They have developed a list of criteria that specify the scope of the public health problem, the ability to control it, and the public health system capacity needed to implement proper control measures (CDC 2012). In the United Kingdom, the Covid-19 pandemic has triggered the creation of a new agency in 2021, the UK Health Security Agency (UKHSA), which is charged with infectious disease surveillance, prevention, and response. It is government agencies like these that decide how threats to the public's health are to be defined.

To declare a population health measure as an indicator of a health burden that requires amelioration, public health researchers, agencies, and politicians must offer a *justificatory/moral* explanation why an intervention is warranted (Figure 9.2, #2a). Of course, this also helps justifying the intervention plan and is, therefore, also a justificatory explanation. Next, a *methodological/procedural* explanation is needed to clarify what sort of intervention is likely to ameliorate the situation and *how* it is supposed to work (Figure 9.2, #2b).

From intervention to evaluation

The expected results will be explained by means of a *prospective anticipatory* explanation before the intervention is initiated and that explanation of expected results is sometimes refined while the intervention is implemented (Figure 9.2, #3a).

Concomitantly, it needs to be explained in what ways the outcome of the intervention will be evaluated. This is a *methodological/analytical* explanation that specifies the technical ways of outcome evaluation (Figure 9.2, #3b).

From evaluation to assessment

When the evaluation is completed, it is time to ask what has been learned. What exactly is the knowledge added by the project? This knowledge gain (if any) is explained in the form of a *meta-epistemological* explanation (Figure 9.2, #4a). Since this is an explanation that increases our knowledge about our knowledge, I count it as a scientific explanation.

One interesting topic in this context is the purported explanatory opacity of some artificial intelligence approaches used in health data analysis (Amann et al. 2020). What can we know about our knowledge gain if it comes from machine learning methods whose results are not interpretable? I have argued elsewhere that there might be ways to use computational models of illness occurrence as providers of etio-prognostic explanations (Dammann, 2021).

The last type of explanation before the workflow cycle arrives back at the beginning is the *prospective/destinatory* explanation of what is to come next (Figure 9.2, #4b). In our current context, this will be an explanation of the next steps (changes to process, especially new forms of assessment, and so on).

Again, the way I use the term *explanation* in this chapter is very broad and goes deliberately beyond the definition of *scientific* explanation, because science is only one component of public health. The types of explanation used in public health I propose and discuss in the next sections include nonscientific explanations that are used for knowledge *transfer*, not in the process of knowledge *generation*.

Types of explanation in public health

As alluded to at the beginning of the previous section, part of my goal is to analyze the types of explanation given in public health. I propose, as summarized in Table 9.1, that four main types of explanation prevail: scientific, justificatory, methodological, and prospective. Each one of these categories has at least two, perhaps more, subcategories. In what follows, I describe these in more detail, using examples from public health practice.

Scientific explanation

Evidence for public health

One of the main ways to collect the necessary evidence is public health surveillance. Public health surveillance is defined as "the ongoing, systematic collection, analysis, and interpretation of health data, essential to the planning, implementation and evaluation of public health practice, closely integrated with the dissemination of these data to those who need to know and linked to prevention and control" (Hall et al. 2012).

The CDC in the United States consider surveillance "the cornerstone of public health practice" (Richards, Iademarco, and Anderson 2014: 472). Surveillance provides data that help "detect and monitor diseases, injuries, and conditions; assess the impact of interventions; and assist in the management of large-scale disease incidents" (Richards, Iademarco, and Anderson 2014: 472). For the detection of *occurrence*, a target condition is defined, and surveillance staff and technology tools are prepared to detect the occurrence of that target condition to an extent higher than expected. Data are accumulated over a defined time period and compared to expected occurrence numbers. For example, if an infectious disease occurs more frequently than expected in a certain area over a certain period of time, this would be considered an outbreak.

However, this evidence is not provided by surveillance alone. Another important source of data is epidemiologic research, the branch of the health sciences that is charged with the design, conduct, and analysis of population-based studies to understand the distribution and determinants of health and disease in populations (Rothman et al. 2021). Contrary to popular belief, recently fueled by its prominent role in the media during the Covid-19 pandemic, epidemiology is not just the science of epidemics. Infectious disease epidemiology is only one branch among many in modern epidemiology. Epidemiologists study the occurrence (prevalence, incidence) of practically *any* health phenomenon in populations under the heading *descriptive epidemiology* and the statistical association (often mislabeled "correlation") between purportedly causal risk factors (exposures) and any kind of illness (outcome) using *analytical epidemiology* methods. Modern epidemiological theory started with predominantly methodological considerations in the 1970s (MacMahon and Pugh 1970) and 1980s (Kleinbaum, Kupper, and Morgenstern 1982; Miettinen 1985; Rothman 1986) and has reached new heights with Nancy Krieger's ecosocial theory of health (Krieger 2001, 2011), Miguel A. Hernán and James M. Robins's framework for causal inference (2020), and Tyler VanderWeele's explanatory approach (2015).

For VanderWeele, an explanation is putting a phenomenon "with a particular context so that the phenomenon is better understood" (VanderWeele 2015: 7), which dovetails with the Merriam-Webster definition of explanation referred to above. His main topic is epidemiological modeling tools for the analysis of mediation, which he briefly defines as "the phenomenon whereby a cause affects its intermediate and the change in the intermediate goes on to affect the outcome" (VanderWeele 2015: 7), and interaction, which "relate[s] to when, and for whom, a cause affects a particular outcome" (VanderWeele 2015: 9). On this view, a *mediator* is just that, an intermediate factor that provides the link between cause and effect. *Interaction*, however, is a somewhat more complex concept, but more important for population health science. In much simplified terms, interaction is a phenomenon of "mixed effects," which results in different magnitudes of influence of cause C on effect E in strata defined by the presence or absence of a third factor F. In other words, the CE relationship R_{CE} among individuals with F differs appreciably from R_{CE} among individuals without F. Stated formally: $(R_{CE}|F) \neq (R_{CE}|\neg F)$. In public health, the importance of this phenomenon is obvious, because one needs to know whether the effect of some intervention should be expected to be different in one subpopulation with F compared to one without F. Identifying factor F in this scenario would obviously have an enormous impact on whether and how the intervention would be implemented. The same holds for clinical (medical) contexts as well, illustrating the general import of clinical epidemiological methods and findings as a basis for medical action. For example, Paul M. Ridker and colleagues conducted a randomized trial of low-dose aspirin in almost 40,000 women aged 45 or older and followed them for ten years regarding cardiovascular events and stroke (Ridker et al. 2005). While the intervention was associated with a risk reduction for myocardial infarction by 34% among women 65 years or older, it did not affect this risk in younger women. This result has obvious consequences for physicians' prescription decisions.

Etiological explanation

Etiological explanations (#1a in Figure 9.2) abound in public health because they unify explanations that refer to the causes of illness and to the mechanisms that provide the connection between causes and the illness they cause. Thus, *causal* explanations are etiological explanations that clarify the causal origin, while *mechanical* explanations clarify the mechanical origin of disease. Taken together, this is what Wesley C. Salmon called a causal-mechanical or etiological explanation (Salmon 1984; see also Dammann 2020). One simple example of an etiological explanation is the explanation of health disparities by reference to socioeconomic status (cause) and stress (mechanism) (Adler and Rehkopf 2008).

The causal-mechanical model represents only one of multiple philosophical accounts of *scientific* explanation (Woodward 2017). In brief, the earlier *deductive-nomological* (or "covering law") model was proposed by Carl Hempel (Hempel 1962). The D-N model, as it is now often abbreviated, states that one or more accepted laws (such as those of thermodynamics) in addition to one or more particular contextual facts about a certain event (a metal lid gets stuck on a glass jar when the jar is put in hot water) *jointly explain* the fact that the metal lid comes off the jar easily once the jar is taken out of the water. Another type of explanation, *unificationist* explanation, was introduced by Michael Friedman, who started his 1974 paper with the question of what connects explanation to scientific understanding (Friedman 1974), a question that Hempel (according to Friedman) shied away from for being psychological and, thus, not to be considered part of logic. Friedman argued that, in essence, providing a scientific explanation is to provide a comprehensive statement that unifies multiple less comprehensive statements. He further argued that since understanding is global, not limited to single instances of phenomena to be explained, we "genuinely increase our understanding of the world" by replacing one statement with a more comprehensive statement, which reduces the total number of accepted statements (Friedman 1974: 19). Friedman's version of unificationist explanation was later modified by Philip Kitcher, who suggested that the number of types of premises accepted as underived can be minimized by reducing the *number* of argument patterns that derive *many* beliefs (Kitcher 1981).

Meta-epistemological explanation

In the above accounts of explanation, an increased intelligibility and, ultimately, understanding is part of the goal. In our framework of explanation in public health, a *meta-epistemological* explanation (#4a in Figure 9.2) is one that increases our knowledge about our knowledge; it increases the number of facts that we know about the number of facts we know. This sounds much more complicated than it is. In our context, a meta-epistemological explanation is nothing more than a clarification of what we have learned from a public health intervention project. This type of explanation would be any explanation that refers to the results of an intervention study that has yielded new knowledge. For example, a community intervention program with the goal to reduce smoking among women yielded results that suggest that community involvement improves the success rate of such program (Secker-Walker, Flynn et al. 2000). Here, the novel piece of information is the community participation bit and any explanation that refers to this bit would count as a meta-epistemological explanation.

Justificatory explanation

These explanations are given for the purpose of action justification. Whoever is in a decision-making position for a public health program will require a solid justification for an action to be taken. The response to the request *What justifies this intervention?* is an explanation that is given to justify or warrant the intervention. Ruth Faden and Sirine Shebaya have argued that the broad mission of public health to protect and improve the health of populations is too broad to appropriately justify some public health interventions (Faden and Shebaya 2019). They identify five justifications that may justify public health interventions: "(1) overall benefit, (2) collective action and efficiency, (3) fairness in the distribution of burdens, (4) prevention of harm (the harm principle), and (5) paternalism."

I will now very briefly refer to three main ways to justify an action in public health: scientific, moral, and economic.

Scientific justification

Scientific justification requires explanations that refer to scientific reasons or desiderata. This type of explanation is not to be confused with scientific explanations (see above). Justificatory explanations of the scientific type simply cite scientific reasons in support of a justificatory statement. In other words, a scientific justificatory explanation refers to a scientific *need* as a justification for action. Perhaps the most frequently employed scientific justificatory explanation is the one given in the background section of scientific grant applications. This usually reads something like: "We want to study the phenomenon P. Previous research has revealed that P is caused by C, but the mechanism M remains to be elucidated. In this application, we propose a series of experiments designed to characterize M."

Moral justification

Moral justification can be provided by offering moral reasons why an action is warranted. Ross Upshur has conveniently summarized the principles to be considered in the justification of public health intervention (Upshur 2002). He discusses the harm, least restrictive means, reciprocity, and transparency principles. These principles can be viewed, individually or together, as reference points for justificatory explanations. The harm principle, rooted in John Stuart Mill's *On Liberty*, holds that personal freedom cannot be rightfully constrained unless such limitations are imposed in order to prevent others from harm. Upshur suggests that the harm principle is "perhaps the foundational principle for public health ethics in a democratic society" (Upshur 2002: 102). For example, mandatory face masks during the most serious phases of the Covid-19 pandemic can be justified by the argument that the mask-associated reduction of personal comfort is far outweighed by the beneficial population effect on disease incidence and mortality. The least restrictive means principle requires that public health policies should have implemented and exhausted less invasive interventions before more draconian measures are initiated. To stay with our previous example, mandatory face masks are considered less restrictive than mandatory sheltering in place. Reciprocity refers to the right of the individual to be compensated for losses due to public health interventions. Transparency covers the need to design decision-making processes in a fair manner that includes all stakeholders, free discourse among them, and the absence of political or financial interests, among others.

Economic justification

Economic justification is the purpose of explanations that cite expected economic gains or losses as reasons why some action should or should not be taken in public health. Comparative economic analysis techniques are involved, such as cost-effectiveness, cost-benefit, cost-utility analyses, and so on. A study from the United Kingdom revealed that decision-makers apparently prefer to base their decisions on more complex and detailed methods rather than on simpler ones (Phillips et al. 2011). The growing field of public health economics (Edwards, Charles, and Lloyd-Williams 2013) is complex and multifaceted and represents a formidable target area for further philosophical inquiry.

Methodological explanation

At first glance, methodological explanations seem to be justifications of *why* certain methods are used. I think, however, that the primary motivation for this type of explanation is to simply describe methodology, just like etiological explanations describe the causal-mechanical genesis of a phenomenon. In public health, methodological explanations explain the details of intervention procedures and data analysis. To explain *why* a particular method is used is a *scientific* justificatory explanation that details scientific reasons for such usage.

Explaining intervention methodology

Any public health intervention will be implemented in a particular way. The creation and provision of an intervention methodology explanation (#2b in Figure 9.2) in the form of a detailed intervention implementation plan is necessary for stakeholders to understand what kind of intervention is planned and what its implementation will mean for them and their constituents.

Public health nursing is one of the areas of public health in which a considerable amount of work has been done to specify what kinds of interventions public health entails. Linda Olson Keller and colleagues have developed a framework for public health intervention known as the Intervention Wheel for population-based public health practice (Keller et al. 1998; Keller et al. 2004). The Wheel is a graphical depiction of its three equally important core aspects: interventions are population-based, they are implemented at the level of the individual/family, community, or system, and there are seventeen different types of public health interventions that are further specified in the model.

Explanation of analytic methods

Once a public health program is implemented, its success (or failure) needs to be evaluated. An analysis plan is needed that explains the methods that are to be used in program evaluation (#3b in Figure 9.2). Bobby Milstein and Scott Wetterhall have proposed a framework for program evaluation that consists of six steps: stakeholder engagement, program description, focusing the evaluation design, evidence gathering, conclusion justification, and ensure usage and lessons learned. Interestingly, the second item (program description) comes rather close to our aforementioned explanation of intervention methodology: "Before stakeholders can talk about evaluating a program, they should agree on what the program is. They must describe the program in enough detail to ensure a solid understanding of its mission, objectives, and strategies" (Milstein and Wetterhall 2016: 222). Part of the explanation of analysis methods should be whether the data to be analyzed are quantitative, qualitative, or mixed methods.

Prospective explanation

Prospective explanations are forward-looking. They explain by reference to future events, not to things that have happened in the past. In other words, both the explanans and the explanandum of prospective explanations are yet to occur. We can offer *anticipatory* explanations in public health in the form of statements like, for example, "We expect this program to reduce the number of opioid overdoses by 10% over the next twelve months." *Destinatory* explanations are visionary statements of what the plans are for the future development of affairs.

Anticipatory explanation

Anticipatory explanations (#3a in Figure 9.2) outline what one expects to be the case under defined circumstances and why. In the public health workflow, they simply explain the results that are expected if a defined intervention is implemented in a certain way. On a superficial level, anticipatory explanations are merely descriptive, serving the purpose of an outline for the uninformed. On a deeper level, they can also serve as a justificatory explanation, when used to mount an argument in support of the initiation of a program.

Destinatory explanation

The final kind of explanation, which we may call *destinatory explanation,* outlines the plan for moving forward after a public health project is completed (#4b in Figure 9.2). It is exemplified by the questions from the audience to the speaker after a presentation at a scientific conference like "Now that you are done with this project, what are your next steps?" or "What else needs to be done to achieve your long-term research goal?"

Destinatory explanations are not teleological explanations (Stout 1996; Wright 1976). The latter explain facts (mainly actions) by means of referring to the actor's reasons to act. The former are explanations of where things are going or are expected to go in the future. While the latter always have a causal connotation (the reason being the cause of the action), the former do not.

Comments

In this chapter, I have departed appreciably from the traditional philosophical concept of explanation as closely and perhaps *exclusively* related to causal inference. Instead, I have offered a smorgasbord of explanations employed for different purposes in public health practice.

One important objection to the framework of explanation types offered in Table 9.1 is that one may say that except for scientific explanations, the other types just are not explanations at all, but justifications, descriptions, predictions, outlines of plans, and so on. In my view, the components of these terms (for example, justification and explanation) are not mutually exclusive, but one specifies what the other does. In this regard, I propose to distinguish between *models* of explanation (for example, the D-N model, the causal-mechanical model, and unificationist models of explanation) and *types* of explanation as those listed in Table 9.1. While models of explanation are defined by how philosophers think explanation works, types of explanation are defined by what purpose they serve.

Of course, my proposed framework of explanation in public health offered in this chapter is just one possible view of public health workflow and the types of explanation used therein. I am certain that many others can be construed and some of these will probably be more helpful than the one presented here. Of note, the framework is *not* intended for usage in other contexts. Most certainly do I not intend to propose a framework for explanation *in general.* It may very well be that some of the classification of explanations depicted in Table 9.1 *can* be used in other contexts. However, such usage would need to be justified before the backdrop of that other context. There is just no one-size-fits-all solution.

Maël Lemoine begins his chapter on explanation in medicine in another handbook in this series with the statement that "the scientific part of medicine seeks explanations" (Lemoine 2017: 296). He continues with a call for inclusion of multiple types of explanation in medicine, such as "molecular, epidemiological, psychiatric, pathophysiological, social, ..." explanations. Two comments, if I may. First, I do not think that there is such a thing as the scientific part of medicine. Medicine has no scientific part. At least, individuals working in medicine *and* science are the exception, not the rule. Indeed, the physician-scientist is a vanishing breed. The vast majority of medics care for patients, organize and optimize that care, and improve it. They *use* scientific data, but they do not *generate* them; they do not *do* the science. This is done by medical and health scientists like epidemiologists, who generate causal explanations, and bioscientists, who generate mechanical explanations (Dammann 2020). Second, Lemoine's list of "types" of explanation is confused in terms of being derived from different classification systems. Molecules are biological entities, psychiatry is part of medicine, and epidemiology, pathophysiology, and sociology are branches of science, and thus activities outside clinical medicine. In the remainder of his chapter, Lemoine distinguishes between deductive-nomological, deductive statistical, and mechanistic models of explanation. While this is certainly a useful approach, I hope that the *purpose*-driven framework of explanation I propose in this chapter will be helpful in providing a purpose-driven roadmap for explanation in public health.

We have to keep in mind what kinds of stakeholders in public health offer the explanation and who are the ones supposed to benefit. Who is the explainer and who is the explainee? Assuming that it will most often be the public health professionals who do the explaining, while the recipients are policymakers and the general public, we may need to consider whether different perceptions of truth and knowledge might affect the explanatory process and success. The attempt to successfully explain a planned public health program—for example, mask wearing in public—to a community whose members subscribe to the notion of "fake news" maybe futile. Public trust is of paramount importance in a healthy public discourse. One important example of philosophical work in this realm is Maya Goldenberg's argument that vaccination hesitancy is not due to science illiteracy but lack of trust in science (Goldenberg 2021).

My discussion in this chapter comes from a Western perspective (I trained as a medical doctor in Germany and as an epidemiologist in the United States). Alex Broadbent and Benjamin Smart have made a cogent argument that in public health policy, "ignoring local social and cultural factors is a mistake" (Broadbent and Smart 2020: 405). On this view, it is objectionable if a public health intervention ignores the specific socio-cultural background of the population it serves. Initiatives such as the decolonization of global health (Büyüm et al. 2020), antiracism efforts in medicine (Paul et al. 2020), and declaring racism a public health crisis in the United States (Paine et al. 2021) will greatly benefit from implementing this insight.

Notes

1 See https://www.merriam-webster.com/thesaurus/explanation (accessed September 15, 2021) and https://www.britannica.com/topic/explanation (accessed July 16, 2021).
2 See https://www.apha.org/what-is-public-health (accessed July 15, 2021).

References

Adler, N. E. and D. H. Rehkopf. 2008. U.S. disparities in health: Descriptions, causes, and mechanisms. *Annual Review of Public Health* 29, no. 1: 235–252. https://doi.org/10.1146/annurev. publhealth.29.020907.090852.

Amann, J., A. Blasimme, E. Vayena, D. Frey, and V. I. Madai. 2020. Explainability for artificial intelligence in healthcare: A multidisciplinary perspective. *BMC Medical Informatics and Decision Making* 20, no. 1: 310. https://doi.org/10.1186/s12911-020-01332-6.

Broadbent, A. and B. Smart. 2020. Kinds of explanation in public health policy. In *Explaining health across the sciences*, ed. J. Sholl and S. Rattan, 405–415. Cham: Springer.

Brownson, R. C., J. E. Fielding, and C. M. Maylahn. 2009. Evidence-based public health: A fundamental concept for public health practice. *Annual Review of Public Health* 30: 175–201. https://doi. org/10.1146/annurev.publhealth.031308.100134.

Büyüm, A. M., C. Kenney, A. Koris, L. Mkumba, and Y. Raveendran. 2020. Decolonising global health: If not now, when? *BMJ Global Health* 5, no. 8: e003394. https://dx.doi.org/10.1136% 2Fbmjgh-2020-003394.

CDC (Centers for Disease Control and Prevention). 2012. Public health surveillance: Preparing for the future. https://www.cdc.gov/surveillance/improving-surveillance/index.html (accessed December 15, 2021).

Dammann, O. 2020. *Etiological explanations: Illness causation theory.* Boca Raton, FL: CRC Press.

Dammann, O. 2021. Agent-based models as etio-prognostic explanations. Argumenta 7: 19–38.

Edwards, R. T., J. M. Charles, and H. Lloyd-Williams. 2013. Public health economics: A systematic review of guidance for the economic evaluation of public health interventions and discussion of key methodological issues. *BMC Public Health* 13: 1001. https://doi.org/10.1186/1471-2458-13-1001.

Faden, R. R. and S. Shebaya. 2019. Public health programs and policies: Ethical justifications. In *The Oxford handbook of public health ethics*, ed. A. C. Mastroianni, J. P. Kahn, and N. E. Kass, 20–32. Oxford: Oxford University Press.

Friedman, M. 1974. Explanation and scientific understanding. *Journal of Philosophy* 71, no. 1: 5–19. https://doi.org/10.2307/2024924.

Goldenberg, M. 2021. *Vaccine hesitancy.* Pittsburgh: University of Pittsburgh Press.

Hall, H. I., A. Correa, P. W. Yoon, C. R. Braden, and Centers for Disease and Prevention. 2012. Lexicon, definitions, and conceptual framework for public health surveillance. *MMWR Surveillance* 61, suppl.: 10–14. https://www.cdc.gov/mmwr/preview/mmwrhtml/su6103a3.htm (accessed December 15, 2021).

Hempel, C. G. 1962. Deductive-nomological versus statistical explanation. In *Scientific explanation, space, and time*, ed. H. Feigl and G. Maxwell, 98–169. Minneapolis: University of Minnesota Press.

Hernán, M. A. and J. M. Robins. 2020. *Causal inference: What if?* Boca Raton, FL: Chapman & Hall/ CRC.

Keller, L. O., S. Strohschein, B. Lia-Hoagberg, and M. Schaffer. 1998. Population-based public health nursing interventions: A model from practice. *Public Health Nursing* 15, no. 3: 207–215. https://doi.org/10.1111/j.1525-1446.1998.tb00341.x.

Keller, L. O., S. Strohschein, B. Lia-Hoagberg and M. A. Schaffer. 2004. Population-based public health interventions: Practice-based and evidence-supported. Part I. *Public Health Nursing* 21, no. 5: 453–468. https://doi.org/10.1111/J.0737-1209.2004.21509.X.

Keyes, K. M. and S. Galea. 2016. *Population health science.* Oxford: Oxford University Press.

Kitcher, P. 1981. Explanatory unification. *Philosophy of Science* 48, no. 4: 507–531. https://www.jstor. org/stable/186834 (accessed December 15, 2021).

Kleinbaum, D. G., L. L. Kupper, and H. Morgenstern. 1982. *Epidemiologic research: Principles and quantitative methods.* Belmont, CA: Lifetime Learning Publications.

Krieger, N. 2001. Theories for social epidemiology in the 21st century: An ecosocial perspective. *International Journal of Epidemiology* 30, no. 4: 668–677. https://doi.org/10.1093/ije/30.4.668.

Krieger, N. 2011. *Epidemiology and the people's health: Theory and context.* New York: Oxford University Press.

Lange, M. 2017. *Because without cause: Non-causal explanation in science and mathematics.* New York: Oxford University Press.

Lemoine, M. 2017. Explanation in medicine. In *The Routledge companion to philosophy of medicine*, ed. M. Solomon, J. R. Simon, and H. Kincaid, 296–309. New York: Routledge.

Lewis, D. 1986. Causal explanation. In *Philosophical papers, vol. 2*, ed. D. Lewis, 214–240. Oxford: Oxford University Press.

Lipton, P. 1991. *Inference to the best explanation.* London: Routledge.

MacMahon, B. and T. F. Pugh. 1970. *Epidemiology: Principles and methods.* Boston, MA: Little.

Miettinen, O. S. 1985. *Theoretical epidemiology.* New York: John Wiley & Sons.

Milstein, B. and S. Wetterhall. 2016. A framework featuring steps and standards for program evaluation. *Health Promotion Practice* 1, no. 3: 221–228. http://dx.doi.org/10.1177/152483990000100304.

Paine, L., P. de la Rocha, A. P. Eyssallenne et al. 2021. Declaring racism a public health crisis in the United States: Cure, poison, or both? *Frontiers in Public Health* 9: 676784. https://doi.org/10.3389/ fpubh.2021.676784.

Paul, D. W., K. R. Knight, A. Campbell, and L. Aronson. 2020. Beyond a moment: Reckoning with our history and embracing antiracism in medicine. *New England Journal of Medicine* 383, no. 15: 1404–1406. https://doi.org/10.1056/nejmp2021812.

Phillips, C. J., R. Fordham, K. Marsh et al. 2011. Exploring the role of economics in prioritization in public health: What do stakeholders think? *European Journal of Public Health* 21, no. 5: 578–584. https://doi.org/10.1093/eurpub/ckq121.

Reutlinger, A. and J. Saatsi. 2018. *Explanation beyond causation: Philosophical perspectives on non-causal explanations.* Oxford: Oxford University Press.

Richards, C. L., M. F. Iademarco, and T. C. Anderson. 2014. A new strategy for public health surveillance at CDC: Improving national surveillance activities and outcomes. *Public Health Reports* 129, no. 6: 472–476. https://dx.doi.org/10.1177%2F003335491412900603.

Ridker, P. M., N. R. Cook, I. M. Lee et al. 2005. A randomized trial of low-dose aspirin in the primary prevention of cardiovascular disease in women. *New England Journal of Medicine* 352, no. 13: 1293–1304. https://doi.org/10.1056/nejmoa050613.

Rothman, K. J. 1986. *Modern epidemiology.* Boston, MA: Little, Brown & Company.

Rothman, K. J., T. L. Lash, T. J. VanderWeele, and S. Haneuse. 2021. *Modern epidemiology.* Philadelphia, PA: Wolters Kluwer.

Salmon, W. C. 1984. *Scientific explanation and the causal structure of the world.* Princeton, NJ: Princeton University Press.

Secker-Walker, R. H., B. S. Flynn, L. J. Solomon, J. M. Skelly, A. L. Dorwaldt, and T. Ashikaga. 2000. Helping women quit smoking: Results of a community intervention program. *American Journal of Public Health* 90, no. 6: 940–946. https://dx.doi.org/10.2105%2Fajph.90.6.940.

Skow, B. 2015. Scientific explanation. In *The Oxford handbook of philosophy of science*, ed. P. Humphreys. Oxford: Oxford University Press. https://doi.org/10.1093/oxfordhb/9780199368815.013.15.

Stout, R. 1996. *Things that happen because they should.* Oxford: Oxford University Press.

Upshur, R. E. 2002. Principles for the justification of public health intervention. *Canadian Journal of Public Health* 93, no. 2: 101–103. https://doi.org/10.1007/bf03404547.

VanderWeele, T. J. 2015. *Explanation in causal inference: Methods for mediation and interaction.* New York: Oxford University Press.

Woodward, James and Lauren Ross, "Scientific Explanation", The Stanford Encyclopedia of Philosophy (Summer 2021 Edition), Edward N. Zalta (ed.), URL = <https://plato.stanford.edu/archives/sum2021/entries/scientific-explanation/>.

Wright, L. 1976. *Teleological explanations: An etiological analysis of goals and functions.* Berkeley: University of California Press.

10

EVIDENCE-BASED MEDICINE AND PUBLIC HEALTH

Mathew Mercuri and Ross E. G. Upshur

Introduction

Evidence-based medicine (EBM) is arguably the dominant framework for contemporary clinical practice. The basic principle of EBM is that clinical decisions should be based on the best available evidence, with "best" determined according to the methodological rigor of the study used to identify the therapeutic effect of specified alternatives. Since introduced in the clinical medicine literature in the early 1990s, the reach of EBM has extended well beyond management of care decisions in the physician-patient encounter. Principles of EBM in many cases now underwrite both the establishment of quality of care metrics and decisions on allocation of health resources. With the early success of EBM, other clinical professions, such as nursing and physiotherapy, have adopted EBM principles in their education and practice (DiCenso, Guyatt, and Ciliska 2005; Jette et al. 2003). We have also seen a rise in the use of "evidence-based" policy language among public institutions, including public health, and the adoption of frameworks for evidence-based decision making.

Framing decisions as "evidence based" implies a sense of objectivity and scrutiny, and leverages lay perceptions of science as a powerful tool to understand, and an impartial judge of, the world around us. It is doubtful that many would prefer that decisions about health or how one's care should be managed should not be based on evidence. However, appeals to evidence do raise questions about what counts as evidence, how different sources are to be integrated, and the process by which evidence is generated and translated to a decision, among others (Mercuri and Baigrie 2019). Although EBM (and by extension, evidence-based policy or practice) has been the target of significant criticism regarding how it deals with these questions, it does continue to garner support by clinicians and public institutions. In this chapter, we will provide a brief review of EBM and the major criticisms of the movement. This will include an overview of the Grading of Recommendations Assessment, Development and Evaluation (GRADE) framework for developing evidence-based recommendations, a process that has been adopted by several key organizations responsible for providing technical knowledge about responding to health issues, such as the World Health Organization (WHO). We will then discuss the role of EBM thinking in public health. That discussion will include an examination of issues that arise when adopting or adhering to standards

DOI: 10.4324/9781315675411-13

of evidence developed for clinical practice by public health decision makers. These issues will be illustrated using a case study of face covering in public as an intervention to mitigate spread of Covid-19.

Evidence-based medicine

What is evidence-based medicine?

Famously described by David Sackett et al. as "the conscientious, explicit, and judicious use of current best evidence in making decisions about the care of the individual patient" (1996: 71), EBM became popular in clinical medicine in the early 1990s when it was presented both as "a new approach to teaching the practice of medicine" and as "a new paradigm for medical practice" (Guyatt et al. 1992: 2420). The impetus for EBM was a concern that many therapies widely used in clinical practice had unproven efficacy. In response, developers of EBM advocated for greater integration of knowledge from clinical epidemiology research into medical decisions and a de-emphasis of "intuition, unsystematic clinical experience, and pathophysiologic rationale as sufficient grounds for clinical decision making" (Guyatt et al. 1992: 2420). The new "EBM" clinician would be taught to apply "formal rules of evidence in evaluating the clinical literature" (Guyatt et al. 1992: 2420).

In the early years of the EBM movement, David Sackett and William Rosenberg (1995) provided a five-step framework for what EBM might look like for a clinician in the course of her daily practice. Upon encountering a clinical problem, the clinician would (1) convert "information needs into answerable questions," (2) track down "the best evidence to answer them," (3) "critically appraise that evidence performance for its validity (closeness to the truth) and usefulness (clinical applicability)," (4) "apply the results of this appraisal in clinical practice," and (5) evaluate their performance (Sackett and Rosenberg 1995: 622).[1] The community has since developed and promoted several tools to help clinicians in these steps, in particular more robust web-based search engines and structured formatting of research papers (for example, in keywords, titles, and abstracts). For the critical appraisal step, "EBM researchers and educators have developed rules of evidence, as epitomized by various schemes of hierarchy of evidence, to help users organize these empirical findings across a gradient of credibility or reliability" (Djulbegovic, Guyatt, and Ashcroft 2009). These "rules of evidence" give weight to observed effect estimates according to the methodological rigor of the studies used to derive them. On the top of the hierarchy are randomized controlled trials (RCTs) and systematic reviews of RCT evidence.

The GRADE framework

The GRADE framework was introduced in 2004 (GRADE Working Group) and is considered an evolution in the EBM movement (Guyatt 2007). The framework provides a roadmap for two activities: (1) assessing the "quality" or "certainty" of evidence to support a claim about an effect of a specified therapy or intervention, and (2) determining a recommendation (and strength of that recommendation) for practice based on the quality/certainty of evidence and other considerations (for example, patients' "values and preferences," resource considerations, equity, and so on). In order to facilitate the first activity, GRADE employs a modified EBM "hierarchy of evidence," which allows for upgrading quality/certainty of evidence derived from lower-level designs (for example, observational methods) and downgrading that derived from higher level designs (for example, RCTs) on the basis of additional considerations (for example, indirectness of evidence, concerns about bias, magnitude of effect, and so on) (Balshem et al. 2011). The strength of the recommendation, as determined through the second activity, provides guidance to the patient, clinician, or policymaker on how to use the recommendation in practice (for example, during the clinical encounter).

The GRADE framework appears to be a response to the initial shortcomings of EBM (Djulbegovic and Guyatt 2017). As the criticisms of EBM will be covered in the next section, we will only highlight a few of them here in the context of the development of GRADE. First, the framework employs a modified hierarchy that is sensitive to the fact that when a study is poorly executed, or where there is good reason to suspect that potential confounding variables have been adequately addressed, a priori commitments to the evidence value of observed effect estimates derived from RCTs or non-randomized observational methods do not hold—hence the provided system for upgrading and downgrading evidence on the basis of additional considerations beyond basic design. Whether the modification adequately addresses criticisms of EBM hierarchies is beyond the scope of our discussion here. Second, the explicit inclusion of additional considerations related to "values and preferences," resources, and so on could be interpreted as an attempt to both mitigate "cookbook" medicine and make EBM actionable—that is, to articulate a process for how one could integrate different sources of evidence and contexts of care when making decisions on how that care will be managed. Again, the extent to which GRADE is satisfactory on such attempts is not our concern here.[2]

The GRADE framework has been adopted by over 100 key organizations around the world (Kavanagh 2009). Many of these organizations, such as the WHO and the National Health Service (United Kingdom), play an important role in informing public health decisions. Thus, GRADE is highly relevant to discussion on EBM and public health. We see that relevance, for example, in some current, highly visible public health responses to the Covid-19 pandemic (for example, mandatory face coverings in public), which we will discuss in a later section.

Criticisms of evidence-based medicine

Several criticisms have been lodged against the EBM movement. These criticisms are well rehearsed in the literature (for example, Norman 1999; Timmermans and Mauck 2005; Upshur and Tracey 2004; Worrall 2002). As such, we will not rehash those arguments or provide significant details here. Rather, we will briefly review some key criticisms that relate to or have an impact on translating EBM thinking to public health. The criticisms of our focus pertain to what counts as "evidence," evidence hierarchies, and external validity of clinical trials.

Studies of clinical populations, such as RCTs, play an important role in assessments of evidence quality and relevance in the EBM practice framework. Knowledge of mechanisms, typically derived from laboratory study, may be considered important, in particular when making claims about whether the results of a clinical trial apply to a target patient or population. This is illustrated in a statement from the *Users' Guides to the Medical Literature*, considered by many the authoritative text on EBM, "A better approach than rigidly applying the study's inclusion and exclusion criteria is to ask whether there is some compelling reason why the results do not apply to the patient" (Guyatt et al. 2008: 103). However, the evidence value of mechanical reasoning is viewed with skepticism due to concerns that such information does not always travel from laboratory to clinic. For example, in the landmark paper outlining the "new paradigm" of EBM, the authors state:

> The study and understanding of basic mechanisms of disease are necessary but insufficient guides for clinical practice. That rationale for diagnoses and treatment, which follow from basic pathophysiologic principles, may in fact be incorrect, leading to inaccurate predictions about the performance of diagnostic tests and the efficacy of treatments.
>
> *(Guyatt et al. 1992: 2421)*

Furthermore, the aforementioned statement in the *Users' Guides* about applying trial results in practice continues with the claim that "you usually will not find a compelling reason, and most often you can generalize the results to your patient with confidence" (Guyatt et al. 2008: 103). In other words, mechanisms can play a role in translating scientific evidence to practice, but clinicians should default to what is known from rigorous study at the level of the clinical populations. However, in thinking about mechanisms, it is important to note the influence of social determinants of health, which becomes important in the context of public health interventions that aim for equitable care for the whole population. The development of the theory of fundamental causes (Link and Phelan 1995; see also Goldberg, this volume), for example, was motivated by the fact that mortality persisted for people of lower socioeconomic status despite intervening on disease and risk factors (Phelan, Link, and Tehranifar 2010). One might not have a compelling reason in disease state or biology but may still have reason to believe that some patients, especially those from marginalized groups, may not benefit from the intervention as suggested in the clinical trial. The EBM literature generally seems to focus on pathophysiologic mechanisms, as is suggested in the quotes provided, although more recent literature on the GRADE framework shows an awareness of equity issues in the development of clinical recommendations (for example, Welch et al. 2017).

Concern about how mechanisms travel from laboratory to clinic appears to have led to a preference for population-level data. However, it was a concern about the impact of unknown confounding variables on the effect estimate that led to evidence hierarchies. The hierarchical structure of evidence in the EBM framework has been the target of significant criticisms. Challenges have been lodged against claims by EBM supporters that randomization adequately controls for known and unknown confounding variables (or is the only way to do so) (for example, Schunemann et al. 2019), RCT evidence entails causal explanations, and evidence derived from designs higher up the hierarchy is "best" in the context of clinical practice (for example, basing practice on RCT data is better than basing it on effect estimates from studies using observational designs). Critics have also noted concerns about the impact of too much emphasis on RCT methods, as they are insufficient for quantifying harms and potentially marginalize patient important outcomes that are not amenable to measurement in RCTs (Stegenga 2018). In response, the EBM community has pivoted to the modified evidence hierarchy promoted in the GRADE framework. Evidence hierarchies might be a useful heuristic tool for clinicians untrained in clinical epidemiology as they engage literature as part of their clinical practice. What is problematic is strict adherence to such hierarchical thinking about evidence as a basis for decisions, especially when trained scientists are available to judge the evidence base. We will illustrate that concern in light of public policy later in this chapter.

External validity (generalizability) of findings is a significant concern when applying research evidence to practice. Advocates of EBM appear to acknowledge this explicitly with respect to laboratory findings but seem to downplay concerns about generalizability of effect estimates derived from RCTs, as is illustrated in the quote from the *Users' Guides* presented above. However, it is not clear why one should have a different attitude about the generalizability of research findings on the basis of study design, as RCT data is also not immune to problems of generalizability. For example, RCTs produce statistical evidence, usually in the form of an average effect—for example, a marginal difference in mean or proportion of a specified outcome between populations in a study. It is not clear what would happen for any individual patient if she were to follow a course of action based on which therapy, for example, showed marginal benefit in a sample population included in the RCT—one cannot know, a priori, if the particular patient will be among those who benefit from the therapy, or among those who will not (Mercuri and Gafni 2018d). Furthermore, it is not clear if a population that might be the target of a policy based on the trial-derived effect estimate is sufficiently similar to that of the trial sample population, such that one can realize a similar outcome, nor can one be sure that the outcomes studied are acceptable or meaningful to those who will receive care consistent with what the trial demonstrated as "best" (Mercuri and Gafni 2018d).[3] Nancy Cartwright and Eileen Munro (2010) highlight the importance of supporting factors when translating RCT findings (or for that matter, any research finding) from the study setting to practice. Given the many ways in which communities can differ from each other (for example, values, preferences, availability and distribution of resources, health status, economy, mobility, education, and so on), understanding which support factors are necessary and present can have significant implications regarding if a study effect is realized in a new setting. That may be especially true for public health interventions, as they often require a wide breadth of support factors and are often one of many potentially competing interests in political discourse and action.

An evidence-based public health (EBPH) based on the principles of EBM is potentially susceptible to all the concerns reviewed here.[4] We will now turn our attention to if and how public health may differ from clinical medicine regarding "evidence-based" and what impact such concerns as reviewed here might have for public health programs that desire to be evidence-based.

Evidence-based medicine and public health

What is evidence-based public health?

While it may be the case that public health has adopted EBM thinking, which we will discuss in more detail in this section, it is important to note that EBM was developed for decisions of clinical medicine. Public health is distinct from clinical medicine in both scope and practice. Clinical medicine is primarily focused on the care of individual patients in the clinical encounter. Public health aims at health of the whole of society and includes, for example, health promotion, disease prevention, sanitation, hygiene, education, and the development and organization of social structures to achieve health. Public health may bring different challenges than does clinical medicine, for example, consideration of others (that is, not only the person who is presenting with a health need) when making decisions about how to intervene. Furthermore, public health practice is often related to governmental organizations such as municipal or federal public health departments rather than individual clinicians.

The concern that drove the demand for EBM also drove the demand for EBPH. As John Kemm suggests, "as in clinical medicine so too in public health there was recognition that practitioners persisted in using interventions, which had been shown to be ineffective"

(2006: 319). Both EBM and public health have strong ties to epidemiology (Muir Gray 1997). Furthermore, Sackett, key in the development of EBM, worked in the US Public Health Service shortly after completing his medical training and later received training in epidemiology, both of which he claims were influential in his desire to bring public health thinking into the clinic.[5] Given such history, it is not surprising that EBM thinking might be adopted (in some ways, back) into public health contexts. However, what EBPH is and how it is similar and/or different than EBM requires some examination. In this section, we will present some proposed definitions of EBPH and a description of what it might look like in practice. We will then examine some of the problems with these definitions and challenges to realizing an evidence-based framework in public health. Finally, we will provide a case study that will further illustrate the challenges of strict application of EBM thinking in public health contexts.

As the EBM movement gained traction, attempts to define EBPH soon appeared in the literature. For example, John Muir Gray (1997) suggested core skills of competent public health professionals similar to those advocated in EBM (for example, searching, appraising, and storing evidence). Using similar language as that seen in definitions of EBM, Milos Jenicek describes EBPH as "the conscientious, explicit, and judicious use of current best evidence in making decisions about the care of communities and populations in the domain of health protection, disease prevention, health maintenance and improvement (health promotion)" (1997: 190). This definition begs several questions related to what is meant by, for example, "conscientious" or "current best evidence." As to the latter question, Jenicek seems to favor data derived from epidemiology study. Scholars on the issue of EBPH acknowledge the need for a wider view on evidence than is often prescribed in EBM, which we will discuss later in this section and in Section "Challenges for an evidence-based public health framework."[6] Ross Brownson, James Gurney, and Garland Land (1999) provide a broader description of EBPH: "The authors define EBPH as the development, implementation, and evaluation of effective programs and policies in public health through application of principles of scientific reasoning including systematic uses of data and information systems and appropriate use of program planning models" (1999: 87). Note that the term "evidence" is not explicitly stated in the definition. The authors refer instead to "data and information systems." This definition goes a step farther than a process of decision making about which programs (or policies) to use, as is suggested in the definitions presented above about EBM and by Jenicek (1997). Rather, it frames EBPH to also include the development and evaluation of such programs (or policies).

Neal Kohatsu, Jennifer Robinson, and James Torner define EBPH as "the process of integrating science-based interventions with community preferences to improve the health of populations" (2004: 418). This definition is remarkable for several reasons. First, there is acknowledgment of "community preferences." That is, there is suggestion that the practice of EBPH includes integrating the preferences of those who are the target of the intervention (that is, the community), although it is not clear how one measures those and if there is indeed a preference that can represent a community (or, if there are several, how they are considered in unison or integrated into a response). It is noteworthy that the addition of community preferences parallels the development of EBM, which, after receiving criticism of promoting "cookbook" medicine, emphasized the role of preferences (in particular, patient "values and preferences") in practice. Second, this definition speaks to "science-based interventions" rather than "best evidence." An often-stated criticism of EBM is its seemingly narrow view on evidence, as is suggested in evidence "hierarchies." Kohatsu, Robinson, and Torner take a broad view on "science based," which "is meant to encompass the range of disciplines, besides epidemiology, that provide the science base for public health, including sociology, psychology, toxicology, molecular biology, anthropology, nutrition, engineering, economics, political science, and others" (2004: 419). Although those disciplines play an important role in our understanding of health, study in the humanities or experience in practice can also be important, notably in helping to address equity issues that are often at the core of public health thinking, raising the issue of to what extent should what counts as evidence be constrained. Overall, it seems that the definitions of EBPH are varied and in some way susceptible to similar criticisms aimed at EBM.

Brownson, Gurney, and Land (1999) offer a "sequential framework for practitioners" that outlines how EBPH might look in practice, similar to the five-step process for EBM outlined by Sackett and Rosenberg (1995). The six "stages" in the EBPH framework are as follows: (1) "develop an initial, concise, operational statement of the issue," (2) "determine what is known through the scientific literature," (3) "quantify the issue," (4) "develop program or policy options," (5) "develop an action plan for the program or policy," and (6) "evaluate the program or policy" (Brownson, Gurney, and Land 1999: 87). Stage two includes a systematic approach to identify and evaluate relevant scientific studies. Here, we see a bit of a departure from EBM thinking in that the evaluation does not include application of an evidence hierarchy. Rather, evaluation or synthesis "can be primarily qualitative" or "quantitative, in the form of a meta-analysis" (Brownson, Gurney, and Land 1999: 91). Compared to EBM frameworks, there also seems to be more emphasis on the evaluation of the program or policy (that is, stage six), which includes application of a wide variety of tools, such as logic models, qualitative designs, participatory planning, and experiments (among others). Others have suggested a more direct adoption of EBM practices, in particular around the activities of assessing the quality of the evidence and determining the policy recommendation. For example, the same year the GRADE framework was first presented in the literature, Kohatsu, Robinson, and Torner state that "one advantage to the GRADE system is that it was designed to be applied across a wide range of interventions and settings, and so should prove useful to both EBM and EBPH" (2004: 420). The WHO appears to agree, as they have adopted GRADE for public health guideline development (World Health Organization 2012),[7] although their use of the system is "often inconsistent with GRADE guidance" (Alexander et al. 2016: 98). One reason for such inconsistency may be the complex nature of public health interventions, where implementation might require deep consideration of context that might rely on evidence sources not favored when applying the GRADE "certainty of evidence" criteria, leading to a need for modification of the framework when in actual practice (see Norris et al. 2019; Siegfried et al. 2017).

Challenges for an evidence-based public health framework

While the effort to align public health decisions and interventions with the best evidence regarding their impact is admirable, there are several barriers that present challenges to realizing EBPH, especially one that is akin to EBM. The barriers pertain to methodological constraints (that is, impacts on internal validity), the complexity of public health interventions and the communities they serve (that is, impacts on generalizability), the acute versus chronic nature of the health risk, and equity concerns, among others. Here, we will offer a brief review of some of these challenges. In the next section, we will illustrate these challenges in a case study on face coverings as a response to the Covid-19 pandemic.

One of the strengths of the EBM mindset is an emphasis on methodological rigor when assessing the evidence base for the impact of an intervention (for example, effect estimate), concerns about evidence hierarchies aside. That is, the evidence value of an effect estimate, which we see as the core of evidence in EBM thinking, is in part determined by the internal validity of the study from which it is derived. While clinical questions are often ideally answered through (or amenable to) RCTs, such methods are difficult to implement or may even be considered inappropriate in the case of public health interventions (Kemm 2006; Victora, Habicht, and Bryce 2004). The public nature of such interventions may create difficulty in defining or implementing a control group, and masking/blinding may not be possible, especially in cases of health promotion. Consider a public "lockdown" intervention to mitigate transmission of an infectious disease—people are certainly aware of if they are in lockdown, and allocating part of the population to a control group might not be politically or ethically tenable (see Rubin et al. 2021).[8] Another methodological challenge is that public health interventions might require longitudinal study, for example, in the case of health promotion or understanding risk factors for chronic disease (for example, the highly influential Framingham study for cardiovascular disease risk (Kannel 1990)). Some questions important to public health often must rely on measurement through self-reporting on surveys, cross-sectional designs, and/or administrative datasets. Such measurement constraints can also impact internal validity. A strict EBM lens on evidence might consider such studies in public health as low quality from which to base decisions. Whether that is a fair assertion is not our purpose here, and such debates about the validity of evidence hierarchies have been taken up in detail by philosophers of medicine elsewhere (for example, Borgerson 2009; Mercuri and Baigrie 2018; Worrall 2002). Next, there is the issue of qualitative methods, which are often the best way to understand the experiences and concerns of people who are the target of some public health program and/or intervention. Such methods have their own theories about validity, different in some ways from notions of validity in RCTs, and it is not clear how they fit into an EBM framework (see Chaisson 2020). The challenges raised here might prompt questions about how public health can be "evidence-based" in the EBM sense, or if it needs its own conception.

Also challenges for realizing EBPH are both the complexity of the communities that public health is to serve and the interventions that might be required to account for that complexity (Kohatsu, Robinson, and Torner 2004). It is well known to philosophers of science that several factors may influence if and how a scientific finding will manifest in another setting. Communities include a mix of values, political structures, resources, and so on, in addition to demographic, biological, and health factors. This mix can create a somewhat unique environment that limits the extent to which different communities are comparable. For an intervention to be successful (or an observation about one to be generalizable to another), it must be sensitive to such factors; for example, the so-called "support factors" must be in place (Cartwright and Munro 2010). That is also true for EBM, although with relatively fewer parties involved in/impacted by the decision, the complexity of many clinical problems might be lesser than what might be seen in public health. Certainly, intervening on a bacterial infection for a patient requires fewer support factors (for example, consent by one person, affordability) than a community-wide program for reducing childhood obesity (for example, which may require buy-in from parents, teachers, children, building of new recreational facilities, improving access to healthy foods, and so on). Therapeutic agents often come in standardized formulas and doses, whereas the features of a public health intervention might need to be tailored to the community and so the intervention itself is not directly comparable between contexts or transportable to a new community.

Public health leaders are occasionally faced with acute problems that can greatly impact the immediate health of the population. An outbreak of an infectious disease is one example.

Such circumstances create additional challenges for realizing EBPH. As Ross Upshur (2012) notes, "public health practitioners and agencies tasked with the mission of protecting and promoting health will always be mediating between the need to take action and the need to gather more information. Action which is evidence based, while desirable, may not be achievable in all circumstances" (2012: 109).

While clinical environments, that are the purview of EBM, offer an opportunity to engage the patient on her preferences when uncertainty in the evidence is present, "such uncertainty in a public health context cannot easily be resolved by soliciting preference for care" (Upshur 2012: 109). An EBPH framework might need to adopt a wider view on evidence or eschew altogether the need for scientific evidence in order to act (for example, adopt a precautionary principle while evidence is pending) or in balancing other competing interests of the community. Such an approach is vitally important, particularly in health protection settings, especially where legal obligations of public health practitioners can differ from those of clinicians—legal obligations are not a core focus of EBM literature.

What is also of consideration in public health is a commitment to equity (Faden, Bernstein, and Shebaya 2020; Valles 2018). Equity issues are not the target of measurement in clinical trials, where the purpose is to determine an unbiased estimate of effect. While the GRADE framework acknowledges other considerations in making clinical recommendations (including equity in more current literature on the topic—see Welch et al. 2017), clinical recommendations are highly sensitive to the quality of evidence of the effect estimate (Djulbegovic et al. 2015). Likewise, critical appraisal exercises, arguably the (traditional) core of EBM practice, are focused on determining threats of bias in effect estimates. Sean Valles (2018) suggests that where public health program options exist, preference should be given to otherwise neglected populations and where we do not know how to proceed, we should err on the side of helping those who are often marginalized (that is, the "Excluded Beneficiary Rule"; see Maglo 2010). Such decisions, while potentially informed by evidence, need not be "evidence based" in the same sense as a claim of therapeutic effectiveness. Furthermore, much of the discussion on equity may leverage literature and study from the humanities and social sciences using methods that are considered low (or not even on) EBM hierarchies of evidence. As such, it is not clear how EBM thinking plays a role in an EBPH in the context of equity.

Case study: Face covering in public to mitigate Covid-19 transmission

The tension between EBM and public health intervention can be illustrated in a case study of the use of face covering (including medical-grade masks) outside of healthcare settings as a public health intervention to reduce transmission of Covid-19. While it is widely accepted in several jurisdictions that face covering is essential to control the pandemic, that was not always the case in its initial stages. On 6 April 2020, the WHO issued a report stating, "there is currently no evidence that wearing a mask (whether medical or other types) by healthy persons in the wider community setting, including universal community masking, can prevent them from infection" (WHO 2020a: 1). Note that the target of the intervention was protection of the wearer—the conversation would later pivot to protection to others from the wearer of the face covering (that is, "source control"). An additional consideration was concerns about supply, that is, public use of medical-grade face masks would divert scarce resources away from healthcare settings that can better benefit from their use. Some governments (in particular, in the Western world where EBM thinking was founded and now permeates public institutions, such as healthcare) were slow to issue public health orders mandating face covering in public spaces, in part due to the "lack" of (highest quality) evidence (by light of EBM standards) to justify such intervention—in stark contrast to orders by governments in East Asia, for example, South Korea, Taiwan, Singapore, Viet Nam, and Hong Kong. A notable exception in the West was the New York State, where Governor Andrew M. Cuomo issued an executive order that included mandatory face covering in public where distancing was not possible.[9] Consider the Government of Canada, whose Chief of Public Health, Theresa Tam, acknowledged "all levels of government are committed to working together towards a shared evidence-based approach to the cautious lifting of public health measures." In reporting to the Canadian House of Commons Standing Committee on Health on 19 May 2020, Tam defended her initial position that the evidence did not support public use of face covering and her apparent turnaround on the issue "based on the evolving science."[10] Tam's commitment to EBM thinking about evidence to base public health recommendations can be seen in the following exchange in the Canada House of Commons:

> Mr. Matt Jeneroux: On that same date, you stated wearing a mask to protect others was ineffective, stating that this view was based on science. On April 6, you said that "A non-medical mask can reduce the chance of your respiratory droplets coming into contact with others or landing on surfaces". Was this decision based on the WHO's recommendations or your own?
>
> Dr. Theresa Tam: This was based on a review of the evidence through the special advisory committee, which I've just talked about, with the other chief medical officers of health. That was based on the evolving science, looking at the role of asymptomatic and presymptomatic transmission and the evolving research that is being published. There was very, very little research being published prior to that, so we kept updating our advice based on the latest information.[11]

While it may be that the science was starting to catch up to the policy needs, recommendations by public health officials did not necessarily translate into policy. From a policy perspective, the issue seemed to gain momentum when the WHO would later shift its position in a 5 June 2020 document supporting the use of face covering in public settings based on "a growing compendium of observational evidence on the use of masks by the general public in several countries, individual values and preferences, as well as the difficulty of physical distancing in many contexts" (WHO 2020b: 6). Several governments who did not initially issue such orders would start to follow suit. For example, the city of Toronto (Canada) introduced a face covering bylaw for all indoor public spaces on 7 July 2020. Likewise, the British government mandated face coverings in shops in England on 24 July 2020.[12] While issuing mandates to the public is ultimately political in nature, there appears to be some threshold of evidence that drives the willingness of governments to enact emergency public health measures or issue laws for the same.

Let us now consider the evidence base examining the use of face coverings that was at issue. The analysis by Trisha Greenhalgh et al. (2020) noted that much of evidence around the use of face coverings was of poor quality, not focused on Covid-19 directly (that is, the target was SARS or influenza), restricted to healthcare settings, and/ or examined surgical and respirator masks (that is, not necessarily the kinds of face coverings that would be more widely used and available to the public). That is, the evidence base suffered from both poor internal and external validity. As a reminder, hierarchies of evidence promoted in the EBM framework privilege information derived from high-quality RCTs (and preferably systematic review and meta-analysis of several RCTs), as effect estimates from those studies are considered to have strong internal validity—and apparently strong external validity, if one were to adhere to the claim by Gordon Guyatt et al. (2008), presented earlier, that one should default in practice to what the RCT demonstrates as effective. We see a similar assessment in a systematic review of the evidence for several public health interventions to reduce Covid-19 transmission, including face masks, produced by Derek Chu et al. (2020). Despite both the observation of a reduction in transmission in all four studies included that examined Covid-19 directly (and 39 studies overall, all of which had effect estimates favoring reduction of events when face masks were used) and a claim that "medical or surgical masks might result in large reduction in virus infection" (Chu et al. 2020: 1979), the authors rated the "certainty" of evidence in the effect as "low" on the basis of the GRADE framework. As expected, the authors identify the need for RCTs on the issue in their conclusion, presumably to raise their "certainty" to "high." Presuming public health officials were to strictly adhere to EBM thinking on evidence in their decisions on public health interventions, the evidence base described in the aforementioned studies might not warrant public use of face coverings to reduce transmission of Covid-19. Perhaps that is what such officials, including the WHO, meant when they said that there was "no evidence" or "very little research published" to support mandating public use of face coverings, and why there was slow uptake in legislating their use. Another interpretation is that officials did not believe that the evidence base warranted a potential diversion of scarce resources away from where they might be most beneficial.

Despite a lack of RCTs, public use of face coverings did become mandated, suggesting that public health decision makers recognize that strict adherence to EBM principles on evidence might negatively impact the health of the public in acute settings, such as the onset of epidemic infectious disease. Greenhalgh (2020) points to a confluence of findings from basic science, epidemiology, mathematical modeling, case studies, and natural experiments that support a reasoned approach to thinking about face covering in public that we believe can be described as "evidence-based"— evidence is more than simply an unbiased estimate of effect size from a RCT. Greenhalgh certainly believed it enough to invoke the precautionary principle in mandating face covering in public.[13] Public health decision makers seemed to follow suit in their own reasoning. For example, the WHO refers to "a growing body of observational evidence" in their 5 June 2020 document, as does Dr Tam refer to the "evolving science" as a basis for their change in policy toward face covering in public. While the decisions by these parties could be explained as entirely political in response to a growing number of public voices calling for accountability and demanding stricter programs (which included face coverings), it is more likely that the burden of evidence did not warrant the need for RCTs in order to act, especially given the minimal harm of the intervention and ease of implementation/low burden on the public. In other words, the threshold for "quality" or "certainty" of evidence is not the same as the threshold for action, although appraisal of evidence was explicitly invoked as an important determinant in the decision-making process with respect to intervening on the public (Bensimon and Upshur 2007). Where the costs or potential harms of an intervention are low, but there is a potential for benefit that is high, the demand for "certainty" in the evidence base might be relatively lower. Interestingly, a recent Danish RCT examining the use of face covering in public showed no effect in reducing Covid-19 infection (Bundgaard et al. 2021). Although that particular study suffered from several limitations, one might wonder if a single, well-executed RCT showing no benefit of face covering in public would be enough to reverse policy now in place.

One might ask whether an acknowledgement by public health decision makers that they appraised the evidence is itself enough to constitute EBPH. Regardless of one's views on that question, the case does highlight several of the challenges for EBPH presented in the previous section. It is doubtful that many would demand RCT evidence before a mandate for face covering be implemented as a public health intervention.[14] Furthermore, developing and implementing such a study is likely not feasible and might be considered undesirable by a community that has seen high uptake, the mentioned Danish study notwithstanding. The case also highlights the interaction between scientific evidence, urgency of the public need, and the political nature of public health intervention. Here, we are reminded of the words of Austin Bradford Hill:

> On fair evidence we might take action on what appears to be an occupational hazard, e.g. we might change from a probably carcinogenic oil to a non-carcinogenic oil in a limited environment and without too much injustice if we are wrong. But we should need very strong evidence before we made people burn a fuel in their homes that they do not like or stop smoking the cigarettes and eating the fats and sugar that they do like. In asking for very strong evidence I would, however, repeat emphatically that this does not imply crossing every "t", and swords with every critic, before we act.
>
> (1965: 300)

Discussion

The EBM movement advocated for greater integration of research evidence into clinical decision making. That was done as a response to the fact that many therapies in use had never been shown to be effective, which raised concern that patients were not getting the best available care or that resources were not used efficiently. Over time, the EBM movement seems to have become synonymous with aligning clinical decisions to trial evidence. While that may not be the intention of the founders (or supporters) of EBM, approaches to operationalize EBM (for example, tying quality metrics to GRADE recommendations; see Djulbegovic, Bennett, and Guyatt 2019) seem to emphasize the evidence base as a primary focus of decision making. As the public has demanded more accountability in their public institutions, those institutions, including public health, have adopted "evidence-based" frameworks for decision making. Certainly, there is an appeal to the notion that decisions should be based on evidence—such an approach might leverage lay views on science as objective and posit decisions as value-free or apolitical. They also allow for practitioners and governments that are responsible to the public to delegate part of that burden to scientists. However, too much dependence on evidence can sometimes compromise the interests of the public—waiting for evidence might not be possible in responding to public health crises. Likewise, strict alignment of decisions with "evidence" is only good if that evidence is sensitive to all the needs, values, and so on, of the public that is to be impacted by a policy or intervention.

The public health portfolio is often broad, covering not only issues of physical disease and mental health, but also lifestyle factors and socioeconomic, cultural, and environmental conditions. While clinical medicine often focuses on optimizing a single outcome (that is, the presenting complaint), public health decisions are often part of a greater political process where several outcomes need to be balanced. In such situations, EBPH might be desirable—political pressures might require demonstration of value before money is spent on a program or freedoms are taken away (Jenicek 1997). However, an EBPH will not necessarily alleviate important considerations of equity that are not so easily determined by the evidence and speak more to values and justice—in some cases, the means of differentiating between competing program options may ultimately fall on equity considerations (see Valles 2018).

Much of the emphasis in EBM and EBPH appears to be on evidence derived from science and social science disciplines. Science is a powerful tool and many decisions on public life and the health of populations and individuals have benefited from findings from scientific study. However, as Baruch Fischhoff notes, "scientists do not normally address decision makers' needs directly" (2020: 140). The inevitable gap between what the science "says" and the policy question must be filled by human judgment. There is also the issue of to what extent scientific evidence should impact policy, public health included (Mercuri 2020; Rubin et al. 2021). Again, public health decisions are ultimately part of a political process, and there is no reason to believe that political life must be constrained by science institutions. As Paul Feyerabend notes, "the sciences do not have the last word on humane matters, knowledge included" (2010: 127). What that might mean for an EBPH framework needs further examination.

Finally, we must be careful to not put too much faith in the evidence or fall prey to reducing public health decisions to technocratic exercises, as might be illustrated in the case study of face covering in public during the recent pandemic where precautionary reasoning warranted their use. As Kemm states, "in policy making the evidence-based approach and the notion that there is a 'best solution' ignores the complexity of the decision-making process" (2006: 322). Public health decisions are often a balancing act, which might have several "best solutions" depending on how different individuals place value on different outcomes. The act of being "evidence-based" does not assure an epistemological or moral high ground for decisions.

Notes

1 Recently, Tikkinen and Guyatt (2020) suggest that few clinicians are able to achieve the skill needed to adequately assess the evidence and now downplay the importance of teaching critical appraisal skills and its necessity for evidence-based practice. It is now suggested that evidence-based practice can be achieved through "secondary sources of evidence – such as trustworthy clinical practice guidelines, and through feedback from clinical mentors" (Tikkinen and Guyatt 2020: 1). If so, then EBM, as originally conceived and promoted for the past three decades, no longer exists (something that seems to have been missed by much of the community advocating for EBM). It seems that authority in clinical practice has shifted from the senior clinician in the pre-EBM era

to the clinician who can critically appraise the literature in the EBM era to the clinical practice guideline in the current era. That shift might explain why there is so much emphasis on the development and uptake of the GRADE framework as part of the EBM portfolio.

2 For a critical examination of the GRADE framework, see Mercuri, Upshur, and Baigrie (2018), Mercuri and Gafni (2018a, 2018b, 2018c), and Mercuri, Baigrie, and Gafni (2021).

3 This leads to a small irony in that EBM may be more useful for population health than for individual patient care as at an aggregate level, who gets the benefit as an individual is largely irrelevant. Thus, concerns about management of care decisions shift from if the therapy is appropriate for optimizing the outcome of an individual to whether the benefits are distributed equitably. In that way, a different concern for bias emerges than what is usually discussed in criticism of EBM in the context of generalizing effect estimates from the clinical study.

4 Implementation science is a field that is working to close some of the gaps in the uptake of evidence-based practice, and the use of research from epidemiology in policy and practice. As part of that goal, scholars in the field are working to resolve some of the issues raised here. Whether such attempts are successful is not a purpose of our examination here. For more on implementation science in the context of epidemiology, see Windle et al. (2019), Neta et al. (2015), and Glasgow et al. (2012).

5 See https://www.jameslindlibrary.org/wp-data/uploads/2019/01/David_L_Sackett_Interview_in_2014_2015.pdf, (accessed April 15, 2021).

6 Marmot and Friel (2008) have pushed back against the strict adoption of EBM thinking in the context of understanding social determinants of health, for example, which is an important consideration in public health interventions. The impact on health of where people are "born, grow, live, work and age; and the inequitable distribution of power, money and resources" (2008: 1095) can be established without RCTs. Social determinants of health should not be ignored because RCT methods are not feasible in their study.

7 An example of the use of GRADE for a public health guideline by the WHO is the "Consolidated Guidelines on The Use of Antiretroviral Drugs for Treating and Preventing HIV Infection: Recommendations for a Public Health Approach" (June 2013), https://apps.who.int/iris/bitstream/handle/10665/85321/9789241505727_eng.pdf;jsessionid=D0F57DDB6AF1822544C-5CA86DE8F473D?sequence=1 (accessed March 4, 2021).

8 What counts as an appropriate control might also be unsound scientifically. For example, during the Covid-19 pandemic, much was made about Sweden's plan to eschew strict population-wide lockdowns like those seen in neighboring countries (Claeson and Hanson 2021). Despite that, Sweden appeared to be faring relatively better with respect to per capita mortality, for example, when compared to many Western European countries that implemented lockdowns (as per the Johns Hopkins University Coronavirus Resource Center data at the time of this writing (https://coronavirus.jhu.edu/data/mortality, accessed April 15, 2021). This might support the notion that lockdowns are not necessary to avoid death from Covid-19. However, one might point to differences between Sweden and many Western European countries in demographics and culture and suggest that Norway might be a better comparator. Indeed, Norway (so far) was more successful than Sweden on incidence and mortality metrics related to the pandemic. The extent to which using Sweden as a control group for the Norwegian lockdown intervention yields evidence that lockdowns work to reduce virus transmission is contingent on if Norway and Sweden are indeed comparable. Of course, this raises questions about which factors are relevant in determining if the groups are comparable and qualities of the intervention (for example: Is it necessarily unique to the population?).

9 https://www.governor.ny.gov/news/no-20217-continuing-temporary-suspension-and-modification-laws-relating-disaster-emergency (accessed April 21, 2021).

10 https://www.ourcommons.ca/DocumentViewer/en/43-1/HESA/meeting-21/evidence (accessed April 21, 2021).

11 https://www.ourcommons.ca/DocumentViewer/en/43-1/HESA/meeting-21/evidence (accessed April 21, 2021).

12 https://www.bma.org.uk/news-and-opinion/government-makes-wearing-face-masks-mandatory (accessed April 21, 2021).

13 The use of the precautionary principle in the context of public health is not new, and the slowness to invoke it in the context of face coverings in Canada is surprising. Reports by the Krevar Commission (Krevar 1997) examining the management of the risk of HIV and hepatitis C transmission

by Canada's blood system and the Campbell Commission (Campbell 2004), reflecting on the country's management of SARS, both were critical of policy leaders' wanting of better evidence before taking further action.

14 Members of the "anti-mask" movement aside, which might be more about a lack of trust in government or elite institutions (scientists and the medical establishment, included) than a desire for RCTs. Certainly, much of the public in our own country (Canada) seems to be pro-face coverings and much of our community did not wait for government to mandate their use before donning a cover.

References

Alexander, P. E., J. P. Brito, I. Neumann et al. 2016. World Health Organization strong recommendations based on low-quality evidence (study quality) are frequent and often inconsistent with GRADE guidance. *Journal of Clinical Epidemiology* 72: 98–106. https://doi.org/10.1016/j.jclinepi.2014.10.011.

Balshem, H., M. Helfand, H. J. Schunemann et al. 2011. GRADE guidelines: 3. Rating the quality of evidence. *Journal of Clinical Epidemiology* 64: 401–406. https://doi.org/10.1016/j.jclinepi.2010.07.015.

Bensimon, C. M. and R. E. G. Upshur. 2007. Evidence and effectiveness in decisionmaking for quarantine. *American Journal of Public Health* 97, suppl. 1: S44–S48. https://dx.doi.org/10.2105%2FAJPH.2005.077305.

Borgerson, K. 2009. Valuing evidence: Bias and the evidence hierarchy of evidence-based medicine. *Perspectives in Biology and Medicine* 52, no. 2: 218–233. https://doi.org/10.1353/pbm.0.0086.

Brownson, R. C., J. G. Gurney, and G. H. Land. 1999. Evidence-based decision making in public health. *Journal of Public Health Management and Practice* 5, no. 5: 86–97. https://doi.org/10.1097/00124784-199909000-00012.

Bundgaard, H., J. S. Bundgaard, D. E. T. Raaschou-Pedersen et al. 2021. Effectiveness of adding a mask recommendation to other public health measures to prevent SARS-CoV-2 infection in Danish mask wearers. *Annals of Internal Medicine* 174, no. 3: 335–343. https://doi.org/10.7326/m20-6817.

Campbell, A. 2004. The SARS Commission interim report: SARS and public health in Ontario. http://www.archives.gov.on.ca/en/e_records/sars/report/v4.html (accessed April 21, 2021).

Cartwright, N. and E. Munro. 2010. The limitations of randomized controlled trials in predicting effectiveness. *Journal of Evaluation in Clinical Practice* 16, no. 2: 260–266. https://doi.org/10.1111/j.1365-2753.2010.01382.x.

Chaisson, K. G. E. 2020. Examining the World Health Organization's governance and response to noncommunicable diseases: A Foucauldian analysis. PhD dissertation. Department of Sociology, University of Calgary. https://prism.ucalgary.ca/handle/1880/111936 (accessed April 21, 2021).

Chu, D. K., E. A. Akl, S. Duda, K. Solo, S. Yaacoub, and H. J. Schunemann. 2020. Physical distancing, face masks, and eye protection to prevent person-to-person transmission of SARS-CoV-2 and Covid-19: A systematic review and meta-analysis. *The Lancet* 395, no. 10242: 1973–1987. https://doi.org/10.1016/ S0140.

Claeson, M. and S. Hanson. 2021. Covid-19 and the Swedish enigma. *The Lancet* 397, no. 10271: 259–261. https://dx.doi.org/10.1016%2FS0140-6736(20)32750-1.

DiCenso, A., G. Guyatt, and D. Ciliska. 2005. *Evidence-based nursing: A guide to clinical practice*. St. Louis, MO: Elsevier Mosby.

Djulbegovic, B., C. L. Bennett, and G. Guyatt. 2019. A unifying framework for improving health care. *Journal of Evaluation in Clinical Practice* 25, no. 3: 358–362. https://doi.org/10.1111/jep.13066.

Djulbegovic, B. and G. H. Guyatt. 2017. Progress in evidence-based medicine: A quarter century on. *The Lancet* 390, no. 10092: 415–423. https://doi.org/10.1016/s0140-6736(16)31592-6.

Djulbegovic, B., G. H. Guyatt, and R. E. Ashcroft. 2009. Epistemological inquiries in evidence-based medicine. *Cancer Control* 16, no. 2: 158–168. https://doi.org/10.1177/107327480901600208.

Djulbegovic, B., A. Kumar, R. M. Kaufman, A. Tobian, and G. H. Guyatt. 2015. Quality of evidence is a key determinant for making a strong GRADE guidelines recommendation. *Journal of Clinical Epidemiology* 68, no. 7: 727–732. https://doi.org/10.1016/j.jclinepi.2014.12.015.

Faden, R., J. Bernstein, and S. Shebaya. 2020. Public health ethics. In *The Stanford encyclopedia of philosophy*, edited by E. N. Zalta. https://plato.stanford.edu/entries/publichealth-ethics/ (accessed April 21, 2021).

Feyerabend, P. 2010. *Against method*. 4th edition. New York: Verso.

Fischhoff, B. 2020. Making decisions in a Covid-19 world. *JAMA* 324, no. 2: 139–140. https://doi.org/10.1001/jama.2020.10178.

Glasgow, R. E., Vinson, C., Chambers, D., Khoury, M. J., Kaplan, R. M., and C. Hunter. 2012. National Institutes of Health approaches to dissemination and implementation science: Current and future directions. *American Journal of Public Health* 102, no. 7: 1274–1281. https://doi.org/10.2105/ajph.2012.300755.

GRADE (Grades of Recommendation, Assessment, Development, and Evaluation) Working Group. 2004. Grading quality of evidence and strength of recommendations. *British Medical Journal* 328: 1490–1494. https://doi.org/10.1136/bmj.328.7454.1490.

Greenhalgh, T. 2020. Face coverings for the public: Laying straw meant to rest. *Journal of Evaluation in Clinical Practice* 26: 1070–1077. https://doi.org/10.1111/jep.13415.

Greenhalgh, T., Schmid, M. B., Czypionka, T., Bassler, D., and L. Gruer. 2020. Face masks for the public during the Covid-19 crisis. *British Medical Journal* 369: 1435. https://doi.org/10.1136/bmj.m1435.

Guyatt, G. 2007. An emerging consensus on grading recommendations? *Chinese Journal of Evidence-Based Medicine* 7, no. 1: 1–8. https://doi.org/10.1136/ebm.11.1.2-a.

Guyatt, G., J. Cairns, D. Churchill et al. 1992. Evidence-based medicine: A new approach to teaching the practice of medicine. *JAMA* 268, no. 17: 2420–2425. https://doi.org/10.1001/jama.1992.03490170092032.

Guyatt, G., D. Rennie, M. Meade, and D. Cook. 2008. *The users' guides to the medical literature: A manual for evidence-based clinical practice*. 2nd edition. New York: McGraw-Hill.

Hill, A. B. 1965. The environment and disease: Association or causation? *Proceedings of the Royal Society of Medicine* 58: 295–300. https://doi.org/10.1177%2F003591576505800503.

Jenicek, M. 1997. Epidemiology, evidence-based medicine, and evidence-based public health. *Journal of Epidemiology* 7, no. 4: 187–197. https://doi.org/10.2188/jea.7.187.

Jette, D. U., K. Bacon, C. Batty et al. 2003. Evidence-based practice: Beliefs, attitudes, knowledge, and behaviours of physical therapists. *Physical Therapy* 83, no. 9: 786–805. https://doi.org/10.1093/ptj/83.9.786.

Kannel, W. B. 1990. Contribution of the Framingham Study to preventative cardiology. *Journal of the American College of Cardiology* 15, no. 1: 206–211. https://doi.org/10.1016/0735-1097(90)90203-2.

Kavanagh, B. P. 2009. The GRADE system for rating clinical guidelines. *PLoS Medicine* 6, no. 9: e1000094. https://doi.org/10.1371/journal.pmed.1000094.

Kemm, J. 2006. The limitations of "evidence-based" public health. *Journal of Evaluation in Clinical Practice* 12, no. 3: 319–324. https://doi.org/10.1111/j.1365-2753.2006.00600.x.

Kohatsu, N. D., J. G. Robinson, and J. C. Torner. 2004. Evidence-based public health: An evolving concept. *American Journal of Preventive Medicine* 27, no. 5: 417–421. https://doi.org/10.1016/j.amepre.2004.07.019.

Krevar, H. 1997. *Final report: Commission of inquiry on the blood system in Canada*. Ottawa: The Commission. https://publications.msss.gouv.qc.ca/msss/en/document-000416/ (accessed April 21, 2021).

Link, B. G. and J. C. Phelan. 1995. Social conditions as fundamental causes of disease. *Journal of Health and Social Behavior* 35: 80–94. https://doi.org/10.2307/2626958.

Maglo, K. N. 2010. Genomics and the conundrum of race: Some epistemic and ethical considerations. *Perspectives in Biology and Medicine* 53, no. 3: 357–372. https://doi.org/10.1353/pbm.0.0171.

Marmot, M. G. and S. Friel. 2008. Global health equity: Evidence for action on the social determinants of health. *Journal of Epidemiology and Community Health* 62, no. 12: 1095–1097. https://doi.org/10.1136/jech.2008.081695.

Mercuri, M. 2020. Just follow the science: A government response to a pandemic. *Journal of Evaluation in Clinical Practice* 26, no. 6: 1575–1578. https://doi.org/10.1111/jep.13491.

Mercuri, M. and B. S. Baigrie. 2018. What confidence should we have in GRADE? *Journal of Evaluation in Clinical Practice* 24, no. 5: 1240–1246. https://doi.org/10.1111/jep.12993.

Mercuri, M. and B. S. Baigrie. 2019. What counts as evidence in an evidence-based world? *Journal of Evaluation in Clinical Practice* 25, no. 4: 533–535. https://doi.org/10.1111/jep.13220.

Mercuri, M., B. S. Baigrie, and A. Gafni. 2021. Patient participation in the clinical encounter and clinical practice guidelines: The case of patients' participation in a GRADEd world. *Studies in History and Philosophy of Science* 85: 192–199. https://doi.org/10.1016/j.shpsa.2020.10.008.

Mercuri, M., B. Baigrie, and R. E. G. Upshur. 2018. Going from evidence to recommendations: Can GRADE get us there? *Journal of Evaluation in Clinical Practice* 24, no. 5: 1232–1239. https://doi.org/10.1111/jep.12857.

Mercuri, M. and A. Gafni. 2018a. The evolution of GRADE (Part 1): Is there a theoretical and/or empirical basis for the GRADE framework? *Journal of Evaluation in Clinical Practice* 24, no. 5: 1203–1210. https://doi.org/10.1111/jep.12998.

Mercuri, M. and A. Gafni. 2018b. The evolution of GRADE (Part 2): Still searching for a theoretical and/or empirical basis for the GRADE framework. *Journal of Evaluation in Clinical Practice* 24, no. 5: 1211–1222. https://doi.org/10.1111/jep.12997.

Mercuri, M. and A. Gafni. 2018c. The evolution of GRADE (Part 3): A framework built on science or faith? *Journal of Evaluation in Clinical Practice* 24, no. 5: 1223–1231. https://doi.org/10.1111/jep.13016.

Mercuri, M. and A. Gafni. 2018d. Reflecting on evidence based medicine, person centered medicine, and small area variations: How contemporary frameworks for medicine address (or not) the needs of the individual patient. *European Journal for Person Centered Healthcare* 6, no. 3: 454–461. http://dx.doi.org/10.5750/ejpch.v6i3.1477.

Muir Gray, J. A. 1997. Evidence-based public health: What level of competence is required? *Journal of Public Health Medicine* 19, no. 1: 65–68. https://doi.org/10.1093/oxfordjournals.pubmed.a024591

Neta, G., R. E. Glasgow, C. R. Carpenter et al. 2015. A framework for enhancing the value of research for dissemination and implementation. *American Journal of Public Health* 105, no. 1: 49–57. https://doi.org/10.2105/ajph.2014.302206.

Norman, G. R. 1999. Examining the assumptions of evidence-based medicine. *Journal of Evaluation in Clinical Practice* 5, no. 2: 139–147. https://doi.org/10.1046/j.1365-2753.1999.00197.x.

Norris, S. L., E. A. Rehfuess, H. Smith et al. 2019. Complex health interventions in complex systems: Improving the process and methods for evidence-informed health decisions. *BMJ Global Health* 4: e000963. https://dx.doi.org/10.1136%2Fbmjgh-2018-000963.

Phelan, J. C., B. G. Link, and P. Tehranifar. 2010. Social conditions as fundamental causes of health inequalities: Theory, evidence, and policy implications. *Journal of Health and Social Behavior* 51, suppl.: S28–S40. https://doi.org/10.1177/0022146510383498.

Rubin, O., N. A. Errett, R. Upshur, and E. Baekkeskov. 2021. The challenges facing evidence-based decision making in the initial response to Covid-19. *Scandinavian Journal of Public Health* 49, no. 7: 790–796. https://doi.org10.1177/1403494821997227.

Sackett, D. L. and W. M. C. Rosenberg. 1995. The need for evidence-based medicine. *Journal of the Royal Society of Medicine* 88: 620–624. https://www.ncbi.nlm.nih.gov/pmc/articles/PMC1295384/pdf/jrsocmed00064-0020.pdf (accessed December 16, 2021).

Sackett, D. L., W. M. C. Rosenberg, J. A. Muir Gray, R. B. Haynes, and W. S. Richardson. 1996. Evidence-based medicine: What it is and what it isn't. *British Medical Journal* 312, no. 7023: 71–72. https://doi.org/10.1136/bmj.312.7023.71.

Schunemann, H. J., C. Cuello, E. A. Akl et al. 2019. GRADE guidelines: 18. How ROBINS-I and other tools to assess risk of bias in nonrandomized studies should be used to rate the certainty of a body of evidence. *Journal of Clinical Epidemiology* 111: 105–114. https://doi.org/10.1016/j.jclinepi.2018.01.012.

Siegfried, N., M. Narasimhan, C. E. Kennedy, A. Welbourn, and A. Yuvraj. 2017. Using GRADE as a framework to guide research on the sexual and reproductive health and rights (SRHR) of women living with HIV: Methodological opportunities and challenges. *AIDS Care* 29, no. 9: 1088–1093. https://doi.org/10.1080/09540121.2017.1317711.

Stegenga, J. 2018. *Medical nihilism*. Oxford: Oxford University Press.

Tikkinen, K. O. and G. H. Guyatt. 2020. Understanding of research results, evidence summaries and their applicability—not critical appraisal—are core skills of medical curriculum. *BMJ Evidence-Based Medicine* 26, no. 5: 231–233. https://doi:10.1136/bmjebm-2020-111542.

Timmermans, S. and A. Mauck. 2005. The promises and pitfalls of evidence-based medicine. *Health Affairs* 24, no. 1: 18–28. https://doi.org/10.1377/hlthaff.24.1.18.

Upshur, R. E. G. 2012. Evidence and ethics in public health: The experience of SARS in Canada. *NSW Public Health Bulletin* 23, no. 5–6: 108–110. https://doi.org/10.1071/nb11044.

Upshur, R. E. G. and C. S. Tracy. 2004. Legitimacy, authority, and hierarchy: Critical challenges for evidence-based medicine. *Brief Treatment and Crisis Intervention* 4, no. 3: 197–204. https://doi.org/10.1093/brief-treatment/mhh018.

Valles, S. A. 2018. *Philosophy of population health: Philosophy for a new public health era.* New York: Routledge.

Victora, C. G., J.-P. Habicht, and J. Bryce. 2004. Evidence-based public health: Moving beyond randomized trials. *American Journal of Public Health* 94, no. 3: 400–405. https://dx.doi.org/10.2105%2Fajph.94.3.400.

Welch, V. A., E. A. Akl, G. Guyatt et al. 2017. GRADE equity guidelines 1: Considering health equity in GRADE guideline development: Introduction and rationale. *Journal of Clinical Epidemiology* 90: 59–67. https://doi.org/10.1016/j.jclinepi.2017.01.014.

WHO (World Health Organization). 2012. WHO handbook for guideline development. https://apps.who.int/iris/rest/bitstreams/651924/retrieve (accessed April 21, 2021).

WHO (World Health Organization). 2020a. Advice on the use of masks in the context of Covid-19: Interim guidance. April 6. https://apps.who.int/iris/bitstream/handle/10665/331693/WHO-2019-nCov-IPC_Masks-2020.3-eng.pdf?sequence=1&isAllowed=y (accessed April 21, 2021).

WHO (World Health Organization). 2020b. Advice on the use of masks in the context of Covid-19: Interim guidance. June 5. https://www.who.int/publications/i/item/advice-on-the-use-of-masks-in-the-community-during-home-care-and-in-healthcare-settings-in-the-context-of-the-novel-coronavirus-(2019-ncov)-outbreak (accessed April 21, 2021).

Windle, M., H. D. Lee, S. T. Cherng et al. 2019. From epidemiologic knowledge to improved health: A vision for translational epidemiology. *American Journal of Epidemiology* 188, no. 12: 2049–2060. https://doi.org/10.1093/aje/kwz085.

Worrall, J. 2002. What evidence in evidence-based medicine? *Philosophy of Science* 69, suppl. 3: S316–S330. https://doi.org/10.1086/341855.

11

PROFILING IN PUBLIC HEALTH

Winnie Ma

Introduction

The World Health Organization (WHO), following Donald Acheson (1988), defines "public health" as "the art and science of preventing disease, prolonging life and promoting health through the organized efforts of society." And in this chapter, I define "profiling" as "forming or holding a belief about an individual on the basis of well-evidenced generalizations about a group or groups to which the individual belongs." Public health, like personal healthcare where individual medical professionals form beliefs about individual patients—especially in public and personal healthcare contexts committed to using the evidence-based medicine (EBM) framework—involves profiling individuals on the basis of their membership in groups. These groups can be defined by various features such as sex, race or ethnicity, age, disability status, and so on. For example, public health campaigns in the United States and the United Kingdom relied on profiling based on features such as ethnicity and socioeconomic status to reach certain individuals and communities because ethnic minority communities were experiencing higher rates of mortality, hospitalization, and serious illness from Covid-19, and lower rates of vaccination.

Much has been written recently by philosophers on the ethical and epistemic permissibility of "stereotyping," closely related to our notion of "profiling," in *non-medical contexts*, where "stereotyping" has been variously defined. Such definitions include "judg[ing] a person by real or apparent group membership" (Beeghly 2021: 2); making "broad ascriptions of salient or in some contextually relevant sense noteworthy properties to particular social groups, and derivatively, to the individuals who compose the group" (Begby 2021: 27); making "false or misleading generalizations about groups held in a manner that renders them largely, though not entirely, immune to counterevidence" (Blum 2004: 251); forming "beliefs about members of social groups that take the form of generalizations" (Johnson 2020: 1197); forming beliefs based on "widely held associations between a given social group and one or more attributes" (Fricker 2007: 30), among other definitions.[1] Much less philosophical work has been done on the ethical and epistemic permissibility of "profiling" as defined here, which involves beliefs about individuals formed on the basis of *well-evidenced* generalizations about the group(s) to which the individual belongs, in *medical contexts,* in either public health or personal healthcare settings.[2] Furthermore, philosophical work on

DOI: 10.4324/9781315675411-14

the epistemology and ethics of "profiling" (defined differently than in the way in which we understand it in this chapter) has focused on profiling in non-medical contexts, and in particular on policing and criminal justice contexts (see, for example, Lever 2017; Lippert-Rasmussen 2006; Risse and Zeckhauser 2004).[3]

Against this background, Katherine Puddifoot's (2019) "Stereotyping Patients," to which this chapter is partly written in response, is an important piece of work on the ethical and epistemic permissibility of stereotyping of patients in personal healthcare contexts.[4] Puddifoot argues that there are good ethical and epistemic reasons both *to* "stereotype" and *not to* stereotype patients in medical contexts. Puddifoot understands "stereotyping" as follows: "Making a judgment about an individual that is influenced by a mental state associating members of a group, to which that individual is perceived as belonging, more strongly than members of other groups with particular traits" (2019: 71).

In this chapter, one of my aims is to extend the discussion of the ethical and epistemic permissibility of stereotyping, and more specifically of *profiling* patients, from the personal healthcare context to the public health context more generally. That is, the question that I am interested in answering in this chapter is this: Is it ethically and epistemically permissible to "profile" patients in biomedical contexts, including both public health and personal healthcare contexts—especially in light of the fact that it at least does not seem to be ethically permissible to profile individuals in the context of police profiling, profiling by banks and insurance companies, academic admissions profiling, and so on?[5]

Much of what is said about the ethical and epistemic permissibility of profiling and stereotyping in this chapter fundamentally depends on exactly how we define these notions. So, in the Section "A definition of 'profiling,'" I stipulate exactly what I mean in this chapter by "profiling," and briefly remark on its relationship to Puddifoot's notion of "stereotyping." Then, in the Section "Is medical and health profiling different?" I raise the question of why many of us seem to intuit that profiling in medicine is ethically and epistemically permissible, whereas we have a different intuition that it is not ethically, at least, permissible to profile in non-medical contexts.

My aim in the second part of this chapter is to support Puddifoot's claim that there are good ethical and epistemic reasons both to profile and not to profile patients. In particular, under the subheading "The epistemic permissibility of profiling," I present an additional reason which Puddifoot (2019) does not consider that makes profiling patients epistemically impermissible—namely, the relevance of Martin Smith's (2018) claim that we ought not form beliefs about individuals on the basis of purely statistical evidence because purely statistical evidence does not *normically support* these beliefs about individuals. And in the next section, "The ethical permissibility of profiling," I present a second additional reason to think that profiling patients is ethically impermissible—namely, Rima Basu and Mark Schroeder's (2019) claim that we can doxastically wrong; that is, we can morally wrong persons just in virtue of the beliefs that we hold about them.

In the third part of this chapter, I consider what the practical implications of the foregoing may be for two rapidly evolving domains. In particular, under the subheading "Profiling and evidence-based medicine," I consider the implications of the above for EBM, given that it relies fundamentally on the practice of profiling patients. I do the same for medical and non-medical algorithms/artificial intelligence (AI) in the following section. I conclude by noting, like Puddifoot (2019), that the picture of the ethical and epistemic permissibility of profiling in biomedical contexts (and beyond) is more complicated than one might have prima facie thought. And I suggest that we may need to reconsider the ethical and epistemic nature of the very foundations of EBM as well as of medical AI, as both rely on profiling to generate diagnoses, predictions, and treatment recommendations.

A definition of "profiling"

In this chapter, I define *profiling* as forming or holding a belief about an individual on the basis of well-evidenced generalizations about a group or groups to which the individual belongs. This notion of profiling is restricted and specific and is both similar to and differs from Puddifoot's notion of stereotyping, above, in several aspects.[6] First, both my notion of profiling and Puddifoot's notion of stereotyping concern the formation or holding of *beliefs* or judgments we form rather than referring to our actions or behaviors. The term "profiling" colloquially connotes *action*, and in particular *police* action. The term "stereotyping" in comparison is associated to a greater extent with belief or internal reasoning. Risse and Zeckhauser, for example, define "profiling" as "any police-initiated action that relies on the race, ethnicity, or national origin and not just on the behavior of an individual" (2004: 136). And Kasper Lippert-Rasmussen says that "racial profiling [...] can be said to occur where, say, there is a greater likelihood that police officers will stop, search, and question people of a certain race because members of this group are believed to be more likely to possess illegal drugs than members of other groups" (2013: 273). In contrast, I am concerned in this chapter with the ethical and epistemic dimensions of profiling, understood as (just) involving the forming and/or holding *beliefs* about an individual.

Second, philosophers have published less on profiling than on stereotyping, perhaps because of the greater connoted specificity and sensitivity of profiling, or the greater concern about action-focused racial profiling by police. Nevertheless, what I mean by "profiling" in this chapter (i) is not restricted to police (or racial) profiling, and includes any kind of belief about individuals based on well-evidenced generalizations about the groups to which they belong; and (ii) might therefore be thought of and used as a more restricted notion of "stereotyping" as "stereotyping" as has been defined by various philosophers, such as Puddifoot (2019), Beeghly (2021, 2015) and others.

Third and perhaps most importantly, I specify (whereas Puddifoot does not) that the generalizations or associations upon which the beliefs about the individual are based are *well-evidenced*.[7] Puddifoot does not specify whether the associations made between groups and traits are based on evidence, or attempt at being based on the evidence. Nor does she specify that the individual needs to actually be a member of the group of which they are perceived as being a member. According to our more restricted notion of "profiling," however, the generalizations upon which the beliefs about individuals are due to their group membership and are well evidenced. This will highlight the interesting, apparent conflicts between ethical and epistemic demands when profiling individuals in a biomedical context, and beyond.

Is medical and health profiling different?

Consider the following imaginary cases of profiling in three different domains—in policing, academia, and medicine.

Police profiling

Officer Smith is a rookie police officer who has just moved to Centreville and has just started working for the 5th Centreville Precinct. And she is told in a morning briefing by her commanding officer (whom Officer Smith knows to be reliable) that the latest statistics available show that 92% of ethnic minority residents compared to 40% of White residents in their precinct have open arrest warrants. The statistics also show that 75% of ethnic minority residents compared to 45% of White residents carry concealed handguns.[8] This briefing is related to her duties to complete arrest warrants and decrease gun possession without permits. Later in the day, she goes on patrol in the precinct and sees a an ethnic minority resident walking his dog down on the sidewalk. In order to decide whether to stop and question the resident about a possible open arrest warrant, as well as whether she should be prepared to draw her weapon, Officer Smith is forced to form some belief about the resident. And Officer Smith forms the belief that it is very likely that this particular an ethnic minority resident has an open arrest warrant and is carrying a concealed handgun.[9]

Profiling professors

You have just arrived at the University of Centerville where you know from reliable employment data that nine out of ten administrators identify as women, and nine out of ten professors identify as men, and there are roughly equal numbers of administrators and professors. You meet a woman wearing a staff ID tag, which means that she is either an administrator or a professor. Based on your statistical evidence, you form the belief that the woman is most likely to be an administrator rather than a professor.[10]

In both of these cases, we have an agent whose statistical evidence appears to support a profiling belief that is also intuitively ethically problematic. That is, to believe that someone is an administrator rather than a professor on the basis of their gender, even when this assumption is apparently supported by one's statistical evidence, is, at least to me, intuitively ethically problematic.[11] (And perhaps this is very intuitively ethically problematic to me because I am a female lecturer in a male-dominated field who is constantly confronted with disbelief when I say that I am a lecturer!) And to believe that someone is much more likely to have an open arrest warrant and to be carrying a concealed weapon on the basis of their ethnicity is also intuitively very ethically problematic, not least because of the ethically problematic consequence that police officers who profile minority ethnic individuals thus are more likely to draw their own weapons. And so the cases give rise to the kind of apparent "ethical-epistemic" dilemmas with which Puddifoot (2017, 2019) is concerned. In these dilemmatic situations, what one ought or is permitted to believe from an epistemic point of view (that is, in accordance with one's evidence) appears to be at odds with what one ought or is permitted to believe from an ethical point of view. That is, it seems that in cases like these, trying to believe truly by believing in accordance with one's evidence will mean believing something that is ethically problematic—for example, given that she is a woman, she probably isn't a professor, or given that he is an ethnic minority, he's more likely to have an open arrest warrant and be carrying a concealed weapon.

Whether these sorts of ethical-epistemic dilemmas occur in non-medical domains such as policing, legal, and criminal domains, in academia, and so on, has been much discussed in the philosophical literature (see, for example, Egan 2011; Gardiner 2018; Gendler 2011; Johnson King and Babic 2020; Kelly and Roedder 2008; Mugg 2013). Less discussed are whether these ethical-epistemic dilemmas occur in the medical/public health domain (although of course Katherine Puddifoot (2017, 2019) has been a trail-blazer on the topic of ethical-epistemic dilemmas in the personal healthcare context). Consider the case below.

Profiling patients: socially stigmatized condition, socially salient group

Dr. Z knows that, statistically, Black men who have sex with men (or MSM), are three times more likely to have HIV/AIDS than White MSM.[12] Dr. Z forms the belief that his

Black patient, Kevin, who reports male-to-male sexual contact, is more likely to have HIV/AIDS than his White patient, Roy, who also reports MSM contact.

Our intuition that there is something ethically problematic going on here and in other similar cases of profiling in the medical domain is often less strong than our intuition regarding there being something ethically problematic about profiling in non-medical domains. Why this is the case is unclear (to me at least) and important to address. One might suggest that the beneficent purpose of medicine—to prevent disease, prolong life, and promote health—makes profiling in medicine (or public health) ethically permissible. It does not seem ethically permissible in the case of police profiling because of its less clearly beneficent purpose for the individual being profiled. Public health officials and medical professionals most often profile patients in order to better identify and target particularly at-risk groups of individuals to prevent disease, form more accurate diagnoses, provide more optimal treatment recommendations, and so on. Police profile individuals in order to be able to better identify and target (for questioning, stop and search, and so on) individuals who are supposedly most likely to have committed or be in the process of committing a crime. The benefit (if there are truly any benefits of police profiling) accrues to others. On the other hand, the individual, profiled patient hopefully receives a benefit in consequence of their being profiled—their health is protected and promoted. The individual profiled by police will generally be in receipt of a harm in consequence of their being profiled. If nothing else, they are treated like persons who deserve to be suspected of criminal activity, something which might be thought to erode their status or their sense of their own status as equal citizens and persons.

However, the ethical picture of profiling in medicine versus by police is more complex than this beneficence objection might suggest. First, while profiling patients in public health and medicine is generally done with a beneficent purpose and may customarily result in the profiled patients being only *benefited (no harms)* in consequence of their being profiled, this is not always the case.

Patients may also be harmed as a result of being profiled in medicine. Take, for example, cases of profiling patients for socially stigmatized medical conditions such as HIV/AIDS, sexually transmitted diseases, various mental health conditions, teenage and unwanted pregnancy, being overweight or obese, and so on. Profiling individuals based on their group membership in relation to such stigmatized conditions could result in various kinds of harms—individuals might, for example, feel morally wronged in virtue of being associated accurately or inaccurately with a socially stigmatized condition, and they might consequently also be treated differently by other members of society in virtue of their being deemed to be more likely to have the stigmatized condition, etc.—despite the beneficent intention to help them. In comparison, we do not find ourselves (too) ethically troubled by profiling a patient for a medical condition that does not bear a social stigma such as diabetes or heart disease. Consider, for example, the following case involving a health condition that does not bear a social stigma:

Profiling patients: socially neutral condition, socially neutral group

Dr. R knows that 75% of all people have attached earlobes, and that the rest have partially or fully detached earlobes. Dr. R forms the belief that her next patient Riva probably has attached earlobes.

Our intuition that something ethically problematic is afoot with these profiling beliefs also seems to be weaker when an individual is not being profiled on the basis of their membership in a *socially salient group*. This term comes from Lippert-Rasmussen (2013: 30) who says that a "group is socially salient if perceived membership of it is important to the structure of social interactions across a wide range of social contexts." When a patient is profiled on the basis of their membership in a socially salient group by public health officials or by medical professionals, and when they are profiled as having or being at risk for a socially stigmatized medical condition, we have a stronger intuition that the patient is not only being benefited in consequence of their being profiled. Being "pigeon-holed" based on membership in a socially salient group and being associated with a socially stigmatized condition may very well be or be experienced as harms arising from being profiled in medicine. That is, with respect to the latter point, one kind of harm that profiling in the medical or public health contexts can lead to is the assignment of social stigma of varying kinds and degrees. And with respect to the former point about pigeon-holing, another kind of harm the profiling can lead to is the feeling that it is being denied that one has the relevant capacity for individual, autonomous self-expression and for living one's life in ways that deviate from the pigeon-holing stereotypes to which one may be subject.

In addition, profiled patients may be harmed if they are profiled in a way so as to deny them access to health benefits that they need or want. Take, for example, potential cases in which minors might wish to be vaccinated despite their guardians' refusal to give their consent, and who are then denied the health benefits of vaccination because they are profiled as minors incapable of making this decision for themselves. Medical profiling can also subject individuals to (at least nudges to undergo) medical scrutiny, screening, and procedures that they do not want or need. Take, for example, late term screening for Down Syndrome in the fetuses of older pregnant women. Medical advice to undergo this screening can be unwanted and emotionally distressing, and can often lead to more invasive testing (De Graaf et al. 2002). The argument here is not that there are not benefits from profiling in medical contexts, but that there are also harms being created and dispensed to individuals.

Being profiled by police, financial institutions and insurance companies, academic admissions committees, and so on, likewise generally has a mix of benefits and harms for the person being profiled. It might be true that, on a spectrum of benefits and harms accrued to the profiled individual in consequence of their being profiled, public health and medicine may lie at the far, beneficent end; profiled individuals accrue greater benefits than harms as a result of their being profiled. And police profiling, conversely, may lie at the opposite, less beneficent end; greater harms accrue to profiled individuals than benefits.

However, police profiling can also result in benefits for profiled individuals such as when profiling is done on individuals at risk of harm—individuals at risk of self-harm, experiencing child neglect, domestic abuse, and so on. Such profiling aims to identify those who need social protection. Profiling by financial institutions, insurance companies, academic admissions committees, and so on might be said to lie somewhere in the middle of the harm-benefit spectrum. The profiling done by these organizations will generally tend to result in *certain* profiled individuals (those with high socioeconomic status, in dominant racial groups, and so on) receiving benefits—loans, insurance coverage and payouts, academic admission, and so on—and other profiled individuals (generally members of marginalized groups) being denied those benefits.

Police departments, as well as financial institutions, insurance companies, and academic admissions committees may object to the characterization of their purposes as less clearly beneficent than that of medicine. The stated mission of the New York Police Department, for example, is to "enhance the quality of life in New York City by working in partnership with the community to enforce the law, preserve peace, protect the people, reduce fear, and maintain order."[13] Whether police departments act in accordance with or live up to their beneficent mission statements, of course, is a very different question. But one might suggest with respect to profiling by police, financial institutions, and so on that we should also consider the benefits accrued to *other* individuals and to the rest of society as a whole perhaps at the cost of profiling particular individuals.

Financial institutions, insurance companies, and academic admissions committees might suggest that profiling individuals is a necessary means to distribute scarce resources and opportunities to the most deserving and capable. Police departments may, again rightly or wrongly, likewise suggest that profiling better enables and may even be a necessary means to protect other members of society, at the cost of the harms of profiling particular individuals. And they may point to the likewise collective rather than individual concerns of public health officials, who similarly must weigh the benefits to society as a whole of public health policies against the harms or costs to profiled individuals. Take, for example, decisions by governments during the Covid-19 pandemic to profile and target certain individuals for shielding, priority vaccination, remote learning, and so on. While this may look like benefitting individuals, it also led to harms being suffered by members of certain social groups in order to protect members of other social groups.

In light of the above discussion, I hope it will be seen that we should not too quickly accept that the medical/public health domain is categorically different with respect to the ethical permissibility of profiling by public health officials and medical professionals from other domains such as policing or finance. Building on this, in the following sections, I consider various reasons to think that *all* of the above medical cases—involving socially stigmatized and socially neutral medical conditions, and generalizations about socially salient and socially neutral groups, may be ethically and epistemically problematic in various ways. On the other hand, I also subsequently offer reasons to think that there are still good ethical and epistemic reasons to profile patients.

The epistemic and ethical permissibility of profiling

The epistemic permissibility of profiling

Puddifoot (2019) presents a plethora of good reasons to think that profiling patients might have various epistemic costs (that is, costs with respect to believing as we ought), as well as epistemic benefits. The reasons she presents for not profiling patients center around the fact that profiling can activate clinicians' implicit biases, which then can lead to various epistemic costs. These include but are not limited to:

i the perpetration of testimonial injustices by clinicians against patients stereotyped as being less credible, which can then lead to knowledge deprivation when clinicians fail to listen to their patients as they ought;
ii leading clinicians to focus on medical conditions of patients that fit stereotypes associated with the patients' social groups, and giving inadequate attention to non-stereotypical conditions that may nevertheless fit with other evidence;
iii distorted perception of the symptoms of stereotyped patients; and so on.

There is one more reason to think that profiling patients is not epistemically permissible that Puddifoot (2019) does not consider. In a series of brilliant papers, Smith (2018, 2021) considers both the *epistemic* and *legal* permissibility of forming beliefs and passing legal judgments on the basis of purely statistical evidence. Smith suggests that profiling would be epistemically impermissible because purely statistical evidence about groups does not *normically support* beliefs about individuals who are members of those groups, where Smith says that "a body of evidence E normically supports a proposition P just in case it generates the need for special explanation in the event that P is false" (Smith 2021: 944). And in order for it to be the case that one is epistemically permitted to believe a proposition *p* or that one is legally permitted to pass a judgment about an individual, one's evidence would need to normically support *p*.

Thus, for example, consider Redmayne's (2008: 282) "Prisoners" case:

> One hundred prisoners are exercising in the prison yard. Ninety-nine of them suddenly join in a planned attack on a prison guard; the hundredth prisoner plays no part. There is no evidence available to show who joined in and who did not.

Redmayne asks, Is the 0.99 probability that a particular prisoner is guilty enough to prove *beyond reasonable doubt* that they are guilty?[14] In this case, according to Smith, one would be neither legally permitted to pass a judgment about, nor epistemically permitted to believe in the guilt of any particular prisoner selected at random. And this is because such a legal judgment or belief about the guilt of a particular prisoner would be solely based on purely statistical evidence, and would therefore lack normic support.

Even more perspicuously, Smith suggests that even in the case of a lottery in which you hold one ticket and have the statistical evidence that there are 1,000,000 tickets, only one of which is winning, you are not epistemically permitted to believe that the ticket you hold is a losing ticket. This is because this statistical evidence does not normically support your belief that your ticket is a losing ticket. That is, if it turned out that your ticket was in fact a winning ticket, you would not need further, special explanation as to how it came to be that your ticket was the winning ticket. It could have just so happened that your ticket was luckily the winning ticket.

On the other hand, let's say you have a trustworthy, reliable friend who gives you testimonial evidence that they've seen the winning lottery numbers and your ticket is not the winning ticket. If it turned out that your belief formed on the basis of your friend's testimony is false because you did win, further, special explanation would be required. And, therefore, this latter "losing ticket" belief based on testimonial evidence would have normic support in Smith's sense, and you'd be permitted to hold it.[15] And note that it is the case that this non-statistical testimonial evidence offers normic support even though the statistical reliability of testimonial evidence generally tends to fall far below 99% or indeed 99.9999%.

The ethical permissibility of profiling

In regard to ethical permissability, Puddifoot (2019) notes that prima facie, intuitively, clinicians ought not profile patients because clinicians ought to be blind to the socially salient group membership of their patients—relevant ethical principles of justice and fairness imply that patients ought not be evaluated or treated differently only on the basis of their racial group, sexual orientation, religion, and so on. At the same time, Puddifoot offers an ethical reason to profile:

> The ethical goal of treating people fairly can sometimes only be achieved via the fulfillment of the epistemic goal of making a correct judgment. Where the epistemic goal requires reflecting on the social group status of a patient in their judgments, there can be an ethical demand on health professionals to be responsive to social group status [that is, to profile patients].
>
> *(2019: 76)*

While I am in agreement with Puddifoot about this possible interplay between ethical and epistemic considerations, I would also suggest for consideration an additional potential ethical cost of profiling patients—namely, as Basu and Schroeder (2019) suggest, that we can morally wrong individuals *just* in virtue of the beliefs we hold about them. That is, Basu and Schroeder (2019) argue that we can *doxastically wrong*: we can morally wrong persons in virtue of the beliefs that we hold about them (*in addition*, that is, to our capacity to morally wrong others with the words we speak, our behaviors, and the actions we take on the basis of our beliefs).

Basu and Schroeder primarily focus on profiling beliefs about individuals formed on the basis of well-evidenced generalizations about their membership in "socially salient groups," such as racial groups, gender groups, religious groups, and so on. They argue that these profiling beliefs about socially salient groups can morally wrong. That is, while acknowledging the deeply *philosophically* controversial nature of the claim that we can doxastically wrong, they nevertheless point to the intuitiveness of the possibility of doxastic wronging in ordinary thought in a variety of contexts (Basu and Schroeder 2019: 182). They leave it open, however, whether *any* profiling belief morally wrongs the subject(s) of that belief, including if the subjects are being profiled on the basis of their membership in groups other than socially salient groups (for example, the group of those individuals with attached earlobes). And they also leave open *why* it is the case that profiling beliefs morally wrong individuals, although Basu (2019b) suggests the Kantian idea that we may wrong others in profiling them by relating to them in the way we ought to relate to objects rather than in the way we ought to relate to persons.

I do not have any fixed opinions in response to the latter question of why it can be morally wrong to profile individuals. Another account that many have found intuitively appealing comes from Benjamin Eidelson (2015). Eidelson suggests that all instances of profiling beliefs (whether or not they concern socially salient group membership) may be ethically costly because in forming such beliefs, we fail to respect and treat profiled persons as *individuals*, where

> X treats Y as an individual if and only if:
> (Character Condition) X gives reasonable weight to evidence of the ways Y has exercised her autonomy in giving shape to her life, where this evidence is reasonably available and relevant to the determination at hand; and
> (Agency Condition) X's judgments concern Y's choices, these judgments are not made in a way that disparages Y's capacity to make those choices as an autonomous agent.
>
> *(2015: 44)*

I now turn to some of the implications of the above for two practices that rely on profiling practices at their core: EBM and medical algorithms.

Applications

Profiling and evidence-based medicine

David L. Sackett et al. describe EBM as the "conscientious, explicit, and judicious use of current best evidence [from systematic research] in making decisions about the care of individual patients" (1996: 71). While the framing here is in terms of decision-making rather than belief, the implication is that good belief-forming practices by practitioners of EBM will involve the formation or holding of beliefs about individual patients on the basis of systematically researched, good evidence about a group or groups to which the individual patient belongs—that is, good EBM practitioners will profile their patients. The power of EBM has been a focus on evidence as the source for treating individuals, but EBM also relies on healthcare workers profiling patients as belonging to the group to which the evidence relates and forming beliefs about the patient as a result.

Importantly, I hope that it is clear that I am not suggesting that EBM clinical practitioners ought not engage in profiling their patients because of the various negative ethical and epistemic reasons discussed above, and therefore, stop practicing EBM full stop. Rather, what I am suggesting, echoing Puddifoot, is that there are potential and hitherto largely ignored epistemic and ethical costs and benefits to profiling patients that EBM practitioners and theorists ought to consider. I am also suggesting, although in a much more preliminary way, that it may be that we ought to weigh up the ethical and epistemic costs and benefits of profiling patients on a patient-by-patient basis in order to determine whether and how we ought to profile each individual patient.

Profiling and medical artificial intelligence

Medical algorithms or medical AI profile patients, forming "beliefs" about likely diagnoses and most appropriate treatments.[16] This, I suggest, raises questions about the ethical and epistemic permissibility of profiling beliefs about patients when they are formed by artificial as opposed to human agents. A medical algorithm, for example, might be programmed to form beliefs about the probability that a patient (call them "Lee") has a certain medical condition (e.g. HIV/AIDS) based on the presence or absence or degree to which the patient is represented as having certain features (e.g. positive HIV test, recurrent infections, as well as sex, sexual orientation, racial group, socioeconomic status)—i.e. is a member of certain social groups picked out by those features. Compare this predictive algorithm to the now infamous Correctional Offender Management Profiling for Alternative Sanctions (COMPAS) algorithm in the United States. COMPAS profiled individuals' risk of criminal recidivism, and was unjustly and inaccurately biased against ethnic minorities, and in particular Black individuals (Larson et al. 2016). The COMPAS algorithm was programmed to form beliefs about the risk an individual would commit crimes again based on the presence or absence or degree to which the individual is represented as having certain features (in this case, racial group membership, among other features). A side by side comparison of medical and criminal predictive algorithms again raises the question of why it is that we seem comfortable, ethically at least, with AI profiling in medical contexts but not in non-medical ones, especially regarding crime and punishment.

Putting aside questions of whether and why medicine might be different from other domains in terms of the ethical and epistemic permissibility of AI profiling, I would like to note two (related) reasons one might think the ethical and epistemic permissibility of profiling by AI in medical and public health contexts may differ in important ways from that of human clinicians. First, it might be suggested that (current) medical AI does not have the degree of *agency* required for moral responsibility for their beliefs.[17] If anything, it might be suggested, it would be the algorithm's human creators who would bear some or most of the moral responsibility for the beliefs formed by their AI.

In response, I would suggest that it is not clear what kind of agency is required for an agent, human or artificial, to be morally responsible for their beliefs. And this is especially the case in light of objections to the claim that *any* agent can be morally responsible for their beliefs. This objection from *doxastic involuntarism* involves the denial that we have the relevant kinds of agential control over what we believe. And, the thought goes, if we do not have the relevant kinds of agential control over what we believe, then, given a widely held principle like Ought-Implies-Can, we cannot be morally responsible for what we believe. Or, at least, the *degree* to which an agent is morally responsible for their beliefs will be correlated with the degree of agential control they have over what they believe.[18]

Second, and on the other hand then, AI is not boundedly rational, or at least is in principle less *boundedly rational* than are human agents.[19] Here, I take "bounded rationality" to refer to the descriptive empirical claim that human beings are cognitively limited with respect to their processing and memory capacities; our cognitive capacity is circumscribed in various ways by various cognitive features. That AI is not or at least is less boundedly rational (that is, AI process information at greater speeds and more accurately, and have larger and more accurate memory capacities) and is less subject to the same sorts of cognitive or doxastic limitations to which human agents are subject implies the following two points. (i) AI are therefore in fact *more* morally responsible, given their lesser cognitive limitations. And (ii) the (more) unbounded cognitive capacities of medical AI could be used by clinicians to mitigate their own bounded rationality—that is, enable human clinicians to make speedier and more accurate judgments supplemented by the greater cognitive processing and memory capacities of AI. The second point (ii) is particularly noteworthy, given, as Puddifoot notes, the time and other resource-constraints clinicians typically find themselves subject to in current clinical practice. These time and other resource-constraints will make it even more necessary and likely for clinicians to make use of the heuristics and stereotypes that are the cognitive bread and butter of boundedly rational human belief-formation (Puddifoot 2019: 80). Furthermore, while AI will of course be subject to a variety of kinds of algorithmic bias, it will not be subject to certain particularly *human* cognitive biases, such as base rate neglect, the gambler's fallacy, confirmation bias, etc., to which even highly trained clinicians will often be subject.

Conclusion

The ethics and epistemology of *profiling*, understood as forming or holding a belief about an individual on the basis of well-evidenced generalizations about a group or groups to which the individual belongs, in public health and medicine more generally are underexplored in comparison to non-medical domains. This is in part because it has been assumed that, because of medicine's beneficent purpose, medical profiling (unlike, for example, police profiling) is ethically unproblematic and even ethically mandated.

What I hope to have done in this chapter is to have extended the limited extant analysis of the ethics and epistemology of stereotyping, in particular by Katherine Puddifoot, and profiling in personal healthcare to public health. I also hope to have supported Puddifoot's claim that the question of the ethical and epistemic permissibility of profiling is more complicated than one might have originally thought. And I hope to have done this by pointing out at least one additional reason to think that profiling patients might be epistemically impermissible, because such profiling lacks the kind of normic support that is possibly required for epistemically permissible belief, as Smith suggests; and at least one additional reason to think that profiling patients might be ethically impermissible, because profiling beliefs themselves (rather than the behaviors and actions taken on the basis of those beliefs) might doxastically wrong patients, as Basu and Schroeder suggest.

In addition, I hope to have encouraged us to have another look at the ethical and epistemic permissibility of profiling practices that form the very foundations of EBM and medical AI. I am not suggesting that these systems—EBM and medical AI—are ethically and epistemically impermissible systems because they fundamentally rely on profiling practices. Nor am I suggesting that we ought not profile patients or individuals more generally. I take it that profiling patients, again assuming our very specific definition of profiling, is sometimes the thing we ought to do overall, both from an ethical and from an epistemic point of view. In the age of Covid-19, for example, given the differential health outcomes of different racialized groups, it seems plausible that health professionals may be both ethically and epistemically obligated to profile ethnic minority patients as being at higher risk of serious illness or death, and therefore in greater need of special attention in their medical care (Centers for Disease Control and Prevention 2020; Office for National Statistics 2021). What I hope to have shed some further light on is just, as Puddifoot argues, that the ethical and epistemic nature of profiling patients is complicated. And we should be careful as we move ahead with EBM practices and especially with medical AI that we conscientiously consider the multifaceted ethical and epistemic natures of profiling in these rapidly evolving domains.

Acknowledgements

I would very much like to thank the editors Sridhar Venkatapuram and Alex Broadbent for their extensive and extremely helpful comments on previous drafts of this chapter. I would also like to thank Trish Greenhalgh for helpful comments on a later draft of this chapter, and audiences at Google and the London Medical Imaging & AI Centre for Value Based Healthcare for helpful feedback. And, last but not least, I want to thank the many wonderful speakers in the Sowerby Philosophy & Medicine Project's colloquium series on "Stereotyping & Medical AI", whose words and work were instrumental in refining my thinking about the ethics of belief of medical profiling. Speakers included, in chronological order, Erin Beeghly, Kathleen Creel, Annette Zimmermann, Will McNeill, Jonathan Gingerich, Georgi Gardiner, David Papineau, Reuben Binns, Robin Carpenter, Zoë Johnson King, Boris Babic, Geoff Keeling, and Rima Basu. Warmest thanks also go to the Sowerby Philosophy & Medicine Project, and in particular Elselijn Kingma, for giving me the opportunity to organize this colloquium series.

Notes

1 Note that these are definitions of "stereotyping" offered by philosophers. For a survey of how psychologists have defined "stereotypes" and "stereotyping," see Beeghly (2015).
2 Moss (2018b: 178) briefly discusses racial profiling, which she defines as "forming opinions about a person on the basis of statistics about members of their racial group," in medical contexts.
3 There is also a very important body of philosophical work on *epistemic injustices*, which Fricker (2007: 1) defines as "wrong[s] done as a result of negative identity-prejudicial stereotypes to someone specifically in their capacity as a knower," in medicine. For an overview of this work, see Carel and Kidd (2017).
4 See also Puddifoot's (2021) *How Stereotypes Deceive Us*, and especially Chapter 5 in the volume, "Where Ethical and Epistemic Demands Meet: Learning from the Role of Stereotyping in Medicine."
5 I have a very particular notion of "profiling" in mind, which I lay out clearly in §2.
6 Even though my notion of profiling differs from Puddifoot's notion of stereotyping in important respects, much—and all of Puddifoot's points discussed in the following sections—of what Puddifoot says regarding the ethical and epistemic permissibility of stereotyping patients applies regarding the ethical and epistemic permissibility of profiling patients.
7 Note that by "well-evidenced", as will become clearer later on the chapter, I do not mean ethically "justified" or "un-biased". Indeed, I take it that disparate base rates of various medical conditions

and, e.g., rates of open arrest warrants, academic admissions, etc., between different socially salient groups are by and large the result of various kinds of bias and injustice, such as structural and
individual racism, sexism, etc.

8 There are, of course, many ways in which our statistical evidence can be biased. Munton (2021),
for example, suggests that statistical evidence can be biased and indeed prejudiced just in virtue
of its taking characteristics like race or gender to be salient. Additional common statistical biases
include *selection bias*, in which surveyed individuals or groups differ systematically from the population of interest, leading to a systematic error in an association or outcome; *ascertainment bias*,
wherein systematic differences in the identification of surveyed individuals lead to a distortion in
the collection of data in a study, among other biases. Let us assume in this case, however, that the
statistical evidence is accurate, and that Officer Smith knows her commanding officer who briefs
her on it to be a trustworthy commander who is aware and as diligent as possible concerning issues
(such as oversurveillance) around biased statistical information, particularly with respect to marginalized ethnic groups.

9 This case is adapted from Basu's (2019a) "Ferguson" case. Basu's "Ferguson" case is, in turn,
loosely based on the Department of Justice's investigation of the Ferguson Police Department
which found that 62% of residents had open arrest warrants, and of those residents, 92% were
Black.

10 This case is adapted from Johnson King and Babic's "Gender Bias Study" (2020: 82).

11 There are also ethically relevant considerations around *stereotype threat* (Steele 1997) and the possibility of self-fulfilling profiling or stereotyping. The latter possibility of self-fulfilling profiling,
stereotyping, and social categorization more generally is an immensely complicated matter. But a
good place to start is with Ian Hacking's (1996) discussion of the "looping effects of human kinds."

12 Although this case is imaginary, it is based roughly on the finding by Millett et al. (2012) that
Black MSM were three times more likely to be HIV positive than were other MSM.

13 The following is the newly adopted Oath of Office of the Minneapolis Police Department (in one
of whose precincts George Floyd was murdered):

> I, [name], do solemnly swear that I will support the Constitution of the United States, the
> Constitution and laws of the State of Minnesota, and the Charter and Ordinances of the City of
> Minneapolis; That I shall, in recognition of my service as a peace keeper, first do no harm, that
> I will upload and safeguard the sanctity of life, and that I will shield and protect my commu-
> nity from those who would seek to cause harm; That I shall intervene in protest, both verbally
> and physically, if I witness anyone violating another's rights; That I recognize those I serve are
> members of the human family worthy of dignity and respect, and my term in office shall be
> guided by my love of service to the community and the grace of humanity.
> (https://www.minneapolismn.gov/government/departments/police/oath/,
> accessed December 16, 2021)

It interestingly includes a pledge to "do no harm" similar to the one in the Hippocratic Oath.

14 The legal standard of proof of guilt being "beyond reasonable doubt" applies to criminal trials.
The legal standard of proof of there being a "preponderance of evidence" in favor of a particular
legal judgment or the legal judgment being true on the "balance of probabilities" is, on the other
hand, the standard of proof applied to civil trials. The latter, less stringent standard of proof applied
to civil trials is said to be met when the probability of the judgment being true exceeds 50%, i.e.
when the judgment is shown to be more likely true than false. Less clear is the probability threshold required for the more stringent "beyond reasonable doubt" standard of proof. However, it is
surely much higher than 50%, and it is almost certainly satisfied by the 99% probability associated
with Redmayne's "Prisoners" case.

15 In certain cases of profiling patients where the moral and/or practical stakes of the profiling belief
are high, moral and pragmatic encroachers—such as Basu (2019c) and Moss (2018a), among many
others—might also argue that because thresholds of evidence required for permissible profiling
beliefs are raised in line with these raised moral and practical stakes, these profiling beliefs become
epistemically impermissible. On the other hand, equally well-evidenced profiling beliefs with
lower or nonexistent moral and practical stakes might be epistemically permitted.

16 The terminology of AI "beliefs," analogous to human beliefs (although exactly how analogous and
how disanalogous AI beliefs are to human beliefs is something that requires further discussion), is
used in the expert literature on AI. See, for example, Hadley (1991) and Perlis (2000).

17 It is also not clear to what extent the ethics of human beliefs can be applied to ethics of AI beliefs. This is a question that I think deserves further investigation.
18 Also important to note is that even if AI cannot be held morally responsible for holding problematic profiling beliefs about patients, patients might very well be and/or feel morally wronged by these profiling beliefs. Lee in the above case might very well be and feel morally wronged by the fact that an AI has formed a judgment about the likelihood of their having or contracting a socially stigmatized medical condition like HIV based on their perceived membership in a particular marginalized racial group.
19 (Future) AI might in fact be helpfully thought of as incarnations of *Homo economicus* or "Econs," the so-called ideally rational agents who do not suffer from limited processing or memory capacities, with whom the boundedly rational *Homo sapiens* are contrasted (Thaler 2015).

References

Acheson, Donald. 1988. *Public health in England: The report of the committee of inquiry into the future development of the public health function.* London: Her Majesty's Stationery Office.
Basu, Rima. 2019a. The wrongs of racist beliefs. *Philosophical Studies* 176: 2497–2515. https://doi.org/ https://doi.org/10.1007/s11098-018-1137-0.
Basu, Rima. 2019b. What we epistemically owe to each other. *Philosophical Studies* 176: 915–931. https://doi.org/10.1007/s11098-018-1219-z.
Basu, Rima. 2019c. Radical moral encroachment: The moral stakes of racist beliefs. *Philosophical Issues* 29, no. 1: 9–23. https://doi.org/10.1111/phis.12137.
Basu, Rima and Mark Schroeder. 2019. Doxastic wronging. In *Pragmatic encroachment in epistemology,* ed. Brian Kim and Matthew McGrath, 181–205. New York: Routledge. https://doi.org/10.4324/ 9781315168197.
Beeghly, Erin. 2015. What is a stereotype? What is stereotyping? *Hypatia* 30, no. 4: 675–691. https:// doi.org/10.1111/hypa.12170.
Beeghly, Erin. 2021. Stereotyping as discrimination: Why thoughts can be discriminatory. *Social Epistemology* June: 1–17. https://doi.org/10.1080/02691728.2021.1930274.
Begby, Endre. 2021. *Prejudice: A study in non-ideal epistemology.* Oxford: Oxford University Press. https://doi.org/10.1093/oso/9780198852834.003.0003.
Blum, Lawrence. 2004. Stereotypes and stereotyping: A moral analysis. *Philosophical Papers* 33, no. 3: 251–289. https://doi.org/10.1080/05568640409485143.
Carel, Havi and Ian James Kidd. 2017. Epistemic injustice in medicine and healthcare. In *The Routledge handbook of epistemic injustice,* ed. Ian James Kidd, José Medina, and Gaile Pohlhaus, 336–346. Abingdon: Routledge. https://doi.org/10.4324/9781315212043.ch32.
Centers for Disease Control and Prevention. 2020. Disparities in deaths from Covid-19: Racial and ethnic health disparities. https://www.cdc.gov/coronavirus/2019-ncov/community/health-equity/racial-ethnic-disparities/disparities-deaths.html#print (accessed December 16, 2021).
De Graaf, Irene M., Tjeerd Tijmstra, Otto P. Bleker, and Jan M. M. van Lith. 2002. Womens' preference in Down Syndrome screening. *Prenatal Diagnosis* 22, no. 7: 624–629. https://doi.org/https:// doi.org/10.1002/pd.358.
Egan, Andy. 2011. Comments on Gendler's "The Epistemic Costs of Implicit Bias." *Philosophical Studies* 156, no. 1: 65–79. http://dx.doi.org/10.1007/s11098-011-9803-5.
Eidelson, Benjamin. 2015. *Discrimination and disrespect.* Oxford: Oxford University Press. https://doi. org/10.1093/acprof:oso/9780198732877.001.0001.
Fricker, Miranda. 2007. *Epistemic injustice: Power and the ethics of knowing.* Oxford: Oxford University Press.
Gardiner, Georgi. 2018. Evidentialism and moral encroachment. In *Believing in accordance with the evidence: New essays on evidentialism,* ed. Kevin McCain, 169–195. Cham: Springer. https://doi. org/10.1007/978-3-319-95993-1.
Gendler, Tamar Szabó. 2011. On the epistemic costs of implicit bias. *Philosophical Studies* 156, no. 1: 33–63. https://doi.org/10.1007/s11098-011-9801-7.
Hacking, Ian. 1996. The looping effects of human kinds. In *Causal Cognition,* ed. Dan Sperber, David Premack, and Ann James Premack, 351–394. Oxford: Oxford University Press. https://doi. org/10.1093/acprof:oso/9780198524021.003.0012.
Hadley, Robert F. 1991. The many uses of "belief" in AI. *Minds and Machines* 1, no. 1: 55–73. https:// doi.org/10.1007/BF00360579.

Johnson, Gabbrielle M. 2020. The structure of bias. *Mind* 129, no. 516: 1193–1236. https://doi.org/10.1093/mind/fzaa011.

Johnson King, Zoë and Boris Babic. 2020. Moral obligation and epistemic risk. In *Oxford studies in normative ethics, Vol. 10*, ed. Mark Timmons, 81–105. Oxford: Oxford University Press. https://doi.org/10.1093/oso/9780198867944.001.0001.

Kelly, Daniel and Erica Roedder. 2008. Racial cognition and the ethics of implicit bias. *Philosophy Compass* 3, no. 3: 522–540. https://doi.org/10.1111/j.1747-9991.2008.00138.x.

Larson, Jeff, Surya Mattu, Lauren Kirchner, and Julia Angwin. 2016. How we analyzed the COMPAS recidivism algorithm. *ProPublica*, May 23. https://www.propublica.org/article/how-we-analyzed-the-compas-recidivism-algorithm (accessed December 16, 2021).

Lever, Annabelle. 2017. Racial profiling and the political philosophy of race. In *The Oxford handbook of philosophy and race*, ed. Naomi Zack, 425–434. New York: Oxford University Press. https://doi.org/10.1093/oxfordhb/9780190236953.001.0001.

Lippert-Rasmussen, Kasper. 2006. Racial profiling versus community. *Journal of Applied Philosophy* 23, no. 2: 191–205. https://doi.org/10.1111/j.1468-5930.2006.00326.x.

Lippert-Rasmussen, Kasper. 2013. *Born free and equal? A philosophical inquiry into the nature of discrimination*. Oxford: Oxford University Press. https://doi.org/10.1093/acprof:oso/9780199796113.001.0001.

Millett, Gregorio A., John L. Peterson, Stephen A. Flores et al. 2012. Comparisons of disparities and risks of HIV infection in black and other men who have sex with men in Canada, UK, and USA: A meta-analysis. *The Lancet* 380, no. 9839: 341–348. https://doi.org/10.1016/S0140-6736(12)60899-X.

Moss, Sarah. 2018a. *Probabilistic knowledge*. Oxford: Oxford University Press. https://doi.org/10.1093/oso/9780198792154.001.0001.

Moss, Sarah. 2018b. Moral encroachment. *Proceedings of the Aristotelian Society* 118, no. 2: 177–205. https://doi.org/10.1093/arisoc/aoy007.

Mugg, Joshua. 2013. What are the cognitive costs of racism? A reply to Gendler. *Philosophical Studies* 166, no. 2: 217–229. https://doi.org/10.1007/s11098-012-0036-z.

Munton, Jessie. 2021. Prejudice as the misattribution of salience. *Analytic Philosophy* 00: 1–19. https://doi.org/10.1111/phib.12250.

Office for National Statistics. 2021. Updating ethnic contrasts in deaths involving the coronavirus (COVID-19), England: 24 January 2020 to 31 March 2021. https://www.ons.gov.uk/releases/updatingethniccontrastsindeathsinvolvingthecoronaviruscovid19englanddeathsoccurring24january2020to-31march2021 (accessed December 16, 2021).

Perlis, Don. 2000. The role(s) of belief in AI. In *Logic-based artificial intelligence*, ed. Jack Minker, 361–374. Boston, MA: Springer. https://doi.org/10.1007/978-1-4615-1567-8_16.

Puddifoot, Katherine. 2017. Dissolving the epistemic/ethical dilemma over implicit bias. *Philosophical Explorations* 20, suppl. 1: 73–93. https://doi.org/10.1080/13869795.2017.1287295.

Puddifoot, Katherine. 2019. Stereotyping patients. *Journal of Social Philosophy* 50, no. 1: 69–90. https://doi.org/10.1111/josp.12269.

Puddifoot, Katherine. 2021. *How stereotypes deceive us*. Oxford: Oxford University Press. https://doi.org/10.1093/oso/9780192845559.001.0001.

Risse, Mathias and Richard Zeckhauser. 2004. Racial profiling. *Philosophy & Public Affairs* 32, no. 2: 131–170. https://doi.org/10.1111/j.1088-4963.2004.00009.x.

Sackett, David L., William M. C. Rosenberg, J. A. Muir Gray, R. Brian Haynes, and W. Scott Richardson. 1996. Evidence based medicine: What it is and what it isn't. *BMJ* 312 (January): 71–72. https://doi.org/10.1136/bmj.312.7023.71.

Smith, Martin. 2018. When does evidence suffice for conviction? *Mind* 127, no. 508: 1193–1218. https://doi.org/10.1093/mind/fzx026.

Smith, Martin. 2021. More on normic support and the criminal standard of proof. *Mind* 130, no. 519: 943–960. https://doi.org/10.1093/mind/fzab005.

Steele, Claude M. 1997. A threat in the air: How stereotypes shape intellectual identity and performance. *American Psychologist* 52, no. 6: 613–629. https://doi.org/10.1037/0003-066x.52.6.613.

Thaler, Richard H. 2015. *Misbehaving: The making of behavioral economics*. New York: W.W. Norton & Company.

12
BIG DATA AND PUBLIC HEALTH

Derek W. Braverman

Introduction

The use of big data in public health raises conceptual and ethical issues. My primary aims in this chapter are to elucidate these issues from the perspective of the philosophy of public health and to describe the big data methods associated with them.

It is often claimed that we live in the era of big data. But despite its status as popular buzzword, "big data" lacks an accepted definition. Big data is standardly characterized with an assortment of pertinent features, most commonly a list of "v-words." Volume and velocity are the two properties most frequently noted: with big data, we can harness a massive amount of information and computing power to generate, process, and analyze data at an incredible pace. Here, I follow Sabina Leonelli's appraisal of big data "as *large* datasets that are produced in a *digital* form and can be analysed through *computational* tools" (2020). Accordingly, in detailing the big data approach in public health, I address the development and use of large data sets as well as the computational tools that make these data sets so valuable.

In the following four sections, I introduce the conceptual and ethical issues that are the focus of this chapter, using recent applications of big data in public health to illuminate them. First, I consider the view that big data enables a new form of research: data-driven research, in which data, rather than our theories or values, guide the research process. To help characterize the disagreement over the possibility of data-driven research, I describe the creation of several enormous data sets of the sort that purportedly facilitate data-driven public health practice. Second, I outline why certain aspects of the big data approach have led to concerns about privacy, especially regarding health information. Third, I turn to a criticism leveled against some of the computational tools used to analyze large data sets: namely, that they are inscrutable insofar as we cannot understand the process whereby these tools analyze data and yield one output as opposed to another, and so these tools offer limited explanatory insight. To clarify this criticism, I describe one of its typical targets, deep-learning algorithms, and specify applications of such algorithms in public health. Fourth, I explore the contention that implementing big data techniques exacerbates health disparities, contrary to one of the main goals of the public health discipline. Finally, I highlight how each of the conceptual and ethical issues detailed in the prior four sections pertains to the use of big data for omics research.

DOI: 10.4324/9781315675411-15

None of these issues are unique to big data in every respect. Indeed, the roles of theories and values in science, the nature and importance of scientific explanation, and the significance of privacy and inequality are all topics of sustained discussion in philosophy. However, the big data approach in public health presents complications for these notable problems and serves as a salient case with considerable practical consequences. I will not attempt to resolve these problems or construct an exhaustive list of big data methods and their associated challenges. Instead, I hope to provide an overview of the relevance of big data for the philosophy of public health by introducing key big data techniques and the prominent issues they raise that are of particular philosophical concern.

Data-driven research

Human theories and values are standardly taken to affect scientific practice, whether explicitly or implicitly. Consider John Snow's classic study of a London cholera outbreak (Snow 1855). Snow had previously hypothesized that cholera could be spread through contaminated drinking water, doubting the prevailing miasma theory that it was spread through "bad air." By mapping cholera deaths against sources of drinking water, Snow discovered that deaths were clustered around the Broad Street water pump. Snow's research was influenced by the contemporary theories of cholera transmission and the value of preventing disease.

Proponents of data-driven research espouse a mode of inquiry in which scientists investigate the clues that emerge through data analysis, with the roles of theories and values minimized. Big data methods are suggested to bolster the viability of this approach by enabling the construction of accurate, extensive data sets and the production of computational tools that can discern patterns within such data sets. So, to study some subject, scientists can use computational tools to analyze the accumulated data on that subject and allow whatever patterns are thereby identified to serve as the driving factor that directs the course of their research. These patterns could provide evidence for or against existing hypotheses and reveal unexpected associations that could generate new avenues for research or prompt the development of new theories. In this way, scientists can "follow the data" with less reliance on theories and values. A putative benefit of this approach is its capacity to circumvent the effects of scientists' personal biases and any blinkering assumptions of entrenched theories (Leonelli 2012, 2020).

The general view that research can be driven by data is compatible with a number of more specific positions. In the context of public health, data-driven research is often promoted as a complement to conventional methods rather than a radical break with them. However, some contend that data-driven research is not merely a supplement to or advancement upon conventional methods, but instead constitutes a new way to engage in scientific inquiry. On this account, big data facilitates research that is discontinuous with standard methods in that the roles of theories and values can be fully eliminated. Some advocates of this approach maintain that it marks the "end of theory" (Anderson 2008; cf. Pigliucci 2009), establishing a new era of science that will entirely supplant the last (Kitchin 2014).

Others argue that it is neither possible nor desirable to circumvent theories and values altogether via big data techniques (Chin-Yee and Upshur 2019; Leonelli 2014, 2020). On this view, scientific practice is inescapably theory- and value-laden: theories and values constrain various aspects of science, including which questions are assessed as worth investigating, which observations are deemed significant, and which hypotheses are taken to be best confirmed by the current evidence. Thus, theories and values affect scientific practice throughout the research process.

Accordingly, the promotion of data-driven research presents several contested issues. First, there is disagreement about the extent to which using big data methods could potentially reduce the influence of theories and values. In particular, there is disagreement about whether their influence could be fully eliminated. Second, setting aside the feasibility of reducing their influence, there is disagreement about the appropriate roles for theories and values in research with big data: if we could reduce their influence, when should we do so? Third, there is disagreement about the roles that theories and values can and should play for specific applications of current big data methods.

In the remainder of this section, I will describe the construction of large data sets in public health to clarify how theories and values may influence how these data sets are constructed and how the patterns discovered in them are used. The roles of theories and values in the creation and implementation of computational tools will be addressed when algorithms are described in the section on explanation and inscrutability.

Surveys are often used in public health for research and surveillance. For example, in psychiatric epidemiology, surveys are conducted to investigate the etiology and monitor the prevalence of mental disorders. Theories and values could influence what information is sought through a survey and therefore what information is ultimately contained in the data set generated from that survey. A survey whose development is guided by the aim of improving well-being among those with mental disorders would likely include different items from a survey guided by the aim of reducing certain disvalued behaviors associated with mental disorders. What items are included in these surveys might also be constrained by theories about how mental disorders affect well-being and behavior.

The existence of competing theories about the nature of mental disorders presents a challenge for surveys by psychiatric epidemiologists. If physicians employ disparate theories of mental disorders in their diagnostic practices, then basing the calculation of mental disorders' prevalence on a survey of diagnostic rates would be unreliable. Such inconsistent practices were identified as the principal reason for a higher rate of schizophrenia found in the United States than the United Kingdom and the inverse relationship for affective disorders (Sharpe et al. 1974). Recognition of these inconsistencies in practice, among myriad other factors, led to the characterization of mental disorders as discrete categories with operationalized diagnostic criteria in the third edition of the American Psychiatric Association's *Diagnostic and Statistical Manual of Mental Disorders* (*DSM-III*), published in 1980 (Hyman 2021). Now, standardized survey tools that measure the presence of each individual diagnostic criterion are used to calculate the prevalence of mental disorders, avoiding the difficulty posed by physicians' inconsistent diagnostic practices. Still, our ability to determine the prevalence of mental disorders from these surveys depends on how well the diagnostic criteria demarcate mental disorders. This problem is especially salient for conditions like mental disorders about which there are diverse theories and whose diagnostic criteria are contested.

In the past two decades, mental health has been propounded as a public health issue, often with a broad notion of mental health cohering with the definition provided by the World Health Organization (WHO): "a state of well-being in which the individual realizes his or her own abilities, can cope with the normal stresses of life, can work productively and fruitfully, and is able to make a contribution to his or her community" (WHO 2013: 6). Accordingly, well-being itself has become a target of public health surveys. There is great variation in how surveys are used to calculate overall well-being, depending, in part, on which theory of well-being is endorsed. The viability of this science of well-being is disputed (Hausman 2015), though Anna Alexandrova (2017) recommends a version in which the roles of theories and values are made explicit and carefully managed.

So, instead of gathering data bit by bit to investigate specific questions, perhaps what is required for the theory- and value-free vision of data-driven research is the construction of accurate, comprehensive data sets. Then, to study some subject, scientists could analyze the relevant data sets, containing exhaustive information about every aspect of that subject and its associations with all other phenomena of scientific interest. This approach is exemplified by the creation of biobanks. The United Kingdom Biobank, for instance, was launched in 2006 as a repository for biomedical research. It already contains detailed genetic and phenotypic information on 500,000 people, and a project is underway to conduct magnetic resonance imaging (MRI) brain scans on 100,000 of them. Biobanks in China and the United States, as well as biobanks established through international collaborations, store data from hundreds of thousands of individuals, too (All of Us Research Program Investigators 2019; Kinkorová and Topolčan 2018).

Researchers can access these biobanks not only to evaluate particular hypotheses, but also to use computational tools to discover patterns. For example, the first 5,000 MRI scans for the United Kingdom Biobank were analyzed to ascertain any structural changes associated with aging; localized differences in white matter and free water were detected. Once the imaging project is complete, data on participants will continue to be updated, so that information such as the eventual diagnosis of a disease can be linked to the data stored in the biobank. It is hoped that the 100,000 MRI scans will contain patterns that reveal early markers or modifiable risk factors: by 2027, it is expected that about 6,000 participants will develop Alzheimer's disease and 2,800 will develop Parkinson's disease (Miller et al. 2016). This research can be classified as data-driven insofar as it does not depend on theories or values, such as those related to aging, neurological disease, and medical imaging. Instead, whatever patterns emerge from the collected data are used to drive inquiry.

Suppose that the analysis of biobank data pinpoints every pattern that is associated with Alzheimer's disease, setting aside, for a moment, any effects of theories and values on the creation of the biobank and the analysis of its data. Even if every pattern could be imparted to us in an unbiased manner, what scientists do with these patterns may be determined, in part, by the scientists' attitudes toward relevant theories. Whether the patterns are judged as evidence for or against some hypothesis about the nature of Alzheimer's disease could depend on scientists' prior confidence in theories about the etiology, symptomology, and typical progression of Alzheimer's disease. Pursuing further study of one pattern instead of another could depend on scientists' prior views about the functions of the genes, neuroanatomy, and environmental factors associated with Alzheimer's disease. Furthermore, a host of values may influence these decisions, including epistemic values about what constitutes a good scientific theory, moral values about the harms produced by Alzheimer's disease and the benefits of generating scientific knowledge, and social and political values that affect how research is funded. Rather than leaving these decisions to individual scientists, perhaps computational tools will be implemented to guide how the patterns identified through the analysis of biobank data are used.

As data are increasingly stored digitally, the process whereby preexisting data from sources like insurance, government, pharmacy, and school records are converted into data sets fit for public health work has been simplified. Electronic health records (EHRs) are a particularly attractive source of data because they contain a wealth of important health information collected longitudinally and linked to the demographic details of many patients. However, a major hurdle for research with EHRs or other sources with preexisting data is interoperability: roughly, the ability to merge data sets and analyze them together with the same tools (Ehrenstein et al. 2017; Jensen, Jensen, and Brunak 2012). Some challenges for achieving interoperability are practical, such as the use of incompatible data formats as well as variation in how people record the same information in EHRs. But interoperability could also be diminished if different theories related to diagnosis and treatment produce different clinical practices between providers. And values related to patient well-being, patient privacy, and the use of EHRs for billing could influence what information is considered worth recording.

The latest iteration of the Global Burden of Diseases, Injuries, and Risk Factors Study (GBD) analyzed data from 86,249 sources, including EHRs and surveys, to investigate 369 diseases and injuries across 204 countries and territories (GBD 2019 Diseases and Injuries Collaborators 2020). The GBD's primary outcome—the burden of diseases and injuries—is measured in disability-adjusted life years (DALYs). This metric combines loss of life and loss of health by assigning each disease and injury a disability weight from 0 to 1, such that 0 represents full health and 1 represents death. Someone's loss of health due to a disease can then be determined by multiplying the number of years lived with that disease by that disease's disability weight. DALYs have been criticized for concretizing the view that the lives of disabled people are less valuable. Some of the disability weights for the most recent GBD are 0.13 for autism spectrum disorder (ASD) without intellectual disability, 0.187 for complete blindness, 0.215 for complete hearing loss, 0.402 for severe motor impairment, and 0.523 for severe anxiety disorders.

Privacy

Though the precise scope of privacy and what makes it valuable are debated, the imperative to protect personal health information is standardly defended. The adequacy of health privacy is a prevalent concern for the big data approach in public health, since it requires the collection and digital storage of detailed health information. As big data techniques have become more widespread, it has become easier for organizations and governmental agencies to access health information from existing databases or to compile and analyze such information themselves. A notable example of this use of big data is the monitoring of employees by employers on factors from productivity to health. Moreover, personal information, especially health information, has become a profitable commodity, as evinced by the data broker industry. Data broker companies gather and sell health data, enabling targeted advertising for items like pharmaceuticals or other health products.

The protection of privacy may be important for maintaining trust in healthcare professionals and systems. Consider, for example, the development of mobile applications (apps) by governmental agencies for tracking Covid-19. This public health intervention relies on uptake by the public for its success in tracking Covid-19, and so it may be rendered less effective by a lack of trust regarding privacy. But some of these apps require that users allow the monitoring of many of their phones' features, such as their contacts, photos, location data, and microphone (Sharma and Bashir 2020).

Privacy concerns are intensified for stigmatized conditions like mental disorders. Recently, the database of a Finnish therapy center was hacked, compromising the EHRs of around 30,000 patients, including children and public figures. These patients received ransom demands with proof that their information had been stolen and a threat to leak their EHRs online. Several months later, the entire database, containing the patients' complete psychotherapy notes and social security numbers, was released online through anonymous file-sharing services. Soon afterward, the therapy center filed for bankruptcy and permanently closed (Ralston 2021).

Given the importance of protecting the privacy of health information, significant efforts are made to secure databases with health information. Often, data is de-identified, minimizing the number of demographic factors linked to health information, to prevent someone who gains access to the data from connecting the health information to specific individuals. However, advances in data analytics have yielded computational tools that make it easier to re-identify individuals from data sets even after de-identification measures have been applied (Rocher, Hendrickx, and De Montjoye 2019).

Explanation and inscrutability

The analysis of massive data sets, now a common practice in public health, would be infeasible without the aid of computational tools. Computerized algorithms that detect patterns present within large data sets are designed to facilitate this process. Some algorithms can make predictions when provided with new data based on their ability to detect patterns, and they are incorporated into automated systems used for public health research and surveillance. These algorithms are therefore crucial for the big data approach, as noted by Ziad Obermeyer and Ezekiel Emanuel:

> By now, it's almost old news: big data will transform medicine. It's essential to remember, however, that data by themselves are useless. To be useful, data must be analyzed, interpreted, and acted on. Thus, it is algorithms—not data sets—that will prove transformative. We believe, therefore, that attention has to shift to new statistical tools from the field of machine learning that will be critical for anyone practicing medicine in the 21st century. [...] Machine learning will dramatically improve the ability of health professionals to establish a prognosis [... and] will improve diagnostic accuracy.
>
> *(2016: 1216–1218)*

Kirsten Martin makes a similar point, though more pessimistically:

> Algorithms silently structure our lives. Not only in determining your search results and the ads you see online, [... but also] what you will pay, what you read, if you get a loan, [...] if and how you are targeted in a presidential election, if you are fired, and most recently, if you are paroled and how you are sentenced. The insights from Big Data do not come from an individual looking at a larger spreadsheet. Algorithms sift through data sets to identify trends and make predictions. While the size of data sets receives much of the attention within the Big Data movement, less understood yet equally important is the reliance on better, faster, and more ubiquitous algorithms to make sense of these ambiguous data sets. Large data sets without algorithms just take up space, are expensive to maintain, and provide a temptation for hackers. Algorithms make data sets valuable.
>
> *(2019: 836)*

Conventional algorithms strictly follow a set of established rules, and so their behaviors are easily explained. However, machine-learning algorithms that can, in a way, learn for themselves have been criticized as inscrutable. To clarify this criticism, I will describe a conventional algorithm before turning to the use of machine-learning algorithms in public health.

The Epidemiological Catchment Area study (Regier et al. 1984) is often cited as a milestone in the history of psychiatric epidemiology for harnessing the operationalized diagnostic criteria of the *DSM-III*. A standardized process was implemented to collect health information from almost 20,000 participants in five cities in the United States, including data indicating the presence or absence of every individual diagnostic criterion for each mental disorder. To analyze this data, an algorithm was coded to apply the *DSM-III* rules for diagnosis. Accordingly, this algorithm took a participant's data on the presence or absence of each individual diagnostic criterion as its inputs and yielded verdicts on whether the participant met sufficient criteria for the diagnosis of each separate mental disorder as its outputs. Thus, conventional algorithms like this one are produced to expedite public health practice. Since they follow a particular set of programmed rules that fully determine their behavior, there is no mystery as to why they produce the outputs they do.

By contrast, the behavior of machine-learning algorithms is less straightforward. A procedure is used to "train" these algorithms, so that they "learn" to identify patterns. In one technique, machine-learning algorithms are initially provided training data with certain associations already tagged. The algorithm learns to detect the pertinent associations from the training data, preparing it to detect similar patterns when presented with novel data. This sort of algorithm can be used to evaluate medical images. Such algorithms are typically trained on a set of medical images associated with expert clinicians' judgments about those images. Algorithms can thereby learn to recognize patterns that indicate, for example, tuberculosis from chest X-rays or glaucoma from retinal images (Litjens et al. 2017). While validation studies may be conducted to test how well a machine-learning algorithm is performing, such as by comparing the algorithm's success rate with that of clinicians, often it is not possible to determine the exact process whereby an output is generated from an input; we cannot definitively establish if algorithms for image analysis are using the same features that clinicians look for when making assessments, or if the algorithms are picking up on other features.

Some suggest that deep-learning algorithms, an increasingly common type of machine-learning algorithm, are poised to glean exceptionally valuable information from EHRs on account of two of their distinctive characteristics (Miotto et al. 2016; Rajkomar et al. 2018; cf. Prosperi et al. 2018). First, these algorithms can be trained unsupervised, meaning that they do not receive any explicit teaching during the training period, such as through tagging associations for recognition by the algorithm. Instead, these algorithms learn from data sets that have not been modified for training. Unsupervised training thus enables data mining, a process in which algorithms discover unknown and sometimes unexpected patterns hidden in massive data sets (Jensen, Jensen and Brunak 2012). Second, deep-learning algorithms can analyze unstructured data, meaning that they can make use of unaltered data in the various forms already present in the relevant data set. So, one algorithm for EHRs could analyze data, including laboratory results, lists of diagnoses and medications, and patient notes with lengthy blocks of text, without a need to standardize or otherwise adjust this data. The development of deep-learning algorithms that receive unsupervised training and analyze unstructured data can therefore bypass difficulties related to training the algorithms and preparing the data sets, typically labor-intensive procedures frequently noted as the most time-consuming aspects of developing such algorithms (Miotto et al. 2016; Rajkomar et al. 2018). Recent deep-learning algorithms created with data sets comprised of EHRs can make predictions for individuals about the onset of disorders, from myocardial infarctions to schizophrenia (Miotto et al. 2016), as well as the outcomes of hospitalizations, such as mortality and length of stay (Rajkomar et al. 2018).

Machine-learning algorithms, especially those trained unsupervised, are criticized as inscrutable, or as black boxes, insofar as we cannot ascertain various aspects of their functioning (Chin-Yee and Upshur 2019; Leonelli 2020; Prosperi et al. 2018). Often, we cannot determine which patterns an algorithm is detecting to produce its outputs or how the algorithm learned to detect those patterns. Accordingly, inscrutability can hinder evaluations of algorithms by impeding tests for reliability. For algorithms that rely on previously unknown patterns, there may be no expert assessment or other gold standard to which the algorithms' performance can be compared. Furthermore, some algorithms, like those that continue to learn and change after implementation in response to new data, cannot be reproduced. For instance, the disputed performance of algorithms for predicting suicide is one important factor in the disagreement about when to use clinical evaluations of suicide risk, algorithms, or a combination of the two (Kessler et al. 2019). Administering risk prediction algorithms for suicide, especially outside of healthcare settings, presents ethical challenges related to privacy and the appropriate response to an algorithm's determination of risk: Facebook's suicide prevention program, which is no longer operating, sent first responders to the homes of around 3,500 people identified to be at risk of suicide based on Facebook's data (Friesen and O'Leary 2019).

Algorithms themselves offer no explanation regarding the nature of the connection between their inputs and outputs. If an algorithm makes excellent predictions from established patterns, then the relationship between those predictions and patterns could be investigated further, as in an assessment of causality, for example. But that option is precluded if the patterns recognized by the algorithm are unknown and cannot be determined. Thus, inscrutability compounds the difficulty of formulating explanations from the behavior of algorithms.

The importance of providing an explanation may depend on the details of the particular case. For example, algorithms used to respond to the opioid crisis by identifying high prescribers could be considered fully successful if they accurately identify high prescribers, even without yielding any explanation as to why some providers prescribe opioids more than others. By contrast, algorithms that predict hospitalization outcomes like mortality or the onset of a disease could be deemed inadequate if they provide no indication of the nature of the connections between their predictions and whatever patterns they detect. If the patterns these algorithms detect remain unknown, the algorithms' ability to make predictions may have little bearing on attempts to understand why these outcomes and diseases occur and on efforts to reduce the prevalence of these outcomes and diseases.

In addition, machine-learning algorithms are a core component of the vision of data-driven research in which theories and values play no role. Unlike conventional algorithms that merely apply rules devised by people, machine-learning algorithms can learn to detect patterns in data sets without any explicit instruction about those patterns. Some proponents of data-driven research suggest that machine-learning algorithms can therefore avoid the influence of theories and values. A common objection to this perspective highlights that our world is replete with bias and inequality, continuously shaped by the actions of people who are influenced by theories and values. Hence, even an ideal algorithm trained on a data set that perfectly reflects the world as it is would learn from a world molded by human theories and values, and so it might recapitulate existing biases and inequalities. A second objection concerns the theories and values of those who construct machine-learning algorithms, such that design choices that affect the behavior of the algorithms are constrained by the designers' theories and values. A third objection suggests that machine-learning algorithms are constitutively theory- or value-laden: even if the prior two objections are circumvented, algorithms might require the recruiting of theories or values to overcome problems of induction and underdetermination (Johnson, forthcoming; Martin 2019).

The recapitulation of racial biases has been prominently discussed for algorithms that assess the risk of violent recidivism. These algorithms estimate individuals' likelihood of being convicted of a violent crime following release from incarceration. They are frequently used to establish the length of sentences and eligibility for parole, among other purposes. Consider OxRec, an algorithm implemented in multiple countries and freely available for use by any system. The smallest allowable shift in any single risk factor can change OxRec's overall assessment for an individual from low to medium risk or from medium to high risk. Many of OxRec's factors, such as immigrant status and disposable income, are correlated with race in locations in which OxRec is used (Van Eijk 2020). OxRec also includes the diagnosis of any mental disorder as a risk factor. The implementation of algorithms like OxRec thus bears on both mental health and violence, two priorities in contemporary public health. The inclusion of factors like immigrant status and mental disorder diagnosis leads to the concern that these algorithms may exacerbate inequalities, such as health inequalities for racial minorities and people with mental disorders, through an increase in the incarceration of people from groups already more likely to be incarcerated (Massoglia and Pridemore 2015).

Risk factors are selected for these algorithms not because of any explanatory or causal connection with violence, but just because of improvements to predictive capacity. So, individuals whose sentences are lengthened, or paroles denied, due to an algorithm's risk assessment, cannot receive any explanation beyond reference to the algorithm. For example, consider someone who receives a longer sentence due to OxRec's assessment of them as high risk, but who would have been assessed as medium risk if they were not an immigrant, or if they had not been diagnosed with a mental disorder. The explanation available to them is that these factors may not dispose individuals to violence, but their inclusion improves OxRec's predictive capacity. In developing such algorithms, a value-laden decision must be made to strike a balance between false positives and false negatives: decreasing the proportion of individuals falsely categorized as at risk requires increasing the proportion of individuals falsely categorized as not at risk.

Health disparities

Reducing health disparities is routinely affirmed as a central goal of public health practice. Big data enables some forms of public health work that are important for addressing health disparities. For example, big data facilitates research to identify or rule out rare, but serious, adverse events, such as those that may not be detected in the trials that are required for the approval of new medications. Since selective serotonin reuptake inhibitors are used in fewer than 2% of pregnancies and congenital disorders occur in about 3% of live births, studies with hundreds of thousands of participants were required to produce convincing evidence against the frequent warnings that antidepressants could harm fetuses (Ehrenstein et al. 2017).

However, some argue that implementing big data techniques in public health exacerbates disparities instead of dissolving them, due to problems in the techniques like algorithmic bias, along with how the techniques are used in practice. Consider the use of commercial algorithms to determine who is selected for hospitals' high-risk care management programs. These algorithms are designed to predict which patients are most at risk for poor health outcomes, based on those patients' current health information. Those identified as most at risk are enrolled in care management programs, providing them with extra care that has been associated with improved outcomes. The health information of around 200,000,000 people in the United States is analyzed by these risk prediction algorithms every year. One of the most widely used of these algorithms was implemented such that everyone classified above the 97th percentile for health risks was automatically eligible for a care management program. A recent study found that the Black patients in the automatically eligible group had, on average, 26.3% more chronic illnesses than the White patients in the automatically eligible group. This disparity was traced to the algorithm's incorporation of patients' healthcare costs as predictors of health risks: for any given severity of health risks, Black patients receive less expensive care than White patients. Resolving this disparity increased the proportion of Black patients within the automatically eligible group from 17.7% to 46.5% (Obermeyer et al. 2019).

A burgeoning strategy whose effect on health disparities is contested is the use of web apps, and especially mobile apps, for public health research, surveillance, and intervention. Mobile apps are used to monitor various activities of patients, including online activity, behaviors like eating and sleeping, and adherence to medical treatment. Data from these apps can be shared with patients' healthcare providers. These data can also be harnessed for digital phenotyping. Digital phenotypes are constructed by identifying associations between a phenotype of interest and online activity, such as social media use and web searches. Digital phenotypes for health conditions, especially mental disorders, are created to support public health surveillance and predict health outcomes (Torous and Baker 2016). Data for digital phenotypes may also be gathered from chatbots—online algorithms that can converse with individuals—trained to provide therapy or improve mental health (Tekin 2021).

Some suggest that the increasing use of web apps for public health practice may worsen health inequalities if access to particular technology becomes a prerequisite for participating in certain forms of research or receiving certain forms of therapy (Brall, Schröder-Bäck, and Maeckelberghe 2019). Moreover, only a subset of mental disorders may be amenable to therapies provided through a web app, but funding for mental health research is limited. However, it is possible that access to web apps will spread across the world faster than access to more traditional therapies. For this reason, web apps could facilitate research with study groups that are more representative of low-income countries than traditional approaches (Torous and Baker 2016). Furthermore, mobile apps that deliver guidance for healthcare decision-making have been developed for use in resource-limited settings. In addition, apps for medical image analysis, incorporating algorithms like those for detecting tuberculosis from chest X-rays, could enhance the capacity to diagnose certain conditions in resource-limited settings (Williams et al. 2021).

Omics

Instead of studying specific genes, proteins, neural connections, and so forth, scientists in the omics disciplines study all instances of those entities in an organism: human genomics investigates our genetic material in its entirety, proteomics investigates all proteins, and connectomics investigates all neural connections and circuits. The advent of genomics was occasioned by the plummeting cost of sequencing a person's whole genome over the past two decades, from around US$100,000,000 to around US$1,000 (Prosperi et al. 2018). Research enabled by advances in sequencing technology resulted in the American College of Medical Genetics and Genomics' publication of a list of 56 actionable genes in 2013, updated to 59 in 2016. Specific variants of these genes are known to produce disorders for which early intervention is possible. Therefore, if one of these variants is detected as a secondary finding on any genetic test, there is compelling reason to inform the individual being tested so that appropriate action may be taken (Kalia et al. 2017). Advances in genetic sequencing have also enabled direct-to-consumer genetic tests, which present privacy concerns when companies can collect and store consumers' genetic information.

In a genome-wide association study (GWAS), the genomes of groups distinguished by some phenotypic feature, often the presence of a medical disorder, are compared to discover associations between genes and that feature. For example, a GWAS used data from the United Kingdom Biobank to identify 64 loci that may underlie coronary artery disease by comparing the genomes of individuals with versus without coronary artery disease (Van der Harst and Verweij 2018). Given the quantity of data required for a GWAS, algorithms are used for processing the information and ascertaining associations, which can pose problems for reliability. In addition, the algorithms used in GWASs to detect associations do not themselves provide any explanation regarding why or in what way genes and phenotypes are associated. The GWAS process itself does not give any hints at a mechanism of action for a gene's role in a phenotype, but once associations are identified, they can be investigated further (Prosperi et al. 2018; Reimers et al. 2019; Turkheimer 2012).

Research to discover biomarkers of mental disorders has become more common in psychiatric omics, though at present no biomarkers are recommended for use in clinical psychiatry. The search for biomarkers—measurable characteristics like genetic, protein, or neural circuit variants—is prompted by hopes that biomarkers could improve various tasks, such as diagnosis or predicting responses to treatment. In a recent study, a machine-learning algorithm identified nine proteins that together predicted ASD diagnosis on *DSM-V* criteria with 83% sensitivity and 84% specificity in the study population. The authors emphasized their findings' importance for diagnosis: ASD is "difficult to assess in younger children. Early diagnosis is critical because not only are intensive behavioral therapy programs effective in decreasing maladaptive behaviors in many children with ASD, the benefits of early intervention are typically greater the earlier the intervention begins" (Hewitson et al. 2021).

This research could be considered theory-laden in being premised on the contested theory that current diagnostic standards for ASD pick out a distinct mental disorder or medically meaningful category (Chapman 2019). Accordingly, it risks reifying that theory of ASD if biomarker panels developed on the basis of associations with the heterogenous criteria of current standards become a routine means of diagnosing ASD; even without clinical implementation or utility, the mere existence of biomarkers for a category can be interpreted as evidence for the significance of that category (Reimers et al. 2019; Turkheimer 2012). As Steven Hyman urges, "certainly a *DSM* diagnosis must never serve as a 'gold standard' against which the utility of a biomarker is judged" (2021: 24). Furthermore, this research could be considered value-laden in being guided by the perspective that early diagnosis facilitates beneficial behavioral interventions, which have received sustained criticism from autistic people and others for doing more harm than good (Wilkenfeld and McCarthy 2020). Finally, only including boys in the study could reinforce the disparities subsequent to the long-standing exclusion of women from biomedical and epidemiological research, which remains common in ASD research (Mandy and Lai 2017).

Conclusion

The use of computational tools, such as deep-learning algorithms, to analyze massive data sets, drawn from sources like surveys, biobanks, and EHRs, has become more common in public health practice. This approach raises issues of interest to philosophers of public health, including the roles of theories and values in data-driven research, the effects of novel methods on privacy and health disparities, and the relevance of inscrutable algorithms to the aim of scientific explanation. Big data in public health is thus an area in which distinctive applications of notable philosophical issues with considerable practical importance can be explored.

References

Alexandrova, A. 2017. *A philosophy for the science of well-being.* New York: Oxford University Press. https://doi.org/10.1093/oso/9780199300518.001.0001.

All of Us Research Program Investigators. 2019. The "All of Us" Research Program. *New England Journal of Medicine* 381, no. 7 (August): 668–676. https://doi.org/10.1056/NEJMsr1809937.

Anderson, C. 2008. The end of theory: The data deluge makes the scientific method obsolete. *Wired Magazine,* June 23. https://www.wired.com/2008/06/pb-theory/.

Brall, C., P. Schröder-Bäck, and E. Maeckelberghe. 2019. Ethical aspects of digital health from a justice point of view. *European Journal of Public Health* 29, suppl. 3 (October): 18–22. https://doi.org/10.1093/eurpub/ckz167.

Chapman, R. 2019. Neurodiversity theory and its discontents: Autism, schizophrenia, and the social model of disability. In *The Bloomsbury companion to philosophy of psychiatry,* ed. Ş. Tekin and R. Bluhm, 371–390. London: Bloomsbury Academic. https://doi.org/10.5040/9781350024090.ch-018.

Chin-Yee, B. and R. Upshur. 2019. Three problems with big data and artificial intelligence in medicine. *Perspectives in Biology and Medicine* 62, no. 2: 237–256. https://doi.org/10.1353/pbm.2019.0012.

Ehrenstein, V., H. Nielsen, A. B. Pedersen, S. P. Johnsen, and L. Pedersen. 2017. Clinical epidemiology in the era of big data: New opportunities, familiar challenges. *Clinical Epidemiology* 9: 245–250. https://doi.org/10.2147/CLEP.S129779.

Friesen, P. and K. O'Leary. 2019. Machine learning and suicide prevention: Considering context as a guide to ethical design. *Developments in Neuroethics and Bioethics* 2: 167–188. https://doi.org/10.1016/bs.dnb.2019.04.006.

GBD (Global Burden of Disease) 2019 Diseases and Injuries Collaborators. 2020. Global burden of 369 diseases and injuries in 204 countries and territories, 1990–2019: A systematic analysis for the Global Burden of Disease Study 2019. *The Lancet* 396, no. 10258 (October): 1204–1222. https://doi.org/10.1016/S0140-6736(20)30925-9.

Hausman, D. M. 2015. *Valuing health: Well-being, freedom, and suffering.* New York: Oxford University Press. https://doi.org/10.1093/acprof:oso/9780190233181.001.0001.

Hewitson, L., J. A. Mathews, M. Devlin, C. Schutte, J. Lee, and D. C. German. 2021. Blood biomarker discovery for autism spectrum disorder: A proteomic analysis. *PLoS ONE* 16, no. 2: e0246581. https://doi.org/10.1371/journal.pone.0246581.

Hyman, S. E. 2021. Psychiatric disorders: Grounded in human biology but not natural kinds. *Perspectives in Biology and Medicine* 64, no. 1: 6–28. https://doi.org/10.1353/pbm.2021.0002.

Jensen, P. B., L. J. Jensen, and S. Brunak. 2012. Mining electronic health records: Towards better research applications and clinical care. *Nature Reviews Genetics* 13, no. 6 (June): 395–405. https://doi.org/10.1038/nrg3208.

Johnson, G.M. Forthcoming. Are algorithms value-free? Feminist theoretical virtues in machine learning. *Journal of Moral Philosophy.* https://philarchive.org/rec/JOHAAV.

Kalia, S. S., K. Adelman, S. J. Bale, et al. 2017. Recommendations for reporting of secondary findings in clinical exome and genome sequencing, 2016 update (ACMG SF v2.0): A policy statement of the American College of Medical Genetics and Genomics. *Genetics in Medicine* 19, no. 2 (February): 249–255. https://doi.org/10.1038/gim.2016.190.

Kessler, R. C., S. L. Bernecker, R. M. Bossarte, et al. 2019. The role of big data analytics in predicting suicide. In *Personalized psychiatry: Big data analytics in mental health,* ed. I. C. Passos, B. Mwangi, and F. Kapczinski, 77–98. Cham: Springer. https://doi.org/10.1007/978-3-030-03553-2_5.

Kinkorová, J., and O. Topolčan. 2018. Biobanks in Horizon 2020: Sustainability and attractive perspectives. *The EPMA Journal* 9, no. 4 (December): 345–353. https://doi.org/10.1007/s13167-018-0153-7.

Kitchin, R. 2014. Big Data, new epistemologies and paradigm shifts. *Big Data & Society* 1: 2053951714528481. https://doi.org/10.1177/2053951714528481.

Leonelli, S, ed. 2012. Data-driven research in the biological and biomedical sciences. Special section, *Studies in History and Philosophy of Science Part C: Studies in History and Philosophy of Biological and Biomedical Sciences* 43, no. 1 (March): 1–87. https://www.sciencedirect.com/journal/studies-in-history-and-philosophy-of-science-part-c-studies-in-history-and-philosophy-of-biological-and-biomedical-sciences/vol/43/issue/1 (accessed December 16, 2021).

Leonelli, S. 2014. What difference does quantity make? On the epistemology of Big Data in biology. *Big Data & Society* 1: 2053951714534395. https://doi.org/10.1177/2053951714534395.

Leonelli, S. 2020. Scientific research and big data. In *The Stanford encyclopedia of philosophy*, ed. E. N. Zalta. https://plato.stanford.edu/entries/science-big-data/.

Litjens, G., T. Kooi, B. E. Bejnordi et al. 2017. A survey on deep learning in medical image analysis. *Medical Image Analysis* 42 (December): 60–88. https://doi.org/10.1016/j.media.2017.07.005.

Mandy, W. and M.-C. Lai, eds. 2017. Women and girls on the autism spectrum. Special issue, *Autism* 21, no. 6 (August): 643–808. https://journals.sagepub.com/toc/auta/21/6 (accessed December 16, 2021).

Martin, K. 2019. Ethical implications and accountability of algorithms. *Journal of Business Ethics* 160, no. 4 (December): 835–850. https://doi.org/10.1007/s10551-018-3921-3.

Massoglia, M. and W. A. Pridemore. 2015. Incarceration and health. *Annual Review of Sociology* 41: 291–310. https://doi.org/10.1146/annurev-soc-073014-112326.

Miller, K. L., F. Alfaro-Almagro, N. K. Bangerter et al. 2016. Multimodal population brain imaging in the UK Biobank prospective epidemiological study. *Nature Neuroscience* 19, no. 11 (November): 1523–1536. https://doi.org/10.1038/nn.4393.

Miotto, R., L. Li, B. A. Kidd, and J. T. Dudley. 2016. Deep patient: An unsupervised representation to predict the future of patients from the electronic health records. *Scientific Reports* 6: 26094. https://doi.org/10.1038/srep26094.

Obermeyer, Z. and E. J. Emanuel. 2016. Predicting the future: Big data, machine learning, and clinical medicine. *New England Journal of Medicine* 375, no. 13 (September): 1216–1219. https://doi.org/10.1056/NEJMp1606181.

Obermeyer, Z., B. Powers, C. Vogeli, and S. Mullainathan. 2019. Dissecting racial bias in an algorithm used to manage the health of populations. *Science* 366, no. 6464 (October): 447–453. https://doi.org/10.1126/science.aax2342.

Pigliucci, M. 2009. The end of theory in science? *EMBO Reports* 10, no. 6 (June): 534. https://doi.org/10.1038/embor.2009.111.

Prosperi, M., J. S. Min, J. Bian, and F. Modave. 2018. Big data hurdles in precision medicine and precision public health. *BMC Medical Informatics and Decision Making* 18: 139. https://doi.org/10.1186/s12911-018-0719-2.

Rajkomar, A., E. Oren, K. Chen et al. 2018. Scalable and accurate deep learning with electronic health records. *npj Digital Medicine* 1: 18. https://doi.org/10.1038/s41746-018-0029-1.

Ralston, W. 2021. They told their therapists everything: Hackers leaked it all. *Wired Magazine*, May 4. https://www.wired.com/story/vastaamo-psychotherapy-patients-hack-data-breach/ (accessed December 16, 2021).

Regier, D. A., J. K. Myers, M. Kramer et al. 1984. The NIMH epidemiologic catchment area program: Historical context, major objectives, and study population characteristics. *Archives of General Psychiatry* 41, no. 10 (October): 934–941. https://doi.org/10.1001/archpsyc.1984.01790210016003.

Reimers, M. A., C. Craver, M. Dozmorov, S-A. Bacanu, and K. S. Kendler. 2019. The coherence problem: Finding meaning in GWAS complexity. *Behavior Genetics* 49, no. 2 (March): 187–195. https://doi.org/10.1007/s10519-018-9935-x.

Rocher, L., J. M. Hendrickx, and Y-A. de Montjoye. 2019. Estimating the success of re-identification in incomplete datasets using generative models. *Nature Communications* 10: 3069. https://doi.org/10.1038/s41467-019-10933-3.

Sharma, T. and M. Bashir. 2020. Use of apps in the Covid-19 response and the loss of privacy protection. *Nature Medicine* 26, no. 8 (August): 1165–1167. https://doi.org/10.1038/s41591-020-0928-y.

Sharpe, L., B. J. Gurland, J. L. Fleiss, R. E. Kendell, J. E. Cooper, and J. R. Copeland. 1974. Comparisons of American, Canadian and British psychiatrists in their diagnostic concepts. *Canadian Psychiatric Association Journal* 19, no. 3 (June): 235–245. https://doi.org/10.1177/070674377401900302.

Snow, J. 1855. *On the mode of communication of cholera*. 2nd edition. London: John Churchill.

Tekin, Ş. 2021. Is big data the new stethoscope? Perils of digital phenotyping to address mental illness. *Philosophy & Technology* 34, no. 3 (September): 447–461. https://doi.org/10.1007/s13347-020-00395-7.

Torous, J. and J. T. Baker. 2016. Why psychiatry needs data science and data science needs psychiatry: Connecting with technology. *JAMA Psychiatry* 73, no. 1 (January): 3–4. https://doi.org/10.1001/jamapsychiatry.2015.2622.

Turkheimer, E. 2012. Genome wide association studies of behavior are social science. In *Philosophy of behavioral biology*, ed. K. S. Plaisance and T. A. C. Reydon, 43–64. Dordrecht: Springer. https://doi.org/10.1007/978-94-007-1951-4_3.

Van der Harst, P. and N. Verweij. 2018. Identification of 64 novel genetic loci provides an expanded view on the genetic architecture of coronary artery disease. *Circulation Research* 122, no. 3 (February): 433–443. https://doi.org/10.1161/CIRCRESAHA.117.312086.

Van Eijk, G. 2020. Inclusion and exclusion through risk-based justice: Analysing combinations of risk assessment from pretrial detention to release. *British Journal of Criminology* 60, no. 4 (July): 1080–1097. https://doi.org/10.1093/bjc/azaa012.

WHO (World Health Organization). 2013. *Mental health action plan 2013–2020*. Geneva: World Health Organization. https://www.who.int/publications/i/item/9789241506021 (accessed December 16, 2021).

Wilkenfeld, D. A. and A. M. McCarthy. 2020. Ethical concerns with applied behavior analysis for autism spectrum "disorder." *Kennedy Institute of Ethics Journal* 30, no. 1 (March): 31–69. https://doi.org/10.1353/ken.2020.0000.

Williams, D., H. Hornung, A. Nadimpalli, and A. Peery. 2021. Deep learning and its application for healthcare delivery in low and middle income countries. *Frontiers in Artificial Intelligence* 4: 553987. https://doi.org/10.3389/frai.2021.553987.

13

MACHINE LEARNING AND PUBLIC HEALTH

Philosophical issues

Thomas Grote and Alex Broadbent

Introduction

The application of artificial intelligence (AI) has a long history in healthcare. However, in recent years, there has been a dramatic surge of interest in using machine learning (ML) algorithms as diagnostic systems or risk-prediction models in clinical environments.[1] Examples range from ML algorithms detecting eye diseases (Gulshan et al. 2016; Yim et al. 2020), as well or even better than clinical experts, to the accurate prediction of acute kidney injury in hospital inpatients (Tomašev et al. 2019).[2]

It is striking that the most frequent examples of ML applications fall into the realm of clinical medicine. Likewise, in the corresponding debate about AI in philosophy of medicine, the emphasis so far lies on the epistemic pitfalls in the collaboration between clinicians and ML algorithms, as well as on issues of patient autonomy (Bjerring and Busch 2020; Grote and Berens 2020). However, especially due to the Covid-19 pandemic, the scope of attention is expanding beyond the clinic. Leading research labs are experimenting with ML methods for epidemiological forecasting and health surveillance (Bengio et al. 2020; Chang et al. 2021; Qian, Alaa, and Van der Schaar 2020). There is reason to be optimistic that ML methods will have more public health applications. Due to social networks, health apps, and smart devices, it has become possible to collect ever-increasing amounts of health-related data on people's lifestyle choices, bodily activity, sleeping and eating behavior, and so on, and this kind of data (sometimes called "big"—see Braverman in this volume) is a good fit for ML approaches. However, since much of the data has been collected for other purposes (for example, identifying consumer preferences), what remains to be settled is how exactly the relevant data can and should be used by ML algorithms to guide public health interventions. Although part of the answer will be technical, philosophical issues also arise, and this chapter offers a guide to some of them.

Setting technical developments aside, we suspect that it is in the public health sector that the larger conceptual and ethical ramifications of ML will really become apparent. Clinical medicine remains mediated by clinicians, whose decisions are a natural target for ML algorithms; and clinicians are trained professionals working within a heavily theorized ethical framework. Public health is much less theorized (as this volume attests) and the implementation of public health interventions is typically more complex, not necessarily enacted by

DOI: 10.4324/9781315675411-16

a single profession with a single code of conduct or hierarchy—in a word, messier. The philosophical issues concerning ML and public health are likely to be complex and will not necessarily bear much relation to those that concern clinical medicine.

Given the lack of prior philosophical literature on ML and public health, this chapter sets out to develop a framework of the key conceptual and ethical issues, by connecting philosophical issues that have already been identified in relation to ML with the aspects of public health we suspect will be salient. In particular, we will focus on the following issues:

1   *Epidemiology and ML:* How might ML methods supplement or even replace traditional epidemiological models? What sorts of public health interventions do ML algorithms facilitate?
2   *Fairness:* How could the use of ML algorithms reinforce/mitigate health disparities?
3   *Privacy:* How can the need for vast amounts of health data be balanced with the privacy rights of citizens?
4   *Googlization:* What novel challenges arise from the intrusion of large tech companies into healthcare?

The chapter is structured as follows. First, we establish terminology and give a brief outline of current research in medical ML. The next section considers potential applications of ML in epidemiology (relating to issue (1) in the list above). We then discuss issues of algorithmic bias and fairness (relating to (2) above). In the following section, we consider issues of data-collection and privacy (relating to (3) above). Finally, we address the political economy of medical ML and its ethical implications (relating to (4) above).

Primer: on machine learning in healthcare

In broad terms, ML algorithms predict an unknown feature (for example, an individual patient's probability of acute kidney injury within a given time frame) from known features (for example, a patient's health records). To establish the mapping between the input and the output, the algorithm generates a model. Crucially, this model is not pre-defined by a developer, specifying how the different input features relate to the output. Rather, this is inferred automatically by the algorithm during the training process, in which it extracts parameters from a training data set. Through this, ML algorithms tend to be more flexible than hand-crafted statistical models or rule-based AI systems when predicting features based on large sets of messy data (Jordan and Mitchell 2015; LeCun, Bengio and Hinton 2015).

The recent surge of interest in applying ML in healthcare can be attributed to three factors: first, medical data are increasingly collected and stored digitally—particularly because of health apps and smart devices, but also through the efforts of researchers to link databases (Bengtsson, Borg, and Rhinard 2019). Second, the computing power of central processing units (CPUs) has grown dramatically. Finally, new classes of algorithms, called deep neural networks (DNNs), have emerged. In deep learning, the model consists of artificial neurons (the basic processing unit) that are hierarchically structured into multiple layers. Deep learning models have been inspired by connectionist models of biological brains, even though there are stark differences in the architecture of deep learning models and biological brains (for an overview, see Buckner 2020). Deep learning has especially exceeded expectations in tasks involving natural language processing and image-recognition, with the latter in particular explaining why it naturally lends itself to applications in healthcare.

Many of the high-profile applications of ML in healthcare can be subsumed under the categories of image-based diagnostic systems and risk-prediction models (see Topol 2019 for a review). In the former case, there are by now dozens of studies reporting on ML algorithms achieving "expert-level" accuracy when detecting diseases by examining medical images. The envisioned role of these algorithms is usually to support clinicians by providing a secondary opinion (Grote and Berens, forthcoming). In the latter case, algorithms are used to monitor patients for the purpose of facilitating timely intervention. While all these developments hold great promise for the application of ML algorithms within clinical settings, there is no such counterpart yet for public health. Indeed, precursors to ML applications in public health, such as Google Flu Trends, have proved somewhat inaccurate—and were abandoned. The basic idea of Google Flu Trends was to predict the influenza activity for different countries by aggregating search queries, which then were compared to a historical baseline of influenza activity in the given region. Inaccuracy resulted from many flu-related searches by people who were not ill but prompted to search by some other "exposure" to the population in question, such as a news story (Butler 2013).

We have already mentioned the "messiness" of public health decision-making, but the contrast bears exploring. There are several reasons why ML algorithms seem to perform better in clinical environments than within a public health context (and further philosophical work might fruitfully clarify these reasons, in a way that could support ML development efforts). ML algorithms tend to be the most efficient if the task that they perform can be easily operationalized and is confined to a narrow domain. In clinical settings, the modalities are usually stable (for example, if the same cameras are used to produce images throughout a hospital), the data has been annotated by medical professionals, and the information provided by the algorithm will be assessed by a clinician (Grote and Berens, forthcoming). In conjunction, these factors act as a professional filter.

By contrast, the domain of public health tends to be less well structured. That said, especially during the global Covid-19 pandemic, public health applications of ML are attracting increasing interest in the computer science community. Pertinent examples involve algorithms used to allocate health resources of hospitals at a national scale (Van der Schaar et al. 2021), epidemiological models to predict patient volume—for the purpose of informing lockdown decisions (Qian, Alaa, and Van der Schaar 2020), and to predict infectiousness for proactive contact tracing (Bengio et al. 2020). We will discuss the wider implications of these developments in subsequent sections.

Despite their staggering predictive capacities, current ML algorithms face some constraints. Two problems that stand out are (non-)interpretability (or opacity) and robustness. The *problem of interpretability* refers to the difficulty of understanding how and why some prediction has been made by an ML algorithm (for reviews, see Doshi-Velez and Kim 2017; Gilpin et al. 2018). It is one thing to base your next chess or Go move on a prediction you do not understand, and quite another to ship vaccines or close a port on that basis. Interpretability failure is due in part to the complexity of deep learning models, which in their current state have billions of parameters. Hence, even if the model parameters were made transparent, the model is bound to be opaque (Creel 2020; Zednik 2019). Opacity (referring to a lack of interpretability) can even arise in simple models, from the fact that there is simply no guide to the interpretation of the model (Sullivan 2020): the computations performed by the network are not programmed by a human, and thus not in any sense given representational content. Therefore, even if a human interpreter can subsequently place a post-hoc interpretation on them, this could be the equivalent of spotting patterns in clouds rather than identifying anything like the "reasoning" that "gave rise to" the answer.

Opacity raises several concerns for the application of ML algorithms within the context of public health. For instance, it is commonly asserted that policymakers should decide according to the best evidence available, although exactly what that is, is another matter (Cartwright and Hardie 2012, 2017). Without understanding why some risk prediction has been made, an assessment of the algorithm's output becomes difficult. Some have argued that public health decision-making in a democratic society requires predictions that have an internalist-style justification, and cannot rely on black boxes (Broadbent 2013). That general proposition may be incorrect: we do not know exactly how anesthetics work, or exactly how tar causes lung cancer; yet, public health policies are sometimes built on such black box causal connections (Broadbent 2011). However, even if the general proposition is incorrect, it may be a matter of degree or context. And the degree of black-boxing in ML-driven public health might still mean that these worries are applicable, where track records are not established, and where the part of the epistemic warrant contained within the black box is large and mysterious (as opposed to being confined to the mechanism of action of a particular pharmaceutical, or the sub-cellular level of cell division). Likewise, opacity might limit the range of possible interventions that follow from said risk prediction, as the underlying causal factors remain elusive. With that in mind, ML researchers are currently exploring ways to render opaque ML algorithms interpretable—most notably by training additional algorithms to post-hoc explain the original model (see Gilpin et al. 2018 for an overview).

The problem of robustness refers to the vulnerability of ML algorithms when deployed in environments differing from training conditions. Many algorithms achieve near-perfect accuracy by overfitting to the training data or by exploiting shortcuts—using antecedent features as predictors (Geirhos et al. 2020). For example, an algorithm might use some artifact (for example, a hook) at the edges of the image as a predictor for pneumonia (Zech et al. 2018). Closely related, ML algorithms are so far unable to capture causal relationships in the data. Once the algorithm gets shown data "outside of the distribution," its performance is likely to decrease significantly. Within the context of public health, the lack of robustness is most concerning with respect to the external validity of ML algorithms. For example, a hypothetical facial recognition algorithm might work well in Tübingen, but this does not mean that it will perform well in Johannesburg. The problem of opacity can compound the problem of robustness: knowing how an algorithm works could be useful (even if neither necessary nor sufficient) for figuring out whether it will work in a new situation.

Machine learning for health monitoring and surveillance

In this section, we discuss the wider implications of using ML algorithms for epidemiological forecasting. The focus here is on the relationship between prediction and causal inference in epidemiological models and how the self-understanding of epidemiology might change through the large-scale use of ML methods.

According to an influential viewpoint paper from Miguel Hernán, John Hsu, and Brian Healy (2019), there are three different types of data-science activities, namely, *description, prediction,* and *causal inference*. In the first case, a data-scientist provides a quantitative summary of features in the world—for example, computing the proportion of individuals with diabetes in a large healthcare database. By contrast, prediction tasks involve a mapping between known features in the world with some unknown feature. Here, a pertinent example would be to predict the risk of hospital admission for patients suffering from Covid-19 based on their health records. Causal inference applications, in turn, involve using features in the data to predict how certain features in the world would change if the world were different—for example, how the mortality in a population would change if they were receiving cancer screening, compared to receiving none. (For more on causal inference, see the chapter in this volume. In relation to ML in particular, see Broadbent and Grote, forthcoming.)

Neat distinctions of this kind are attractive but may be misleading, and it is important for philosophical inquiry to subject distinctions of this kind to critique. Can the world be simply described, with no causal interpretation at all? Does not causal inference imply some degree of prediction, especially if by "causal inference" we mean a counterfactual-based approach (Broadbent 2015; Hernán and Robins 2020)? ML puts these distinctions under particular pressure because it is insensitive to them, and this raises the question—philosophical in character, practical in consequence—of whether they must be enforced on ML.

Among the three types of data-science activities, causal inference enjoys a special status. First, causal inference is intimately linked to the self-understanding of epidemiology, as it is traditionally defined in terms of distribution and determinants of disease—with "determinants" taken to be causes (Broadbent 2013). Second, it is often assumed that causal inference is epistemically superior for important public health purposes, specifically when seeking to understand the outcome of a contemplated intervention. In establishing a causal link between cancer screening and a mortality reduction, policymakers and healthcare professionals are enabled not merely to foretell how things will go in the future, but to develop reliable preventive measures to change the future for the better. An accurate prediction without a causal inference could be the result of more than one causal relationship, including some that do not result in a change in the outcome of interest, as when one pushes the needle of a barometer in hopes of averting a storm.

While ML methods are commonly used for description and prediction tasks, causal inference is—so far—beyond their reach. Furthermore, some proponents of formalizing causal inference (which is a movement unto itself in a number of sciences) are happy to point out the flaws of ML-based prediction models, which they consider merely an exercise in curve-fitting (Pearl and Mackenzie 2018). This raises the question of what exactly the epistemic merits are of ML algorithms in public health, and at the same time puts pressure on formal causal inference frameworks, which seem to be pushing in exactly the opposite direction, methodologically speaking: toward isolating differences in an emulation of the experimental method, and away from complexity, feedback loops, and all the other things that a DNN could make use of.

The idea of ML projects coming up with all kinds of predictive models but nothing that can be used to actually intervene and improve healthcare is, of course, not attractive. This would suggest that a causal constraint on ML research—requiring it to uncover causal structure, or else play a supporting role in a larger causal inference—could save a lot of time and effort. However, it is worth countenancing some of the difficulties that face formal causal inference and contrasting these with the potential of ML applications in those domains. First of all, causal inference requires generating a hypothesis, and selecting variables. But the conceptual framework may be quite inadequate, which could be part of the problem. Is obesity one thing or many? How many kinds of diabetes are there? What is race? If one must settle such questions before investigating a public health problem, as causal inference frameworks require, then one might go wrong before even looking at the data. Such variables are also not readily open to counterfactual treatment: what does it mean to suppose that a given individual might have been of a different race, or even income level? What parts of their history must we adjust to bring about these changes—or must we leave history untouched, and thus model a bizarre, "jerky" world, in which people's skins change color and incomes double or halve instantaneously? The effects of such changes are clearly not what we are after when seeking to assess the impact of race or income on an outcome. The systems in which such features of human life have their effects are also commonly complex, with feedback loops and other features that generally violate the conditions required by formal causal inference frameworks.

The rise of smart devices and health apps yields data concerning a person's psychological state, activity level, eating patterns, and so on—which then can be linked to traditional outcome measures. But most of these linkages will be far short of a causal inference, and it is far from clear that separating them all out and conducting causal research is feasible, let alone the best way to proceed to identify public health interventions. Identifying causal relationships in these heterogeneous types of data can be reminiscent of the search for a needle in a haystack. While ML algorithms so far will not capture causal relationships, they excel in detecting meaningful statistical relationships in heterogeneous data and knowing about these when devising public health interventions is surely positive. Yet, causally constraining ML suggests that we would be better off not knowing.

To better understand the opportunities that ML might provide for public health, consider two examples of ML algorithms, used for the purpose of epidemiological forecasting and health surveillance, developed in response to Covid-19. The first one from Zhaozhi Qian, Ahmed Alaa, and Mihaela van der Schaar (2020) predicts the lockdown policy effects of Covid-19 fatalities in a global context. The basic idea of the algorithm is to treat each country as a distinct data point and then learn the country-specific effects of different policies for the Covid-19 fatality rate. For each country, the algorithm considers social, economic, demographic, environmental, and public health indicators. While models to study the transmission dynamics of viruses are well established in epidemiology—with the SEIR (susceptible, exposed, infectious, removed) model being the most prominent example—Qian, Alaa, and Van der Schaar's model claims to have various advantages over traditional epidemiological models. In particular, it outperforms them with regard to predictive accuracy. More importantly, it can predict the effect of counterfactual lockdown policies—how the fatality rate would change in light of a different hypothetical policy. Hence, the algorithm might be pivotal in informing policymakers on the effects of lockdown strategies. Notably, the authors did not use deep learning techniques, but combined a mechanistic SEIR model with a data-driven Bayesian ML-model.

The other example is an algorithm used for digital contact tracing, developed by Yoshua Bengio et al. (2020). In principle, what the authors did was to train an algorithm to estimate an individual's infectiousness for Covid-19 and to provide a graded risk estimate to other people who have been in contact with that individual. To this end, the algorithm uses a large set of features, potentially available on a smartphone, including an individual's symptoms, preexisting conditions, age, and lifestyle choices. Again, while contact tracing apps have been commonly used by many countries during the pandemic, the algorithm poses an advancement over existing technologies. First, most contact tracing apps model infections as a binary event: if an individual has been infected, it is being recommended to send all his contacts to quarantine. By contrast, Bengio et al.'s algorithm makes probabilistic estimates—enabling more fine-grained recommendations. Moreover, the algorithm also includes privacy-preserving tools, trying to protect the data of individuals from central authorities, who could abuse the relevant information.

The list of potential applications of ML for epidemiological forecasting or health surveillance is non-exhaustive. It must also be emphasized that the algorithms have not been tested in ecologically valid settings. Nevertheless, we are confident that these examples will allow us to draw some initial conclusions of their benefit and limitations for public health. First, both examples are extensions of existing tools in epidemiology, whose predictive capacities are enhanced by ML methods. Moreover, for both applications, the emphasis lies in prediction, as opposed to uncovering causal factors of some health outcome. More sharply put, in both cases, the authors highlight an increase in predictive accuracy as the major advantage over existing health monitoring and health surveillance tools. By contrast, little emphasis is being put on the interpretability/explanation of the models.

What are the wider implications for epidemiology due to the rise of ML applications for health monitoring and surveillance? The answer is inevitably speculative, given that ML applications for epidemiology are still in their infancy. A possible option is that we will see a shift in epidemiological modeling, with prediction trumping over explanation. The alternative might be that researchers will try to blend the predictive prowess of ML algorithms with causal inference: either the algorithm learns to discover causal relationships (known as "causal structure learning" (Schölkopf et al. 2021), or the model is made interpretable by way of coarse-grained causal graphs (Blakely et al. 2020; Naimi and Balzer 2018). While such a blend might be considered the best of both worlds, its technical feasibility remains to be established (see Schölkopf et al. 2021 for a good overview of causal inference methods in deep learning).

Fairness

A major concern in utilizing ML algorithms is that they might lead to unfair treatment of social minority groups (women, certain races, or people of low socioeconomic status). The susceptibility of algorithms to social biases is well documented in computer vision, natural language processing as well as in the domain of criminal justice (Angwin et al. 2016; Buolamwini and Gebru 2018). First studies indicate that the same problems carry over to healthcare (Chang et al. 2021; Obermeyer et al. 2019). Hence, there is a serious threat that the use of ML algorithms exacerbates existing injustices in healthcare.

There are various factors that contribute to unfair algorithmic treatment, with the most pertinent one being data bias: either members of groups that are less visible to researchers, for example, due to being a local minority, are underrepresented in the data or the data shows strong social bias. An algorithm trained with such biased data is likely to underfit for said groups, while overfitting for others. Besides biases in the data, it is also the framing of the problem that the algorithm is supposed to solve, which can put minorities, or groups that are less visible in the data for whatever reason, at a disadvantage (Biddle 2020; Obermeyer et al. 2019).

The desire to reduce this risk has animated an interdisciplinary research program, named Fair ML, which is concerned with defining (mathematical) fairness criteria—for example, equalized odds, calibration, or predictive parity (see Barocas, Hardt, and Narayanan 2019 for a review). The underlying problem, however, is that fairness is not a uniform concept, and non-equivalent notions of fairness will be satisfied by different outcomes in at least some situations. Any account of algorithmic fairness therefore has to take into account the specifics of the medical domain exceedingly well and would have to make considered choices of value.

The problem of algorithmic discrimination in healthcare is showcased by a study from Ziad Obermeyer et al. (2019). The researchers examined an algorithm used to identify which patients will derive most benefit from high-risk care management programs—involving extra primary care appointments or dedicated nurses. For the algorithm, this amounts to a prediction problem: patients with the greatest needs are likely to benefit the most from the program. To make these predictions, the algorithm uses a large set of insurance claims data, containing demographic features, insurance type, medical history, medications, and detailed costs. Notably, "race" was not a feature in the data. The primary objective of the study was to investigate differences in the predictions regarding White and Black patients (the race of data subjects was known to the investigators through the patients' health record, which they also had access to).

A special feature of the study is that the researchers had access to a vast data set, containing information about the algorithm's predictions, its objective function, model, patient data, as well as outcome data. This allowed them to map the inputs and outputs of the algorithm. In total, the study had data from 6,000 patients, self-identifying as Black and 43,000 patients, who self-identified as White, including their risk scores for each patient-year. To measure bias in the algorithm's prediction, the study used "calibration" as a metric of fairness, basically stating that for a risk score to be fair for Black and White patients, it needs to mean the same thing for both groups. Accordingly, the study compared how well the risk scores are calibrated across race with regard to health outcomes. In this vein, the study found that for the same level of algorithm-predicted risk, Black patients are significantly sicker than Whites.

The miscalibration of Black and White patients can be attributed to the fact that the algorithm took the total medical expenditures of patients to predict their health needs. Medical expenditure tracks both health and wealth (among other things). There is a strong correlation between an *individual* patient's health costs and the severity of her illness because the sicker an individual is, the more care she typically needs (or at least is motivated to pay for). However, the ability to pay varies between individuals, and also between groups. Because Black patients in this study were, on average, poorer than Whites, they tended to spend less on healthcare for a given level of illness, effectively leading the algorithm to confuse health status with wealth status and therefore to pronounce sicker Black patients equally as healthy as less sick White patients.

Similarly, race-related biases in the clinician-patient relationship might result in more preventive care measures being recommended to White patients. At the same time, Obermeyer et al. (2019) found that the bias in the prediction can be mitigated by the algorithm using a different predictor (for example, health or avoidable costs). In sum, the study paradigmatically illustrates the different mechanisms through which unfair algorithmic treatment can arise for vulnerable social groups within healthcare. That said, the study does not capture the whole complexity of mitigating biases in a healthcare algorithm—which the researchers acknowledge—particularly because their analysis is confined to Black and White patients. In real world settings, the sex of the patients and additional racial categories would have to be accounted for, just as intersectional categories (for example, Black females might be treated differently by the algorithm than Black males). Overall, this adds to the challenge of uncovering and mitigating the pathways leading to discriminatory treatment.

However, another study by Emma Pierson et al. (2021) shows how ML algorithms might be utilized to mitigate health disparities. Here, the researchers set out to address the problem of higher pain levels experienced by Black osteoarthritis patients at the same "grade" of osteoarthritis according to standard measures. They trained an algorithm to predict the severity of osteoarthritis, training a deep learning algorithm to predict pain from knee X-rays. The Kellgren-Lawrence grade (KLG), a standard radiographic measure for osteoarthritis severity, was developed in the 1950s in White British populations. Pierson and her colleagues trained an algorithm to generate an alternative measure, while using a data set of radiographic images with a higher than usual representation of women, Black people, and people with a low socioeconomic status (although it is hard to imagine that many of them had it harder than the postwar coalminers on which KLG was originally calibrated). They claim that their new radiographic pain measure accounted much better for pain disparities in said groups than KLG. Whether their approach stands the test of time in the way that KLG has, the principle of developing algorithms to update old classification and diagnostic methods has obvious potential applications to reducing various kinds of unfairness.

While the two studies highlight mechanisms of algorithmic unfairness and possible ways for counteracting it, there is still a clear need for a deeper involvement of public health ethics. Most notably, while the different fairness criteria have been loosely inspired by philosophical theories of justice (see Binns 2018), they are by no means full-fledged normative theories. In our view, an important desideratum is to systematically analyze how issues of algorithmic fairness relate to familiar debates between utilitarian and egalitarian approaches to distributional questions in public health (Daniels 2008; Powers and Faden 2008). Consider the algorithm from the aforementioned studies: should their primary aim be to maximize some net good (health)—at the risk of exacerbating health disparities—or should egalitarian concerns regarding race, gender, and socioeconomic status claim center stage (Faden, Bernstein, and Shebaya 2020)? For instance, could it be morally permissible to use an alternative pain measure, which performs better for social minority groups if it is less accurate for White people? Importantly, any such analysis should not limit itself to considering ML algorithms in isolation, but rather address the wider institutional context within which the algorithms are used and how the risk estimates provided by the algorithm affect the final decisions made by medical professionals (Grote and Keeling, forthcoming).

Connected with this is the question how biases in the data can be mitigated, so that it happens to be representative of the target phenomenon. This is a multifaceted problem, given that bias in the data can take many forms. However, allow us to point us out two issues that we deem crucial. The first concerns the use of racial categories, whose epistemic value is heavily contested in different branches of medicine (Valles 2018; Vyas, Eisenstein, and Jones 2020), and particularly in epidemiology (VanderWeele and Robinson 2014). Here, one worry is that racial categories could act as confounding factors, thus leading the algorithm astray. Relatedly, including racial categories might cause representational harm: they could be used to justify unequal treatment of different social groups, thus *naturalizing* injustices in healthcare. The second issue relates to the fair representation of social minority groups in the data. This problem has a long history in medicine, especially due to the underrepresentation of social minority groups in clinical trials and due to socioeconomic barriers in accessing healthcare services (Khan et al. 2020). While underrepresentation could be mitigated through affirmative action policies (for example, social minority groups are incentivized to ex-proportionally share their medical data), this might also impose an unequal burden on them—due to privacy risks, discussed below.

Privacy

The promise of ML for healthcare is inevitably linked to the availability of huge volumes of data. For health monitoring and surveillance algorithms to be effective, it is a prerequisite that the majority of the population uses relevant health apps. East-Asian countries such as Taiwan and South Korea have been hugely successful in containing the first wave of Covid-19 spread—at the cost of their citizens' privacy. For citizens, this risks the potential for social stigma if members of their community know that they have been infected (Zastrow 2020). Crucially, it also gives rise to the worry that governments obtain unduly information on their citizens' private lives, undermining their political freedom.

However, privacy issues in digital technologies are not confined to health monitoring and surveillance technologies. Besides the Covid-19 pandemic, it is especially the prospect of precision medicine that hinges on the availability of large quantities of biomedical data. Likewise, to ensure that the predictive accuracy of a health management algorithm is equal for different social groups, it is pivotal that data from marginalized populations are collected equitably (Price and Cohen 2019). At the same time, the need for medical data raises serious concerns for citizens' informational privacy.

According to an influential view, informational privacy is essentially a kind of control (Menges 2020). In determining how and to what extent to disclose sensitive information regarding private matters, a person has control on how to present themselves to others. Conversely, a loss of privacy allows others to intrude in a person's life. Thus, the moral value of privacy is closely linked to the preservation of a person's autonomy and intimacy (DeCew 2018; Rössler 2004).

Privacy issues are well established in medicine: for instance, confidentiality is considered a key component in the patient–clinician relationship and there is a close link to the protection of privacy and abortion rights (Allen 2021). That said, the advent of Big Data and ML algorithms brings genuine challenges. To provide motivation for the problem, consider digital tracing apps, used to contain the spread of Covid-19. Many require numerous types of access to "contacts, photos, media, files, location data, the camera, the device ID, call information, the Wi-Fi connection, the microphone, full network access, the Google service configuration, and the ability to change network connectivity and audio settings, to name just a few types of access" (Sharma and Bashir 2020, 1666). As a result, various privacy issues arise, including security risks, informed consent, and corporate encroachment, which we discuss below.

Security risks: If health-related data is being leaked to the public, this imposes severe risks on data subjects. For instance, if an employer learns that an employee has a history of depression, this might jeopardize her career prospects. Moreover, as a result of health apps, data is being collected that provides deep insights into the private lives of citizens—how many steps they move (and where), what they eat, what their sleeping patterns are, alcohol consumption, and so on. Crucially, the data not only provides information on health-related matters, but it can also be used to infer consumer behavior or political orientation (Vayena et al. 2015). Hence, the data could be exploited for targeted online manipulation. Lastly, even if the data has been properly anonymized or pseudonymized, there is an underlying worry that ML methods can be used to re-identify people.

Informed consent: It is well established that people hardly ever read the terms of agreement for apps or digital devices. Closely related to this point, the highly abstract nature of privacy issues and relevant harms makes it challenging to comprehend what exactly it is that one is consenting to. Another particular tricky issue concerns the reuse of medical data outside the actual study that a research subject consented to (Barocas and Nissenbaum 2014).

Corporate encroachment: The use of digital health monitoring and surveillance technologies creates dependencies between the public health sector and large tech companies. For instance, Google and Apple partnered in enabling contact tracing for the Covid-19 pandemic—and to assist in privacy and security. As a result, companies holding a monopoly in the digital domain gain access to the sphere of health and medicine—and ultimately to the health data of citizens (Sharon 2020).

While some of these issues can be dealt with through technological *fixes* (for example, privacy-preserving ML methods), or by redesigning informed consent procedures, there are also some substantive normative issues. In particular, it is about how the goods of health and privacy should be weighed. For instance, in the case of data-driven biomedical research, some scholars are exploring the idea of (posthumous) data donation (Krutzinna and Floridi 2019). Most fundamentally, it must be considered how health concerns and privacy rights should be balanced in cases of conflict. Is it possible to design health monitoring and surveillance technologies that account for the privacy rights of citizens? In what situations, if any, should it be permissible for health concerns to override privacy rights? What justifies the axiological priority of health over privacy concerns? While the current debate is standing in the shade of the Covid-19 pandemic, we believe that addressing these questions will prove pressing, even in a (hopefully not too distant) post-pandemic future.

The Googlization of healthcare

What is particularly striking about the advent of ML algorithms is that it is a revolution of healthcare from the outside—as opposed to from within. Looking at many of the breakthrough papers in the field, it is apparent that many of them have been authored by corporate research labs—most pertinently, Google and DeepMind but also Apple and Microsoft. To some extent, the predominance of corporate research labs can be attributed to their superior financial resources over academic institutions: the hardware required to train the algorithms, medical professionals, and especially ML developers are all very expensive. However, the real bottleneck lies in the availability of medical data. Unlike basic research in computer vision, where huge quantities of data can be accessed through publicly available repositories, the access to medical data is heavily restricted because of privacy concerns. Here, large corporations receive privileged access to medical data through collaborations with healthcare institutions. For instance, in the period between 2015 and 2016, DeepMind collaborated with the United Kingdom's National Health Service (NHS) to develop a risk-prediction model for kidney injury. This collaboration has been heavily criticized as it gave the company access to the full health records of 1.6 million people without consulting relevant public bodies, and without the informed consent of individual patients being required. Indeed, the patients were not at all aware that their data were being shared (Powles and Hodson 2017; Sharon 2018).

The privileged access to medical data is also tantamount to a competitive edge. In this way, large tech companies are emerging as a major force in the multibillion-dollar healthcare sector, which so far has been ruled by the pharmaceutical industry. While the challenge to Big Pharma might be welcomed by some, the worry arises that Big Tech could then become the new gatekeeper in the healthcare sector and compound the existing role that financial interests play in directing health research with the problems of "digital capitalism" (Sharon 2016). The perils of industry-funded research have been receiving increased interest by philosophers of science and scholars in science and technology (see Holman and Elliot 2018 for an overview). Here, recurring themes are objectivity, transparency, and reproducibility: for instance, Bennett Holman and Kevin Elliot (2017) use game-theoretic models to show how industry-funded research in medicine introduces intransigent biases in the scientific community—for example, which topics to work on, or how to evaluate the trustworthiness in individual studies—without intentionally corrupting individual researchers. Likewise, it is well documented that there is a reporting bias in randomized controlled trials (RCTs), as only those studies demonstrating a positive effect in a given intervention are being published. It is still uncertain to what extent the same problems hold true for ML research in healthcare, given that only very few RCTs have been conducted yet on medical ML algorithms (see Topol 2020 for an overview). However, particularly the privileged access to medical data raises challenges in replicating ML algorithms. To what extent these issues can be mitigated through more pronounced reporting standards in trials for ML systems still needs to be established.

Another problem we see is in the way scientific results are communicated to the public, considering that many of the high-profile publications of ML applications in healthcare are accompanied by press releases, blog posts, or even videos produced by the public relations (PR) departments of the relevant companies. These publications walk a fine line between science communication and PR work—at the risk of painting an overly rosy picture of the advancements of ML. This potentially poses a threat to public trust in ML applications within healthcare.

Setting ML research aside, the crux of the matter is the larger repercussions for the healthcare sector as a result of the involvement of leading tech companies. In an influential paper, Tamar Sharon (2018) raises concerns about tech companies becoming the new gatekeepers of valuable health data sets and the fact that companies that already control many parts of our personal lives might start setting healthcare agendas. Lastly, the increased influence of technology companies is also important from a justice-related point of view: if much of the relevant research is based on data generated by wearables or health apps, or if public health interventions try targeting citizens through smartphones, then people who cannot afford these devices will be excluded.

Conclusion

In this chapter, we have tried to give an overview of advances in ML, which are potentially shaping the future of public health. To this end, we considered the role of ML in epidemiology, issues of fairness, privacy, and the influence of Big Tech companies on the tech sector. Our considerations are not exhaustive, and neither is it our aim to end this chapter with a pessimistic outlook. However, it is important that a philosophical analysis should not be merely confined to investigating the epistemic advantages of ML algorithms, but also needs to take into account the political economy of implementing said algorithms in healthcare and in public health.

Notes

1 We focus specifically on ML rather than AI more broadly. Much of what we say will apply to AI in general, but the field is so broad that we do not want to overgeneralize. We see ML as being the specific area where public health is likely to be impacted soon, and thus where philosophical questions are most urgent.
2 These algorithms might be seen as useful tools for medical professionals, supporting more accurate diagnoses and timely interventions. But the implementation of ML algorithms might also be seen as revolution from the outside, because the main drivers of medical ML research are large tech companies such as Google or Microsoft, which traditionally do not have a place in biomedical research.

References

Allen, A. 2021. Privacy and medicine. *The Stanford encyclopedia of philosophy* (Spring 2021 edition), ed. Edward N. Zalta. https://plato.stanford.edu/archives/spr2021/entries/privacy-medicine/ (accessed December 16, 2021).
Angwin, J., J. Larson, S. Mattu, and L. Kirchner. 2016. Machine bias: There's software used across the country to predict future criminals. And it's biased against blacks. In *Propublica*. https://www.propublica.org/article/machine-bias-risk-assessments-in-criminal-sentencing (accessed December 16, 2021).

Barocas, S., M. Hardt, and A. Narayanan. 2019. Fairness and machine learning. http://www.fairml-book.org (accessed December 16, 2021).

Barocas, S. and H. Nissenbaum. 2014. Big data's end run around procedural privacy protections. *Communications of the ACM* 57, no. 11: 31–33. http://dx.doi.org/10.1145/2668897.

Bengio, Y., P. Gupta, T. Maharaj et al. 2020. Predicting infectiousness for proactive contact tracing. https://arxiv.org/abs/2010.12536 (accessed December 16, 2021).

Bengtsson, L., S. Borg, and M. Rhinard. 2019. Assembling European health security: Epidemic intelligence and the hunt for cross-border health threats. *Security Dialogue* 50, no. 2: 115–130. https://doi.org/10.1177%2F0967010618813063.

Binns, R. 2018. Fairness in machine learning: Lessons from political philosophy. In *Proceedings of the 1st conference on fairness, accountability and transparency, vol. 81. New York, NY, USA: PMLR (Proceedings of Machine Learning Research)*, ed. Sorelle A. Friedler and Christo Wilson, 149–159. http://proceedings.mlr.press/v81/binns18a.html (accessed December 16, 2021).

Bjerring, J. C. and J. Busch. 2020. Artificial intelligence and patient-centered decision-making. *Philosophy & Technology*. https://doi.org/10.1007/s13347-019-00391-6.

Blakely, T., J. Lynch, K. Simons, R. Bentley, and S. Rose. 2020. Reflection on modern methods: When worlds collide—prediction, machine learning and causal inference. *International Journal of Epidemiology* 49, no. 6: 2058–2064. https://doi.org/10.1093/ije/dyz132.

Broadbent, A. 2011. Causal inference in epidemiology: Mechanisms, black boxes, and contrasts. In *Causation in the sciences*, ed. P. Mckay Illari, F. Russo, and J. Williamson. Oxford: Oxford University Press. https://doi.org/10.1093/acprof:oso/9780199574131.003.0003.

Broadbent, A. 2013. *Philosophy of epidemiology*. London: Palgrave Macmillan.

Broadbent, A. 2015. Causation and prediction in epidemiology: A guide to the "methodological revolution". *Studies in History and Philosophy of Science Part C: Studies in History and Philosophy of Biological and Biomedical Sciences* 54: 72–80. https://doi.org/10.1016/j.shpsc.2015.06.004.

Broadbent, A., Grote, T. 2022. Can Robots Do Epidemiology? Machine Learning, Causal Inference, and Predicting the Outcomes of Public Health Interventions. *Philos. Technol.* 35, no. 14. https://doi.org/10.1007/s13347-022-00509-3

Buckner, C. 2019. Deep learning: A philosophical introduction. *Philosophy Compass* 14, no. 10: e12625. https://doi.org/10.1111/phc3.12625.

Buolamwini, J. and T. Gebru. 2018. Gender shades: Intersectional accuracy disparities in commercial gender classification. In *Proceedings of the 1st conference on fairness, accountability and transparency, vol. 81. New York, NY, USA: PMLR (Proceedings of Machine Learning Research)*, ed. Sorelle A. Friedler and Christo Wilson, 77–91. http://proceedings.mlr.press/v81/buolamwini18a.html (accessed December 16, 2021).

Biddle, J. 2020. On Predicting recidivism: Epistemic risk, tradeoffs, and values in machine learning. *Canadian Journal of Philosophy*, First view: 1–21. https://doi.org/10.1017/can.2020.27.

Butler, D. 2013. When Google got flu wrong. *Nature* 494, no. 7436: 155–156. https://doi.org/10.1038/494155a.

Cartwright, N. and J. Hardie. 2012. *Evidence-based policy: A practical guide to doing it better*. Oxford: Oxford University Press.

Cartwright, N. and J. Hardie. 2017. Predicting what will happen when you intervene. *Clinical Social Work Journal* 45, no. 3: 270–279. https://doi.org/10.1007/s10615-016-0615-0.

Chang, S., E. Pierson, P. W. Koh et al. 2021. Mobility network models of Covid-19 explain inequities and inform reopening. *Nature* 589, no. 7840: 82–87. https://doi.org/10.1038/s41586-020-2923-3.

Creel, K. A. 2020. Transparency in complex computational systems. *Philosophy of Science* 87, no. 4: 568–589. https://doi.org/10.1086/709729.

Daniels, N. 2008. *Just health*. Cambridge: Cambridge University Press.

DeCew, J. 2018. Privacy. In *The Stanford encyclopedia of philosophy* (Spring 2018 edition), ed. Edward N. Zalta. https://plato.stanford.edu/archives/spr2018/entries/privacy/ (accessed December 16, 2021).

Doshi-Velez, F. and B. Kim. 2017. Towards a rigorous science of interpretable machine learning. https://arxiv.org/abs/1702.08608 (accessed December 16, 2021).

Faden, R., J. Bernstein, and S. Shebaya. 2020. Public health ethics. In *The Stanford encyclopedia of philosophy* (Fall 2020 edition), ed. Edward N. Zalta. https://plato.stanford.edu/archives/fall2020/entries/publichealth-ethics/ (accessed December 16, 2021).

Geirhos, Robert, Jörn-Henrik Jacobsen, Claudio Michaelis et al. 2020. Shortcut learning in deep neural networks. *Nature Machine Intelligence* 2, no. 11: 665–673. https://doi.org/10.1038/s42256-020-00257-z.

Gilpin, L. H., David Bau, Ben Z. Yuan, Ayesha Bajwa, Michael Specter, and Lalana Kagal. 2018. Explaining explanations: An overview of interpretability of machine learning. https://arxiv.org/pdf/1806.00069.pdf (accessed December 16, 2021).

Grote, T. and P. Berens. 2020. On the ethics of algorithmic decision-making in healthcare. *Journal of Medical Ethics* 46, no. 3: 205–211. https://doi.org/10.1136/medethics-2019-105586.

Grote, T. and P. Berens. Forthcoming. Uncertainty, evidence, and the integration of machine learning into medical practice. *Journal of Medicine and Philosophy.*

Grote, T. and G. Keeling. 2022 On algorithmic fairness in medical practice. *Cambridge Quarterly of Healthcare Ethics (31), no. 1: 83-94.* https://doi:10.1017/S0963180121000839

Gulshan, V., L. Peng, M. Coram et al. 2016. Development and validation of a deep learning algorithm for detection of diabetic retinopathy in retinal fundus photographs. *JAMA* 316, no. 22: 2402–2410. https://doi.org/10.1001/jama.2016.17216.

Hernán, M. A., J. Hsu, and B. Healy. 2019. A second chance to get causal inference right: A classification of data science tasks. *CHANCE* 32, no. 1: 42–49. https://doi.org/10.1080/09332480.2019.1579578.

Hernán, M. A. and J. Robins. 2020. *Causal inference: What if?* Boca Raton, FL: Chapman & Hall/CRC.

Holman, B. and K. C. Elliott. 2018. The promise and perils of industry-funded science. *Philosophy Compass* 13, no. 11: e12544. https://doi.org/10.1111/phc3.12544.

Jordan, M. I. and T. M. Mitchell. 2015. Machine learning: Trends, perspectives, and prospects. *Science* 349, no. 6245. https://doi.org/10.1126/science.aaa8415.

Khan, S. U., M. Z. Khan, S. Raghu et al. 2020. Participation of women and older participants in randomized clinical trials of lipid-lowering therapies: A systematic review. *JAMA Network Open* 3 no. 5: e205202–e205202. https://doi.org/10.1001/jamanetworkopen.2020.5202.

Krutzinna, J. and L. Floridi, eds. 2019. *The ethics of medical data donation.* Cham: Springer.

LeCun, Y., Y. Bengio, and G. Hinton. 2015. Deep learning. *Nature* 521, no. 7553: 436–444. https://doi.org/10.1038/nature14539.

Menges, L. 2020. A defense of privacy as control. *Journal of Ethics* 25, no. 4: 1–18. https://doi.org/10.1007/s10892-020-09351-1.

Naimi, A. I. and L. B. Balzer. 2018. Stacked generalization: An introduction to super learning. *European Journal of Epidemiology* 33, no. 5: 459–464. https://doi.org/10.1007/s10654-018-0390-z.

Obermeyer, Z., B. Powers, C. Vogeli, and S. Mullainathan. 2019. Dissecting racial bias in an algorithm used to manage the health of populations. *Science* 366, no. 6464: 447. https://doi.org/10.1126/science.aax2342.

Pearl, J. and D. Mackenzie. 2018. *The book of why: The new science of cause and effect.* New York: Basic Books.

Pierson, E., D. M. Cutler, J. Leskovec, S. Mullainathan, and Z. Obermeyer. 2021. An algorithmic approach to reducing unexplained pain disparities in underserved populations. *Nature Medicine* 27, no. 1: 136–140. https://doi.org/10.1038/s41591-020-01192-7.

Powers, M. and R. Faden. 2008. *Social justice: The moral foundations of public health and health policy.* Oxford: Oxford University Press.

Powles, J. and H. Hodson. 2017. Google DeepMind and healthcare in an age of algorithms. *Health and Technology* 7, no. 4: 351–367. https://doi.org/10.1007/s12553-017-0179-1.

Price, W. N. and I. G. Cohen. 2019. Privacy in the age of medical big data. *Nature Medicine* 25, no. 1: 37–43. https://doi.org/10.1038/s41591-018-0272-7.

Qian, Z., A. M. Alaa, and M. van der Schaar. 2020. When and how to lift the lockdown? Global Covid-19 scenario analysis and policy assessment using compartmental Gaussian processes. *Advances in Neural Information Processing Systems* 34. https://arxiv.org/abs/2005.08837 (accessed December 16, 2021).

Rössler, B. 2004. *The value of privacy.* London: Polity.

Schölkopf, B., F. Locatello, S. Bauer et al. 2021. Toward causal representation learning. *Proceedings of the IEEE* 109, no. 5: 612–634. https://doi.org/10.1109/JPROC.2021.3058954.

Sharma, T. and M. Bashir. 2020. Use of apps in the Covid-19 response and the loss of privacy protection. *Nature Medicine* 26, no. 8: 1165–1167. https://doi.org/10.1038/s41591-020-0928-y.

Sharon, T. 2016. The Googlization of health research: From disruptive innovation to disruptive ethics. *Personalized Medicine* 13, no. 6: 563–574. https://doi.org/10.2217/pme-2016-0057.

Sharon, T. 2018. When digital health meets digital capitalism, how many common goods are at stake? *Big Data & Society* 5, no. 2: 2053951718819032. https://doi.org/10.1177/2053951718819032.

Sharon, T. 2020. Blind-sided by privacy? Digital contact tracing, the Apple/Google API and big tech's newfound role as global health policy makers. *Ethics and Information Technology* 23, suppl. 1: 45–57. https://doi.org/10.1007/s10676-020-09547-x.

Sullivan, E. 2020. Understanding from machine learning models. *British Journal for the Philosophy of Science.* https://doi.org/10.1093/bjps/axz035.

Tomašev, N., X. Glorot, J. W. Rae et al. 2019. A clinically applicable approach to continuous prediction of future acute kidney injury. *Nature* 572, no. 7767: 116–119. https://doi.org/10.1038/s41586-019-1390-1.

Topol, E. J. 2019. High-performance medicine: The convergence of human and artificial intelligence. *Nature Medicine* 25, no. 1: 44–56. https://doi.org/10.1038/s41591-018-0300-7.

Topol, E. J. 2020. Welcoming new guidelines for AI clinical research. *Nature Medicine* 26, no. 9: 1318–1320. https://doi.org/10.1038/s41591-020-1042-x.

Valles, S. 2018. *Philosophy of population health: Philosophy for a new public health era.* New York: Routledge.

Van der Schaar, M., A. M. Alaa, A. Floto et al. 2021. How artificial intelligence and machine learning can help healthcare systems respond to Covid-19. *Machine Learning* 110, no. 1: 1–14. https://doi.org/10.1007/s10994-020-05928-x.

VanderWeele, T. J. and W. R. Robinson. 2014. On the causal interpretation of race in regressions adjusting for confounding and mediating variables. *Epidemiology* 25, no. 4: 473–484. https://doi.org/10.1097/EDE.0000000000000105.

Vayena, E., M. Salathé, L. C. Madoff, and J. S. Brownstein. 2015. Ethical challenges of big data in public health. *PLOS Computational Biology* 11, no. 2: e1003904. https://doi.org/10.1371/journal.pcbi.1003904.

Vyas, D. A., L. G. Eisenstein, and D. S. Jones. 2020. Hidden in plain sight: Reconsidering the use of race correction in clinical algorithms. *New England Journal of Medicine* 383, no. 9: 874–882. https://doi.org/10.1056/NEJMms2004740.

Yim, J., R. Chopra, T. Spitz et al. 2020. Predicting conversion to wet age-related macular degeneration using deep learning. *Nature Medicine* 26, no. 6: 892–899. https://doi.org/10.1038/s41591-020-0867-7.

Zastrow, M. 2020. South Korea is reporting intimate details of Covid-19 cases: Has it helped? *Nature.* https://doi.org/10.1038/d41586-020-00740-y.

Zech, J. R., M. A. Badgeley, M. Liu, A. B. Costa, J. J. Titano, and E. K. Oermann. 2018. Variable generalization performance of a deep learning model to detect pneumonia in chest radiographs: A cross-sectional study. *PLOS Medicine* 15, no. 11: e1002683. https://doi.org/10.1371/journal.pmed.1002683.

Zednik, C. 2019. Solving the black box problem: A normative framework for explainable artificial intelligence. *Philosophy & Technology.* https://doi.org/10.1007/s13347-019-00382-7.

PART 3

Distribution and inequalities

14

CAPABILITIES, HUMAN FLOURISHING, AND THE HEALTH GAP

Michael Marmot

Introduction

Amartya Sen's insights have been important to my work in at least four ways: providing intellectual justification for my empirical findings that health can be an "outcome" of social and economic processes; providing insight into the debate on relative or absolute inequality; emphasizing the central place of freedoms or agency in human well-being; and alerting me to the importance of the question of "inequality of what." The last is shameful to admit for someone who had been pursuing research on inequalities in health for two decades before I met Sen in person and in his writings. Could I really be obsessed with health inequalities without recognizing that there was more than one way to think about inequality?

In this Amartya Sen Lecture, I will start by sketching briefly how these seminal ideas of Sen influence what I do.[1] More accurately, I should say how Sen's ideas influence how I think about what I do. For, as just stated, I had been doing it for some time before I encountered Sen's fundamental contributions—I am a doctor and medical scientist, after all. In particular, my research on health inequalities has focused on the social gradient in health, its general-izability, how to understand its causes, and what to do about it. I have pursued this research since 1976 when I began work on the first Whitehall study (Marmot et al. 1978b), and to think about health inequalities more generally (Marmot et al. 1978a). Although I had not used the term "social determinants of health" until later (Marmot et al. 1999), my research on health inequalities fitted that description, along with the research on health of migrants (Marmot, Adelstein, and Bulusu 1984; Marmot and Syme 1976).

I will then illustrate the approach in more detail, drawing on my book, *The Health Gap* (Marmot 2015).

Social determinants of health, inequalities in health, and Amartya Sen

Causal arrows

In 1978, I published my initial paper from the Whitehall Study of British Civil Servants (Marmot et al. 1978b). It was my first clear demonstration of the social gradient in health. Men were classified by their grade of employment and deaths tracked over time. There was an inti-mate relation between employment status and risk of death: the lower the grade of employment,

DOI: 10.4324/9781315675411-18

the higher the mortality rate. This social gradient in health has exercised me ever since—in research, to understand the causes of the social gradient; and in policy, to use evidence to take action on the social determinants of health in order to improve population health and to achieve a fairer distribution of health. In particular, the challenge was to recognize not only that poverty and ill-health are highly correlated, they are, but that the social gradient applies to people who are not poor. People in the middle of the social hierarchy have worse health than those at the top, but better health than those below them. It is easy to think of the various ways poverty can cause ill-health; less easy to think why, among people who are not poor, being a bit above the middle of the social hierarchy is better for your health than being a bit below.

All of this research and policy is based on the overarching view that the causal direction is from social circumstances to health. Such a view is, of course, not the starting assumption of most economists who teach their students that the causal direction is from health to wealth or income. I spent a great deal of space and time discussing this counterview in my book, *Status Syndrome* (Marmot 2004), and elsewhere (Marmot 2013).

In my experience, if your starting assumption is that the causal arrow usually goes from health to wealth that is what you find in your studies. If your starting assumption is that social conditions are determinants of health—here, I share this with health researchers from Hippocrates through Ramazzini, Virchow, Durkheim, and William Farr to those in modern public health—then that is what you find in your studies. It is a frustrating clash of views because data analyses seem not to settle the problem.

Amartya Sen, unusually among economists, but not uniquely, was entirely sympathetic to my view that the social gradient in health was caused by differential exposure to social circumstances through the life course. Indeed, he invited me to various discussions to develop this view.

This debate also applies to inequalities between countries. The Commission on Macroeconomics and Health, for example, urged control of major killing diseases in order to achieve economic growth (Sachs 2001). From my days as an ignorant medical student, I had been speculating that the health of a society was a reflection of how well a society met the needs of its citizens. It was a revelation to come across Amartya Sen expressing this view (Sen 1995). Certainly, my motivation to study medicine was not that if we cured people, they might get rich. Nor was my transition to public health because I thought controlling disease would help societies get richer. No, my view was that we should be improving society, socially and economically, to get better health—not the other way round. Dickensian conditions caused ill-health; it was not that ill-health caused Dickensian conditions of living and working. Amartya Sen, of course, convinced me that the causal direction could go both ways. That said, he became a member of the Commission on Social Determinants of Health (CSDH), which I chaired (Commission on the Social Determinants of Health 2008). I will say more of that in what follows. Before I do, though, Robert Fogel's views are interesting. He thought that improved nutrition led to economic growth, largely because without calories people could not work (Fogel 2000). This could be taken as evidence by both sides of the argument. In my view, nutrition is one of the mechanisms by which the social determinants of health operate—here I am consistent with Thomas McKeown (1976). Alternatively, if the way nutrition contributed to economic growth were through lowered susceptibility to infectious disease, the arrow could be assumed to go the other way. The current sobering observation, though, relates to the Preston Curve (see below): above a national income of about $13,000 per person, adjusting for purchasing power, there is little relation between national income and life expectancy. The relation doesn't go either way, in these richer countries. Or, to put in my terms, to improve health, we need to improve society, not only increase national income.

Relative or absolute inequality

I mentioned Dickens above. Tales of women dying in childbirth; children dying in squalor; young adults with tuberculosis; starvation and unsanitary living conditions; debtors' prisons; and dark satanic mills—there is no difficulty understanding how poverty of material conditions can lead to ill-health and premature death. But the gradient is different. Why, in modern Britain, should civil servants in the middle of the occupational hierarchy have higher death rates than those above them, but lower death rates than those below them? It is difficult to think of being in the middle of the gradient as being somewhat deprived, materially, in ways that damage health. These civil servants all have housing with plumbing and heating, stable jobs in decent offices, and money enough to put food on the table; yet, there is a social gradient in health.

And not just in civil servants. Figure 14.1 shows the social gradient in health in the population of England. The top graph is life expectancy, the bottom disability-free life expectancy. Each dot represents a neighborhood classified on an index of multiple deprivation. The less deprived the neighborhood, the greater the life expectancy and disability-free life expectancy. The gradient runs all the way from top to bottom. Health improved in general over a decade, but the slope of the gradient did not change.

At the bottom of the hierarchy, even in a rich country such as the UK in the first decades of the twenty-first century, material deprivation can damage health. Resort to food banks or choosing between heating your dwelling or eating can certainly be bad for health. But people in the middle can heat *and* eat; why is their health worse than those at the top? This has to relate, surely, to relative inequalities. I seem to be arguing then that absolute inequalities are important when it comes to poverty of material conditions, relative when people are above that threshold of absolute deprivation.

Then I read in Amartya Sen's *Inequality Reexamined:* "Relative inequality in the space of incomes can yield absolute deprivation in the space of capabilities" (Sen 1992: 115).

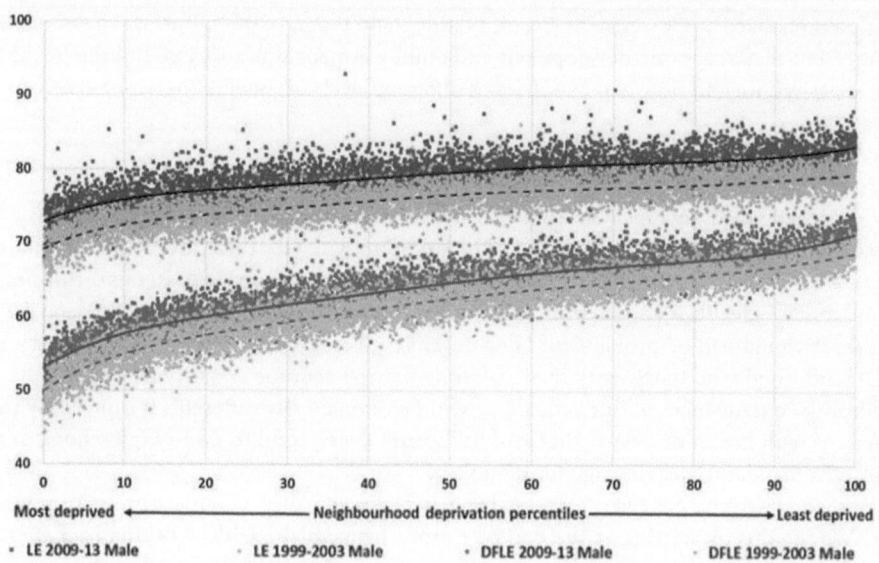

Figure 14.1 Life expectancy and disability-free life expectancy (DFLE) at birth, males by neighborhood deprivation, England, 1999–2003 and 2009–2013 (UCL Institute for Health Equity)

My reformulation of this concise statement: it is not so much what you have, but what you can do with what you have that is important for health. In a low-income country, low income matters because of lack of basic necessities for health and life. In a high-income country, the poor are fantastically rich by global standards, adjusting for purchasing power. But relatively low income matters in so far as it interferes with capabilities—all the things that are necessary for good health, even after the basic needs for food, shelter, and sanitation have been met. One of those central capabilities is having control over your life, and that led me to:

Freedoms and agency

Here, too, I felt like Molière's Bourgeois Gentleman who discovered that he had been talking prose for decades. I had been emphasizing empirical research showing the importance of how much control one had to the risk of getting heart disease or mental illness when I "discovered" Sen. Or, more accurately, he detected me.

One of the puzzles about the social gradient in heart disease was that it contradicted conventional wisdom about stress and the heart. "Everyone knew" that it was more stressful to be in a high-status job and such executive stress was responsible for heart attacks in high-status men. Except that it wasn't true. As the Whitehall studies showed, and numerous studies have confirmed, the lower the employment level, the higher the risk of heart disease and a range of other diseases. The solution to this conundrum came in the form of a model of stress at work that said it was not just demand that was important but also how much control one had over the work (Karasek and Theorell 1990). In the Whitehall II study of civil servants, we showed that low control at work predicted heart disease incidence and, statistically, contributed to the social gradient in heart disease (Marmot 2004).

Perhaps it is something of a stretch to go from low control at work predicting heart disease in British civil servants to a general theory of empowerment as underlying global health inequalities, but the authority of Sen helped. His *Development as Freedom* put agency in central place (Sen 1999). Similarly, Nicholas Stern, former chief economist at the World Bank, emphasized empowerment (Stern, Dethier, and Rogers 2004). Putting these together, I suggested that economic development and empowerment was a way of linking health inequalities within and between countries at different levels of income (Marmot 2006).

Inequality of what?

I have never heard anyone who subscribes to democracy, politician or academic, say that equality of opportunity is a bad thing. The question is whether the conversation should stop there. I have two comments. First, as a doctor, I am interested not only in opportunities but in outcomes—health is an outcome. If genuine equality of opportunity led to inequality in health, it would still be problematic. For example, tossing a coin to decide who stays on in high school and who starts work in a coal mine may be genuine equality of opportunity but the health consequences of this "equality" will be dramatically different. It is precisely those concerns with health outcomes that lead us to want every child to go to high school, and to applaud a mandatory leaving age for school.

A second serious concern is that what passes for equality of opportunity is anything but. We see this by starting at the end of a process, unequal health; working back we may well find that equality of opportunity is a chimera. For example, the higher the income of parents, the greater the life chances of their children, which, in turn, lead to inequalities in health. In certain quarters, such focus on outcomes is dammed as consequentialist. Sen's robust defense of examining capabilities and functionings gives succor to those of us who recognize the central place of health as an outcome.

Philosopher Michael Sandel (2010) suggests three approaches to social justice: maximizing welfare, promoting freedom, and rewarding virtue. Influenced by Sen's formulation of freedoms, and my own work on control or empowerment, I give great emphasis to freedoms. But I emphasize that is not a libertarian notion of freedoms where individuals are left alone but we need social action to create the surrounding social conditions, to quote Sen, for people to lead lives they have reason to value.

The health gap: the challenge of an unequal world

The book I published in 2015 with the above title weaves together three strands of work: a conceptual approach that incorporates what I have just sketched above; an account of empirical work setting out the evidence on social determinants of health equity, explaining the gradient in particular; and a call to action to create fairer societies, based on the best evidence on what can be done.

Social justice and health: creating fairer societies

"Social injustice is killing on a grand scale" is my message to policymakers. So much so that, as a chair, I put it on the cover of the report of the World Health Organization (WHO) CSDH, *Closing the Gap in a Generation* (Commission on the Social Determinants of Health 2008). Our view was that inequalities in health between social groups that are judged to be avoidable by reasonable means, and are not avoided, are unfair—hence health inequities. Our conceptual framework is shown in Figure 14.2. Health and the unfair distribution of health are the outcomes.

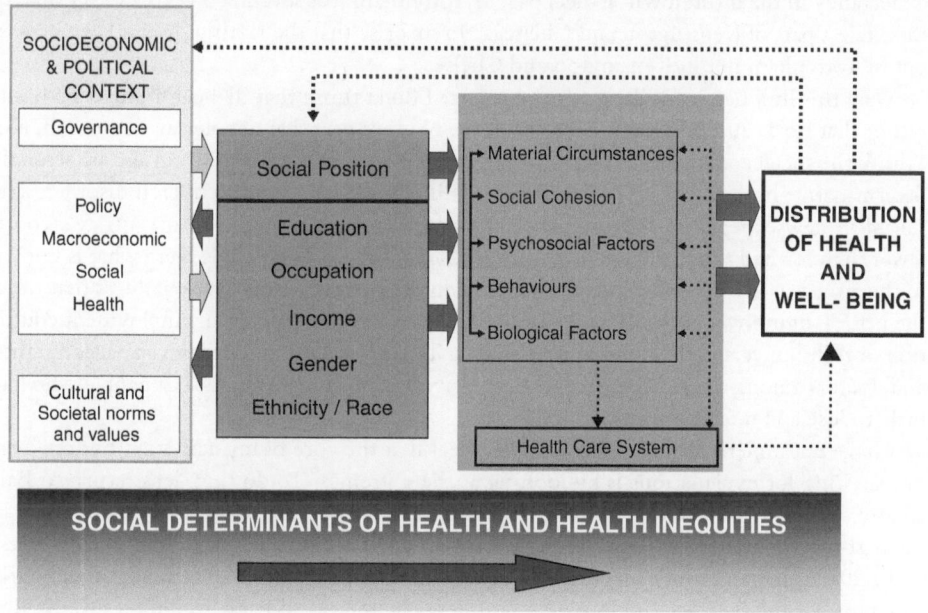

Figure 14.2   Commission on the Social Determinants of Health conceptual framework (World Health Organization)

The starting point for most people when they contemplate inequities in health is a focus on inequities in healthcare. There are undoubted inequities in healthcare, and these must be addressed through universal health coverage, but the social determinants of health framework make makes clear that we have to address the causes of ill-health. This is the message with which I begin *The Health Gap*: what good does it do to treat people and send them back to the conditions that made them sick?

Social determinants, health, and civil unrest

Variations in the conditions that make people sick are in grim display in the US city of Baltimore in Maryland. Such conditions do not lead only to ill-health. In early 2015, Baltimore erupted. Civil unrest broke out. The precipitant of the riots was the killing of a Black man in police custody. Or should I say one more killing of a Black man by the police. But the underlying cause of the riot was inequality of social and economic conditions.

I said Baltimore erupted, but it was one part of Baltimore, the poor inner city, that erupted. I had been studying health inequalities in Baltimore before there was civil unrest. In the poor part, where the riots broke out, life expectancy for men was 63 years. In the richest part, it was 83 years. A twenty-year difference in life expectancy in one city. If you live in the rich part of Baltimore and want to see what it is like to live in a place with male life expectancy of 63, you could fly to Ethiopia. Easier is to travel a short way across town. Life expectancy for men in the poorest part of Baltimore is the same as in Ethiopia, two years shorter than the Indian average.

A link between riots and ill-health is not unique to Baltimore. In summer 2011 in London, riots broke out. They started in Tottenham in North London. Eerily, the precipitant was the killing of a Black man by the police. As with Baltimore, the underlying cause was inequality. I had been pointing to figures on health differences in London. For men, life expectancy in the most down-at-heel part of Tottenham was seventeen years shorter than in the ritziest part of Kensington and Chelsea. No surprise that the rioting should have broken out in Tottenham not in Kensington and Chelsea.

Why this link between ill-health and crime? I don't think that ill-health causes civil unrest or that riots cause ill-health—except in the obvious way that people can be injured. No, I think the social conditions in which people are born, grow, live, work, and age are strongly determinative both of risk of ill-health and of likelihood of engaging in civil disorder. The *Guardian* newspaper reported that of 1,000 rioters going through the magistrate's court, fewer than 9% had a job or were in training; 91% of these young people were what is known in the jargon as NEET—not in employment education or training. Nationally, at that time, the NEET figure was about 10%. A stark contrast: 91% of rioters not in employment education or training versus 10% among non-rioters. There were no trainee lawyers, accountants, and doctors among the rioters, or plumbers, drivers, and shop assistants, but people who had little to lose and uncertain futures.

I have put understanding the gradient in health at the core of my activities, but one way of searching for explanations is by looking at the extremes. To do that, let's return to Baltimore, where men in the worst-off part, Upton Druid, have life expectancy of 63; men in the best-off, Roland Park, have life expectancy of 83. The comparisons of the two are stark.

In 2010, median family income was $17,000 in Upton Druid; $90,000 in Roland Park. In Upton Druid, 50% are single-parent families; 7% in Roland Park. In Upton Druid, 90% of the young people don't go to college; in Roland Park, 75% complete college. In Upton Druid, one third of people aged ten to seventeen are arrested each year for a juvenile disorder. One third each year means that the chance of getting to age seventeen without a criminal record is quite slim. In Roland Park, it was not one third each year but one in fifty.

In theory, the slate is wiped clean at eighteen, no criminal record. In theory. You apply for a job and you are asked if you have ever been in trouble with the police. I suppose you could lie, but that is hardly a good qualification for getting a job. Or you could tell the truth which, given your record, is not a good qualification for getting a job.

Then, there is the American disease: guns. In Upton Druid, over a four-year period, there were 100 non-fatal shootings per 10,000 residents and 40 homicides. In Roland Park, there were no non-fatal shootings and four homicides, one tenth of the rate in Upton Druid.

What these comparisons make clear is that we need to look at the whole of life from early childhood to older age and the life chances that differ so dramatically between areas even within one city. And we need to look at the differences in life chances precisely because the health outcomes are so different.

It is also worth adding that, in some quarters, the poor are blamed for their own ill-health. The argument seems to be that knowledge of the harms of smoking, poor diet, obesity, and alcohol misuse are widely available. If the poor persist in these behaviors, they have no one to blame but themselves. I invite someone who holds this view to go to Upton Druid, and tell a youth who has just been released from police custody, and as a result can't get a job, that he really shouldn't smoke as it might cause heart disease or cancer when he's in his fifties. To put it delicately, he would be given short shrift. We need to address the social determinants of behaviors and of ill-health.

Evidence-based policy on social determinants of health and heath equity

The WHO CSDH was global in scope. We said that it was vitally important for countries, and perhaps cities, to adapt the recommendations of the CSDH into evidence-based policies adapted to national and local contexts. The British government invited me to conduct such a review for one country, England. The Marmot Review, so-called, was published as *Fair Society Healthy Lives* (Marmot 2010). We had six domains of recommendations, the evidence for each of which is dealt with in *The Health Gap* (Marmot 2015):

- Give every child the best start in life
- Education and life-long learning
- Employment and working conditions
- Ensure everyone has at least the minimum income necessary for a healthy life
- Healthy and sustainable places in which to live and work
- Taking a social determinants approach to prevention.

I will illustrate some key points in what follows. Central to my agenda is that the "Marmot Six" provide explanations *and* a basis for action to reduce the social gradient in health as well as to interrupt the link between poverty and ill-health. In each of these six domains, we see social gradients in determinants of health. In what follows, I give examples of the first four. Not that the last two are unimportant. There is ample evidence that inequalities in local environments, including air quality, housing, transport, access to green space, and amenities, will all make contributions to inequalities in health. There is much focus on individual behaviors such as diet and smoking, particularly. One cannot understand the public health impact of these without exploring the social determinants of these behaviors and resultant inequalities.

Give every child the best start in life

What happens to children in the early years has a profound effect on their life chances and hence their health as adults. At the heart of it is empowerment, developing the capacities for, *and* having the conditions that allow, enjoyment of basic freedoms that give life meaning. Early child experiences have a determining influence on that development. Early child development is influenced in part by quality of parenting or caring from others, which, in turn, are influenced by the circumstances in which parenting takes place.

The higher the income of parents, and the more education, the better do their children score on measures of early child development. We have been monitoring early child development in Britain and find that the more economically deprived a neighborhood is, the lower the proportion of children, at age five, that have a good level of development: cognitive, linguistic, social, emotional, and behavioral. There is a clear relationship: more deprivation means worse early child development. But that's not all there is. Pick any given level of deprivation, and you will see that some local areas are doing better than others—they have a higher proportion of children ready for school.

These findings serve as a political litmus test. People on the right politically blame poor parenting; those on the left say it is poverty and deprivation. I say they're both correct. The social conditions in which parents are trying to raise their children affect their ability to be "good" parents.

To test out the contribution of parenting activities to the social gradient in child development, a group of us at University College London analyzed data from the Millennium Birth Cohort Study, a national study in England. Looking at fifths of household income, we saw a clear gradient: the lower the income, the worse the early child development. We then asked mothers of children aged three: was it important to talk to a child? About 20% of mothers denied that talking to a child was important. And this followed the social gradient—the lower the income, the more likely were mothers to deny the importance of talking to a child. We asked: is it important to cuddle a child? Is there anything in the world more fulfilling than cuddling a child? About 20% of mothers denied that it was important to cuddle a child aged three. Talking, cuddling, playing, reading, singing—all those "normal" parenting activities—showed a social gradient: the lower the income, the less frequent these activities.

Our analyses suggested that about a third of the social gradient in linguistic development and about half of the differences in social and emotional development could be attributed to differences in parenting (Kelly 2011).

Think about these findings in relation to a family living in material deprivation. A well-meaning child expert says: you should read bed-time stories to your children. The response might be: I would if I were sure I had a bed, let alone a book. Remember the gradient, though. Families in the middle of the income range were, to be sure, engaging more with their children than the poor, but were engaging less than those with more income.

Finding that good child development is less common in deprived areas suggests one strategy for improving early child development: reduce deprivation and, more generally, inequality. Finding that for a given level of deprivation some areas are doing better than others suggests a complementary strategy: support parents and families. There is evidence of benefit from both strategies.

One measure of deprivation and inequality is child poverty. We can compare countries by looking at the proportion of children living in families whose income is less than 50% of the median. Of course, no society takes poverty as a given. The finance minister can use the tax system to redistribute income. He (ministers of finance are rarely she) can also apportion benefits to the needy: the so-called social transfers. Some countries use these mechanisms more than others and thus policy can have marked differences in its effect on child poverty. I was writing about this for an American publication and wanted to compare the US with another country. I thought if I took Sweden as my comparator, Americans would say Sweden?! A Marxist-Leninist hellhole. So I chose Australia. To some Americans, Australia sounds a bit like Texas. Or perhaps California.

In the US before actions by the minister of finance, 25% of children were in poverty, defined as households at less than 50% of the median national income. In Australia, 28% were in poverty. In the US, after taxes and transfers, poverty levels were reduced just a little, from 25% to 23%. But in Australia, poverty levels dropped from 28% to 11% (Marmot 2015).

The editor of the US publication for which I was writing said: "I think we should take this section out. I think you are talking about redistribution and there is no appetite for that in the US."

I replied: "I *am* talking about redistribution. If there is no appetite for it in America, that is precisely why we should leave it in."

The editor said: "OK. But I don't get it. I know what taxes are. But what are transfers?"

> They're benefits paid.
>
> "Let me see if I understand this," said the editor. "You are saying that in Australia middle-income earners, let's say, pay taxes and that money provides money and services to poorer people?"
>
> Absolutely.
>
> "Really," he said, "some countries actually do that!"

Australia uses taxes and transfers to reduce inequality and child poverty to a far greater extent than the US does. Many countries have a fairer distribution of income and lower child poverty than Australia. In Report Card 13, the latest report on inequalities in child well-being from the United Nations Children's Fund (UNICEF), Australia ranks behind fifteen other countries on child poverty (UNICEF 2016). These countries include Korea and Slovenia as well as the usual suspects: the Nordic countries, Switzerland, Netherlands, Germany, and France.

The complementary strategy is supporting families and children, whatever the level of deprivation. Not long ago, I got on my bicycle and peddled off to Hackney, traditionally a very deprived area in East London. Now, it shows the economic and social gradient in pure culture, ranging from pockets of deprivation all the way to rapidly gentrifying areas where house prices are beyond the reach of mere university graduates. I showed graphs of the link between deprivation and both poor early child development and poor school performance. The head of education said that these figures don't apply in Hackney. She said: "We tell ourselves everyday: poverty is not destiny! We have broken the link between deprivation and poor early child development."

Indeed, they have. One way of looking at family poverty in Britain is to use eligibility for free school meals as a marker for poverty. These children, eligible for free school meals, score worse than the average on various measures of development at the end of the first, reception (kindergarten), year of school. In Hackney, though, the gap is tiny. The difference in early child development between the deprived children and the average is hardly discernible. In more affluent parts of England, however, the gap is huge. Poverty is not destiny. Having quality pre-school services and educationalists who are committed to bringing the performance level of deprived children up to that of the average makes a major difference.

My guess is that in more affluent parts of the country, where deprived children are more of a rarity, they are not geared up to deal with the problem. Poverty is not destiny.[2]

Education

There is much to say on education, the second domain of the Marmot Review. Here, I will confine myself to the observation that first, early child development is a potent predictor of subsequent performance in the education system. Children who score higher on measures of early child development, readiness for school, fare better during their school careers. Further, the Organisation for Economic Co-operation and Development (OECD) showed that PISA scores (Program on International Student Assessment) on maths and science at age fifteen are consistently higher in children who attended pre-school (OECD 2013).

Second, the same sets of drivers of good early child development are also drivers of good school performance: family effects, general socioeconomic forces, and quality of schools and teachers.

Education, of course, is a vital step on the path of achieving both the capacity to control your life, and the conditions of income, employment, and living conditions that make such control more possible.

Employment and working conditions

Empowerment implies having developed appropriate personal resources *and* enjoying the conditions that enable control over one's life. Good early child development and education are key to the first, personal resources. Good employment and working conditions are among the determinants of the second, conditions that allow personal control to be exercised.

In the report of the CSDH, we said that inequities in power, money and resources drive inequities in the conditions of daily life, which, in turn, drive health inequities (Commission on the Social Determinants of Health 2008). Work and employment is one area where inequities in power, money, and resources all play out.

The ultimate work-related disempowerment is unemployment. Of course, when there is an economic downturn, unemployment is not randomly distributed. The more years of education, the lower the likelihood of unemployment, of young people in particular. It is a paradigmatic example of the intersection of effects from early life and current conditions in influencing empowerment. Nor does unemployment strike randomly among populations. Unemployment among 15- to 24-year-olds in Spain was as high as 58%. It is now "only" 43%. In Greece, the figures are even higher, 50% of young people unemployed; in Italy 37%. Society's implied promise to these young people has been broken—grow up, go to school, study, prepare, and then it will be your turn to embark into the world of work, earn your living, and do what every generation has done before.

Globally, the Great Recession of 2007–2009 was disastrous for employment. The International Labour Organisation (ILO) estimates that in 2013 there were over 200 million people unemployed in the world. An economic crisis begun in Wall Street and the City of London is depriving young people of work in North Africa and the Middle East, parts of Latin America and the Caribbean, as well as Southern Europe.

Elsewhere, the real unemployment is hidden. In a country like India, more than 80% of working people are in the "informal" sector. If the economy turns down, they do not go and register with their unemployment office—there is no such thing. They pick up rubbish, clean latrines, and take whatever demeaning work is available. The alternative to work is not unemployment benefits. It is starvation if they do not do whatever it takes to earn a tiny amount of money.

Not usually given to hyperbole, I have described this youth unemployment as a public health time bomb. Unemployment is bad for health and it blights lives. Young people who leave school for the scrapheap are in danger of never getting the habit of work—potentially, they face a lifetime on the margin.

Unemployment is particularly bad for mental health. Some of our politicians claim that unemployment is a lifestyle choice. If so, it is an odd one as it puts people at an increased risk of depression and suicide.

David Stuckler from Bocconi University looked at figures for Europe and showed that a rise in a country's unemployment rate was correlated with a rise in that country's suicide rate. A dramatic finding, though, was that the size of the effect varied according to how generous a country was in its spending on social protection—which included unemployment benefits, active labor market programs, family support, and healthcare (Stuckler et al. 2009).

The analysis was a bit complex, but the conclusion was straightforward: unemployment damages mental health so severely that it can even lead to suicide, but government policies can make a difference.

Work, too, can be disempowering. Earlier, I described findings from the Whitehall II study of British civil servants that low control was related in a graded way to position in the employment hierarchy: the lower the position, the less control entailed in the job. This systematic link accounts in part for progressively higher rates of heart disease and mental illness, the lower the position in the hierarchy.

There is a large body of research that points to the pathogenic effects of psychosocial work characteristics: high demand and low control, imbalance between effort and rewards, organizational injustice, shift work, job insecurity. Each of these has been shown to be linked with an increased risk of ill-health. Each of these tends to follow the social gradient: progressively worse the lower the social position (Marmot 2015).

Inequities in money

I endorsed Amartya Sen's formulation that relative inequalities in income can yield absolute inequalities in capabilities. An important part of the evidence base on health inequalities is that there is more to life than money: early child development, education, living and working conditions are all important. But money will be at the back of at least some of these, particularly at lower levels of income. I have, for example, made clear that child poverty is a potent driver of early child development. Policies to reduce child poverty, *ceteris paribus*, are likely to improve early child development and have a long-term favorable impact on health equity.

One way to reduce poverty should be through work. But inequities in money, alongside inequities in power, play out in the workplace. In the UK, the Joseph Rowntree Foundation monitors in-work poverty—a household below the minimum income threshold where at least one adult is working.[3] In work, poverty has been rising for the last decade—it now exceeds poverty in households where adults are retired or otherwise without work.

In the US, as recovery from the global financial crisis proceeded, for every dollar of economic growth, 92 cents went to the top 1%.

Work, then, should be, but is no longer the way out of poverty. There has been a subliminal message, sometimes more overt, on both sides of the Atlantic that people who are poor are work-shy and hence have themselves to blame. The evidence just cited suggests not that people are poor because they are somehow feckless, but because they are lowly paid.

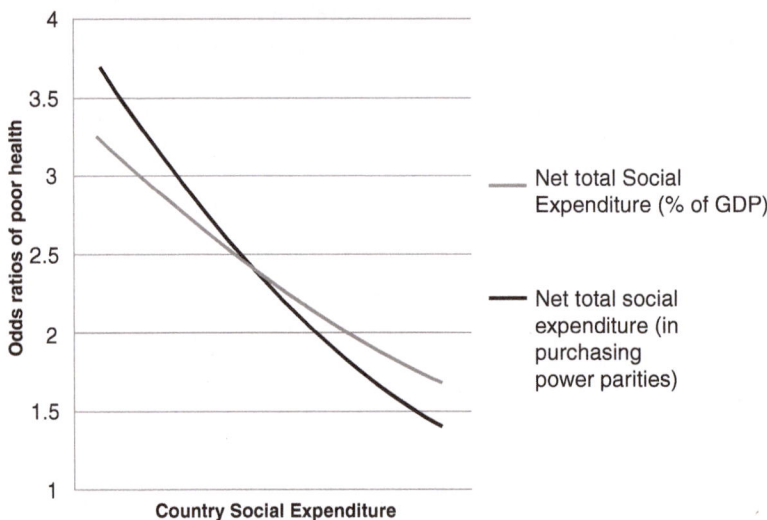

Relative inequalities in health, primary vs. tertiary (women)

Figure 14.3 Shocking news: Welfare spending improves health and reduces inequality (Lundberg et al. 2012)

Part of the narrative about the work-shy is that we should spend less on benefits, on welfare, and hence encourage people back to work. I am in little doubt that work is a better option than subsisting on benefits. But when work is not an option, benefits are important. I reported Stuckler's work showing that the more active a country is with its active labor market programs, including unemployment benefits, the weaker the link between unemployment rates and suicide.

More generally, the more generous a country is in its social spending, the better the health and the narrower the health inequalities. This relationship is shown for European countries in Figure 14.3. The odds of poor health for women with primary education, compared to women with tertiary education, get progressively smaller the more generous the country's social expenditure (Lundberg et al. 2012).

We have lots of evidence, but can we really make a difference to health equity?

There are three answers to this question—all positive. First, one way of posing the question is to reflect that all societies have socioeconomic inequalities. If these give rise to health inequalities, then is it not inevitable that there should be a social gradient in health? Indeed, but the slope of the gradient varies. Figure 14.4 (reproduced in Marmot 2015) shows life expectancy at 50 by level of education for fifteen European countries. As is commonly the case, inequalities in health are smaller in women than in men. Focusing on the men, the gap in life expectancy between those with only primary education and those with tertiary education varies widely across countries: small in Sweden, wide in the former communist countries of

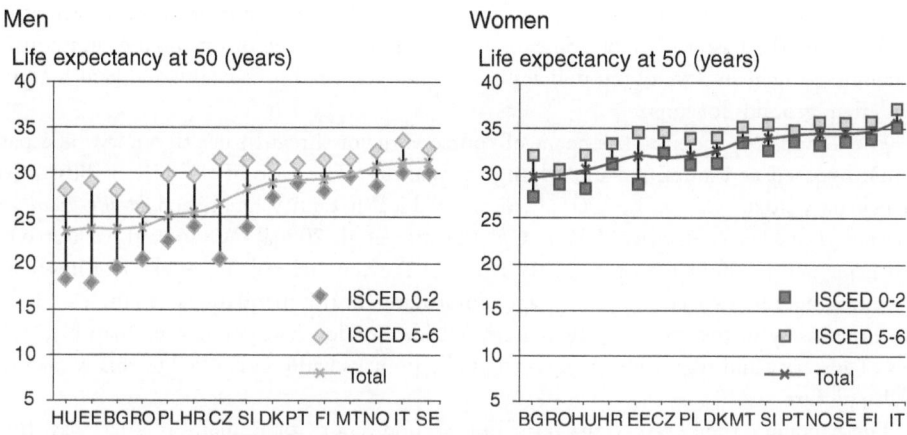

Figure 14.4   Life expectancy for men and women at age 50 (Eurostat 2013)

Central and Eastern Europe. We do not have to accept a steep social gradient as a given. It can be shallow as in Sweden, Italy, Norway, and Malta.

The second answer to the question of whether we can make a difference is that the magnitude of the gradient varies over time. In Brazil, for example, in the 1970s, there was a steep social gradient in stunting—slow growth of children in the first year of life (Victora et al. 2011). Over the next three decades, the gradient became progressively flatter to the point of being barely detectable, a striking social advance.

Third, there have been major reductions in health inequalities between countries. Countries such as Peru, Colombia, and Brazil, which in the 1950s had male life expectancy in the 50s, now have male life expectancy hovering around the 70s; for women, it is higher.

These three answers to the question of whether we can reduce health inequalities and make advances toward health equity are what I describe as my evidence-based optimism. Armed with the evidence and a commitment to social justice and creating the conditions for people to have control over their lives, we can make progress toward health equity.

Postscript, Autumn 2021

A common response when confronted with health inequities, and the realization that they arise not simply from inequalities in access to care, but from the way society is organized, is to be overwhelmed. If health inequity is related to inequity in deep structures of society, perhaps it is too complicated to address. The framework and evidence presented above, influenced by Amartya Sen, provide a structure into which to fit the evidence on social determinants of health and health equity. The recommendations flowing out of this synthesis of evidence, such as the six in the English Marmot Review (above), are manageable in scale. Reduction in child poverty, for example, is a discreet policy that can be implemented easily and is likely to have rapidly beneficial results.

The picture since the WHO CSDH has been mixed—strongly encouraging in some quarters, profoundly challenging in others. On the plus side is the real and developing interest in social determinants of health. Following the WHO CSDH, I have led WHO

Commissions on Social Determinants of Health in WHO's Regions of Euro, the Americas (PAHO) and the Eastern Mediterranean. The fact that these regions wanted to put considerable investment in developing policies on social determinants of health and health equity gives firm grounds for hope.

The Covid-19 pandemic has been, of course, a major threat to health equity. The pandemic exposed and amplified underlying inequalities. The case of the UK is illustrative. In February 2020, we, at the UCL Institute of Health Equity, published *Health Equity in England: The Marmot Review 10 Years On* (Marmot et al. 2020a). We looked back at what had happened in the wake of the 2010 Marmot Review, described above. The news was discouraging. Life expectancy had stopped improving, health inequalities had increased, and life expectancy in the most deprived areas outside London had got worse. Plausibly, policies of austerity and regressive changes to public policies had contributed to this worsening health picture.

The pandemic then crashed upon us. Our second report for England in 2020 was: *Build Back Fairer: The COVID-19 Marmot Review* (Marmot et al. 2020b). We documented the steep social gradient in Covid-19 mortality and increased inequalities in many of the key social determinants of health, notably the increased educational divide and food insecurity. We drew attention to the fact that in the decade prior to the pandemic, the UK had among the worst health improvement of any rich country; during the first half-year of the pandemic, it had the highest excess mortality—a similar picture to the US. We speculated that there may be four levels of explanation for the link between poor health improvement before the pandemic and poor performance during it: quality of governance and political culture; high social and economic inequalities; disinvestment from public services; and poor population health status.

We called our report, *Build Back Fairer*, as we did a subsequent report in the Eastern Mediterranean and Greater Manchester (Marmot et al. 2021). I want to finish this postscript with Greater Manchester, because it illustrates an important point. While national governments are an appropriate level for action on social determinants of health, they are not the only locus for action. Greater Manchester invited us to work with them because the political leadership judged that a city region was a good level at which to take action to improve the conditions in which people are born, grow, live, work, and age. The Eastern Mediterranean report also argues for action at the supranational level. In all cases, what we need is a commitment to social justice and action on the evidence to achieve it.

Notes

1 A version of this chapter was first presented at the Amartya Sen Lecture, at the Human Development and Capability Association Conference in Tokyo in 2016.
2 See the Institute of Health Equity's Monitoring Report—https://www.instituteofhealthequity.org/projects/marmot-indicators-2015 (accessed December 5, 2016).
3 See http://www.jrf.org.uk/data/work-poverty-levels (accessed November 6, 2016).

References

Commission on the Social Determinants of Health. 2008. *Closing the gap in a generation: Health equity through action on the social determinants of health; Final report of the Commission on Social Determinants of Health.* Geneva: World Health Organization.

Eurostat. 2013. *Europe in figures: Eurostat yearbook 2012*. European Commission. https://ec.europa.eu/eurostat/web/products-statistical-books/-/ks-cd-12-001 (accessed December 16, 2021).

Fogel, R. W. 2000. *The fourth great awakening and the future of egalitarianism*. Chicago, IL: University of Chicago Press.

Karasek, R. and T. Theorell. 1990. *Healthy work: Stress, productivity, and the reconstruction of working life*. New York: Basic Books.

Kelly, Y., A. Sacker, B. E. Del, M. Francesconi, and M. Marmot. 2011. What role for the home learning environment and parenting in reducing the socioeconomic gradient in child development? Findings from the Millennium Cohort Study. *ArchDisChild* 96, no. 9: 832–837. https://doi.org/10.1136/adc.2010.195917.

Lundberg, O., E. Dahl, J. Fritzell, J. Palme, and O. Sjoberg. 2012. *Social protection policies, income and health inequalities*. Geneva: World Health Organization. https://www.euro.who.int/—data/assets/pdf_file/0006/302874/TG-GDP-taxes-income-welfare-final-report.pdf (accessed December 16, 2021).

Marmot, M. 2004. *Status syndrome: How your social standing directly affects your health and life expectancy*. London: Bloomsbury.

Marmot, M. 2006. Health in an unequal world. *The Lancet* 368, no. 9552: 2081–2094. https://doi.org/10.1016/s0140-6736(06)69746-8.

Marmot, M. 2010. *Fair society, healthy lives: The Marmot review; Strategic review of health inequalities in England post-2010*. Florence: Leo S. Olschki.

Marmot, M. 2013. Fair society healthy lives. In *Inequalities in health: Concepts, measures and ethics*, ed. N. H. S. Eyal, O. Norheim, and D. Wikler, 282–298. New York: Oxford University Press.

Marmot, M. 2015. *The health gap*. London: Bloomsbury.

Marmot, M. G., A. M. Adelstein, and L. Bulusu. 1984. Lessons from the study of immigrant mortality. *The Lancet* 1, no. 8392: 1455–1458. https://doi.org/10.1016/s0140-6736(84)91943-3.

Marmot, M. G., A. M. Adelstein, N. Robinson, and G. Rose. 1978a. The changing social class distribution of heart disease. *British Medical Journal* 2, no. 6145: 1109–1112. https://dx.doi.org/10.1136%2Fbmj.2.6145.1109.

Marmot, M., J. Allen, T. Boyce, P. Goldblatt, and J. Morrison. 2020a. *Health equity in England: The Marmot review 10 years on*. London: Institute of Health Equity.

Marmot, M., J. Allen, T. Boyce, P. Goldblatt, and J. Morrison. 2021. *Build back fairer in Greater Manchester: Health equity and dignified lives*. London: Institute of Health Equity.

Marmot, M., J. Allen, P. Goldblatt, E. Herd, and J. Morrison. 2020b. *Build back fairer: The COVID-19 Marmot review: The pandemic, socioeconomic and health inequalities in England*. London: Institute of Health Equity.

Marmot, M. G., G. Rose, M. Shipley, and P. J. S. Hamilton. 1978b. Employment grade and coronary heart disease in British civil servants. *Journal of Epidemiology and Community Health* 32, no. 4: 244–249. https://doi.org/10.1136/jech.32.4.244.

Marmot, M., J. Siegrist, T. Theorell, and A. Feeny. 1999. Health and the psychosocial environment at work. In *Social determinants of health*, ed. M. Marmot, and R. G. Wilkinson, 105–131. New York: Oxford University Press.

Marmot, M. G. and S. L. Syme. 1976. Acculturation and coronary heart disease in Japanese Americans. *American Journal of Epidemiology* 104, no. 3: 225–247. https://doi.org/10.1093/oxfordjournals.aje.a112296.

McKeown, T. 1976. *The role of medicine: Dream, mirage or nemesis?* London: Nuffield Provincial Hospitals Trust.

OECD (Organisation for Economic Co-operation and Development). 2013. *PISA 2012 results: Excellence through equity; Giving every student the chance to succeed*, vol. II. Paris: OECD Publishing.

Sachs, J. 2001. *Macroeconomics and health: Investing in health for economic development; Report of the Commission on Macroeconomics and Health*. Geneva: World Health Organization.

Sandel, M. J. 2010. *Justice: What's the right thing to do?* New York: Farrar, Straus and Giroux.

Sen, A. 1992. *Inequality reexamined*. Oxford: Oxford University Press.

Sen, A. 1995. Mortality as an indicator of economic success and failure. UNICEF Innocenti Lecture, Florence.

Sen, A. 1999. *Development as freedom*. Oxford: Oxford University Press.

Stern, N., J. J. Dethier, and H. Rogers. 2004. *Growth and empowerment: Making development happen*. Cambridge, MA: MIT Press.

Stuckler, D., S. Basu, M. Suhrcke, A. Coutts, and M. McKee. 2009. The public health effect of economic crises and alternative policy responses in Europe: An empirical analysis. *The Lancet* 374, no. 9686: 315–323. https://doi.org/10.1016/s0140-6736(09)61124-7.

UNICEF (United Nations Children's Fund). 2016. *Fairness for children: A league table of inequality in child well-being in rich countries.* Innocenti Report Card 13. Florence: UNICEF Office of Research.

Victora, C.G., E. M. Aquino, M. do Carmo Leal, C. A. Monteiro, F. C. Barros, and C. L. Szwarcwald. 2011. Maternal and child health in Brazil: Progress and challenges. *The Lancet* 28, no. 377: 1863–1876. https://doi.org/10.1016/s0140-6736(11)60138-4.

15

MEASURING SOCIAL POSITION IN HEALTH INEQUALITY RESEARCH

Mel Bartley

Introduction

For some time, it has been recognized that research on the social determinants of health is handicapped greatly by the use of poorly defined and understood measures of social position (Krieger, Williams, and Moss 1997; Liberatos, Link, and Kelsey 1988). So it is dismaying that decades later, leading scholars publishing in respected journals are still making comments such as: "Socioeconomic status (SES) is a central measure in social epidemiology, but its use is complicated by the fact that scholars have not agreed on a definition, and probably never will" (Oakes and Andrade 2014: 40), with the result that "different conceptual approaches to SEP and the resultant measurement of it have generated a complex picture including conflicting findings" (Elgar et al. 2015).

In addition to this recognition that socioeconomic status lacks conceptual clarity, Carles Muntaner points out: "Most studies use socioeconomic status indicators such as educational level, occupational class, or even income without any serious consideration of the social mechanisms that link exposure and outcome. This makes for weak ability to examine causality and thereby to propose effective interventions" (Muntaner 2013: 853). M. Maria Glymour, Cheryl R. Clark, and Kristen K. Patton add: "Good measurement of SES at individual, family, and community levels remains a major challenge" (2014: 92) and argue that "to translate this evidence into effective public-health interventions, we need more conclusive evidence on the causal components of highly correlated socioeconomic measures and on the major mediators of inequalities" (Glymour, Clark, and Patton 2014: 92).

This chapter seeks to provide some clarity on what is and is not plausible reasoning regarding the ways in which different dimensions of inequality can plausibly be related to health.

Ideas about social inequality vary widely between nations and cultures. They form a part of the everyday common sense of social life and are deeply embedded in consciousness. What Nancy Kreiger, David R. Williams, and N. E. Moss (1997) and John Goldthorpe (Goldthorpe 1997), Gordon Marshall (Marshall 1997a), and David Rose and colleagues (Rose and Pevalin 2005) called for was a way to measure one dimension of inequality, social class, in a manner that could be replicated and validated across time and place (Rose, Harrison, and Pevalin 2010). This chapter will trace some of the history of inequality measures used in health research, and reflect on the importance of taking a more rigorous approach to measurement.

DOI: 10.4324/9781315675411-19

The Registrar-General's Social Class classification was the measure used in the classical British reports on health inequality between the 1920s and 1990s. This series was the foundation for the present-day research on health inequality, and its use also contributes to the basic explanation for present confusions in research. Understanding a little of this history may help clarify some of the confusion that surrounds the measurement of social position.

Social class measurement in Britain: some history

Marshall et al. have described the Registrar-General's social class schema in the following way: "The scheme embodies the now obsolete and discredited conceptual model of the nineteenth century eugenicists: namely, that of society as a hierarchy of inherited natural abilities, these being reflected in the skill level of different occupations" (1988: 19).

This set of unstated and untested nineteenth-century assumptions underlies one of the most common theoretical frameworks for health inequality research. This framework is itself usually implicit. It combines Francis Galton's ideas on the distribution of "genetic fitness" with the American sociologist Talcott Parsons' functionalist theory of social stratification (Parsons 1953)—well explained by Michael J. Oakes and Peter H. Rossi (2003).

The functionalist theory of social inequality views societies as able to ensure that their most able and energetic members are placed in the jobs most important to the working of the society. These jobs include political and commercial leadership as well as the major professions such as law, church, and the military officer corps. In order to attract the most able into these roles, the rewards of high income and high status are offered (Davis and Moore 1945). Accordingly, the fact that an individual has a high-income and a high-status job is taken as a measure of their underlying *individual* characteristics such as intelligence, conscientiousness, self-efficacy, and so on. In turn, these ideas date back to the work of Galton and the Eugenicists in Britain who saw social structure as a natural order based on the *genetic worth* of individuals as depicted in Figure 15.1.

From this theoretical basis, it is easy to go on to the idea that health inequalities can never be ameliorated, but rather that "increased opportunities for social selection [...] may have made the lower social groups more homogeneous with regard to personal characteristics like low cognitive ability and less favourable personality profiles" (Mackenbach 2012: 766). According to this point of view, intelligence, self-efficacy, and so on are the determinants of health-related behaviors, which, in turn, generate health inequality.

Although this is a rather depressing portrait of society for those interested in public health, it is not an untestable theory and could form one of the *narratives* recommended by Richard Breen and David Rottman (Breen and Rottman 1995). A narrative sets out a clear chain of events and factors that plausibly connect a position in society, clearly defined, to a health outcome. For example, social class and social status are closely correlated. But as we know that status groups resemble each other in many behaviors, such as diet and leisure activity, it makes more sense to emphasize the status dimension when trying to explain social inequality in diseases more closely linked to behavior. In contrast, it is plausible that diseases more closely linked to work stress can be better explained using occupational class. These differences are empirically observed (Bartley et al. 1999; Sacker et al. 2001). Making explicit these differences also leads us to question the pervasive and indiscriminate use of *high* and *low* to describe all measures of social position (social class, social status, socioeconomic status). Although such terms are rarely defined in epidemiology, one suspects that what is *high* or *low* is in some form or another referring to the concept of genetic *worthiness* depicted

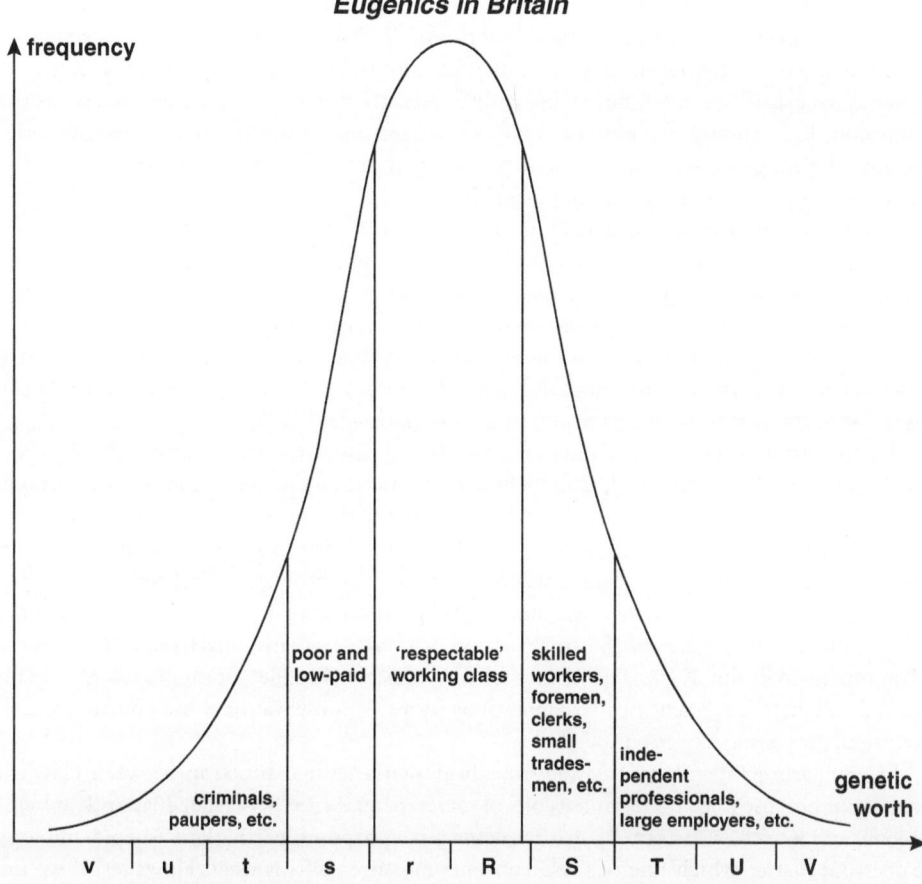

Figure 15.1 Francis Galton's representation of social inequality in the early twentieth century. Creative Commons 4.0 International. https://creativecommons.org/licenses/by/4.0/

in Galton's diagram, and exemplified in recent attempts to discover genetic foundations for both educational attainment and social class (Belsky et al. 2016; Davies et al. 2015; Krapohl and Plomin 2015).

   T. H. C. Stevenson, a leading public health official at the time of Galton, developed a five-level social class schema which we would now recognize as the Registrar-General's classification based on these eugenicist beliefs (see Table 15.1).

Table 15.1 Classification of the Registrar-General's Social Classes (RGSCs) of 1931

Class number	Description
I	Professional
II	Managerial
III	Routine non-manual and skilled manual
IV	Semi-skilled manual
V	Unskilled manual

Leete and Fox (1977) and Szreter (1984) record the way in which the five classes of Stevenson's schema came to be understood in terms of the five divisions in Galton's distribution of "genetic worth" (MacKenzie 1979, 1981). Despite the fact that Stevenson was not a eugenicist, his classification left health inequality researchers with a tangled web of conceptual confusion. Even though we now have clearly defined and measured social class categories, eugenic thinking and structural-functionalism, its more recent manifestation, continue to befuddle those of us working in public health research.

The term "socioeconomic status" unfortunately exacerbates the confusion between the sociological concepts of social status, social class, and income and wealth. In epidemiology, though not in sociology, education is also often used as a measure of position in the social structure, which further adds to the confusion. To make matters worse, sometimes these measures are used as if they were interchangeable (Torssander and Erikson 2010), partly based on Paul Lazarsfeld's argument that these diverse social facts all produce similar associations with a range of social and health outcomes (Lazarsfeld 1939).

The few studies, which have tested the validity of this assumption, such as that by Siegfried Geyer et al. (Geyer et al. 2006), find that education, income, and an occupational measure of social class are only moderately correlated with one another and do not show the same degree of relationship with specific health outcomes. For example, education was more closely related to diabetes incidence, whereas income was more closely related to mortality.

These conceptual problems regarding social position have been summarized in terms of the difficulty they pose for the construction of *plausible narratives* (Marshall 1997b; Rose, Harrison, and Pevalin 2010). This is another way of expressing the notion of a *causal chain* but stated in perhaps less scientifically contentious terms. In observational life course research, we use the term *causality* at our peril.

In comparison, sociology has traditionally drawn a clear distinction between class and status. But because both these dimensions of social inequality are correlated, as both are with income and wealth, it can appear that for descriptive purposes, particularly in epidemiology, it does not matter which one of these concepts/measurements is used. However, if we understand the conceptual basis of the different measures, we are likely to greatly accelerate our efforts of explanation. This chapter aims to address this work of clarification: first by being clear on the definition of the most commonly used measures of social inequality that are social status or prestige, social class, income and wealth; and second by illustrating how these measures of social inequality may implicate different pathways likely to influence health. Once these conceptual issues are clarified, it becomes easily evident that distinct dimensions of inequality will implicate aetiological pathways composed of different mixtures of material, psychosocial, cultural, and behavioral factors. For example, as status is known to be a greater influence on tastes and behaviors, it is no surprise that a measure of social position based on status gives us stronger associations with risk factors such as smoking and diet, whereas a measure such as the NC-SEC based on employment relations and conditions shows stronger relationships to risk factors such as work stress, work control, and occupational hazard exposure.

Social status (prestige)

Status is inherently hierarchical, but any specific form of status exists only within the culture which sustains it and of which it is a part. So what can be a source of self-satisfaction or humiliation in one context will be meaningless in others.

The term "socioeconomic status" is used so frequently in epidemiology that it might lead one to believe that status is the most common measure in its studies. In fact, this is not true

(Featherman and Hauser 1976). Social status or prestige is very hard to measure. It has been described as a measure of "social honor," the degree of respect to which members of an occupation (status is usually attached to occupations in developed industrial nations) are generally regarded as entitled (Weber 1982). However, status hierarchies are specific to cultures and vary greatly across nations and sub-national geographical units.

Status is easiest to measure in caste societies such as the Hindu communities in India and elsewhere in the world. Everyone in these societies knows what the castes are, which ones are superior to which other ones, and to which caste they themselves belong. Members of a higher caste impose *social distance*, by refusing to eat with, worship with or marry members of a lower caste. Caste is associated with the traditional occupations of families, and not necessarily those professions practiced by the members of the current generation (Beteille 1992). They might be a computer professional, but their caste would be linked to the traditional occupation of their families.

Figure 15.2 shows a very simplified version of the Hindu caste system found in India. As you can see, the caste groups are associated with different types of occupation (priest, warrior, merchant) but this does not mean every member must work in that occupation. Rather, a member of a caste is regarded as descended from ancestors who once exercised a certain type of occupation. The organizing idea of this caste hierarchy is being purer/more virtuous and spiritually closer to the Divine. The highest status is accorded to those descended from priestly ancestors, and traditionally those who devote their lives to prayer and study, providing religious services, rather than amassing earthly power or wealth. In this diagram, the castes are represented as corresponding to parts of a *social body*. While this caste system may seem unique to Indian society, in fact, caste-like phenomena exist in more or less all societies.

The first attempt to measure social status in the United States in the early twentieth century took the form of studies of small towns, such as the anonymous "Midddletown" (in fact, Muncie, Indiana) (Lynd and Lynd 1929) and New Haven (Hollingshead and Redlich 1958),

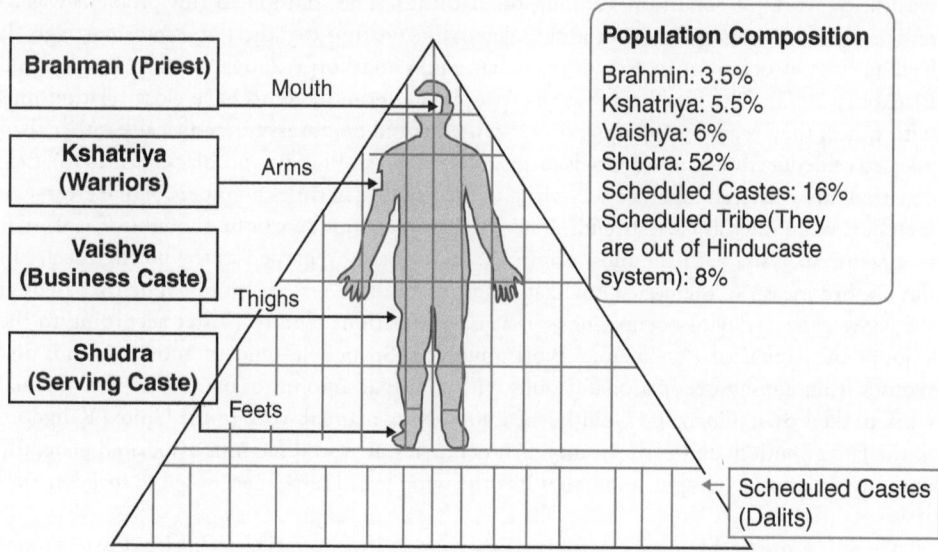

Figure 15.2 Hindu castes. Markville History. http://schools.yrdsb.ca/markville.ss/history/religion/caste_system_overview.html

where everyone knew everyone else, rather like the Indian villages where some of the most detailed studies of caste were conducted. In these small communities, it was possible to ask about the reputation of individuals and families, so the method itself became known as a *reputational* method (Nam and Terrie 1982; Oakes and Rossi 2003). Occupations were rated according to the prestige ascribed to individual incumbents by their fellow citizens. However, when large-scale surveys started to be carried out, it was obviously no longer possible to do this kind of detailed exercise (Duncan 1961; Stewart, Prandy, and Blackburn 1973). Instead, a sample of the population, sometimes called a panel of judges, were given a list of occupations and asked to rank these in order of their prestige. Obviously, there are enormous problems in developing measures of prestige for very large numbers of diverse occupations: how many judges should be used for the ranking to be valid, and how many of the myriad occupations in a society is it fair or sensible to ask them to rank or to score? The original study of this kind was carried out by the National Opinion Research Centre in the United States in 1947 and asked respondents to rank 90 occupations. But there are many hundreds of occupations in any society. One way around this, and used in the American research, was to find out the average income and education level of the jobs which had been given a score, and to use this data to impute a score to all other occupations (Duncan 1961; Hollingshead 1971; Nam and Terrie 1982).

It is clear from these accounts of the development of status measures in the United States that neither income nor education was what really interested the researchers; they were simply using these facts as a feasible way to get at the *social judgments* of the characteristics of both the occupations and their incumbents which conferred high or low prestige. However, this process led increasingly to the practice of using combined income and education as the sole measure of social position, and calling this *socio-economic status* (Featherman and Hauser 1976).

More recently, British scholars criticized the practice of asking people to rank occupations on the grounds that it was not at all clear what criteria the judges had in mind. If ranking an army general above a miner, for example, judges might have been thinking about income, wealth, or working conditions, among other things. The solution to this problem was to return to the ethnographic criteria of co-mensality (eating together) and intermarriage, as well as close associations in friendship (Chan and Goldthorpe 2004; Stewart, Prandy, and Blackburn 1973). The idea here was that people are more likely to have close relationships with others they regard as of equal status, which could be observed empirically rather than guessed or deduced (Chan and Goldthorpe 2004; Stewart, Prandy, and Blackburn 1973). Occupations are clustered together according to the number of times members of one cross-cite members of another as close friends. The clustering technique can be thought of as similar to a factor analysis, with the most dominant factor being regarded as the prestige scale. In the Oxford measure, the conceptualization of the prestige scale is more explicitly based on the *degree of manuality* of occupations—that is, occupations tend to cluster according to the amount of manual or non-manual work involved. So people tend to choose friends and spouses from among occupational groups with a similar amount of manual or non-manual work to their own (Chan and Goldthorpe 2004). Non-manual work in the United Kingdom in the late twentieth and early twenty-first centuries, it would seem, is associated generally with higher prestige, despite anomalies like the widespread respect accorded to surgeons and artists.

There is a reasonably clear plausible narrative that links prestige to health. Caste groups display their relative prestige by distancing themselves from forms of activity and people considered unclean or unworthy. They also mark their social status by bodily adornment, clothing, and various other aspects of what sociologists of industrial societies might call *lifestyle*. These include dietary practices and attitudes toward mood-altering substances like alcohol, caffeine, tobacco, and cocaine. There are strong similarities between the displays of prestige in both more and less traditional societies (Bourdieu 1984). In both cases, individuals mark their actual prestige, and attempt to increase it, by confining themselves to what are considered worthy activities, and attempting to associate only with others who are perceived as of appropriate rank (Chan and Goldthorpe 2007). An essential part of the claim to prestige includes the adoption of certain forms of lifestyle. A *cultural* theory of the relationship between prestige and lifestyle makes more sense of the social distribution of smoking and exercise, for example, than a theory based purely on income, as neither non-smoking nor physical exercise need cost any money. In contrast, being a non-smoker and certain forms of exercise are more or less obligatory in certain high- and medium-status social circles.

It is this possibility, of using measures of social position to construct a chain of risks and resources (Marshall 1997a; Rose and O'Reilly 1998), which makes it possible to take forward more quickly our attempts at understanding health inequality. Not because any one of the measures is superior to the others, but because we can see that inequality can be of different kinds and may influence health in different ways. As the originators of the Cambridge score have observed: "It may be that policemen and skilled workers [...] interact with each other as equals, yet their relations to the productive system are different and this can have important behavioural consequences under certain conditions" (Stewart, Prandy, and Blackburn 1980: 28). So, we can, for example, test whether lower prestige is associated with diet or tobacco smoking even within groups with similar incomes. There are rich possibilities for developing more complex and sensitive causal models which, at the same time, are more likely to be useful for health policy (Sacker et al. 2001; Torssander and Erikson 2010).

Despite their conceptual clarity and empirical validation, these status measures have not been widely adopted in health studies. Instead, both the study of status and the functionalist eugenic tradition have left a persistent thread for epidemiology in the use of education as a measure of social position. Education and income, as we have seen, are embodied in the functionalist perspective which regards the education system as the main way in which the genetically fitter are channeled into the higher-paying jobs with higher status and superior working conditions.

Social class

It is reasonable to base any analysis of the social structure on occupational conditions because the best hours of most days of the best years of most lives are spent at work. Within social research, conceptualizing social position as social class derives from Weberian theory, which identifies members of the classes essentially through the "life chances" available to them as a result of their occupation (Weber 1978). Max Weber's theory of social inequality is partly based on Karl Marx's idea that social classes are determined primarily by the rights and power that people have over various components of the means of production (labor power, capital, land), to which Weber adds the degree of access to resources relatively scarce and valuable in a society, such as goods and services, which determine people's material living conditions and shape relationships at work and in society at large (Wright 2005).

Modern social class schemas tend to have two organizing principles: ownership of productive resources (land, companies) and employment relations and conditions. Ownership of assets such as property, factories, or firms (or large numbers of shares in any of these) is what determines whether a person needs to work at all or whether she or he is the owner of a business, land, or other assets sufficient to make working for a wage or salary unnecessary. The second feature of social class of generally agreed significance is the relationship of all those who do have to work for a living to those who own and manage the establishments in which they work, those who supervise their work, and also to any others whose work they, in turn, may manage or supervise (Rose, Harrison, and Pevalin 2010).

The most widely used social class measure in the United Kingdom derives from Goldthorpe and colleagues' work. The EGP (Erikson-Goldthorpe-Portocarrero) or Comparative Analysis of Social Mobility in Industrial Nations (CASMIN) schema is described as combining:

> occupational categories whose members would appear, in the light of the available evidence, to be typically comparable, on the one hand, in terms of their sources and levels of income, their degree of economic security and chances of economic advancement [market situation]; and, on the other hand in their location within the systems of authority and control governing the processes of production in which they are engaged, and hence in their degree of autonomy in performing their work-tasks and roles [work situation].
>
> *(Goldthorpe, Llewellyn, and Payne 1980: 54)*

It is important to note that individuals are not allocated to social classes on the basis of individual ancestry or characteristics, with the corollary that these classes would exist even if all individuals were descended from similar parents and had identical personal characteristics. Classes have been compared to rooms in a hotel, which exist and have their stable characteristics regardless of the different individuals who may occupy them. Knowing a person's social class tell us nothing about features such as their height, education level, income, cultural preferences, leisure activities, and so on. These characteristics may be correlated with social class, but they are not part of its definition or measurement.

The EGP schema contains seven classes, of which three are subdivided:

I Higher-grade professionals, administrators, and officials; managers in large industrial establishments; large proprietors

II Lower-grade professionals, administrators, and officials, higher-grade technicians; managers in small industrial establishments; supervisors of non-manual employees

IIIa Routine non-manual employees, higher grade (administration and commerce)

IIIb Routine non-manual employees, lower grade (sales and services)

IVa Small proprietors, artisans, and so on, with employees

IVb Small proprietors, artisans, and so on, without employees

IVc Farmers and smallholders; other self-employed workers in primary production

V Lower-grade technicians; supervisors of manual workers

VI Skilled manual workers

VIIa Semi-skilled and unskilled manual workers (not in agriculture, and so on)

VIIb Agricultural and other workers in primary production.

In Britain, the EGP schema was the basis for the National Statistics Socio-Economic Classification or NS-SEC, developed as the official social classification used in government reports such as the 2001 and 2011 decennial censuses of England and Wales and of Scotland and the annual health surveys (Coxon and Fisher 2002; Rose and Pevalin 2003). The conceptual basis of the NS-SEC is very similar to that of the EGP, based on the relations and conditions of employment. The NS-SEC differs from the EGP schema in that it does not use *manual*

Box 15.1 Criteria for the "service relationship score"

1   the timing of payment for work (monthly versus weekly, daily or hourly);
2   the presence of regular increments;
3   job security (over or under one month);
4   how much autonomy the worker has in deciding when to start and leave work;
5   promotion opportunities;
6   degree of influence over planning of work;
7   level of influence over designing their own work tasks (Rose and Pevalin 2003: 51–55).

---

versus non-manual work as a criterion. This makes it more distinct from prestige (although the two measures co-vary). Accordingly, the EGP classes IIIa and IIIb are allocated to NS-SEC social classes 3 and 6, according to the extent to which the work is *routine* (rather than non-manual). Another major advantage of the NS-SEC over the EGP schema is that the criteria for allocating occupations to the different classes have been made even more explicit, as can be seen in Box 15.1.

Extensive empirical work went into deciding which occupations to put in each social class. Questions covering each of the seven criteria were asked of some 60,000 citizens in the United Kingdom's Labour Force Survey of 1997. Occupations could then be allocated into social classes according to the typical answers of members of each occupation to these questions (Mills and Evans 2003).

Because it is used for a wide range of official statistics as well as for research, the NS-SEC in its *full* form has a large number of categories which can be combined in different ways according to the purpose at hand. A seven-category version is most frequently used in reports and studies, as in Box 15.2.

Box 15.2 The NS-SEC

1   Higher managerial and professional occupations, including employers in large firms, higher managers, professionals whether they are employees or self-employed
2   Lower managerial and professional occupations and higher technical occupations
3   Intermediate occupations (clerical, administrative, sales workers with no involvement in general planning or supervision but high levels of job security, some career prospects and some autonomy over their own work schedule)
4   Small employers and self-employed workers
5   Lower technical occupations (with little responsibility for planning own work), lower supervisory occupations (with supervisory responsibility but no overall planning role and less autonomy over own work schedule)
6   Semi-routine occupations (moderate levels of job security; little career prospects; no pay increments; some degree of autonomy over their own work)
7   Routine occupations (low job security; no career prospects; closely supervised routine work) (Rose and Pevalin 2003: 24).

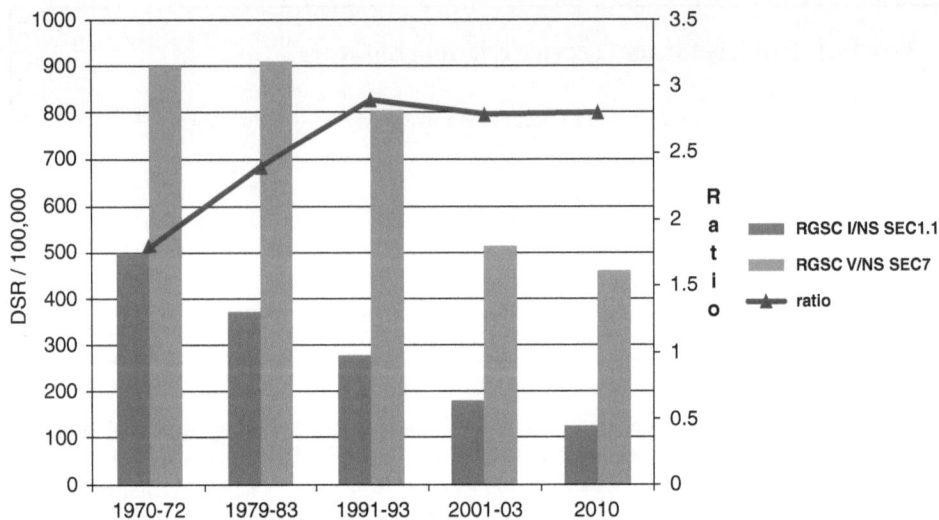

Figure 15.3 Social class differences in mortality using old and new classifications (Bartley 2017: 31)

The NS-SEC is not based on any consideration of status or prestige. The distinction between *higher* and *lower* managers and technical workers is based purely on the seven criteria—for example, *higher* managers have command over a *larger number of employees* and *higher* technical workers have *more responsibility for planning their own work*. The convention is emerging of referring to "*more advantaged* and *less advantaged* employment conditions" due to the criteria of job security and career prospects. But neither the EGP nor the NS-SEC is strictly hierarchical (unlike the status measures). Most importantly, the self-employed and small employers lie outside any continuum of advantage and disadvantage in employment conditions.

The NS-SEC is used for all official statistics in the United Kingdom, including those related to health. It has the advantage that, due to its clear conceptual foundation and extensive work of validation, the analyst knows exactly what is being measured. NS-SEC classes 1 and 7 are quite large compared to the RGSC's Professional (I) and Unskilled Manual (V), which also gives the measure better statistical properties. In theoretical terms, it is also striking that the NS-SEC gives a gradient in life expectancy of very similar magnitude to the older measure (Fitzpatrick and Dollamore 1999; Langford and Johnson 2010; Office for National Statistics 2012) that isolated smaller *extreme* groups at the top and bottom.

Figure 15.3 shows trends in mortality inequality in England and Wales between 1970 and 2010, that is, before and after the introduction of the NS-SEC. Although mortality rates (standardized for age) fell sharply in all social classes, the change over from the RG schema to the NS-SEC was not accompanied by any decrease in the ratio.

Income and wealth

Income is often seen as the least problematic measure of socioeconomic position, with a straightforward meaning. Nevertheless, there is a long debate concerning the direction of the association between income and health, as it has been hypothesized that it could be due mainly to reverse causation, that is, to the negative effect of bad health on earnings, rather than the opposite (Smith 1999). The direct association, however, has been confirmed in several longitudinal studies which adjusted for health status at baseline, demonstrating that lower income was still significantly associated with increased mortality and morbidity, although with attenuated risks (Benzeval and Judge 2001; Lynch et al. 1997; Smith 1999).

We need to also keep in mind that while some research has focused on absolute income, and what it will buy, others have focused on wealth, and others on relative income. The most sophisticated version of the *absolute income* approach is the work of Jerry Morris and his colleagues on a *minimum income for healthy living* (MIHL) (Morris et al. 2000, 2007; Morris and Deeming 2004). Morris reviewed the literature on diet, housing, exercise, social partic-ipation, and such like in relation to life expectancy to produce a basket of goods that could be regarded as the minimum necessary for health at different stages of life. In a life course perspective, the amount of time spent with an income lower than the MIHL would be ex-pected to increase in a cumulative manner the risk of poor health and shorter life expectancy.

Morris and others' techniques of assessing a *healthy living* level or a *decency standard* are a great step forward. But they do not deal with the problem that relative income may be important for health as well as absolute income (Lynch et al. 2000). Nor do they deal with the fact that life expectancy within any particular nation appears to increase right across the entire income distribution; it is not a question of a low-income group that has worse health and everyone else who is equally healthy and long-lived (Adler et al. 1994); and there does not seem to be a *threshold* amount above which income no longer influences health. This makes it look as if there may be something about relative income that is important. When we compare nations and look at national life expectancy figures in relation to average incomes, the results are regarded by some as supporting the causal importance of relative income. Data at the national level show the Preston Curve in which a nation's average life expectancy in-creases pretty rapidly up to about US$7,000 per annum; above which, some have argued that it is income distribution rather than absolute income per capita that is important to higher life expectancy.

It also needs to be mentioned here that studies like those of Richard Wilkinson and Kate Pickett (Pickett and Wilkinson 2014; Wilkinson and Pickett 2009) which correlate a nation's or region's life expectancy with the level of its income inequality are not studies of health inequality between social groups—they are studies of income inequality's relationship to the health of whole populations. Wilkinson and Picket have shown in many papers and books that life expectancy, as shown in Figure 15.4, is not related to income per head above around US$15,000. Rather, it is more convincingly related to the *distribution* of income (Pickett and Wilkinson 2014; Wilkinson 1986, 1992). The person earning, say, US$20,000 per annum at purchasing power parity will live longer than another person with the same income, if they live in a nation where the difference between top and bottom earners is smaller. In this way, Wilkinson and Pickett argue, income inequality is related to the health of all individuals. Social classes, status groups, or groups defined according to education do not enter into their main arguments at all.

Wealth is also a powerful predictor of illness and life expectancy, although very seldom available in studies. It can be regarded as essentially a product of income adequacy over the life course, so its predictive power is not surprising. As wealth is often inherited, it is also a marker for childhood conditions. However, the great majority of people in any study will have either no wealth or a modest and non-liquid amount fixed in one or two necessities. One is the amount saved into a pension scheme to sustain life during the decade or two of life between labor market exit and death. The median pension pot in the United Kingdom is around UK£26,000 in total, or around €28,000, which is enough to enhance living stan-dards only modestly for this length of time, particularly given the additional costs of chronic

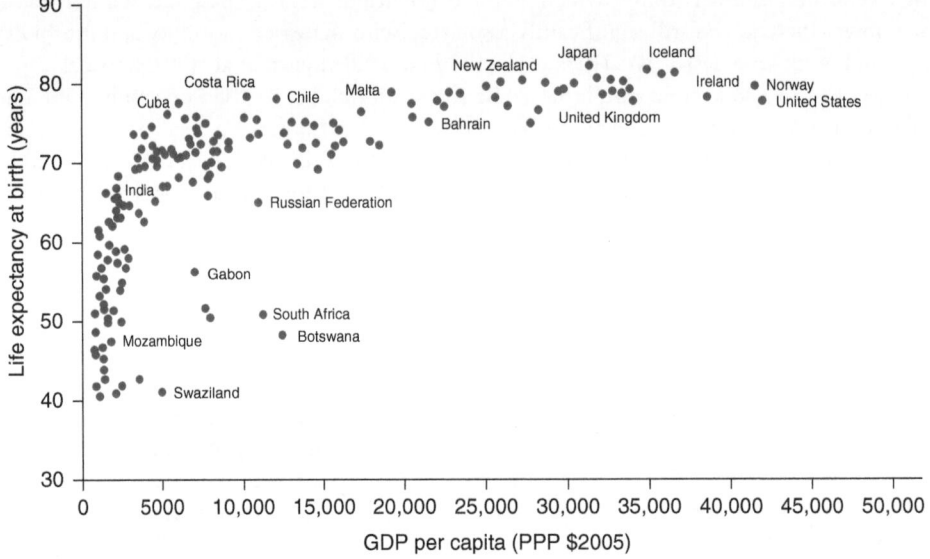

Figure 15.4   The Preston Curve: Life expectancy in countries with different levels of income. http://depthofprocessing.blogspot.co.uk/2009/11/maps-of-life-expectancy.html (accessed December 22, 2021)

illness, incapacity, and infirmity. The second is the value of the person's home, but the need for *a* roof over one's head combined often with a yet-to-be-repaid mortgage prevent this being a liquid financial resource.

Education

Increasingly, education is used as a marker of social position in health studies (Elo 2009; Ernstsen, Bjerkeset, and Krokstad 2010; Torssander and Erikson 2010). It might seem strange not to deal with education in the same way as class, status, income, and wealth.

Education has strong relationships to many measures of health (Mirowsky and Ross 2003). It has the virtue that as in most cases people finish their education in early adulthood at the latest, there is far less time for reverse causation (health determining education) to take place. Also, precisely because most education takes place before the individual lives independently, it is a strong marker for social and economic inequality over the life course (Mirowsky and Ross 2003). But education is a very different kind of measure to other indicators of social position, for a number of reasons:

1   It does not in itself confer a social class. If the whole population had the same level of education in a modern industrial society, there would still be social classes in pretty much the same way.
2   Education is one of the pathways into certain occupations and hence into a class position. But it is well known that the same level of education does not give an equal admission to an occupation in all gender or ethnic groups (Egerton and Halsey 1993).
3   In different nations and age cohorts, there are widely differing proportions who leave school at various ages or who gain certain qualifications. And once again these very

differences are influenced by gender, ethnicity, and parental social position (Chen et al. 2013).

4   A simple measure of educational level does not reflect existing variation in education quality and prestige across schools, leading to quite different employment and income opportunities in those from elite schools to similarly educated people from non-elite schools.

Education may be regarded as a very approximate or probabilistic indicator of class and income. It is possible that educational level per se confers prestige independently of income or occupation. Would a carpenter with a university degree have access to social relationships that were barred to carpenters without degrees? We have little data on this kind of question. But research in any topic needs indicators of the key concepts which are clear in their meaning. Keeping education separate from class, status, and income helps to maintain this clarity.

In addition, the use of education as a marker of adult social position prevents us from developing narratives of very important kinds. Education takes place across two critical periods of the life course, childhood and adolescence, during which children are socialized for distribution across the social class structure. Educational outcomes are known to be influenced by aspects of the home environment which may well also be important factors in health (Chandola et al. 2006; Fujiwara and Kawachi 2009). There may be personal characteristics as well which play a role in both educational and health outcomes (Jokela, Batty et al. 2009, Jokela, Elovainio et al. 2009). These processes need to be explored explicitly if we are to attain an understanding of health inequality that is useful for policy purposes.

One of the related dangers when using education as a measure of social position arises from the implicit, unstated influence in social epidemiology of Parsonian structural-functionalism, as discussed above. A lot of confusion can arise from this. Both eugenic and functionalist theories regard educational attainment as the outcome of personal, probably genetic, levels of intelligence. But a modern "causal narrative" needs to be able to test all these assumptions with separate, well-validated measures of each construct. In the words of Rose, Harrison, and Pevalin (2010): "Without a clear conceptual rationale, we shall not be able to understand the causal pathways which lead to regular patterns revealed by the use of a [social position measure] in research that is, the processes that generate empirical regularities."

Conclusion

For many decades, official documentation of health inequality in England and Wales relied on the Registrar-General's social class schema, a measure with no classificatory criteria, no stable definition (and therefore no possible test of validity), and unknown reliability. Subsequently, myriad studies repeated the finding of a *health gradient,* using many different measures. This was considered to give strong evidence that health inequality existed, as it did not seem to matter what measure one used.

However, we are now very far from a situation where all that is required is repeated descriptive work. Both scientific and policy considerations have for some time called for explanations to be provided. This has given rise to new work using validated measures of different dimensions of social inequality in combination with measures of plausible pathways. The increasing volume of longitudinal and life course data available makes this kind of work increasingly feasible.

As technology makes it possible to measure biomarkers at smaller and smaller resolutions, theoretical and conceptual clarity about the pathways and mechanisms between the social structure and the molecules, cells and tissues of the body becomes more important than ever. Measuring social position according to employment relations and conditions contributes to this endeavor because it has the virtue of such clarity. Social class stops being a *black box*. We know what it does measure, and we know what it does not measure. Perhaps most importantly, we have a measure thoroughly purged of implicit quasi-eugenic theories that can damage our efforts at understanding.

References

Adler, N. E., T. Boyce, M. A. Chesney et al. 1994. Socioeconomic status and health: The challenge of the gradient. *American Psychologist* 49, no. 1: 15–24. https://doi.org/10.1037//0003-066x.49.1.15.

Bartley, M. 2017. *Health inequality: An introduction to concepts, theories and methods.* 2nd edition. Cambridge: Polity.

Bartley, M., A. Sacker, D. Firth, and R. Fitzpatrick. 1999. Understanding social variation in cardiovascular risk factors in women and men: The advantage of theoretically based measures. *Social Science & Medicine* 49, no. 6: 831–845. https://doi.org/10.1016/s0277-9536(99)00192-6.

Belsky, D. W., T. E. Moffitt, D. L. Corcoran et al. 2016. The genetics of success: How single-nucleotide polymorphisms associated with educational attainment relate to life-course development. *Psychological Science* 27, no. 7: 957–972. https://doi.org/10.1177/0956797616643070.

Benzeval, M. and K. Judge. 2001. Income and health: The time dimension. *Social Science & Medicine* 52, no. 9: 1371–1390. https://doi.org/10.1016/s0277-9536(00)00244-6.

Beteille, A. 1992. Caste in a south indian village. In *Social stratification*, ed. D. Gupta, 142–162. Delhi: Oxford University Press.

Bourdieu, P. 1984. *Distinction.* London: Routledge.

Breen, R. and D. Rottman. 1995. Class analysis and class theory. *Sociology* 29, no. 3: 453–473. https://doi.org/10.1093/esr/jch033.

Chan, T. W. and J. H. Goldthorpe. 2004. Is there a status order in contemporary British society? Evidence from the occupational structure of friendship. *European Sociological Review* 20, no. 5: 383–401. https://doi.org/10.1093/esr/jch033.

Chandola, T., P. Clarke, J. Morris, and D. Blane. 2006. Pathways between education and health: A causal modelling approach. *Journal of the Royal Statistical Society: Series A (Statistics in Society)* 169, no. 2: 337–359. https://doi.org/10.1111/j.1467-985X.2006.00411.x.

Chen, J. T., J. Beckfield, P. D. Waterman, and N. Krieger. 2013. Can changes in the distributions of and associations between education and income bias temporal comparisons of health disparities? An exploration with causal graphs and simulations. *American Journal of Epidemiology* 177, no. 9: 870–881. https://doi.org/10.1093/aje/kwt041.

Coxon, A. P. M. and K. Fisher. 2002. Criterion validity and occupational classification: The seven economic relations and the ns-sec. In *A researcher's guide to the national statistics socio-economic classification,* ed. D. Rose and D. J. Pevalin, 107–130. London: Sage.

Davies, N. M., G. Hemani, N. J. Timpson, F. Windmeijer, and G. Davey Smith. 2015. The role of common genetic variation in educational attainment and income: Evidence from the national child development study. *Scientific Reports* 5: 16509. https://doi.org/doi: 10.1038/srep16509.

Davis, K. and W. E. Moore. 1945. Some principles of stratification. *American Sociological Review* 10, no. 2: 242–249. https://doi.org/10.2307/2085643.

Duncan, O. D. 1961. A socioeconomic status for all occupations. In *Occupations and social status*, ed. J. A. J. Reiss, 109–138. New York: Free Press.

Egerton, M. and A. H. Halsey. 1993. Trends by social class and gender in access to higher education in Britain. *Oxford Review of Education* 19, no. 2: 183–196. https://doi.org/10.1080/0305498930190205.

Elgar, F. J., B. McKinnon, T. Torsheim et al. 2015. Patterns of socioeconomic inequality in adolescent health differ according to the measure of socioeconomic position. *Social Indicators Research* 127, no. 3: 1169–1180. https://doi.org/10.1007/s11205-015-0994-6.

Elo, I. T. 2009. Social class differentials in health and mortality: Patterns and explanations in comparative perspective. *Annual Review of Sociology* 35: 553–572. https://doi.org/10.1146/annurev-soc-070308-115929.

Ernstsen, L., O. Bjerkeset, and S. Krokstad. 2010. Educational inequalities in ischaemic heart disease mortality in 44,000 Norwegian women and men: The influence of psychosocial and behavioural factors. The Hunt Study. *Scandinavian Journal of Public Health* 38, no. 7: 678–685. https://doi.org/10.1177/1403494810380300.

Featherman, D. L. and R. M. Hauser. 1976. Prestige or socioeconomic scales in the study of occupational achievement? *Sociological Methods and Research* 4, no. 4: 403–422. https://doi.org/10.1177/004912417600400401.

Fitzpatrick, J. and G. Dollamore. 1999. Examining adult mortality rates using the national statistics socio-economic classification. *Health Statistics Quarterly* 2: 33–40.

Fujiwara, T. and I. Kawachi. 2009. Is education causally related to better health? A twin fixed-effect study in the USA. *International Journal of Epidemiology* 38, no. 5: 1310–1322. https://doi.org/10.1093/ije/dyp226.

Geyer, S., Ö. Hemström, R. Peter, and D. Vågerö. 2006. Education, income, and occupational class cannot be used interchangeably in social epidemiology: Empirical evidence against a common practice. *Journal of Epidemiology and Community Health* 60, no. 9: 804–810. http://dx.doi.org/10.1136/jech.2005.041319.

Glymour, M. M., C. R. Clark, and K. K. Patton. 2014. Socioeconomic determinants of cardiovascular disease: Recent findings and future directions. *Current Epidemiology Reports* 1, no. 2: 89–97. https://doi.org/10.1007/s40471-014-0010-8.

Goldthorpe, J. H. 1997. The 'Goldthorpe' class schema: Some observations on conceptual and operational issues in relation to the ESRC review of government social classification. In *Constructing classes: Toward a new social classification for the UK,* ed. D. Rose and K. O'Reilly, 40–48. Swindon: ONS/ESRC.

Goldthorpe, J. H., C. Llewellyn, and C. Payne. 1980. *Social mobility and class structure in modern Britain.* Oxford: Clarendon Press.

Hollingshead, A. B. 1971. Commentary on "the indiscriminate state of social class measurement". *Social Forces* 49, no. 4: 563–567. https://doi.org/10.2307/2576737.

Hollingshead, A. B. and F. C. Redlich. 1958. The social structure in historical perspective. In *Social class and mental illness,* ed. A. B. Hollingshead and F. C. Redlich, 47–65. London: John Wiley and Sons.

Jokela, M., G. D. Batty, I. J. Deary, C. R. Gale, and M. Kivimaki. 2009. Low childhood IQ and early adult mortality: The role of explanatory factors in the 1958 British birth cohort. *Pediatrics* 124, no. 3: e380–388. https://doi.org/10.1542/peds.2009-0334.

Jokela, M., M. Elovainio, A. Singh-Manoux, and M. Kivimaki. 2009. IQ, socioeconomic status, and early death: The US national longitudinal survey of youth. *Psychosomatic Medicine* 71, no. 3: 322–328. https://doi.org/10.1097/PSY.0b013e31819b69f6.

Krapohl, E. and R. Plomin. 2016. Genetic link between family socioeconomic status and children's educational achievement estimated from genome-wide SNPS. *Molecular Psychiatry* 21, no. 3: 437–443. https://doi.org/10.1038/mp.2015.2.

Krieger, N., D. R. Williams, and N. E. Moss. 1997. Measuring social class in US public health research: Concepts, methodologies, and guidelines. *Annual Review of Public Health* 18: 341–378. https://doi.org/10.1146/annurev.publhealth.18.1.341.

Langford, A. and B. Johnson. 2010. Trends in social inequalities in male mortality, 2001–08: Intercensal estimates for England and Wales. *Health Statistics Quarterly* 47: 5–32. https://doi.org/10.1057/hsq.2010.14.

Lazarsfeld, P. F. 1939. Interchangeability of indices in the measurement of economic influences. *Journal of Applied Psychology* 23, no. 1: 33–45. https://doi.org/10.1037/h0056732.

Leete, R. and A. J. Fox. 1977. Registrar general's social classes: Origins and uses. *Population Trends* 8: 1–7.

Liberatos, P., B. G. Link, and J. L. Kelsey. 1988. The measurement of social class in epidemiology. *Epidemiologic Reviews* 10: 87–121. https://doi.org/10.1093/oxfordjournals.epirev.a036030.

Lynch, J., N. Krause, G. A. Kaplan, J. Tuomilehto, and J. T. Salonen. 1997. Workplace conditions, socioeconomic status, and the risk of mortality and acute myocardial infarction: The Kuopio Ischemic Heart Disease Risk Factor Study. *American Journal of Public Health* 87, no. 4: 617–622. https://doi.org/10.2105/AJPH.87.4.617.

Lynch, J. W., G. D. Smith, G. A. Kaplan, and J. S. House. 2000. Income inequality and mortality: Importance to health of individual income, psychosocial environment, or material conditions. *BMJ* 320: 1200–1204. https://doi.org/10.1136/bmj.320.7243.1200.

Lynd, R. S. and H. M. Lynd. 1929. *Middletown: A study in contemporary American culture*. London: Constable.

Mackenbach, J. P. 2012. The persistence of health inequalities in modern welfare states: The explanation of a paradox. *Social Science & Medicine* 75, no. 4: 761–769. https://doi.org/10.1016/j.socscimed.2012.02.031.

MacKenzie, D. 1979. Eugenics and the rise of mathematical statistics in Britain. In *Demystifying social statistics*, ed. J. Irvine, I. Miles, and J. Evans, 39–50. London: Pluto Press.

MacKenzie, D. 1981. *Statistics in Britain, 1865–1930: The social construction of scientific knowledge*. Edinburgh: Edinburgh University Press.

Marshall, G. 1997a. Class and class analysis in the 1990s. In *Repositioning class: Social inequality in industrial societies*, 1–30. London: Sage.

Marshall, G. 1997b. Repositioning class: Social inequality in industrial societies. In *Repositioning class: Social inequality in industrial societies*. London: Sage.

Marshall, G., D. Rose, H. Newby, and C. Vogler. 1988. *Social class in modern Britain*. London: Hutchinson.

Mills, C. and G. Evans. 2003. Employment relations, employment conditions and the NS-SEC. In *A researcher's guide to the national statistics socio-economic classification*, ed. D. Rose and D. J. Pevalin, 77–106. London: Sage.

Mirowsky, J. and C. E. Ross. 2003. *Education, social status and health*. New York: Aldine de Gruyter.

Morris, J. N. and C. Deeming. 2004. Minimum incomes for healthy living (MIHL): Next thrust in UK social policy? *Policy and Politics* 32, no. 4: 441–454. https://doi.org/10.1332/0305573042009507.

Morris, J. N., A. J. M. Donkin, D. Wonderling, P. Wilkinson, and E. A. Dowler. 2000. A minimum income for healthy living. *Journal of Epidemiology and Community Health* 54, no. 12: 885–889. https://doi.org/10.1136/jech.54.12.885.

Morris, J. N., P. Wilkinson, A. D. Dangour, C. Deeming, and A. Fletcher. 2007. Defining a minimum income for healthy living (MIHL): Older age, England. *International Journal of Epidemiology* 36, no. 6: 1300–1307. https://doi.org/10.1093/ije/dym129.

Muntaner, C. 2013. Invited commentary: On the future of social epidemiology—A case for scientific realism. *American Journal of Epidemiology* 178, no. 6: 852–857. https://doi.org/10.1093/aje/kwt143.

Nam, C. B. and W. E. Terrie. 1982. Measurement of socioeconomic status from United States census data. In *Measuring social judgements: The factorial survey approach*, ed. P. H. Rosse and S. L. Nock, 95–118. Beverley Hills, CA: Sage.

Oakes, J. M. and K. N. Andrade. 2014. Methodologic innovations and advances in social epidemiology. *Current Epidemiology Reports* 1, no. 1: 38–44. https://doi.org/10.1007/s40471-014-0005-5.

Oakes, J. M. and P. H. Rossi. 2003. The measurement of SES in health research: Current practice and steps toward a new approach. *Social Science & Medicine* 56, no. 4: 769–784. https://doi.org/10.1016/S0277-9536(02)00073-4.

Office for National Statistics. 2012. *Intercensal mortality rates by NSSEC, 2001–2010*. London: Office for National Statistics.

Parsons, T. 1953. A revised analytical approach to the theory of social stratification. In *Essays in sociological theory*, 30–42, ed. T. Parsons. New York: Free Press.

Pickett, K. E. and R. G. Wilkinson. 2014. Income inequality and health: A causal review. *Social Science & Medicine* 128: 316–326. https://doi.org/10.1016/j.socscimed.2014.12.031.

Rose, D., E. Harrison, and D. Pevalin. 2010. The European socio-economic classification: A prolegomenon. In *Social class in Europe*, ed. D. Rose and E. Harrison, 4–57. London: Routledge.

Rose, D. and K. O'Reilly. 1998. Final report of the ESRC review of government social classifications. In *Final report of the ESRC review of government social classifications*. Swindon: ESRC/ONS.

Rose, D. and J. Pevalin, eds. 2003. *A researcher's guide to the national statistics socio-economic classification*. London: Sage.

Rose, D. and D. J. Pevalin. 2005. *The national statistics socio-economic classification: Origins, development and use*. Colchester: Palgrave Macmillan.

Sacker, A., M. Bartley, D. Firth, and R. Fitzpatrick. 2001. Dimensions of social inequality in the health of women in England: Occupational, material and behavioural pathways. *Social Science & Medicine* 52, no. 5: 763–781. https://doi.org/10.1016/S0277-9536(00)00176-3.

Smith, J. P. 1999. Healthy bodies and thick wallets: The dual relation between health and economic status. *Journal of Economic Perspectives* 13, no. 2: 144. https://doi.org/10.1257/jep.13.2.145.

Stewart, A., K. Prandy, and R. M. Blackburn. 1973. Measuring the class structure. *Nature* 245, no. 5426: 415–417. https://doi.org/10.1038/245415a0.

Stewart, A., K. Prandy, and R. M. Blackburn. 1980. The measurement of stratification. In *Social stratification and occupations*, 17–70. London: Macmillan.

Szreter, S. 1984. The genesis of the registrar-general's social classification of occupations. *British Journal of Sociology*: 522–546. https://doi.org/10.2307/590433.

Torssander, J. and R. Erikson. 2010. Stratification and mortality: A comparison of education, class, status, and income. *European Sociological Review* 26, no. 4: 465–474. https://doi.org/10.1093/esr/jcp034.

Weber, M. 1978. *Economy and society, vols 1 & 2*. Berkeley: University of California Press.

Weber, M. 1982. Selections from economy and society vols 1 and 2; and general economic theory. In *Classes, power and conflict*, ed. A. Giddens and D. Held, 60–86. London: Macmillan.

Wilkinson, R. G. 1986. Income and mortality. In *Class and health: Research and longitudinal data*, ed. R. G. Wilkinson. London: Tavistock.

Wilkinson, R. G. 1992. For debate: Income-distribution and life expectancy. *British Medical Journal* 304, no. 6820: 165–168. https://doi.org/10.1136/bmj.304.6820.165.

Wilkinson, R. G. and K. Pickett. 2009. *The spirit level*. London: Penguin.

Wright, E. O. 2005. *Approaches to class analysis*. New York: Cambridge University Press.

16

RACE AND RACISM IN PUBLIC HEALTH

M. A. Diamond-Hunter

Introduction

In dealing with the philosophical foundations of public health, it seems to be correct that, as discussed by H. G. Nijhuis and L. J. van der Maesen (1994: 1), "philosophical foundations such as underlying ontological notions are rarely part of public health discussions, but these are always implicit and lie behind the arguments and reasoning of different viewpoints or traditions." The discussion of race and racism in public health (and in associated biomedical and health-related research) also has important underlying ontological notions, and what is interesting about these is that it has direct downstream effects upon the empirical research that is undertaken, along with the specific public health policy implementations that are suggested in light of the evidence gathered from said research outputs. Besides being something of academic interest, the philosophical examination of public health is important for making changes to the field, given the fact that the world remains dynamic—especially when socially important categorizations and descriptors like *race* and *racism* are involved. Nijhuis and van der Maesen also argue that "in the complex modern social world of public health, a better understanding of the philosophical foundations of the professional orientation of the public health expert may help in making the right choices" (1994: 3). While contemporary social complexities provide the motivation and urgency for addressing issues in public health, it should be taken as straightforward that public health issues concerning race and racism are a pressing subset of these concerns. This is alluded to—explicitly and implicitly—in the work produced by practitioners of public health and cognate biomedical disciplines. A cursory glance at the news surrounding movements for racial justice should be plenty of real-world evidence to back the claim that philosophers, public health practitioners, epidemiologists, social scientists, and others within the umbrella of public health and biomedical-related research should wrestle with these issues.

One way in which the connections between philosophy and public health manifest is given by D. L. Weed (1999), who discusses the ways in which ontological, ethical, and epistemological considerations are behind a number of public health decisions. For any particular public health decision, there are presupposed or implicit premises, with some examples, including the nature of evidence used in public health and how it was generated through empirical (qualitative; quantitative; historical; mixed-methods) means; whether the concepts

DOI: 10.4324/9781315675411-20

used in public health either actually capture something about a collection of individuals, or are used as placeholders for yet-to-be-developed concepts; and whether there are rules of inference between purported groupings and individuals that can be descriptive rather than proscriptive. This chapter aims to bring to the fore some of the ontological presuppositions that undergird the concepts of *race* and *racism* as they are used in public health. Included are discussions of differing accounts for race in public health, the ways in which racism is understood to be a public health issue, and where future research in public health, as it relates to the concepts of *race* and *racism,* is headed.

Before proceeding, a word of explication: throughout the chapter, while the focus on public health is paramount, there are also connections drawn between public health and biomedicine, broadly construed. This is not because of a particular conflation between the two; rather, this is because the two are deeply interconnected in various ways. In other words, the boundary between the two is more akin to a fuzzy boundary between sets rather than a crisp boundary (Smithson and Verkuilen 2006). Weed elucidates reasons for why the two are largely connected:

> Interestingly, interventions in medicine and public health arise from the same large pot of scientific research in biological, epidemiological, and behavioural disciplines, and with rare exceptions the conceptual and methodologic issues are so similar that it is very difficult to discern whether or not substantive differences exist between epistemological frameworks for medicine on the one hand and public health on the other.
>
> *(2004: 528)*

The connections between public health and other cognate studies that fall under the broad umbrella of biomedicine (namely, epidemiology) are also discussed by Alex Broadbent (2013). He defines epidemiology as "the study of the distribution and determinants of disease and other health states in human populations by means of group comparisons for the purpose of improving population health" (2013: 1). The final example of connections between public health, biomedicine, and other disciplines is given by Stephen Gillam:

> The disciplines that underpin public health include medicine and other clinical areas, epidemiology, demography, statistics, economics, sociology, psychology, ethics, leadership, policy and management. Public health specialists typically work with many other disciplines whose activities impact on the population's health [...] The science of public health is concerned with using these disciplines to make a diagnosis of a population's, rather than an individual's, health problems, establishing the causes and effects of those problems, and determining effective interventions. The art of public health is to create and use opportunities to implement effective solutions to population health and healthcare problems.
>
> *(2016: 5)*

The ways in which public health, epidemiology, and other biomedical disciplines are all oriented toward mitigating and improving the health of human beings writ large, along with the overlapping connections and fruitful interactions between them, provide justification for seeing them as deeply connected, even though there are differences between them (the extent to the types of solutions and policy positions advocated for based upon the scope of their empirical work, for example).

How are *race* and *racism* defined?

This is one of the more difficult philosophical and practical issues for public health. This is especially so given that some definitions in use in other aspects of biomedicine (epidemiology, genetics) are different than those used in public health, and yet there is a definite interaction between them. According to *A Dictionary of Public Health, race* is defined in the following way:

> In biology, vital statistics, epidemiology, and several other disciplines, [race] designates identifiable groups for classification purposes. Social scientists challenge the biological concept of race, asserting that it reflects ideological and culturally determined values rather than verifiable or classifiable criteria. In the United States, the word has an emotive connotation that makes its use politically volatile in some contexts. The dictionary definition "a major division of humankind having distinct physical characteristics" is generally valid and useful for simple statistical classification. A "racial" classification of humans is difficult, if not meaningless, because of genetic overlaps, but some risk factors are so strongly correlated with characteristics (mainly socioeconomic factors) customarily identified as "racial" that it would be foolish not to use them in statistical analyses.
>
> *(Porta and Last 2018)*

With respect to public health and epidemiology, the term *race* has been defined in all sorts of ways. In the United States (US), for example, the focus of how *race* is defined has rested upon classification by the categories found in the US Census (Baer et al. 2013: 212). This categorization follows what is dictated by the Office of Management and Budget (OMB) in their 1997 standards on race and ethnicity. The five categories of racial groups given by the US Census are White; Black or African-American; American Indian or Alaska Native; Asian; and Native Hawaiian or Other Pacific Islander. Additionally, the US Census offers two choices of ethnicities: Hispanic or Latino; or Not Hispanic or Latino.[1] In conjunction with these categories, the National Institutes of Health (NIH) (2001) mandated that all researchers report the racial/ethnic backgrounds of study participants based upon the categories in the US Census. Per §289-2a, investigators who apply for NIH grants are required to ensure that "members of minority groups are included as subjects" and are reported in research (National Institute of Health 2007).

In the United Kingdom, the term *race* is conflated with the term *ethnicity*. The most recent census, taken in 2021, identifies the following ethnic groups: White (which includes English; Welsh; Scottish; Northern Irish; British; Irish; Gypsy or Irish Traveller; Roma; and Any Other White Background); Mixed or Multiple Ethnic Groups (which includes White and Black Caribbean; White and Black African; White and Asian; and Any Other Mixed or Multiple Background); Asian/Asian British (which includes Indian; Pakistani; Bangladeshi; Chinese; and Any Other Asian Background); the category Black, Black British, Caribbean or African (which includes African; Caribbean; and Any Other Black, Black British, or Caribbean Background); and finally, Other ethnic group (which includes Arab; and Any other ethnic group [write in]).[2]

Outside of the United Kingdom and the US, race has different instantiations in different geopolitical contexts. Examples of the differences found across Latin America are found in Mara Loveman (2014), which provides detailed documentation in which racial categorizations differ across countries and across time, highlighting the sociopolitical reasons for why (or why not) certain racial categories have been used for institutional purposes. Empirical evidence is also provided by official census documentation of places like Canada, New Zealand, Australia, and South Africa (to name a few).

The term "racism" appears to be easier to define than the term *race* and the use of *racism* can also seem to be more standardized and uniform than the previous term. As defined by Miquel Porta and John M. Last (2018), "racism" is a collection of

> attitudes and behaviours based on a belief that people in a particular group or class are inherently different from and inferior to others and that it is therefore justifiable to discriminate against them; to stigmatize, persecute, and victimize them; to deny them access to services available to others; and, at the most extreme, to torture and murder them. Racism may be overt and individual or covert and institutionalized. Racism always has adverse health consequences for the group that is stigmatized and discriminated against, even in the absence of overt violence, and has adverse psychological consequences for the group that discriminates.

David R. Williams, Jourdyn A. Lawrence, and Brigette A. Davis (2019) define racism as

> an organized social system in which the dominant racial group, based on an ideology of inferiority, categorizes and ranks people into social groups called "races" and uses its power to devalue, disempower, and differentially allocate valued societal resources and opportunities to groups defined as inferior [...] A characteristic of racism is that its structure and ideology can persist in governmental and institutional policies in the absence of individual actors who are explicitly racially prejudiced.
>
> *(2019: 106)*

While the latter definition differs from the former (specifically concerning the inclusion of a dominant racial group, which under some understandings may make it incompatible with the former), what seems to overlap with these definitions is that racism involves more than just interpersonal prejudicial treatment. Rather, it should be noted that racism is seen as operating on marginalized or stigmatized groups through practices and institutions. A further explication regarding the difference between *structural* and *institutional* racism is found in Zinzi D. Bailey et al. (2017):

> Many academics use structural racism and institutional racism interchangeably, but we consider these terms as two separate concepts.
>
> Structural racism refers to "the totality of ways in which societies foster [racial] discrimination, via mutually reinforcing [inequitable] systems [...] (e.g., in housing, education, employment, earnings, benefits, credit, media, health care, criminal justice, etc.) that in turn reinforce discriminatory beliefs, values, and distribution of resources", reflected in history, culture, and interconnected institutions. This definition is similar to the "über discrimination" described by Reskin.
>
> Within this comprehensive definition, institutional racism refers specifically to racially adverse "discriminatory policies and practices carried out [... within and between individual] state or non-state institutions" on the basis of racialised group membership.
>
> Some of these institutional policies and practices explicitly name race (e.g., de jure Jim Crow laws, which required schools and medical facilities to be racially segregated, and restricted certain neighbourhoods to be white-only), but many do not (e.g., employer

practices of screening applications on seemingly neutral codes, such as telephone area codes or ZIP codes, because of presumptions about which racial groups live where).

(Bailey et al. 2017: 1455)

The definitions of racism discussed above do not necessarily define or describe particular individuals as being racist. What is emphasized, however, is that the targets of these unjustly discriminatory institutions and practices face adverse health outcomes because of their actual (or even perceived) targeting. With respect to public health, the ways in which social structures help to perpetuate racism (mainly as found in institutions, but not always) and the development of adverse health outcomes as a result provide impetus for it to be changed by public health practitioners and others who are connected to broader biomedical concerns (clinicians, researchers, social scientists, demographers, policymakers and analysts, historians of medicine, philosophers, and concerned individuals).

Race in public health and biomedicine

The use of *race* in public health may be seen to fall under two different general thoughts that follow from discussions and debates in biomedicine broadly understood. Namely, the first position is that *race* should be used in biomedicine (and, by extension, public health); the second is that it should not be used. This kind of dichotomous thinking obscures more of the nuanced positions found in the literature. The framing of positions in public health—which is arguably part of a biomedical framework, per Sean Valles (2020)—should be recalibrated in the following way: (1) using race in biomedicine because race is biologically real; (2) using race in biomedicine even though it is *not* biologically real; (3) using race in biomedicine because it is an important *social* category; (4) agnosticism on whether or not to use race in biomedicine; (5) reconsidering the use of race in biomedicine on a conditionalized basis; (6) the use of race in biomedicine on an instrumentalist basis; and (7) the abandonment of the use of race.

Using *race* as a biological reality

Proponents of the first position—that race should be used in public health and biomedicine because it reflects a biological reality—include Esteban González Burchard et al. (2003) and Luisa N. Borrell et al. (2021). Burchard et al. take it that recent work by Noah A. Rosenberg et al. (2002) helps to provide the empirical evidence that supports their position: namely, that there are five major racial groups, which are defined as the ones given from the 2000 US Census (Black or African-American; White; Asian, Native Hawaiian or Other Pacific Islander; and American Indian or Alaskan Native) (Burchard et al. 2003: 1171). The risk for not using *race* in public health (and biomedical research that supports public health) is three-fold: the first is that ignoring race would be detrimental to the persons and populations that need specific interventions; the second is that knowledge of a person's genetic ancestry may facilitate testing and other potential interventions; the third is that racial groups and persons are under-represented across clinical studies, and including them will help with potential future public health interventions and policy developments based upon epidemiological research. Specifically, Burchard et al. state: "Only by focusing attention on these issues can we hope to understand better the variations among racial and ethnic groups in the prevalence and severity of diseases and in responses to treatment. Such understanding provides the opportunity to develop strategies for the improvement of health outcomes for everyone" (2003: 1174–1175).

Borrell et al. (2021), in line with Burchard et al. (2003), argue for the use of race in bio-medical research that supports public health aims. In their approach, Borrell et al. take it that "it may seem reasonable to assume that all racial/ethnic differences in disease incidence and outcomes derive from socioeconomic differences. However, race is also directly associated with genetic ancestry and therefore indirectly related to genetic variants that may affect disease and health outcomes" (2021: 475).

The difference between Borrell et al. (2021) and Burchard et al. (2003) appears in the recognition that race captures different information than genetic ancestry; namely, that in practice, race is either a self-identified category, socially ascribed, or—at least in the context of the US—assigned by members of institutions (hospital staff, police, and so on) on a naïve basis (Borrell et al. 2021: 475). This differs from genetic ancestry, which is taken to be the origin population of an individual. As far as motivation for why Borrell et al. wish to continue to use race in bio-medical research that supports public health, they state that using race will continue to help researchers and public health professionals to "address health inequities […] given the emergence of precision medicine and persistent salience of overt racism, abandoning race/ethnicity without substituting better disease predictors not only is irresponsible but also ignores the reality of U.S. social stratification and its implications for population health" (Borrell et al. 2021: 479).

Using *race* as a non-biological entity

This position can be seen in Koffi N. Maglo's article "Genomics and the Conundrum of Race," in which Maglo provides an argument that "race in the biomedical sciences appears to be more of a convenient designator for multiple presumed layers of human population structures and, in public health settings, a multipurpose managerial tool" (2010: 358). Maglo's position is one that is

> an alternative to the belief that race is a fact of nature, as well as an alternative to 'eliminativism,' or calls for a straightforward elimination of the concept from biomedicine […] Even if the view that race has a biological reality and scientific validity is false, eliminativism may still be unjustified.
>
> *(2010: 358)*

For Maglo, the use of *race* in biomedical and public health contexts can be permissible, even if *race* is not a fact of the natural world. Maglo contends that there is an unresolved question regarding which discretionary level of population substructure actually corresponds to human biological races (2010: 361). Human beings have a number of different population substructures (ranging from multiple groupings of two humans all the way up to the entire human species being one population), and there seems to be no way to say which one of them is *the* way to have human biological races, especially when these different population structures are all biologically significant.

The alternative framework Maglo suggests is informed by the fact that particular scientific concepts, even if they have been shown to have conceptual issues, can nevertheless be used for solving particular empirical issues. One example of this is the use of Newtonian mechanics; it is taken that this framework for the physical world is largely helpful for getting a plane from Bogotá to Chennai, but it is not helpful for dealing with objects with masses near the extremes. For Maglo, "the utility of race does not necessarily require the reality or even the validity of race as a fundamental biological category" (2010: 362). Race, as Maglo discusses, should be seen more as a tool for pragmatic purposes and given particular ethical considerations—in the same way that the concepts *occupation* and *socioeconomic status* may serve as useful variables in biomedicine without necessarily being biological categories themselves (2010: 360).

Using *race* as an important social category

This seems to be the consensus view for contemporary public health practice, as well as that of other fields that fall under the biomedical framework, including epidemiology, sociology, demography, human genetics, and others. This position seems to be so deeply established that to provide a recapitulation of the important articles, books, chapters, and other official statements (by public health bodies, institutions, and professional societies) would be exhaustingly long, and would rehash wide swathes of academic research. Even though this is a position that has been defended on numerous occasions, there are potential philosophical and methodological concerns for the future use of *race* as an important social category, as how it is realized, understood, and deployed in empirical research is not necessarily as straightforward as it may seem—as we will see below.

Agnosticism regarding the use of *race*

The agnostic position can be attributed to Quayshawn Spencer's (2018) article "A Racial Classification for Medical Genetics." This position may seem counter-intuitive, given Spencer's previous (and most recent) defenses of race as a biological reality (2012, 2014, 2016; Spencer et al. 2019). Given these defenses, Spencer highlights a dilemma regarding the use of race in biomedicine and public health. While the argument developed in Spencer (2018) implies that there is at least one racial classification that is useful for medical genetics, the argument itself does not imply

> that medical researchers or clinicians should actually use this racial classification in clinical practice or medical research, nor does this fact guide us in how we should use this racial classification in medicine if we should use it at all. Also, it really is a dilemma whether we should use any racial classification in a genetic way in medicine.
>
> *(Spencer 2018: 1034)*

For Spencer, there are pressing pros and cons regarding the use of *race* within biomedical frameworks. With respect to the negatives, Spencer identifies work done by Brian M. Donovan (2014) that provides evidence where just the act of reading about human genetic diseases in racial terms "significantly raises one's probability of developing an 'essentialist' conception of race, which itself is correlated with developing racist attitudes" (Spencer 2018: 1034). Further empirical evidence regarding the connections between essentialization and discriminatory attitudes and/or practices include Nick Haslam, Louis Rothschild, and Donald Ernst (2000); Deborah A. Prentice and Dale T. Miller (2007); Kristin Pauker, Nalini Ambady, and Evan P. Apfelbaum (2010); and Johannes Keller (2005). Donovan states that

> while modern biological evidence does not support many essentialist beliefs, those who essentialize race tend to believe that races are discrete and that genes explain perceived differences between races. This belief structure tends to be associated with stereotyping, prejudiced attitudes, and a decreased motivation to redress racial inequality or socialize across racial boundaries.
>
> *(2014: 467)*

Given the empirical evidence provided above, it seems clear why there may be hesitation for using the concept of *race* within biomedical frameworks.

Spencer does identify positives for using *race* within biomedicine and public health. For Spencer, "organizing observational data in racial terms may allow medical researchers to more quickly find the genetic causes of and treatments for genetic disorders" (2018: 1034). In addition, the use of race would also allow for tracking the health effects of racism (2018: 1014). Spencer states unequivocally that there is uncertainty regarding the ethical dilemma of whether or not to use race in biomedicine and public health, even though there is at least one classification that is available for use (2018: 1034).

Reconsidering and conditional use of *race*

The idea that the use of *race* in public health and related biomedical fields should be reconsidered can be seen as a fairly developed and established position. The ways in which it should be reconsidered vary, but what unites the positions here is that the naïve use of race in public health (and other related biomedical fields) needs to be seriously reconsidered.

Ludovica Lorusso and Fabio Bacchini argue that racial categories based on self-identification have a useful role to play in research that examines the etiology of complex diseases (2015: 57). An appropriate use of self-identified races in research that helps to inform public health is one where

> self-identified races may be critically used as proxies for a risk-related environmental and epigenetic variation in the context of the United States. Self-identified race is what we need to capture the complexity of the effects of present and past racism on people's health and investigate risk-related external and internal exposures, gene-environment interactions, and epigenetic events. Our point is that a promising category of studies into the etiology of complex diseases [focuses] on non-genetic causal factors [...]
>
> *(Lorusso and Bacchini 2015: 57)*

Part of the reason why Lorusso and Bacchini come to this position is because of conceptual and methodological critiques of what they describe as *race-based studies* (RBS). RBS are defined by Lorusso and Bacchini as studies that investigate complex diseases while employing *race* as a relevant variable in their study design; these studies assume that race either an important or reliable proxy for at least some causal factors (specified or not) that leads to negative health outcomes for individuals (Lorusso and Bacchini 2015: 57). This is in distinction to *race-neutral studies* (RNS), which (a) study the etiology of complex diseases while not employing race as a relevant variable; (b) do not focus upon the racial differences in disease risk when investigating determinants of disease; and (c) therefore avoid considering race as a proxy for any causal factors on the pathway leading to disease (2015: 57). For Lorusso and Bacchini, RBS also include a particular hypothesis: that self-identified races are proxies for a specific genetic ancestry that is, in turn, associated with specific genetic variants contributing to the risk of complex diseases.

Their critique of this particular hypothesis rests on a number of challenges. The first is that racial self-identification relies on a number of contextual factors (geopolitical residence; salient institutional categories available to the person; and other sociopolitical factors), and as such is difficult (at best) to disentangle in any uniform way. The second is that the possibility of identifying different genetic ancestries for human beings that is both correct and unambiguous is itself difficult, especially when the groupings are artifacts of the models and algorithms used for generating populations which individuals are deemed to be a "best fit." The third challenge to the genetic hypothesis is that it appears to be no empirical support for the kind of risk-related variants that are unambiguously connected to particular groupings based on genetic ancestry that are unambiguous and exclusive.

To better understand how race is connected to public health, epidemiology, and other biomedical research, Lorusso and Bacchini argue that self-identified races are useful proxies for risk-related exposomes and epigenomes. They provide the reasoning for this as follows:

> At the population level, fluid patterns of racial self-identification continuously adapt to patterns of heterogeneous assortments of risk-related factors; and vice versa. The result is a consistent tendency for the two configurations to overlap, which endlessly coevolve and reinforce each other. As a consequence, self-identified races turn out to be excellent proxies for complex variation in risk-related environmental, psychological, cultural and social factors that it would be hard to fully account for in any other way.
>
> (Lorusso and Bacchini 2015: 60)

This can be understood as a type of looping effect: there is ample evidence that racial self-identification tracks aspects of deficiencies in positive health-related resource access (or over-abundances of negative health-related exposures)—whether as a result of structural, systemic, or interpersonal reasons; and the types of access to health-related resources and valence of health-related exposures reinforce the racial self-identification of the individual. Given this, Lorusso and Bacchini note that "the use of self-identified races has a potential important critical function as well, since it might remind us that racial discrimination and racial prejudice do have concrete, remarkable biological consequences on people, their minds and their bodies" (2015: 62).

This does come with a particular warning: that while the use of self-identified race may be beneficial for public health, epidemiology, and other types of biomedical research, their continued use may help to entrench or amplify particular understandings of diseases as racialized. The use of race may be seen as bringing critical attention to *racism* and its effects upon racialized persons, but it can also reinforce already pernicious stereotypes and false beliefs about the connections between these self-identified races and negative health outcomes. Lorusso and Bacchini therefore offer a note of caution: "We should be prepared to dismiss self-identified races if we suspect that the inequalities caused by racism are reinforced rather than weakened as an overall effect of their employment" (2015: 63). This line of reasoning—that race should be reconsidered as a variable in public health and other health-related studies—is echoed by Raj Bhopal, who says: "Data on race and ethnic group have both harmed and benefited minority populations, and will continue to do so, yet without the data the need for services cannot be established" (2015: 1375).

The move to reconsider the use of race also has found footing within other biomedical-related discussions. Valles (2012) discusses issues for using race within public health. Focusing on two case studies—the first being the generic claim that "African-Americans are at an elevated risk of hypertension," and the second being that "Caucasians are at elevated risk of cystic fibrosis"—Valles argues that the use of race is too broad. Specifically, he contends that these unmodified racial categories create

> the unique situation in which low-risk subpopulations have had their interests marginalized during the propagation of broad claims about race-wide disease risks. Hence, we have two distinct problems that overlap in practice: the problem of ignoring low-risk

islands within seas of high risk (so to speak) and the problem of privileging mere race when delineating which populations have public health risks. Together, the two problems combine to impede the dissemination of more nuanced data about heterogeneity of risk within racial groups.

(Valles 2012: 405)

Valles raises an important issue: that the misapplication of broad racial descriptors for public health population groups not only harms racialized minority groups, but also harms racialized majority groups. In this case, the solution that Valles proposes addresses a number of issues that arise when using overly broad racial terminology in public health contexts:

Of all the possible levels of population specificity, race is probably the choice that introduces the most unintended harm, primarily due to its tacit reinforcement of biological race essentialism. Adding one more level of specificity beyond mere race would leave the target population delineations simple enough to be accessible to laypeople and also limit the socially detrimental side-effects of using racial categories in medicine. In fact, it offers an opportunity to combat prejudice through undercutting essentialism.

(Valles 2012: 408)

Darshali A. Vyas, Leo G. Eisenstein, and David S. Jones highlight a partial list of race-adjusted algorithms used in clinical practice—some whose justifications for using different calculations are traced to biased data or flawed racial-science presuppositions (2020: 879). They conclude:

The clinical tools we use daily should reflect these new insights to remain scientifically rigorous. Equally important is the project of making medicine a more antiracist field. This involves revisiting how clinicians conceptualize race to begin with. One step in this process is reconsidering race correction in order to ensure that our clinical practices do not perpetuate the very inequities we aim to repair.

(Vyas, Eisenstein, and Jones 2020: 880–881)

While the ways in which the use of *race* should be reconsidered vary among the authors discussed here, it is important to note that what needs to be reconsidered is the way in which race is used as a blunt tool or generic descriptor, instead of being something more precise and nuanced.

Instrumental use of *race*

The view that race can be understood instrumentally is a newer position, which I have advocated elsewhere (Diamond-Hunter 2020). Ontologically speaking, this is an antirealist position that rejects both the notions that *race* is a biological reality that easily maps onto social-scientific classificatory schema, and that race is a logically coherent social construction. *Race,* however, should be treated in an instrumental fashion. Specifically, this means that the use of *race* is akin to using a conceptual tool—one that rejects realist commitments (like those found in Burchard et al. [2003] and Borrell et al. [2021]), and where values play an integral part of the use of the tool. The tool includes *methodological values* (including commitments to well-defined, operationalizable concepts, and methodological transparency) as well as *epistemic and communicative values* (including appropriate restrictions on the domain of inquiry, the non-conflation of models with the actual world, and a clear commitment to limits of generalizability). The downstream effects of using this tool include non-stigmatization of vulnerable populations, mitigation of conceptual confusion, and truncating of overly broad claims. One example of this would be using *post code* (or *zip code*, depending on the relevant context) as a conceptual tool for mitigating disparities in public health. One can use this tool for developing testable hypotheses, gathering exploratory data, and for measuring the effectiveness of public health interventions while avoiding the notion that *post code* is somehow a coherent biological reality or a logically consistent social construction that covers all domains.

What specifically separates the position I have advocated from that of Maglo? This is a fair question, which merits an answer. One major difference is that, unlike Maglo, I argue that the class of views that take race to be socially constructed are logically inconsistent. According to my view, for any social constructionist account, the account will be both too restrictive and too permissive. The account will, given its criteria, include individuals as members of a group whom *prima facie* would not be included—while simultaneously excluding individuals as members of that same group whom *prima facie* would be included. Maglo does not rule out a coherent and logically consistent way of having socially constructed races; I do. Additionally, I do not utilize the ethical considerations that Maglo posits for correct usage. Rather, I take it that epistemological and methodological values (noted above) are integral to the use of race as a tool. The place of ethical considerations, for me, is important—it just comes at a different place in the development of an empirical project.

What gives my particular position backing is reflected by the empirical evidence that the use of racial categorizations is not logically consistent nor is deployed consistently. One example of this is taken from Bhopal, which notes that there may be issues in both developing a technical terminology and providing uniformity: "As this paper shows even basic work such as defining terms is problematic, and the challenges are compounded by the pace of social change, and scientific practice [...] There are other issues, for example, whether international understanding and agreement on these concepts and terms, is achievable" (2004: 444–445).

Bhopal also highlights the ways in which *race* has been used inconsistently within biomedical and public health studies. With respect to racial classifications found in the health sciences, he notes:

> Classifications vary across times and places, reflecting both the pragmatic nature of the process of their creation and the varying purposes for which they were designed [...] The classification process is, inevitably, arbitrary, subjective, context specific, purpose driven, and imprecise. The process is atheoretical in that there is no coherent, valid genetic or social theory that underpins classifications.
>
> *(2015: 1373–1374)*

In addition to Bhopal, Judith B. Kaplan and Trude Bennett (2003) also discuss the ways in which the use of *race* in public health and biomedicine has been inconsistent or non-standardized. This is not only because researchers themselves have at times loosely substituted terms or conflated terms like *race*, *ethnicity*, and *ancestry*, but because the presuppositions regarding *race* as a descriptor are mistaken. Kaplan and Bennett note that racial identity is not always fixed, nor easily determined—this is reflected in the changes in the US Census categories, as well as the ways in which people may change their racial self-identification across time (2003: 2709). Additionally, racial concepts and categories are not as precise as they are taken to be. Kaplan and Bennett note that "the racial/ethnic categories commonly used in biomedical sciences and epidemiology are broad and overlapping. Individuals do not fit neatly into these categories, and these broad groupings can obscure significant within-group heterogeneity" (2003: 2710).[3]

Given the well-documented inconsistencies, conflations, and other issues in the deployment of *race* as a variable (causal, inferential, and/or descriptor), along with the ways in which *race* clearly varies across geopolitical contexts, time, institutions, and for individuals during their lifespan, the position that *race* should be understood instrumentally seems to have plenty of empirical evidence to support it. The benefits of seeing it this way include having minimalist ontological commitments while retaining the flexibility that the dynamism of the concept demands (as evidenced above). One of the potential challenges for this view is how it may be tied to *identity* but it seems (at least for public health and other biomedical endeavors) that is a question for a potential application of the view that is outside the remit of this discussion. A second challenge for this view is that racial groups or categorizations are different across different geopolitical contexts. Perhaps there are more specific racial terms that are better applied to restricted domains or contexts, instead of generic racial terms for *all* contexts. Perhaps this could be borne out through empirical research but an initial response for this is that a contextualist move, while admirable (and more focused than using, say, the 2000 US Census racial categorizations for the entire globe—which can potentially be seen as ethnocentric, or a strong case of hubris), falls privy to complications where multiple contexts overlap.

Abandoning *race*

The position that the use of *race* should be abandoned in public health is advanced by Paula Braveman and Tyan Parker Dominguez (2021), who argue for abandoning the term *race* as a way for categorizing human beings, while simultaneously retaining the term *racism* as a way to identify and dismantle systems of unjust treatment. Initially, this may appear to be counter-intuitive—or at the very least a difficult needle to thread. As a substitution, Braveman and Parker Dominguez prefer to use the term *ethnic group* or *ethnicity* as a replacement for *race*. They provide a detailed rationale for doing so, based on the discriminatory treatment that racialized groups (groups that have either been treated as or been presupposed as distinct biological groups) have faced in the context of the US. Braveman and Parker Dominguez argue that the use of *ethnicity* avoids the implicit connotation of biological differences, while also being a useful category for studying these groups—namely, because "racism [...] holds profound implications for health and well-being" (2021). While noting that they are not the first to call for the abandonment of the use of race—acknowledging that Ashley Montagu (1945) and Hannah Bradby (1995) have also done so—they re-emphasize that the abandonment of *race* does not entail the avoidance of cataloguing or studying discrepancies due to perceived group membership. Braveman and Parker Dominguez state:

> Because of the profound impact of racism on health and well-being, we must continue to collect data on these socially constructed categories that have been called "races." We should not, however, continue to unintentionally or intentionally *racialize* people—i.e., to regard people as if they represent fundamentally distinct groups—by using that term.
> *(2021)*

In line with other positions in this chapter, Braveman and Parker Dominguez (2021) take it that *racism* is a causal factor for negative health outcomes. Specifically, structural (or systemic) racism—the unjust systems or structures that systematically set racialized groups at a disadvantage—is the origin of potential causal pathways where health discrepancies are found. Braveman and Parker Dominguez reveal how structural or systemic racism manifests in negative health outcomes for members of marginalized racial groups. The structures or systems that unjustly discriminate against these groups lead to unfair treatment and differential access to resources and opportunities. Examples include not only the interpersonal, but differences in treatment with respect to employment hiring and pay; less economic mobility, which, in turn, restricts access to schools and other educational opportunities; and poorer public services. The differential access to resources and unfair treatment lead to exposure to health-harming conditions, as well as prohibit exposure to health-promoting conditions; and (over) exposure to health-harming (or insufficient exposure to health-promoting) conditions, in turn, manifests in triggering biological mechanisms (chronic stress, inflammation of the immune system) that lead to deleterious health outcomes.

Braveman and Parker Dominguez acknowledge that the abandoning of *race* and substituting it for *ethnic group* or *ethnicity* is not the end-goal for mitigating health disparities found for members of racialized groups. As a matter of fact, they note that abandoning the term will not (either primarily, or by itself) eliminate racism (in structural, systematic, or interpersonal form). Nevertheless, Braveman and Parker Dominguez (2021) argue that it is still highly important to abandon its use:

> Abandoning "race" should be part—admittedly a small part—of a strategy to intensify and broaden actions against racism. While abandoning "race," we should not only retain the term "racism" but also mount more intensive efforts to identify and dismantle it. In particular, we need to focus on systemic or structural racism, often invisible but posing the greatest barriers to justice and health because it is the root source of the varied manifestations of racial discrimination observed in multiple domains [...] the public health crisis produced by racism requires fighting vigorously in many arenas, including conceptual and semantic spheres. Abandoning "race" is not a panacea but may be a useful adjunct to other crucial efforts to dismantle racism in all of its forms.

Part of the reasoning to abandon the term is to reject the notion that race is a biological feature of the world, while recognizing that it is the actions based upon a mistaken belief (that *race* is biologically real) that have led to the kind of public health disparities we see today. In some senses, this is analogous to the recognition that people can organize others (and be organized themselves) according to fictional entities; while the entities themselves do not exist in the actual world, the effects that organizing around them has on people (and groups) are real. Braveman and Parker Dominguez do take the issue of *racism* and the negative health outcomes it produces seriously, and their move to abandon race is an attempt to put the focus upon the social structures and systems that perpetuate public health disparities.

Empirically speaking, the move away from *race* and toward *ethnicity* is well documented (even if places like the US are behind the rest of the world in this regard) (Afshari and Bhopal 2010). The move to abandon *race* as an important variable also finds footing in other aspects of biomedical research. Michael D. Yudell et al. (2016) argue that the use of *race* in human genetics should be substituted by other technical terms like *ancestry* or *population*. What lies behind the impetus for replacing *race* is that the authors "believe the use of biological concepts of race in human genetic research—so disputed and so mired in confusion—is problematic at best and harmful at worst" (Yudell et al. 2016: 564). Recently, Dorothy E. Roberts (2021: 17) has argued that the use of race should be abolished from diagnostic algorithms, such as those used for estimating kidney function, among others. Adrienne Milner and Sandra Jumbe (2020) also argue that the acronym for Black, Asian, and Minority Ethnic (BAME) persons should be abandoned in the context of the United Kingdom. Even though there may be subtle differences between the positions held by Yudell et al. and that of Braveman and Parker Dominguez, both share the view that *race* should cease to be used in public health and biomedical frameworks.

Racism as a public health issue

The development and understanding that racism can be a public health issue is one that has gathered steam across (at least) the last two decades, even though, as Krieger (2003) notes, "concerns about health consequences of racism clearly are not new; to suggest otherwise is to misstate the historical record" (2003: 195). In the context of the US, this has become a major point of discussion. Dara D. Mendez et al. (2020) note that as of October 2020, there were 125 resolutions and/or declarations relating to racism as a public health crisis. According to the *American Public Health Association*, as of August 2021, there have been 209 recorded declarations of racism as a public health crisis in 37 states; Milwaukee County, in Wisconsin, became the first community to declare it as such in 2018. Other professional associations within the biomedical world have also recognized that racism is a public health issue. In a statement approved by the board of regents of the American College of Physicians (2017): "Hate crimes directed against individuals based upon their race, ethnic origin, ancestry [...] are a public health issue." The American Medical Association specifically recognizes that "racism negatively impacts and exacerbates health inequities among historically marginalized communities" and argues that "declaring racism as an urgent public health threat is a step in the right direction toward advancing equity in medicine and public health, while creating pathways for truth, healing, and reconciliation" (O'Reilly 2020). The US Centers for Disease Control and Prevention (CDC) has also produced a statement that identifies racism as a public health issue. Specifically, the CDC states:

> Racism—both interpersonal and structural—negatively affects the mental and physical health of millions of people, preventing them from attaining their highest level of health, and consequently, affecting the health of our nation.
>
> A growing body of research shows that centuries of racism in this country has had a profound and negative impact on communities of color. The impact is pervasive and deeply embedded in our society—affecting where one lives, learns, works, worships and plays and creating inequities in access to a range of social and economic benefits—such as housing, education, wealth, and employment. These conditions—often referred to as social determinants of health—are key drivers of health inequities within communities of color, placing those within these populations at greater risk for poor health outcomes.
>
> *(CDC 2021)*

In Canada, the Association Canadienne de Santé Publique/Canadian Public Health Association stated the following with regard to racism being a public health issue:

> Canada remains a nation where a person's colour, religion, culture or ethnic origin are determinants of health that result in inequities in social inclusion, economic outcomes, personal health, and access to and quality of health and social services. These effects are

especially evident for racialized and Indigenous peoples [...] Complicating this scenario are government and non-governmental systems that impose barriers on those in need which limits their ability to obtain the services and benefits that are easily available to most Canadians. Steps must be taken to eliminate these systemic barriers.

(Canadian Public Health Association 2018)

Outside of official statements and proclamations by various biomedical institutions and professional bodies, the topic of racism as a public health issue has come up in numerous publications geared toward the general public. In the US, articles have been produced with titles and headlines such as "What 'Racism is a Public Health Issue' Means" (Thulin 2020), "Dozens of City Governments Declare Racism a Public Health Crisis" (Mock 2020), and "Racism Is Undeniably a Public Health Issue" (Eschner 2020).

Racism as a public health crisis has also pushed individual practitioners to speak out about how it affects the health outcomes of millions of people. Jennifer Jee-Lyn García and Mienah Zulfacar Sharif (2015) provide commentary and potential solutions for mitigating and reducing the effects of racism in the public health sphere. Michele K. Evans et al. (2020) provide evidence of how racism as an issue affects both clinical practice and public health interventions.[4] In line with the empirical evidence just mentioned, the editor and deputy editor of the *JAMA Network Open* recently issued a call for papers to help address this issue. Specifically, they state that there is a need for

papers that contribute to the evidence base on prevention and the effects of systemic racism on health and health care. We are interested in papers that apply rigorous science to examine who is affected, the mechanisms of how racism translates into poor health and health care, and how racism and its effects can be addressed at the primary, secondary, and tertiary levels of prevention. Studies that use rigorous science, including randomized and non-randomized clinical trials that assess interventions, observational studies, and systematic reviews and meta-analyses are needed to make progress in this area.

(Rivara and Fihn 2020: 1)

Perhaps unsurprisingly, the connections between Covid-19 and racism have been discussed in the popular press, in governmental technical reports, and in academic publications. Public Health England produced a report detailing the disparities in risk and outcomes of Covid-19, providing evidence that "suggests that COVID-19 may have a disproportionate impact on people from Black, Asian and minority ethnic (BAME) groups" (2020). In the article "Why Racism, Not Race, Is a Risk Factor for Dying of Covid-19," public health specialist, epidemiologist, and family physician Dr. Camara Phyllis Jones was interviewed to discuss racism as a risk factor for Covid-19 mortality (Wallis 2020). The links between Covid-19 and racism have been recently discussed in the academic literature by Delan Devakumar, Sunil S. Bhopal, and Geordan Shannon (2020), Devakumar et al. (2020), and Bentley (2020).

The increasing consensus that racism is a public health issue is borne out through institutions of higher education across the US. On the website of Tulane University's School of Public Health and Tropical Medicine (2021), a post titled "Why Racism is a Public Health Issue" states that "as a major cause of health inequity, racism violates a core mission of public health professionals: creating conditions that give all people the opportunity to achieve their best health." At the website of the School of Public Health at the University of Michigan, a post by the Dean of the School of Public Health states:

It has never been more apparent that racism is a public health crisis [...] Systemic racial inequities in our country shape many aspects of people's lives and health—from the jobs they hold and the places they live, to the air they breathe, the water they drink, the food they can buy, and the levels of stress they suffer because of their income, their personal safety, and the racism they may experience on a daily basis.

(DuBois Bowman 2020)

The Dean of Brown University's School of Public Health states:

Racism is a deep, systemic, and longstanding problem in America and we, as a public health community, must use every tool we have to confront it in all its forms [...] We not only must condemn these acts of racism, we must take action that will, now and over time, reduce its pernicious effects on the lives, health, and well-being of Black Americans.

(Ashish n.d.)

Purdue University's Department of Public Health makes the following statement:

Racism is a public health crisis. The Department of Public Health recognizes and is committed to responding to the devastating harms that racism, injustice, discrimination, colonialism, and police violence have on the safety and health of Black Americans and other communities of color. Social determinants of health, including racism-propelled adverse socioeconomic conditions, are key drivers of health disparities. The disproportionate burden of COVID-19 on Black and Latinx communities is just the latest example of how structural and systemic racism leads to devastating health outcomes.

Health is a fundamental human right for all people. Our department commits to upholding this right, applying rigorous science and de- signing evidence-based solutions to dismantle oppressive policies and systems that lead to racial disparities in health, and training future generations of diverse, inclusive, and anti-racist Public Health leaders.

(Purdue University Department of Public Health n.d.)

The above examples are in no way outliers, or a niche trend—a whole host of universities in the US take this position, including Ohio State University,[5] George Washington University,[6] Emory University,[7] and Harvard University.[8] The University of California, Los Angeles (UCLA), which has its own Center for the Study of Racism, Social Justice, and Health, sees as part of its mission to target "racism as a public health issue."[9]

This declaration, or realization, of the connections between racism and public health concerns is also, notably, not restricted to one particular geopolitical region. With respect to institutional statements, Public Health England published a technical report on ways to understand and reduce ethnic inequalities in health (2018). Additionally, member institutions of the Association of Schools of Public Health in the European Region (ASPHER) published their own statement regarding racism and discrimination in public health. While the published statement specifically addresses racism and discrimination with regard to Covid-19, their response also covers broader concerns:

The amalgamation of different forms of inequalities resulting from racism and socio-economic disadvantages signals an urgent need to protect the health of vulnerable groups. On the one hand, social inequalities which the pandemic reinforces need to be tackled; on the other hand, inappropriate government policy responses to it must be addressed…Racism and discrimination are public health issues, globally and in Europe. They are contributing factors to the COVID-19 crisis. As public health researchers and practitioners, we must be aware of this. We need to take the necessary actions to address racism and discrimination in order to attain health equity.

(Akbulut et al. 2020: 727–728)

While it is commendable that colleges and universities, and departments of public health are identifying the need to combat racism as a pressing public health issue, those institutions themselves are (or have been), to some extent, part of the problem. As Lisa Wandschneider et al. (2020) discuss how, in addition to combating racism in general society:

> public health schools need to consider an upstream stage of action: they need to turn their gaze inwards and check how they themselves maintain racist structures in internal policies and actions […] Recognising that these schools are not immune to racism is an essential first step to building anti-racist action within the institution.

There is also ample empirical evidence that racism itself is a public health issue in contexts outside of the US. Heather Came (2014) provides a mixed-methods study that discusses the ways in which institutional racism affects public health policy in New Zealand. Came notes:

> The study identified sites of racism across the policy making processes despite a raft of controls across the system to prevent discrimination. Racism was detected within decision making process and within the (mis)handling of evidence that informs policy […] It seems this pattern of behaviour has survived changes in government and can be tracked across successive race relations policy platforms whether it be colonisation, assimilation, biculturalism or neo-liberalism […] The cumulative effect of these sites of racism is the development of mono-cultural health policy which marginalizes Māori perspectives and paradigms within health policy.

> *(Came 2014: 218)*[10]

Adding to the empirical evidence that racism (and its effects upon racialized groups) is a public health issue, there have been a host of studies done to examine the effects of racism upon minoritized groups. Studies include racism and its effects in the general European region (Hamed et al. 2020), a comparative study between Brazil and South Africa (De Souza et al. 2020), and a comparative study between Australia, Canada, and New Zealand (Mitrou et al. 2014).[11]

Race and racism in public health: How to proceed?

If one takes the evidence given to this point of the ways in which historical events, policies, and institutions have affected the public health of racialized groups, one of the concerns should be how to proceed with the stated goals of reducing health disparities. One of the benefits of having collaborative interactions between public health practitioners, philosophers, epidemiologists, public policy professionals, and social scientists is that these future concerns can (to some degree) be anticipated and discussed. While this does not mean that we (as a collective body of interested persons) will be able to necessarily solve all problems before they arise, it does suggest that we can take the evidence that we have about the world around us and provide speculative or theorized future issues and concerns to engage with our collective intellectual capacity. From the overlapping standpoint of a philosopher of science and philosopher of race, there are a number of potential avenues that can be pursued.

One avenue would be from a methodological and disciplinary standardization standpoint. Given that the concept of *race* has been (and continues to be) contested with respect to its metaphysical standing, perhaps what can be done is to develop a way of standardizing a *racialized* group. This seems to allow for the flexibility for the metaphysical debates to play out while utilizing a concept that could be compossible with any underlying ontological stance (biological realism; social constructionism; antirealism; instrumentalism). How this would work in practice, with numerous public health bodies and governmental agencies coordinating would be a challenge—but not one that would be impossible to overcome. Even if there is no one universally accepted standard, the inclusion of conceptual parameters and criteria for classifying something as a *racialized* group in the methodology of empirically oriented public health (and biomedical) research could help immensely. This could be borne out through a richer understanding of public health crises comparatively—across sociopolitical contexts, with respect to retrospective public health studies, and to projecting and measuring the efficacy of public health interventions. These types of recommendations have been recently discussed by Jacquelynn Orr et al. (2021) and Krieger (2021) and are excellent steps in bringing the methodological issues surrounding categorizations of *race* and *racism* to the fore.

The avenue mentioned above is motivated by the ways in which racial classifications and their purported referents have changed across time and context. A notable instantiation of this dynamism is the concept of *mixed-race*, which portends to provide new and important complications for dealing with *race* and *racism* in public health—for our understanding of how that affects individuals, institutions, and populations themselves. Threads of this development can be found in Comstock, Castillo, and Lindsay (2004); Aspinall, Song, and Hashem (2006); Aspinall (2009, 2018); Valles, Bhopal, and Aspinall (2015); Tabb (2015); Roth (2016); and Ellison et al. (2017). While there is a broader literature regarding the concept of *mixed-race* and mixed-race categorizations, the focus for the current discussion is how, exactly, this will be dealt with from a philosophical and public health standpoint—which remains an open line of inquiry.

There are plenty of other avenues to be pursued with respect to race and racism in public health, of which philosophers, practitioners, researchers, governmental agencies, policy professionals, and all who are interested in improving the health outcomes of all persons, can contribute. Ranging from advancements in the assessment of health disparities for racialized groups; to developing and implementing strong methodological practices for gathering data and information regarding race, racism, and public health—whether qualitative, quantitative, historical, or emerging methods; carefully considering and reckoning with ethical considerations for direct public health interventions; refining and developing better understandings of concepts used in public health (Krieger 2012); and building or restructuring organizations and institutions so that they are not only attuned to mitigating current malpractices, but are able to deal with past injustices and are aimed at mitigating future injustices with respect to race and racism. While these are big questions, the need for dealing with them in light of contemporary and historical racial injustices is eminent. Too much is at stake for those who are currently suffering and for those who are currently on trajectories of developing negative health outcomes for all of us to be complacent.

Conclusion

This chapter aimed to bring to the fore some of the ontological presuppositions that undergird the concepts of *race* and *racism* as they are used in public health. While outlining a number of positions that are held, it should be noted that while the ontological commitments for *race* (as it is used in public health and biomedical research) are varied, all of the positions take it that addressing health inequalities (or health disparities) remains an important and pressing problem—especially in light of the recent social movements for the lives and dignity of those who have, are, and continue to be marginalized due to their perceived or purported racial membership. The task for public health to respond to this is in no way an easy one, especially since the concepts of *race*—and, to some extent, *racism*—have been utilized in ways that have been either conceptually confused or methodologically inconsistent. In order to make headway on these pressing issues, of which affect millions of people around the world, one important part of this is to make some progress on providing robust, logically consistent, and empirically applicable concepts that will help researchers and public health practitioners with the empirical work needed to monitor better interventions for all involved.

Notes

1 From a purely logical standpoint, the latter choice should be interpreted as "neither Hispanic nor Latino."
2 https://www.ons.gov.uk/file?uri=/census/censustransformationprogramme/ questiondevelopment/census2021paperquestionnaires/householdenglandpdf.pdf (accessed November 21, 2021).
3 In addition to these examples, other publications that bring attention to the inconsistent ways in which race is used include Vyas, Eisenstein, and Jones (2020); Yudell et al. (2016, 2020); Hahn and Stroup (1994); Ford and Kelly (2005); Valles, Bhopal, and Aspinal (2015); Paradies (2006); Mays et al. (2003); Whaley (2003); Maglo (2010); Krieger (2000); Comstock, Castillo, and Lindsay (2004); Moubarac (2013); Baer et al. (2013); and Braveman and Parker Dominguez (2021).
4 Other recent publications that have provided evidence for the connections between racism and health outcomes (or the issues that those connections create for marginalized groups) include Krieger (1990); Krieger et al. (1993); Noh and Kaspar (2003); Gee et al. (2009); Satcher and Higginbotham (2008); Pascoe and Richman (2009); Shavers et al. (2012); Phelan and Link (2015); Bailey et al. (2017); Feagin and Bennefield (2014); Paradies et al. (2015); Williams (2018); Thomas (2019); Trent, Dooley, and Dougé (2019); Williams, Lawrence, and Davis (2019); Yearby and Mohapatra (2020); Hardeman et al. (2018); and Yashadhana et al. (2020).
5 https://cph.osu.edu/news/2020/06/racism-public-health (accessed November 13, 2021).
6 https://onlinepublichealth.gwu.edu/resources/racism-public-health-crisis/ (accessed November 13, 2021).
7 https://www.sph.emory.edu/about/community-diversity/anti-race-social-justice/index.html (accessed November 13, 2021).
8 https://www.hsph.harvard.edu/news/racism-is-a-public-health-crisis/ (accessed November 13, 2021).
9 https://ph.ucla.edu/research/centers/center-study-racism-social-justice-health (accessed November 13, 2021).
10 Other studies from the region include Cave et al. (2020); Harris (2006); Harris, Cormack, and Stanley (2018); Harris, Stanley, and Cormack (2018); Paradies et al. (2009); Kairuz et al. (2020); Larson et al. (2007); Ziersch et al. (2011); Came et al. (2018); Bilal, Chan, and Somerset (2019); and Talamaivao et al. (2020).
11 Single-country studies include those done in Brazil (Hogan et al. 2018; Chauhan et al. 2018), the United Kingdom (Bécares, Kapadia, and Nazroo 2020; Nazroo 2004), Sweden (Bradby et al. 2019; Wamala et al. 2007), Canada (Datta et al. 2021; Dryden and Nnorom 2021; El-Mowafi et al. 2021; Gajaria, Guzder, and Rasasingham 2021; Levy, Ansara, and Stover 2013; Leyland

et al. 2016; Mahabir et al. 2021; Monchalin, Smylie, and Nowgesic 2019; Tuyisenge and Goldenberg 2021), Mexico (Dörr and Dietz 2020; Marquez-Velarde, Jones, and Keith 2020; Ortiz-Hernandez, Ayala-Guzman, and Perez-Salgado 2020), France (Rivenbark and Ichou 2020), and Spain (Agudelo-Suárez et al. 2009; Pérez-Urdiales et al. 2019).

References

Afshari, R. and R. S. Bhopal. 2010. Ethnicity has overtaken race in medical science: Medline-based comparison of trends in the USA and the rest of the world, 1965–2005. *International Journal of Epidemiology* 39, no. 6: 1682–1684. https://doi.org/10.1093/ije/dyp382.

Agudelo-Suárez, A., D. Gil-González, E. Ronda-Pérez et al. 2009. Discrimination, work and health in immigrant populations in Spain. *Social Science & Medicine* 68, no. 10: 1866–1874. https://doi.org/10.1016/j.socscimed.2009.02.046.

Akbulut, N., N. Limaro, L. Wandschneider et al. 2020. ASPHER statement on racism and health: Racism and discrimination obstruct public health's pursuit of health equity. *International Journal of Public Health* 65, no. 6: 727–729. https://dx.doi.org/10.1007%2Fs00038-020-01442-y.

American College of Physicians. 2017. Position statement on recognizing hate crimes as a public health issue. Technical report. https://www.acponline.org/acp policy/policies/hate crimes_public_health_issue_2017.pdf (accessed December 18, 2021).

American Public Health Association. 2021. Analysis: Declarations of racism as a public health crisis. Technical report. https://apha.org/-/media/Files/PDF/topics/racism/Racism_Declarations_Analysis.ashx (accessed December 18, 2021).

Ashish, K. Jha. n.d. Actions to confront anti-black racism. https://www.brown.edu/academics/public-health/diversity/actions (accessed November 10, 2021).

Aspinall, P. J. 2009. Short report: Concepts, terminology and classifications for the "mixed" ethnic or racial group in the United Kingdom. *Journal of Epidemiology & Community Health* 64, no. 6: 557–560. http://www.jstor.org/stable/20721248 (accessed December 18, 2021).

Aspinall, P. J. 2018. Measuring the health patterns of the "mixed/multiple" ethnic group in Britain: Data quality problems, reporting issues, and implications for policy. *International Journal of Social Research Methodology* 21, no. 3: 359–371. https://doi.org/10.1080/13645579.2017.1399623.

Aspinall, P. J., M. Song, and F. Hashem. 2006. Mixed race in Britain: A survey of the preferences of mixed race people for terminology and classifications. Technical report. Centre for Health Services Studies, Canterbury. https://kar.kent.ac.uk/24465/ (accessed December 18, 2021).

Baer, R. D., E. Arteaga, K. Dyer et al. 2013. Concepts of race and ethnicity among health researchers: Patterns and implications. *Ethnicity and Health* 18, no. 2: 211–225. https://doi.org/10.1080/13557858.2012.713091.

Bailey, Z. D., N. Krieger, M. Agénor, J. Graves, N. Linos, and M. T. Bassett. 2017. Structural racism and health inequities in the USA: Evidence and interventions. *The Lancet* 389, no. 10077: 1453–1463. https://doi.org/10.1016/s0140-6736(17)30569-x.

Bécares, L., D. Kapadia, and J. Nazroo. 2020. Neglect of older ethnic minority people in UK research and policy. *BMJ*: m212. https://doi.org/10.1136/bmj.m212.

Bentley, G. R. 2020. Don't blame the BAME: Ethnic and structural inequalities in susceptibilities to Covid-19. *American Journal of Human Biology*. https://doi.org/10.1002/ajhb.23478

Bhopal, R. 2004. Glossary of terms relating to ethnicity and race: For reflection and debate. *Journal of Epidemiology & Community Health* 58: 441–445. http://dx.doi.org/10.1136/jech.2003.013466.

Bhopal, R. 2015. Ethnicity, race, epidemiology, and public health. In *Oxford textbook of global public health, vol. 3*, 6th edition, ed. R. Detels, M. Gulliford, Q. Abdool Karim, and C. C. Tan, 1371–1381. Oxford: Oxford University Press.

Bilal, P. I., C. K. Y. Chan, and S. M. Somerset. 2019. Acculturation and perceived ethnic discrimination predict elevated blood glucose level in sub-Saharan African immigrants in Australia. *Journal of Immigrant and Minority Health* 22, no. 4: 771–777. https://doi.org/10.1007/s10903-019-00958-7.

Borrell, L. N., J. R. Elhawary, E. Fuentes-Afflick et al. 2021. Race and genetic ancestry in medicine: A time for reckoning with racism. *New England Journal of Medicine* 384, no. 5: 474–480. https://doi.org/10.1056/nejmms2029562.

Bradby, H. 1995. Ethnicity: Not a black and white issue—A research note. *Sociology of Health & Illness* 17, no. 3: 405–417. http://dx.doi.org/10.1111/1467-9566.ep10933332.

Bradby, H., S. Thapar-Björkert, S. Hamed, and B. M. Ahlberg. 2019. Undoing the unspeakable: Researching racism in Swedish healthcare using a participatory process to build dialogue. *Health Research Policy and Systems* 17, no. 1. https://doi.org/10.1186/s12961-019-0443-0.

Braveman, P. and T. Parker Dominguez. 2021. Abandon "race." Focus on racism. *Frontiers in Public Health* 9: 689462. https://dx.doi.org/10.3389%2Ffpubh.2021.689462.

Broadbent, A. 2013. *Philosophy of epidemiology*. London: Palgrave Macmillan.

Burchard, E. G., E. Ziv, N. Coyle et al. 2003. The importance of race and ethnic background in biomedical research and clinical practice. *New England Journal of Medicine* 348, no. 12: 1170–1175. https://doi.org/10.1056/nejmsb025007.

Came, H. 2014. Sites of institutional racism in public health policy making in New Zealand. *Social Science & Medicine* 106: 214–220. https://doi.org/10.1016/j.socscimed.2014.01.055.

Came, H., C. Doole, B. McKenna, and T. McCreanor. 2018. Institutional racism in public health contracting: Findings of a nationwide survey from New Zealand. *Social Science & Medicine* 199: 132–139. https://doi.org/10.1016/j.socscimed.2017.06.002.

Canadian Public Health Association. 2018. Racism and public health. https://www.cpha.ca/racism-and-public-health (accessed November 13, 2021).

Cave, L., M. N. Cooper, S. R. Zubrick, and C. C. J. Shepherd. 2020. Racial discrimination and allostatic load among first nations Australians: A nationally representative cross-sectional study. *BMC Public Health* 20, no. 1. https://doi.org/10.1186/s12889-020-09978-7.

CDC (Centers for Disease Control and Prevention). 2021. Racism and health: Racism is a serious threat to the public's health. https://www.cdc.gov/healthequity/racism-disparities/index.html (accessed November 10, 2021).

Chauhan, A., G. de Wildt, M. da Cunha Lopes Virmond et al. 2018. Perceptions and experiences regarding the impact of race on the quality of healthcare in southeast Brazil: A qualitative study. *Ethnicity & Health* 25, no. 3: 436–452. https://doi.org/10.1080/13557858.2018.1431206.

Comstock, R. D., E. M. Castillo, and S. P. Lindsay. 2004. Four-year review of the use of race and ethnicity in epidemiologic and public health research. *American Journal of Epidemiology* 159, no. 6: 611–619. https://doi.org/10.1093/aje/kwh084.

Datta, G., A. Siddiqi, and A. Lofters. 2021. Transforming race-based health research in Canada. *Canadian Medical Association Journal* 193, no. 3: E99–E100. https://doi.org/10.1503/cmaj.201742.

De Souza, I. M., G. D. Hughes, B. E. van Wyk, V. Mathews, and E. M. de Araújo. 2020. Comparative analysis of the constitution and implementation of race/skin color field in health information systems: Brazil and South Africa. *Journal of Racial and Ethnic Health Disparities* 8, no. 2: 350–362. https://doi.org/10.1007/s40615-020-00789-5.

Devakumar, D., S. S. Bhopal, and G. Shannon. 2020. Covid-19: The great equaliser. *Journal of the Royal Society of Medicine* 113, no. 6: 234–235. https://doi.org/10.1177/0141076820925434.

Devakumar, D., S. Selvarajah, G. Shannon et al. 2020. Racism, the public health crisis we can no longer ignore. *The Lancet* 395, no. 10242: e112–e113. https://dx.doi.org/10.1016%2FS0140-6736(20)31371-4.

Diamond-Hunter, M. A. 2020. An instrumentalist account of race and its applicability to the empirical sciences. PhD diss., University of California, Davis.

Donovan, B. M. 2014. Playing with fire? The impact of the hidden curriculum in school genetics on essentialist conceptions of race. *Journal of Research in Science Teaching* 51, no. 4: 462–496. https://doi.org/10.1002/tea.21138.

Dörr, N. M. and G. Dietz. 2020. Racism against Totonaco women in Veracruz: Intercultural competences for health professionals are necessary. *PLOS One* 15, no. 1: e0227149. https://doi.org/10.1371/journal.pone.0227149.

Dryden, O. and O. Nnorom. Time to dismantle systemic anti-black racism in medicine in Canada. *Canadian Medical Association Journal* 193, no. 2: E55–E57. https://doi.org/10.1503/cmaj.201579.

DuBois Bowman, F. 2020. Public health's role in addressing racism. https://publichealth.umich.edu/pursuit/2020posts/public-healths-role-in-addressing-racism.html (accessed November 10, 2021).

Ellison, G. T., P. J. Aspinall, A. Smart, and S. Salway. 2017. The ambiguities of "race" in UK science, social policy and political discourse. *Journal of Anthropological Sciences* 95: 299–306. http://dx.doi.org/10.4436/JASS.95018.

El-Mowafi, I. M., A. Yalahow, D. Idriss-Wheeler, and S. Yaya. 2021. The politest form of racism: Sexual and reproductive health and rights paradigm in Canada. *Reproductive Health* 18, no. 1. https://doi.org/10.1186/s12978-021-01117-8.

Eschner, K. 2020. Racism is undeniably a public health issue. *Popular Science*. https://www.popsci. com/story/health/racism-public-health/ (accessed November 10, 2021).

Evans, M. K., L. Rosenbaum, D. Malina, S. Morrissey, and E. J. Rubin. 2020. Diagnosing and treating systemic racism. *New England Journal of Medicine* 383, no. 3: 274–276. https://doi.org/10.1056/ nejme2021693.

Feagin, J. and Z. Bennefield. 2014. Systemic racism and U.S. health care. *Social Science & Medicine* 103: 7–14. https://doi.org/10.1016/j.socscimed.2013.09.006.

Ford, M. E. and P. A. Kelly. 2005. Conceptualizing and categorizing race and ethnicity in health services research. *Health Services Research* 40, no. 5 (Part 2): 1658–1675. https://dx.doi.org/10.1111%2Fj. 1475-6773.2005.00449.x.

Gajaria, A., J. Guzder, and R. Rasasingham. 2021. What's race got to do with it? A proposed framework to address racism's impacts on child and adolescent mental health in Canada. *Journal of the Canadian Academy of Child and Adolescent Psychiatry* 30, no. 2: 131–137. https://www.ncbi.nlm.nih. gov/pmc/articles/PMC8056965/ (accessed December 18, 2021).

García, J. J.-L. and M. Z. Sharif. 2015. Black lives matter: A commentary on racism and public health. *American Journal of Public Health* 105, no. 8: e27–e30. https://dx.doi.org/10.2105%2FAJPH.2015.302706.

Gee, G. C., A. Ro, S. Shariff-Marco, and D. Chae. 2009. Racial discrimination and health among Asian Americans: Evidence, assessment, and directions for future research. *Epidemiologic Reviews* 31, no. 1: 130–151. https://doi.org/10.1093/epirev/mxp009.

Gillam, S. 2016. *Essential public health*. 2nd edition. Cambridge: Cambridge University Press.

Hahn, R. A. and D. F. Stroup. 1994. Race and ethnicity in public health surveillance: Criteria for the scientific use of social categories. *Public Health Reports* 109, no. 1: 7–15. https://www.ncbi. nlm.nih.gov/pmc/articles/PMC1402237/pdf/pubhealthrep00062-0009.pdf (accessed December 17, 2021).

Hamed, S., S. Thapar-Björkert, H. Bradby, and B. Maina Ahlberg. 2020. Racism in European health care: Structural violence and beyond. *Qualitative Health Research* 30, no. 11: 1662–1673. https://doi. org/10.1177/1049732320931430.

Hardeman, R. R., K. A. Murphy, J. Karbeah, and K. B. Kozhimannil. 2018. Naming institutionalized racism in the public health literature: A systematic literature review. *Public Health Reports* 133, no. 3: 240–249. https://doi.org/10.1177/0033354918760574.

Harris, R., M. Tobias, M. Jeffreys, K. Waldegrave, S. Karlsen, and J. Nazroo. 2006. Racism and health: The relationship between experience of racial discrimination and health in New Zealand. *Social Science & Medicine* 63, no. 6: 1428–1441. https://doi.org/10.1016/j.socscimed.2006.04.009.

Harris, R. B., D. M. Cormack, and J. Stanley. 2018. Experience of racism and associations with unmet need and healthcare satisfaction: The 2011/12 adult New Zealand health survey. *Australian and New Zealand Journal of Public Health* 43, no. 1: 75–80. https://doi.org/10.1111/1753-6405.12835.

Harris, R. B., J. Stanley, and D. M. Cormack. 2018. Racism and health in New Zealand: Prevalence over time and associations between recent experience of racism and health and wellbeing measures using national survey data. *PLoS One* 13, no. 5: e0196476. https://doi.org/10.1371/journal. pone.0196476.

Haslam, N., L. Rothschild, and D. Ernst. 2000. Essentialist beliefs about social categories. *British Journal of Social Psychology* 39, no. 1: 113–127. https://doi.org/10.1348/014466600164363.

Hogan, V. K., E. M. de Araujo, K. L. Caldwell, S. N. Gonzalez-Nahm, and K. Z. Black. 2018. "We black women have to kill a lion everyday": An intersectional analysis of racism and social determinants of health in Brazil. *Social Science & Medicine* 199: 96–105. https://doi.org/10.1016/j. socscimed.2017.07.008.

Kairuz, C. A., L. M. Casanelia, K. Bennett-Brook, J. Coombes, and U. N. Yadav. 2020. Impact of racism and discrimination on the physical and mental health among Aboriginal and Torres Strait Islander peoples living in Australia: A protocol for a scoping review. *Systematic Reviews* 9, no. 1: 223. https://doi.org/10.1186/s13643-020-01480-w.

Kaplan, J. B. and T. Bennett. 2003. Use of race and ethnicity in biomedical publication. *JAMA* 289, no. 20: 2709. https://doi.org/10.1001/jama.289.20.2709.

Keller, J. 2005. In genes we trust: The biological component of psychological essentialism and its relationship to mechanisms of motivated social cognition. *Journal of Personality and Social Psychology* 88, 4: 686–702. https://doi.org/10.1037/0022-3514.88.4.686.

Krieger, N. 1990. Racial and gender discrimination: Risk factors for high blood pressure? *Social Science & Medicine* 30, no. 12: 1273–1281. https://doi.org/10.1016/0277-9536(90)90307-e.

Krieger, N. 2000. Counting accountably: Implications of the new approaches to classifying race/ethnicity in the 2000 census. *American Journal of Public Health* 90, no. 11: 1687–1689. https://dx.doi.org/10.2105%2Fajph.90.11.1687.

Krieger, N. 2003. Does racism harm health? Did child abuse exist before 1962? On explicit questions, critical science, and current controversies: An ecosocial perspective. *American Journal of Public Health* 93, no. 2: 194–199. https://doi.org/10.2105/ajph.93.2.194.

Krieger, N. 2012. Who and what is a "population"? Historical debates, current controversies, and implications for understanding "population health" and rectifying health inequities. *The Milbank Quarterly* 90, no. 4: 634–681. https://doi.org/10.1111/j.1468-0009.2012.00678.x.

Krieger, N. 2021. Structural racism, health inequities, and the two-edged sword of data: Structural problems require structural solutions. *Frontiers in Public Health* 9. https://doi.org/10.3389/fpubh.2021.655447.

Krieger, N., D. L. Rowley, A. A. Herman, B. Avery, and M. T. Phillips. 1993. Racism, sexism, and social class: Implications for studies of health, disease, and well-being. *American Journal of Preventative Medicine* 9, no. 6: 82–122. https://doi.org/10.1016/S0749-3797%2818%2930666-4.

Larson, A., M. Gillies, P. J. Howard, and J. Coffin. 2007. It's enough to make you sick: The impact of racism on the health of Aboriginal Australians. *Australian and New Zealand Journal of Public Health* 31, no. 4: 322–329. https://doi.org/10.1111/j.1753-6405.2007.00079.x.

Levy, J., D. Ansara, and A. Stover. 2013. Racialization and health inequities in Toronto. Technical Report. Toronto Public Health. https://www.toronto.ca/legdocs/mmis/2013/hl/bgrd/backgroundfile-62904.pdf (accessed December 18, 2021).

Leyland, A., J. Smylie, M. Cole et al. 2016. Health and health care implications of systemic racism on indigenous peoples in Canada. Technical Report. Le Collège des Médecins de Famille du Canada/The College of Family Physicians of Canada. https://www.cfpc.ca/systemic-racism (accessed December 18, 2021).

Lorusso, L. and F. Bacchini. 2015. A reconsideration of the role of self-identified races in epidemiology and biomedical research. *Studies in History and Philosophy of Science Part C: Studies in History and Philosophy of Biological and Biomedical Sciences* 52: 56–64. https://doi.org/10.1016/j.shpsc.2015.02.004.

Loveman, M. 2014. *National colors: Racial classification and the state in Latin America*. Oxford: Oxford University Press.

Maglo, K. N. 2010. Genomics and the conundrum of race: Some epistemic and ethical considerations. *Perspectives in Biology and Medicine* 53, no. 3: 357–372. https://doi.org/10.1353/pbm.0.0171.

Mahabir, D. F., P. O'Campo, A. Lofters, K. Shankardass, C. Salmon, and C. Muntaner. 2021. Experiences of everyday racism in Toronto's health care system: A concept mapping study. *International Journal for Equity in Health* 20, no. 1: 74. https://doi.org/10.1186/s12939-021-01410-9.

Marquez-Velarde, G., N. E. Jones, and V. M. Keith. 2020. Racial stratification in self-rated health among Black Mexicans and White Mexicans. *SSM Population Health* 10: 100509. https://doi.org/10.1016/j.ssmph.2019.100509.

Mays, V. M., N. A. Ponce, D. L. Washington, and S. D. Cochran. 2003. Classification of race and ethnicity: Implications for public health. *Annual Review of Public Health* 24: 83–110. https://doi.org/10.1146/annurev.publhealth.24.100901.140927.

Mendez, D. D., J. Scott, L. Adodoadji, C. Toval, M. McNeil, and M. Sindhu. 2021. Racism as public health crisis: Assessment and review of municipal declarations and resolutions across the United States. *Frontiers in Public Health* 9: 686807. https://dx.doi.org/10.3389%2Ffpubh.2021.686807.

Milner, A. and S. Jumbe. 2020. Using the right words to address racial disparities in Covid-19. *The Lancet Public Health* 5, no. 8: e419–e420. https://doi.org/10.1016/s2468-2667(20)30162-6.

Mitrou, F., M. Cooke, D. Lawrence et al. 2014. Gaps in indigenous disadvantage not closing: A census cohort study of social determinants of health in Australia, Canada, and New Zealand from 1981–2006. *BMC Public Health* 14, no. 1. https://doi.org/10.1186/1471-2458-14-201.

Mock, B. 2020. Dozens of city governments declare racism a public health crisis. *Bloomberg City Lab*. https://www.bloomberg.com/news/articles/2020-07-13/dozens-of-cities-dub-racism-a-public-health-crisis (accessed November 27, 2021).

Monchalin, R., J. Smylie, and E. Nowgesic. 2019. "I guess I shouldn't come back here": Racism and discrimination as a barrier to accessing health and social services for urban Métis women in Toronto, Canada. *Journal of Racial and Ethnic Health Disparities* 7, no. 2: 251–261. https://doi.org/10.1007/s40615-019-00653-1.

Montagu, A. 1945. *Man's most dangerous myth: The fallacy of race*. 2nd edition. New York: Columbia University Press.

Moubarac, J-C. 2013. Persisting problems related to race and ethnicity in public health and epidemiology research. *Revista de Saude Publica* 47, no. 1: 105–116. https://doi.org/10.1590/s0034-89102013000100014.

National Institutes of Health. 2001. NIH policy and guidelines on the inclusion of women and minorities as subjects in clinical research. https://grants.nih.gov/policy/inclusion/women-and-
minorities/guidelines.htm (accessed December 17, 2021).

National Institutes of Health. 2007. Title 42: Public health and welfare. Technical report. https://www.
gpo.gov/fdsys/pkg/USCODE-2011-title42/pdf/USCODE-2011-title42-chap6A-subchapIII-
partH-sec289a-2.pdf (accessed November 23, 2020).

Nazroo, J. Y. 2004. Ethnic disparities in aging health: What can we learn from the United Kingdom?
In *Critical perspectives on racial and ethnic differences in health in late life,* ed. N. B. Anderson, R. A.
Bulatao, and B. Cohen, 667–702. Washington, DC: National Academies Press.

Nijhuis, H. G. and L. J. van der Maesen. 1994. The philosophical foundations of public health: An
invitation to debate. *Journal of Epidemiology and Community Health* 48, no. 1: 1–3. https://dx.doi.
org/10.1136%2Fjech.48.1.1-a.

Noh, S. and V. Kaspar. 2003. Perceived discrimination and depression: Moderating effects of coping,
acculturation, and ethnic support. *American Journal of Public Health* 93, no. 2: 232–238. https://
dx.doi.org/10.2105%2Fajph.93.2.232.

O'Reilly, K. B. 2020. AMA: Racism is a threat to public health. https://www.ama-assn.org/delivering-
care/health-equity/ama-racism-threat-public-health (accessed November 13, 2021).

Orr, J. Y., M. S. Shaw, R. Bland, G. Hobor, and A. L. Plough. 2021. Addressing racism in research
can transform public health. *American Journal of Public Health* 111, suppl. 3: S182–S184. https://ajph.
aphapublications.org/doi/full/10.2105/AJPH.2021.306542 (accessed December 18. 2021).

Ortiz-Hernandez, L., C. I. Ayala-Guzman, and D. Perez-Salgado. 2020. Health inequities associated
with skin color and ethnicity in Mexico. *Latin American and Caribbean Ethnic Studies* 15, no. 1:
70–85. https://doi.org/10.1080/17442222.2020.1714846.

Paradies, Y. 2006. A systematic review of empirical research on self-reported racism and health. *International Journal of Epidemiology* 35, no. 4: 888–901. https://doi.org/10.1093/ije/dyl056.

Paradies, Y., J. Ben, N. Denson et al. 2015. Racism as a determinant of health: A systematic review and
meta-analysis. *PLoS One* 10, no. 9: e0138511. https://dx.doi.org/10.1371%2Fjournal.pone.0138511.

Paradies, Y., L. Chandrakumar, N. Klocker et al. 2009. Building on our strengths: A framework to
reduce racial discrimination and promote diversity in Victoria. Technical report. Victorian Health
Promotion Foundation. https://ro.uow.edu.au/scipapers/4674 (accessed November 13, 2021).

Pascoe, E. A. and L. S. Richman. 2009. Perceived discrimination and health: A meta-analytic review.
Psychological Bulletin 135, no. 4: 531–554. https://dx.doi.org/10.1037%2Fa0016059.

Pauker, K., N. Ambady, and E. P. Apfelbaum. 2010. Race salience and essentialist thinking in racial stereotype development. *Child Development* 81, no. 6: 1799–1813. https://dx.doi.org/10.1111%2Fj.1467-
8624.2010.01511.x.

Pérez-Urdiales, I., I. Goicolea, M. S. Sebastián, A. Irazusta, and I. Linander. 2019. Sub-Saharan African immigrant women's experiences of (lack of) access to appropriate healthcare in the public
health system in the Basque country, Spain. *International Journal for Equity in Health* 18, no. 1: 59.
https://doi.org/10.1186/s12939-019-0958-6.

Phelan, J. C. and B. G. Link. 2015. Is racism a fundamental cause of inequalities in health? *Annual
Review of Sociology* 41, no. 1: 311–330. https://doi.org/10.1146/annurev-soc-073014-112305.

Porta, M. and J. M. Last. 2018. *A dictionary of public health.* 2nd edition. Oxford: Oxford University
Press. https://doi.org/10.1093/acref/9780191844386.001.0001.

Prentice, D. A. and T. D. Miller. 2007. Psychological essentialism of human categories. *Current Directions
in Psychological Science* 16, no. 4: 202–206. https://doi.org/10.1111%2Fj.1467-8721.2007.00504.x.

Public Health England. 2018. Local action on health inequalities: Understanding and reducing ethnic inequalities in health. Technical Report. https://www.instituteofhealthequity.org/resources- reports/
local-action-on-health-inequalities-understanding-and-reducing- ethnic-inequalities-in-health-/
understanding-and-reducing-ethnic- inequalities-in-health.pdf (accessed November 15, 2021).

Public Health England. 2020. COVID-19: Review of disparities in risks and outcomes. Technical report. https://www.gov.uk/government/publications/covid-19-review-of-disparities-in-risks-and-
outcomes (accessed November 15, 2021).

Purdue University Department of Public Health. n.d. Racism is a public health crisis. https://www.
purdue.edu/hhs/public-health/diversity/racism-is-a-public-health-crisis.php (accessed November
13, 2021).

Rivara, F. P. and S. D. Fihn. 2020. Call for papers on prevention and the effects of systemic racism in health. *JAMA Network Open* 3, no. 8: e2016825. https://doi.org/10.1001/jamanetworkopen.2020.16825.

Rivenbark, J. G. and M. Ichou. 2020. Discrimination in healthcare as a barrier to care: Experiences of socially disadvantaged populations in France from a nationally representative survey. *BMC Public Health* 20, no. 1. https://doi.org/10.1186/s12889-019-8124-z.

Roberts, D. E. 2021. Abolish race correction. *The Lancet* 397, no. 10268: 17–18. https://doi.org/10.1016/s0140-6736(20)32716-1.

Rosenberg, N. A., J. K. Pritchard, J. L. Weber et al. 2002. Genetic structure of human populations. *Science* 298, no. 5602: 2381–2385. https://doi.org/10.1126/science.1078311.

Roth, W. D. 2016. The multiple dimensions of race. *Ethnic and Racial Studies* 39, no. 8: 1310–1338. https://doi.org/10.1080/01419870.2016.1140793.

Satcher, D. and E. J. Higginbotham. 2008. The public health approach to eliminating disparities in health. *American Journal of Public Health* 98, no. 3: 400–403. https://dx.doi.org/10.2105%2Fajph.98.supplement_1.s8.

Shavers, V. L., P. Fagan, D. Jones et al. 2012. The state of research on racial/ethnic discrimination in the receipt of health care. *American Journal of Public Health* 102, no. 5: 953–966. https://doi.org/10.2105/ajph.2012.300773.

Smithson, M. and J. Verkuilen. 2006. *Fuzzy set theory: Applications in the social sciences*. London: Sage.

Spencer, Q. 2012. What "biological racial realism" should mean. *Philosophical Studies* 159, no. 2: 181–204. https://doi.org/10.1007/s11098-011-9697-2.

Spencer, Q. 2014. A radical solution to the race problem. *Philosophy of Science* 81, no. 5: 1025–1038. http://dx.doi.org/10.1086/677694.

Spencer, Q. 2016. Do humans have continental populations? *Philosophy of Science* 83, no. 5: 791–802. https://doi.org/10.1086/687864.

Spencer, Q. N. J. 2018. A racial classification for medical genetics. *Philosophical Studies* 175, no. 5: 1013–1037. https://doi.org/10.1007/S11098-018-1072-0.

Spencer, Q., J. Glasgow, S. Haslanger, and C. Jeffers. 2019. *What is race? Four philosophical views*. Oxford: Oxford University Press, 2019.

Tabb, K. M. 2015. Changes in racial categorization over time and health status: An examination of multiracial young adults in the USA. *Ethnicity & Health* 21, no. 2: 146–157. https://doi.org/10.1080/13557858.2015.1042431.

Talamaivao, N., R. Harris, D. Cormack, S.-J. Paine, and P. King. 2020. Racism and health in Aotearoa New Zealand: A systematic review of quantitative studies. *New Zealand Medical Journal* 133, no. 1521. https://journal.nzma.org.nz/journal-articles/racism-and-health-in-aotearoa-new-zealand-a-systematic-review-of-quantitative-studies (accessed December 18, 2021).

Thomas, S. B. 2019. Racial and ethnic disparities as a public health ethics issue. In *The Oxford handbook of public health ethics*, ed. A. C. Mastroianni, J. P. Kahn, and N. E. Kass, 276–289. Oxford: Oxford University Press.

Thulin, L. 2020. What "racism is a public health issue" means. *Smithsonian Magazine* https://www.smithsonianmag.com/science-nature/what-racism-public-health-issue-means-180975326/ (accessed November 23, 2021).

Trent, M., D. G. Dooley, and J. Dougé. 2019. The impact of racism on child and adolescent health. *Pediatrics* 144, no. 2: e20191765. https://doi.org/10.1542/peds.2019-1765.

Tulane University's School of Public Health and Tropical Medicine. 2021. Why racism is a public health issue. https://publichealth.tulane.edu/blog/racism-public-health/ (accessed November 13, 2021).

Tuyisenge, G. and S. M. Goldenberg. 2021. Covid-19, structural racism, and migrant health in Canada. *The Lancet* 397, no. 10275: 650–652. https://doi.org/10.1016/s0140-6736(21)00215-4.

Valles, S. 2020. Philosophy of biomedicine. In *The Stanford encyclopedia of philosophy (Summer 2020)*, ed. E. N. Zalta. https://plato.stanford.edu/entries/biomedicine/ (accessed December 17, 2021).

Valles, S. A. 2012. Heterogeneity of risk within racial groups, a challenge for public health programs. *Preventive Medicine* 55, no. 5: 405–408. https://doi.org/10.1016/j.ypmed.2012.08.022.

Valles, S., R. Bhopal, and P. Aspinall. 2015. Census categories for mixed race and mixed ethnicity: Impacts on data collection and analysis in the US, UK and NZ. *Public Health* 129: 266–270. https://doi.org/10.1016/j.puhe.2014.12.017.

Vyas, D. A., L. G. Eisenstein, and D. S. Jones. 2020. Hidden in plain sight: Reconsidering the use of race correction in clinical algorithms. *New England Journal of Medicine* 383, no. 9: 874–882. https://doi.org/10.1056/nejmms2004740.

Wallis, C. 2020. Why racism, not race, is a risk factor for dying of Covid-19. *Scientific American*. https://www.scientificamerican.com/article/why-racism-not-race-is-a-risk-factor-for-dying-of-covid-191/ (accessed November 22, 2021).

Wamala, S., J. Merlo, G. Bostrom, C. Hogstedt, and G. Agren. 2007. Socioeconomic disadvantage and primary non-adherence with medication in Sweden. *International Journal for Quality in Health Care* 19, no. 3:134–140. https://doi.org/10.1093/intqhc/mzm011.

Wandschneider, L., Y. Namer, N. Akbulut, and O. Razum. 2020. Fighting racism in schools of public health. *The Lancet* 396, no. 10260: e66. https://doi.org/10.1016/s0140-6736(20)32157-7.

Weed, D. L. 1999. Towards a philosophy of public health. *Journal of Epidemiology and Community Health* 53, no. 2: 99–104. https://dx.doi.org/10.1136%2Fjech.53.2.99.

Weed, D. L. 2004. *Handbook of bioethics: Taking stock of the field from a philosophical perspective.* Dordrecht: Springer.

Whaley, A. L. 2003. Ethnicity/race, ethics and epidemiology. *Journal of the National Medical Association* 95, no. 8: 736–742. http://www.ncbi.nlm.nih.gov/pmc/articles/pmc2594561/ (accessed December 17, 2021).

Williams, D. R. 2018. Stress and the mental health of populations of color: Advancing our understanding of race-related stressors. *Journal of Health and Social Behavior* 59, no. 4: 466–485. https://dx.doi.org/10.1177%2F0022146518814251.

Williams, D. R., J. A. Lawrence, and B. A. Davis. 2019. Racism and health: Evidence and needed research. *Annual Review of Public Health* 40, no. 1: 105–125. https://doi.org/10.1146/annurev-publhealth-040218-043750.

Yashadhana, A., N. Pollard-Wharton, A. B. Zwi, and B. Biles. 2020. Indigenous Australians at increased risk of Covid-19 due to existing health and socioeconomic inequities. *The Lancet Regional Health – Western Pacific* 1: 100007. https://dx.doi.org/10.1016%2Fj.lanwpc.2020.100007.

Yearby, R. and S. Mohapatra. 2020. Law, structural racism, and the Covid-19 pandemic. *Journal of Law and the Biosciences* 7, no. 1. https://doi.org/10.1093/jlb/lsaa036.

Yudell, M., D. Roberts, R. DeSalle, and S. Tishkoff. 2016. Taking race out of human genetics. *Science* 351, no. 6273: 564–565. https://doi.org/10.1126/science.aac4951.

Yudell, M., D. Roberts, R. DeSalle, and S. Tishkoff. 2020. NIH must confront the use of race in science. *Science* 369, no. 6509: 1313–1314. https://doi.org/10.1126/science.abd4842.

Ziersch, A. M., G. Gallaher, F. Baum, and M. Bentley. 2011. Responding to racism: Insights on how racism can damage health from an urban study of Australian Aboriginal people. *Social Science & Medicine* 73, no. 7: 1045–1053. https://doi.org/10.1016/j.socscimed.2011.06.058.

17

SEX AND GENDER BLIND SPOTS AND BIASES IN HEALTH RESEARCH

Avni Amin, Lavanya Vijayasingham, and Jacqui Stevenson

Introduction: why sex and gender biases are a problem in health research

Sex, gender, and gender inequality are known determinants of health, with well-established differentiated and unequal risks and outcomes across multiple health issues and in health systems responses. Biological (that is, sex) differences produce health differences mostly between males and females. There are also effects of gender norms, socialization, roles, and differentials in power relations that contribute to differential health risks/exposures, access to health information and outcomes and inequities between and among women, men, and people of other gender identities. Gender differences and inequalities play out in intimate relationships, families, communities, and institutions through the influence of social, cultural, economic, and political factors. The impact of gender has been well established in a robust body of literature on determinants of health (Heise et al. 2019; Mauvais-Jarvis et al. 2020). Both sex and gender can modify the outcomes of diagnostic procedures and of preventive and treatment interventions in public health.

Problematically, in public health—including pre-clinical, clinical, epidemiological, behavioural, and health systems research—while the need for considering sex and gender is recognized, the practice of systematically doing so has lagged far behind. Failure to properly address sex and gender is endemic in the production of public health evidence and knowledge, calling into question the scientific rigour and generalizability of the research (Ruiz-Cantero et al. 2007), as well as raising ethical challenges related to equity and social justice.

Disaggregation of data by sex is an important first step in integrating sex and gender in health research. Calls for disaggregation of data by sex have been made for the last three decades. However, a substantial proportion of human trials continue to not report data by sex, including most recently, with respect to Covid-19 studies where only 4% of registered studies reported a plan to include sex or gender as an analytical variable (Brady et al. 2021; Sugimoto et al. 2019; Welch et al. 2017). Moreover, women are underrepresented in clinical trials on several health conditions. In a global study on sex bias in clinical studies, in at least seven out of eleven disease categories, women were underrepresented in clinical trials (Feldman et al. 2019). Even where women are represented in sufficient numbers in proportion to disease prevalence, data are often not analysed by sex to understand the effects (for example, severity,

DOI: 10.4324/9781315675411-21

rate of progress, sex-specific side effects, or effectiveness) separately in females and males (Ravindran et al. 2020). Lastly, conditions that predominantly or specifically affect women continue to be under-researched, such as endometriosis, menstrual disorders, migraines, and autoimmune disorders (Eisenstein 2020; Mann et al. 2018; Rogers et al. 2009).

Several studies have examined the reasons for persistent gaps in integrating sex and gender and the male bias in health research, which includes the underinvestment in research on women's health (Holdcroft 2016). These studies point to the subjectivities of knowledge generation, in turn, influenced by a historical legacy of bias in medicine and public health. In sum, the male body and men's lived experiences have been considered the standard, or norm, and the knowledge generated about it as transferable to and representative of the female body in non-reproductive system-based medical studies. The generalizability of knowledge derived from the male body and experience is thought to justify the neglect of the nuances of the female body, and women's lived experiences outside of female reproductive health issues.

Barriers to integrating sex and gender into health research are many and diverse (Day et al. 2016; Kalenga et al. 2020). First is a conflation of the distinct concepts of sex and gender. Second is the lack of knowledge and practical skills/capacities of how to apply the concepts to health research and the related interpretation of its impact on the evidence produced. Treating considerations of sex and gender as extra or optional asserts the concepts as being non-essential or lower order in causal explanations. Third, researchers perceive that women's bodies are too complex or that because of their childbearing potential they must be protected as reasons for not including women or focusing on health conditions affecting women (Mazure and Jones 2015; Pascual et al. 2021). Fourth, there is a lack of demand and enforcement of integration of sex and gender into research by research funders, publishers, institutions, and pharmaceutical regulators (Day et al. 2016; Hankivsky et al. 2018). These barriers are related to research and development (R&D) institutions and systems that are male-led and patriarchal (Global Health 50/50 2021).

This chapter seeks to address three questions. First, why do sex and gender matter in the production of scientific evidence or research on health, including medicine and public health? Second, what are emerging areas of medical and public health research and innovation where sex and gender considerations need to be explicitly addressed from the outset? Third, how can sex and gender be systematically embedded into production of scientific knowledge and generation of evidence in medicine and public health? We foreground the response to these three questions by highlighting how sex and gender are defined and the contributions of intersectional feminist theories in providing an analytical framework to examine the subjectivities of scientific evidence production.

Defining sex and gender and their application to health research

Sex and gender are distinct concepts and should be applied precisely. The use of these two terms interchangeably perpetuates confusion and leads to incorrect analyses. Sex is widely defined and understood as the biological and physiological characteristics that distinguish males and females. And sex is thought to have independent and cumulative effects on disease pathology, progression, health outcomes, and inequities through genetic, cellular, and physiological pathways. Sex is usually understood in binary terms—as genetic differences between females and males based on the former carrying two X chromosomes and the latter carrying an X and a Y chromosome. There is an increasing recognition that sex is not an absolute binary category and includes intersex individuals with variations in sex chromosomes, genes, internal reproductive organs, and hormones and secondary sex characteristics such as external genitalia. Intersex persons have been estimated to make up 1–2% of the population. The estimations can depend on the diagnostic criteria and cultural stigma, which can prevent disclosure (Carpenter 2016; Fausto-Sterling 2000; Jones 2018).

Differences in risk of acquiring diseases, pathology, morbidity, response to treatment, and mortality are found to be linked to the sex-differentiated biological aspects of the human body, including the presence or absence, and the expressions of specific alleles on the X and Y chromosomes, as well as broader molecular, physiological, and biochemical differences (Maan et al. 2017; Schurz et al. 2019). For example, it is known that females are more likely to have better immediate and long-term immunity to infections—a phenomenon that is thought to be linked to having two X chromosomes (Schurz et al. 2019). The phenotypic differentiation of sex characteristics—that is, genitalia and gonadal hormones—also manifests differently, with females having a dominance of oestrogen to varying degrees and males having a dominance of testosterone to varying degrees. Apart from sex-specific diseases (for example, testicular cancer in males or ovarian, uterine, and cervical cancers in females), it is generally recognized that oestrogen and androgen receptors play a role in shaping the progression and manifestations of diseases in females differently than in males and across the life course (Mauvais-Jarvis et al. 2020).

Gender, however, has several definitions and multiple meanings, but is widely understood to be socially constructed. It influences exposure to risks, diseases, and illness; health behaviours, uptake of and access to information and services, therapeutics, and health technologies; and how societies and health systems respond to those who are ill. Gender has been defined in at least three distinct ways. The first and the most widely described definition of gender is "a set of socially constructed roles and expectations or norms that go along with being biologically male and female, which manifest in terms of different attitudes, beliefs, norms, socialization of roles, and division of labour" (World Health Organization 2011). The second definition describes gender as "power relations that privilege men over women" (World Health Organization 2021b).

A third description is gender identity, which is a related concept to gender, but one that is unhelpfully and increasingly conflated with the term gender. Gender identity refers to a "person's innate, deeply felt internal and individual experience of gender, which may or may not correspond to the person's physiology or designated sex at birth" (World Health Organization 2021b). The categories of gender identity include cis women, cis men, trans women, trans men, or gender queer/fluid (World Health Organization 2021b). The recognition of non-binary gender identities is becoming more frequent in public health literature. Estimates of what percentage of the population identifies as transgender and gender queer/fluid depend on whether countries recognize trans and non-binary gender identities, the variation in definitions of transgender (for example, based on self-identification, or those requesting hormone therapy or surgery), and societal attitudes towards non-binary, including transgender identities. Some estimates suggest a prevalence of 0.3% to 0.5% for people who identify as transgender (Reisner et al. 2016).

The first and second definitions of gender are the ones most often used in global development and health agendas and United Nations' standard-setting frameworks, including the Sustainable Development Goals (SDGs), which have a specific goal (SDG 5) focusing on gender equality and women's empowerment. However, the increasing conflation of gender as "roles, norms and power relations" with gender as "identity" is producing tensions in how gender is conceptualized and raising challenges in how it is measured and used in health research. Measuring and using the term "gender" incorrectly as "identity" categories inhibit the ability of public health research to examine the social and relational factors, such as norms and power relations, which act as determinants of health. It can lead to depoliticizing gender discrimination and unequal power relations that privilege cis men over all others. For example, there has been some limited exploration of power in terms of social status, cultural norms, economic resources, and political factors as determinants of health in some topics such as HIV and sexual and reproductive health (SRH) (Schaaf et al. 2021), but less so in others. Distinguishing between gender and gender identity, and centring and focusing on power differentials/inequalities, allows for intersectional analysis and can minimize the challenges of framing gender as being about competing vulnerabilities (Allotey and Remme 2020).

Contributions of intersectional feminist theories, including feminist technoscience

Feminist theories have been instrumental in explaining sex and gender constructs. Earlier theories of feminism conceptualized the distinction between sex as biologically constructed and gender as socially constructed. These conceptualizations of sex and gender continue to dominate much of the mainstream perspectives in medicine and public health (GWAnet 2021). However, feminist theories from the last twenty years have challenged this distinction, arguing that the human body is both biologically and socially constructed (Fausto-Sterling 1993). This view is contested and less applied in mainstream medical and public health literature (Torgrimson and Minson 2005).

Since the 1980s, several feminist theorists have criticized the dominance of White, middle-class perspectives that excluded the lived realities of Black women and women from different classes and ethnicities. Feminists from the global south also critiqued Western feminism for failing to account for how colonialism and racism intersected with sexism. These critiques informed to various degrees what is today referred to as intersectional feminism (Crenshaw 1989). Adding to intersectional feminist theories is "queer feminism", which highlights the need to consider non-binary gender identities. The intersectional feminist perspective recognizes that apart from sex and/or gender, discrimination based on race, ethnicity, class, age, sexual orientation, and gender identity, among other attributes, produces multiple and overlapping forms of inequalities and disadvantage. The language and concept of intersectionality is increasingly being mentioned in global health research, but its widespread use in research is still to be taken up systematically and the challenge is to make it operational (Hankivsky et al. 2010). The relevance and importance of an intersectional perspective in research are that even where data are disaggregated by sex, it would be erroneous to infer or treat all females/women or males/men as similar. Further disaggregation of data, analysis of sub-categories, and/or research with specific populations based on age, ethnicity, gender identities, sexual orientation, socioeconomic status, and disability status are needed.

The application of feminism to critique the male bias of biomedical and technical sciences has led to feminist technoscience. This provides a conceptual and analytic framework to probe the influence of sex and gender in the production of scientific knowledge, and its consequent application to technology development (Åsberg and Lykke 2010; Zeiler 2020). In feminist technoscience, there is a dual assertion that there is no such thing as neutral or value-free science, and neither should its application be distanced from the values of those who produce the research (Åsberg and Lykke 2010; Zeiler 2020). Recognizing the importance of power in influencing the production of knowledge, including decisions made related to it, feminist technoscience approaches require that researchers ask and answer who is doing the science, who does it benefit, whose bodies it includes, and whose interests are served (Åsberg and Lykke 2010; De Lange et al. 2021). This approach contrasts with the prevailing view of the epistemology of science, which claims that scientific knowledge can and should be objective and biases, including gender biases, can be removed (Nelson and Nelson 1996).

Feminist technoscience further frames the endeavours of scientific research and technology as emerging from hierarchical systems that are essentially masculinist in ideology in their desire for dominance and control. It calls into question the scientific validity and ethical justification of assuming the norm or standard of the male as representative of all human beings in health research, and as the default participant-subject from which all effects are measured (Pascual et al. 2021). It also articulates the fusing together of science, technology, and capitalism as a way to further concentrate wealth, as well as to monopolize reproduction and labour in ways that are worsening various forms of inequalities and human deprivations. In offering these critiques, feminist technoscience urges more reflexivity in theory being used in mainstream science and research (Weber 2006).

Why does sex and gender bias in health research lead to poor science and health inequities?

Sex and gender blindness and bias in public health research lead to poor science in terms of findings that are not generalizable and contribute to worse health outcomes and inequities. The relative importance of sex and gender varies across type of disease, illnesses, and health conditions. For example, regarding infectious diseases, including Covid-19, pathogens may infect anyone, but the susceptibility to disease may vary by sex, age, and gender roles. Sex-specific diseases such as endometriosis, cervical or breast cancer, or prostate cancers are largely a function of biology, although gender plays a role in shaping access to health services. Other diseases, such as cardiovascular disease, have been largely driven by behaviours or lifestyles and predominantly affect men because of gendered behaviours such as smoking and drinking, although women are also increasingly affected (Mauvais-Jarvis et al. 2020). However, it has become clear that sex hormones also affect how cardiovascular disease manifests in women and men differently at different age groups. Risk factors to various diseases and impairments, such as violence or alcohol use, are influenced by gender norms (although biology plays a role in how alcohol is absorbed by men and women differently) (Cislaghi et al. 2020). In sum, biology shared by all sexes, biology unique to sexes, and gender norms, roles, and power relations have different effects along the pathway from risks to exposure to disease progression to outcomes.

Gender blindness in research is based on assumptions that health risks and situations are similar for women and men, when in fact they are not. In the case of physical health problems, observed differences are underestimated. For example, this occurs when trials conducted in one population group (often men) are generalized to the whole population (Eisenstein 2020; Mann et al. 2018). In pre-clinical cell and animal studies, drug treatments are primarily tested in male cells and animals, even though it has been well established that there are sex differences in the responses of male and female animals and cells. A review showed that 90% of pharmacological studies in cells were using male-only cell lines (Hughes 2007). Even where studies include females and males, they either fail to report or analyse the data separately or ignore the differences. For example, another review showed that only 22% of animal studies specified the sex of the subject (Hughes 2007; Yoon et al. 2014). Similarly, while women are half of the population currently living with HIV, a 2016 review found that they made up only 19% of participants in antiretroviral studies and 38% in vaccination trials, and results were not analysed separately (Curno et al. 2016).

In contrast, gender bias, or double standards, in research has been demonstrated where illnesses in men are investigated and treated more extensively than in women with the same severity of symptoms. Illness in men is often considered as physiological and in women often dismissed as psychosomatic. For example, greater research investment has been made in conditions affecting men (for example, erectile dysfunction) than those affecting women (for example, menstrual disorders and endometriosis) (Nieuwenhoven and Klinge 2010). Gender bias is also apparent when it is assumed that there are differences between women and men, when in fact there may be similarities. This is the case with emotionally and self-expressed health problems (that is, similar responses or situations are treated or evaluated differently based on sex). In this case, there is an overestimation of observed differences. For example, because of assumptions that depression largely occurs among women, researchers looking at hospitalized patients (where women were overrepresented) developed diagnostic scales for depression that counted descriptions that fit women, missing out on symptoms more particular to men (for example, misuse of alcohol or drug abuse). This further perpetuated notions among clinicians that depression largely affected women, contributing to underdiagnosis of depression in men (Hamberg 2008). Boxes 17.1–17.4 provide examples of four health conditions that illustrate manifestations and consequences of sex and gender blindness and bias.

Box 17.1 Cardiovascular disease: undertreated due to undifferentiated diagnoses and lack of data from women

Sex and gender differences in cardiovascular disease (CVD) risks, onset, diagnosis presentations, and management outcomes are increasingly being studied. While women have some of the same risk factors as men, there are also additional factors such as menopause, pre-term delivery, gestational diabetes, hypertension during pregnancy, depression, breast cancer treatments, and systemic autoimmune disease (Baetta et al. 2018; Garcia et al. 2016; O'Neil et al. 2018). Women's oestrogen levels in reproductive age are considered to be protective, and a reason for later onset of CVD, but this difference is reducing in recent times, potentially due to changes in age of menopause and in lifestyle (O'Neil et al. 2018). Women also tend to have a higher prevalence of persistent angina, non-obstructive coronary disease, and stress-induced cardiomyopathy (Taqueti and Bairey Merz 2017). They are about twice as likely as men to develop heart failure (Baetta et al. 2018).

Gender norms and roles are also risk factors. Socialization of boys to pursue physical activity is protective, while many girls do not engage in sport or activity beyond school (O'Neil et al. 2018). There are several reasons for this, including lack of safety in public spaces, high levels of unpaid care work, and time poverty to engage in rest and protective behaviours. Long hours of care work appear to be a risk factor for nonfatal CVD in middle-aged women, but not men (O'Neil et al. 2018).

Much of the research on CVD has focused on men, with the assumption that clinical findings are transferable to women (that is, gender blind research) (Baetta et al. 2018; Peters et al. 2016). For example, in 31 trials for congestive heart failure conducted between 1987 and 2012, women made up only 25% of the participants (Vitale et al. 2017). A consequence of being under-represented in trials is that women are not provided with nuanced or optimal management strategies, and face challenges in access to life-saving interventions. Overall, women tend to receive fewer interventions that prevent recurrence of cardiac events than men (Smolina et al. 2015; Walli-Attaei et al. 2020). Women's "atypical" presentations delay their diagnoses (Eindhoven et al. 2018; Smolina et al. 2015). They less frequently receive and adhere to therapies such as aspirin and statin drugs (Eindhoven et al. 2018).

Box 17.2 Interactions of sex, gender, and age in Covid-19 outcomes

In general, men are known to be biologically more susceptible to infectious disease and severity in terms of complications. Data from the early days of the Covid-19 pandemic indicated a sex difference in hospitalizations and deaths (Klein et al. 2020; Wolfe et al. 2021). The angiotensin-converting enzyme 2, which binds to the SARS-COV2 virus, is found in higher quantities in men, and was highlighted as a probable contributor to the severe outcomes among men (Klein et al. 2020). Gendered behaviours provide additional explanations for men's increased risk of acquiring SARS-COV2, including their lower rates of handwashing, higher rates of smoking and alcohol misuse, and related to that, higher comorbidities for severe Covid-19 symptoms (Betron et al. 2020). However, women's higher risk of exposure to SARS-COV2 is linked to their gender roles as carers. Women comprise 70% of the health work force (Boniol et al. 2019). They are more likely to be working in care homes, and at home, to be caring for the elderly and the sick.

However, the relationship of sex, gender, and Covid-19 is not straightforward. Research shows sex-differentiated presentations of Covid-19 immune response, virus shedding, and in manifestations of longer-term complications that are also linked to age (Wolfe et al. 2021). Oestrogen in women of reproductive ages is found to be protective in terms of severity. The gaps in severity between older men and women are reduced as compared to those in reproductive age, in part explained by reductions in oestrogen (Pivonello et al. 2020). There is some indication that more women experience longer-term post-Covid conditions, including symptoms that are similar to chronic fatigue syndrome (Evans et al. 2021; Sigfrid et al. 2021; Sudre et al. 2021; Wolfe et al. 2021). Women are also known to mount a higher immune response to vaccinations (Flanagan et al. 2017; Klein and Morgan 2020; Klein and Pekosz 2014). However, rare, early, and real-world Covid-19 vaccination outcomes are also showing women-disproportionate adverse events (Shimabukuro 2021), which has not been taken into account in vaccine research in dosing studies, or reporting of safety outcomes (Vijayasingham et al. 2021).

Box 17.3 Violence: distinct and separate risk factors for women's and men's health outcomes

Interpersonal violence is ranked fifth among the causes of disability adjusted life years (DALYs) for adolescent boys and young men (10–24 years) (GBD 2019 Diseases and Injuries Collaborators 2020). An analysis of sex differences from 2017 global burden of disease (GBD) estimates shows that male-to-female ratio for DALYS due to interpersonal violence is 3.77 to 1 (Cislaghi et al. 2020; Hawkes and Buse 2013). However, concluding that men face a higher burden of interpersonal violence based on the sex differences in DALYs can lead to an erroneous conclusion, as the choice of outcome masks the different nature and impacts of violence experienced by men and women (World Health Organization 1999). One health consequence factored into DALYS is injuries. However, injuries are not the main consequence for women and girls experiencing violence. Instead, women face disproportionate impacts related to sexual and reproductive health (World Health Organization 2013), which are not factored into the DALYS. Hence, interpersonal violence can be underestimated as an important risk factor for women's health.

And yet, World Health Organization (WHO) estimates based on surveys conducted with women show that physical and/or sexual violence by an intimate partner or sexual violence by someone other than a partner affects nearly 1 in 3 women globally (World Health Organization 2021c). Intimate partner violence leads to a two-fold likelihood of women experiencing depression, a 1.5-fold increase in acquiring sexually transmitted infections, a 16% increase in women giving birth to low-birth-weight babies and two-fold increase in the likelihood of women having induced abortions (often in unsafe conditions) (World Health Organization 2013). Distinct from the violence faced by men who do not necessarily get stigmatized, women experience violence at the hands of their intimate partners and in their homes where they should feel most protected. Societies stigmatize women subjected to violence and hence, most do not report to authorities. Violence statistics therefore grossly undercount and underrepresent women. Violence against women and against men should be understood as two distinct public health problems with distinct consequences and outcomes.

Box 17.4 Endometriosis: a sex-specific neglected condition affecting women

Endometriosis affects 10% (190 million) of women of reproductive age, with debilitating effects ranging from severe pain during periods, sexual intercourse, or bowel movements to chronic pelvic pain and infertility (Word Health Organization 2021a). Causes of endometriosis are several, but mainly related to oestrogen. Although endometriosis has been described over several decades, to date, little is known about how to treat it. Millions of women struggle with endometriosis in silence. It affects their daily functioning and causes them loss in time for work, leisure, and other activities. A key barrier in managing endometriosis has been the limited funding for research on effective treatments in comparison to research investments in other diseases with similar burden and impact, such as diabetes (Rogers et al. 2009). For example, in the United States, endometriosis receives $1 of research funding for every $200 invested in diabetes (COYA Partners 2020). One explanation is that women's health needs are not always perceived as having a market with a return on investment by predominantly male investors (Stengel 2020). Prevailing attitudes that dismiss and stigmatize when it comes to women's health have also played a role in the underinvestment in research and diagnosis. For example, there is tendency for the public and providers to dismiss endometriosis as something that women should bear as painful periods rather than a debilitating condition. Very often, women with endometriosis spend many years seeing multiple providers before getting an accurate diagnosis (COYA Partners 2020).

Emerging issues when integrating sex and gender in health research

The life-course perspective

The impacts of sex and gender on health vary considerably across the life course. We highlight the lack of knowledge that is reflected from underrepresentation of two life-course cohorts—older and pregnant women. First, regarding older women, women live more years than men, and these years are often lived with higher levels of morbidities and disabilities (Institute for Health Metrics and Evaluation 2018). Sex-specific health risks change with age (Baden et al. 2014). However, we know much less about how sex and gender interact to affect the health of older women (Rochon et al. 2020). This is a matter of urgency, considering an ageing population globally, where older people, particularly women, are living longer. For example, a report from the United States has highlighted that while women represented two-thirds of Alzheimer's patients, there is much less information about how hormonal changes as well as social including gender-related factors affect the brain (Baird et al. 2021).

The second group, pregnant women, have been long excluded in clinical trials due to ethical concerns for potential impacts on the pregnancy and foetus (Mazure and Jones 2015; Tannenbaum and Day 2017). Despite advocacy and regulatory calls, pregnant women continue to be excluded from clinical trials for many medicines, even once safety profiles have been established. A cross-sectional study of 558 industry-sponsored phase 4 (post-market) studies (2011–2012) of medicines not categorized as potentially teratogenic (that is, having a negative influence on foetal development) found that 95% of studies still excluded pregnant women (Shields and Lyerly 2013). More recently, a high proportion of registered Covid-19 treatment trials (above 75%) have excluded pregnant women or listed pregnancy as exclusion criteria (Taylor et al. 2020). Their exclusion is despite the fact pregnant women are at a high risk of severe Covid-19 illness (Ciapponi et al. 2021). For innovators, the liabilities and costs associated with testing in pregnant women may be perceived to be high (Amir et al. 2020). To rectify this historical exclusion, the 2016 international guidelines from the Council for International Organizations of Medical Sciences (CIOMS) provide guidance on how to include pregnant women in therapeutic trials ethically and safely (World Health Organization and Council for International Organizations of Medical Sciences 2017).

Understanding the health needs of transgender and intersex populations

There are big gaps when it comes to our knowledge of health issues affecting intersex and transgender persons. Transgender people face higher levels of adverse health outcomes compared to the general population (Reisner et al. 2016). For example, transgender people are approximately thirteen times more likely to be HIV-positive than other adults of reproductive age. Transgender populations also face higher risks of other sexually transmitted infections, poor mental health, and substance abuse. This evidence is limited to some geographic regions (mostly the United States and some from Canada, Europe, India, and Australia) (Reisner et al. 2016). Much less is known about other sexual and reproductive health needs and concerns, other health issues, as well as experiences of violence and access to and experiences of health services among transgender populations, particularly in low- and middle-income countries. Those who seek gender-affirming or transition-related healthcare face access barriers in many parts of the world. In the United States, many are denied gender-affirming surgery or hormonal treatment as part of normal health insurance coverage, despite the fact that gender-affirming care is found to be cost-effective in the long term (Learmonth et al. 2018).

Throughout history and across cultures, intersex people have experienced stigmatization, discrimination, and social exclusion (Carpenter 2016; Jones 2018). They have often faced unnecessary medical treatment because they continue to be classified in medical terms as people with disorders of sex development, which can be traumatizing for them (Jones 2018). A systematic review of healthcare inequalities affecting intersex persons highlights that for those who have undergone hormonal treatment or surgery, often as minors, to align their bodies with typical male/female sex characteristics, several healthcare needs emerge, ranging from problematic sexual experiences to feelings of being trapped in rigid binary gender identities. Regardless of hormonal treatment or surgery, mental health is a significant concern in relation to being stigmatized (Zeeman and Aranda 2020). The gaps in knowledge of the health needs of intersex and transgender populations call for specific research with attention to methods to reach them and include them in safe ways. Several research funders have provided guidelines to include intersex, non-binary (including transgender) persons in research in order to build the evidence about their health needs (Bauer 2021; Kirwan et al. 2021; Reisner et al. 2016).

Understanding the role of epigenetics in mediating the influence of gender on health inequities

Another emerging area that can help to elaborate pathways by which sex and gender interact to affect health is epigenetics. Epigenetics studies explain how the expression of genes into observable characteristics in the body varies in response to different environmental influences (Cortes et al. 2019). Of relevance here are observational studies in humans and experimental animal studies showing that discrimination based on gender can produce biological changes in the body—that is, in the neural architecture, gene expression, cellular ageing, inflammatory processes, and changes. These changes reflect the body's response to stress brought on by the cumulative effects of discrimination. Adversity and disadvantage "embed in the body" so that before birth, epigenetic markers are switched on. For example, a study of mothers and newborns in the eastern Democratic Republic of Congo showed that conflict-related stress was a strong predictor of newborn birth weight and epigenetic changes in the mother and the child (Rodney and Mulligan 2014). Of all conflict-related stressors—the experience of rape had the most profound impact, accounting for 31% of differences in birth weight (Heise et al. 2019; Rodney and Mulligan 2014). Similarly, exposure to stress early in life leaves epigenetic signature in the brain—particularly the pre-frontal cortex. For example, studies conducted with rodents show that early life maltreatment or neglect changes expression of certain genes associated with immune response, mood, and social behaviours in adulthood (Cortes et al. 2019). Environmental endocrine disrupters that are commonly found in cosmetics, scented lotions, nail polish, and feminine care products have been shown in adolescent rodents to alter social and fear behaviours. Differences in levels of endocrine disrupters in the urine of men and women have been observed in adolescence. This is also the age at which girls in many societies, influenced by gendered expectations of beauty, often start experimenting with cosmetics, highlighting the potential of these chemicals having epigenetic consequences (Cortes et al. 2019). These examples emphasize the need to explore and address the harmful impacts of the environment, which is gendered, on altered gene expression and on the health of the individual.

Addressing sex and gender biases in the use of artificial intelligence for healthcare

Health technologies based on artificial intelligence (AI) have a critical role to play in the identification of biomedically relevant patterns that can facilitate tailored preventive and therapeutic interventions for individuals. The collection and analysis of health data from AI technologies can either worsen or potentially mitigate the negative impacts of sex and gender biases (Cirillo et al. 2020; Van Daal et al. 2020). AI technologies include digital biomarkers, big data analytics, robotics, natural language processing, and 3-D bioprinting technologies. An example of sex bias in the application of AI is in the development of digital biomarkers for early detection of Parkinson's disease. Digital biomarkers are portable, wearable, implantable, and even ingestible devices that collect health data from human-computer interactions (for example, swipes), physical activity (for example, dexterity), and voice variations. Data collected from digital biomarkers are used to explain, influence, or predict health outcomes. The development of digital biomarkers for the early detection of Parkinson's disease was based on research with a male-disproportionate data set (Cirillo et al. 2020). As a result, the algorithm was more accurate in detecting symptoms in men with Parkinson's disease (for example, rigidity and rapid eye movement) as compared to women (for example, depression and involuntary movements) (Miller and Cronin-Golomb 2010).

Another AI tool is big data analytics, which involves developing diagnostic algorithms to analyse large data sets containing information about patterns of health conditions and behaviours (Cirillo et al. 2020). Analysis of a large data set involving management of Covid-19 cases by health professionals from an examination of 1.4 million electronic health records in Spain in 2020 helped to identify sex-dependent characteristics of patients and gender bias in healthcare responses. While younger females were significantly more affected by Covid-19 than their male counterparts in the same age group and females showed more frequent ear, nose, and throat symptoms, basic diagnostic tests such as blood tests or imaging were less used in females than their male counterparts. This led the authors to conclude that there was an inherent gender bias in the health system impacting care for women with Covid-19 (Ancochea et al. 2020). The examples described in this section highlight the potential for AI technologies to reduce sex and gender biases in healthcare by increasing awareness in the scientific and technology communities; developing algorithms to detect or explain sex and gender biases; and improving the quality of life for patients of all sexes and gender identities (Cirillo et al. 2020).

The way forward: how sex and gender can be systematically embedded in health research

There have been long-standing calls for integration of sex and gender into health research. However, progress has been slow due to various barriers. Overcoming these barriers requires changes in individual capacities and behaviours of researchers; institutions responsible for conducting, funding, and publishing research; and in structural mechanisms to incentivize change and hold the health research community accountable.

At the individual level, researchers not only conflate concepts of sex and gender, but also do not know how to apply these concepts (Van Hagen et al. 2021). Literature has flagged the lack of capacities in applying sex and gender into designing research questions, selecting appropriate frameworks and methods, sampling and recruiting the appropriate participants, constituting a multidisciplinary team, and having appropriate analysis methods (Day et al. 2016; Runnels et al. 2014). A number of tools and training materials have already been developed to build such capacities for researchers, including in conducting intersectional gender analysis of data (Canadian Institutes of Health Research Government of Canada 2015; Day et al. 2016; McGregor et al. 2016; World Health Organization 2020; World Health Organization and UNAIDS 2016). However, a survey of 45 research funders shows that only 5 of them provide concrete guidelines on how to apply sex and gender concepts in funding proposals (Hankivsky et al. 2018). Hence, there is a clear need to establish guidelines for inclusion of sex and gender in health research, and to improve the uptake of existing resources by researchers. Such guidelines need to emphasize sex and gender as fundamental to producing quality, rigorous, ethical, and plausible science, rather than it being supplementary or optional (Day et al. 2016).

At the institutional level, changing who is doing, managing, funding, publishing, and teaching research so that more women and feminists are in science leadership has the potential of producing public health science that is more inclusive of sex and gender considerations (Nelson and Nelson 1996). The underrepresentation of women in science leadership has been identified as a factor contributing to research that is male-biased (Coe et al. 2019; Shannon et al. 2019). To correct this, calls have been made to appoint women in leadership roles in scientific institutions and to enhance mentoring opportunities for women scientists (Coe et al. 2019; Sugimoto et al. 2019).

Equally important is to query the content of what is being taught in schools of medicine and public health in ways that reinforces male bias. For example, textbooks in medicine and epidemiology have long depicted male bodies or the Caucasian male as the reference standard—socializing students into seeing these as the norm (Parker et al. 2017; Regensteiner et al. 2019; Verdonk et al. 2005). Changing this norm requires embedding concepts such as sex, gender, and intersectionality in medical and public health education and research curricula; teaching courses that enable students to learn about the social, political, and ethical aspects of medicine and public health; and encouraging students to be reflexive about their own power and role in perpetuating stereotypes and bias in research (Hamberg 2008; Kalenga et al. 2020; Regensteiner et al. 2019; Verdonk et al. 2005; World Health Organization 2007).

Research funders and publishers can shape norms for integrating sex and gender in research. Few research funding agencies pay attention to the inclusion of sex and gender in funding applications and even fewer make this a mandatory requirement (Hankivsky et al. 2018). Even where funding agencies such as the National Institutes for Health (NIH) in the United States have issued guidance on the inclusion of sex and gender for their research applicants since 1993, only 26% of their trials in 2015 reported results by sex, or included sex as a covariate in the analysis (Geller et al. 2018). When it comes to publishing research, despite several top journals adopting guidelines (SAGER, Sex and Gender Equity in Research) requiring authors to report separately for male and female study participants, their enforcement is lagging (Clayton and Tannenbaum 2016; Heidari et al. 2016). A systematic review of Covid-19 trials examining whether SAGER guidelines were used in the publication of studies found that only 31% had approximately half-female participants and only 12% disaggregated their main outcomes by sex (Palmer-Ross et al. 2021). There is a clear need for better enforcement of SAGER guidelines by journals to ensure that researchers report how their results address sex and gender considerations.

At a structural level, incentivizing change requires making the case for the economic and societal costs and benefits of integrating sex and gender in health research and holding Research and Development institutions accountable. One of the main arguments of the pharmaceutical industry to exclude women from trials is that it is costly to do so (Liu and DiPietro Mager 2016; Stengel 2020). Countering this narrative requires reframing the exclusion of sex and gender in research as a waste of resources and an economic burden to societies, or investments in research on women's health as a good return on investment. For example, a report on Alzheimer's disease among women in the United States shows that doubling the research investment of 12% of the budget dedicated to women to obtain a minimal 0.01% improvement in healthy life expectancy has a potential return on investment of 224% in terms of reduced disease burden, costs of nursing home care, and improved quality of life (Baird et al. 2021). Drug regulators need to set and enforce standards for the industry to include women in clinical studies and publicly present the data disaggregated by sex, so that differences in outcomes by sex can be factored into cost-effectiveness analysis and inform decisions around what products are included in health benefits and insurance packages for women and men (Ravindran et al. 2020). Accountability is required to foster research that promotes the goals of gender equality. In public health, social movements (including feminist movements) have played a critical role in holding institutions and researchers accountable. A notable example is the HIV/AIDS and the feminist movements that pushed for investments in research on female-controlled HIV-prevention methods (Forbes 2013; Germain and Liljestrand 2009). Another example is the partnerships between researchers and feminist activists, forged to document the magnitude and impacts of violence against women, which led to the WHO multi-country study on domestic violence and women's health (García-Moreno et al. 2005; World Health Organization and Program for Appropriate Technology in Health (PATH) 2005).

There is an urgent need to take actions to address patriarchal Research and Development systems to counter the long legacy of male bias in medical and public health science. At the same time, we need to ask research questions about how sex and gender are likely to impact several emerging trends. These include demographic transitions leading to an ageing population; social transitions leading to increasing recognition of non-binary gender identities; technological transitions involving digitization of healthcare delivery; and climate change/environmental transitions influencing epigenetics. The landmark "Beijing Platform for Action on Women", adopted in 1995, called for sex disaggregation of data and research on women's health (United Nations 1995). The calls for sex disaggregation of data continue today, but this is just the beginning in the quest to understand how sex and gender interact and how gender inequalities intersect with other socioeconomic inequalities to affect health inequities, particularly among women. The Covid-19 pandemic has shown that it is possible to mobilize vast sums of funding for medical and public health research in a short period of time and to innovative in putting out vaccines within a year of the beginning of the pandemic. We would like to end with a call for improved accountability of research funders, institutions, scientists, journals, and regulators to show a similar and urgent commitment towards integrating sex and gender in health research—now, during the pandemic—as well as in the future.

Acknowledgments

The authors thank Mariam Otmani Del Barrio from the Special Programme for Research and Training in Tropical Diseases (TDR), and Claudia García-Moreno and Ian Askew from the Department of Sexual and Reproductive Health and Research at the World Health Organization for their feedback on this chapter.

Avni Amin and Jacqui Stevenson are funded by the Special Programme for Research on Human Reproduction (HRP), housed in the Department of Sexual and Reproductive Health and Research.

Avni Amin and Lavanya Vijayasingham developed the outline for this chapter. Avni Amin drafted the following sections: introduction, defining sex and gender, examples in Box 17.1, 17.3, and 17.4, and the emerging areas section focused on the life course, addressing intersex and transgender and understanding the role of epigenetics. Lavanya Vijayasingham drafted the following sections: contributions of feminist technoscience and addressing bias in artificial intelligence. Jacqui Stevenson drafted the abstract, reviewed and revised multiple drafts, including the final section on the way forward.

Disclaimer

The views expressed in this chapter represent those of the authors and do not reflect the views of the institutions they represent.

References

Allotey, P. and M. Remme. 2020. Gender equality should not be about competing vulnerabilities. https://blogs.bmj.com/bmj/2020/04/17/gender-equality-should-not-be-about-competing-vulnerabilities/ (accessed September 7, 2021).

Amir, L. H., L. E. Grzeskowiak, and R. L. Kam. 2020. Ethical issues in use of medications during lactation. *Journal of Human Lactation* 36, no. 1: 34–39. https://doi.org/10.1177/0890334419888156.

Ancochea, J., J. L. Izquierdo, Savana COVID-19 Research Group, and J. B. Soriano. 2020. Evidence of gender bias in the diagnosis and management of COVID-19 patients: A big data analysis of electronic health records (preprint). *Infectious Diseases (except HIV/AIDS)*. https://doi.org/10.1101/2020.07.20.20157735.

Åsberg, C. and N. Lykke. 2010. Feminist technoscience studies. *European Journal of Women's Studies* 17, no. 4: 299–305. https://doi.org/10.1177/1350506810377692.

Baden, R., J. K. Rockstroh, and M. Buti. 2014. Natural history and management of hepatitis C: Does sex play a role? *Journal of Infectious Diseases* 209, suppl. 3: S81–S85. https://doi.org/10.1093/infdis/jiu057.

Baetta, R., M. Pontremoli, A. Martinez Fernandez, C. M. Spickett, and C. Banfi. 2018. Proteomics in cardiovascular diseases: Unveiling sex and gender differences in the era of precision medicine. *Journal of Proteomics* 173: 62–76. https://doi.org/10.1016/j.jprot.2017.11.012.

Baird, M.D., M. A. Zaber, A. W. Dick et al. 2021. *Societal impact of research funding for women's health in Alzheimer's disease and Alzheimer's disease-related dementias*. RAND Corporation. https://doi.org/10.7249/RR-A708-1.

Bauer, G. 2021. Quantitative intersectional study design and primary data collection. Meet the Methods Series. https://cihr-irsc.gc.ca/e/documents/intersectional-study-design-data-collection_EN.pdf (accessed December 20, 2021).

Betron, M., A. Gottert, J. Pulerwitz, D, Shattuck, and N. Stevanovic-Fenn. 2020. Men and Covid-19: Adding a gender lens. *Global Public Health*: 1–3. https://doi.org/10.1080/17441692.2020.1769702.

Boniol, M., M. McIsaac, L. Xu, T. Wuliji, K. Diallo, and J. Campbell. 2019. Gender equity in the health workforce: Analysis of 104 countries. Working paper 1. Geneva: World Health Organization.

Brady, E., M. W. Nielsen, J. P. Andersen, and S. Oertelt-Prigione. 2021. Lack of consideration of sex and gender in Covid-19 clinical studies. *Nature Communications* 12, no. 1: 4015. https://doi.org/10.1038/s41467-021-24265-8.

Canadian Institutes of Health Research Government of Canada. 2015. Online training modules: Integrating sex & gender in health research. https://cihr-irsc.gc.ca/e/49347.html (accessed December 20, 2021).

Carpenter, M. 2016. The human rights of intersex people: Addressing harmful practices and rhetoric of change. *Reproductive Health Matters* 24, no. 47: 74–84. https://doi.org/10.1016/j.rhm.2016.06.003.

Ciapponi, A., A. Bardach, D. Comandé et al. 2021. Covid-19 and pregnancy: An umbrella review of clinical presentation, vertical transmission, and maternal and perinatal outcomes. *PLOS ONE* 16, no. 6: e0253974. https://doi.org/10.1371/journal.pone.0253974.

Cirillo, D., S. Catuara-Solarz, C. Morey et al. 2020. Sex and gender differences and biases in artificial intelligence for biomedicine and healthcare. *npj Digital Medicine* 3: 1–11. https://doi.org/10.1038/s41746-020-0288-5.

Cislaghi, B., A. M. Weber, G. R. Gupta, and G. L. Darmstadt. 2020. Gender equality and global health: Intersecting political challenges. *Journal of Global Health* 10, no. 1: 010701. https://doi.org/10.7189/jogh.10.010701.

Clayton, J.A. and C. Tannenbaum. 2016. Reporting sex, gender, or both in clinical research? *JAMA* 316, no. 18: 1863–1864. https://doi.org/10.1001/jama.2016.16405.

Coe, I.R., R. Wiley, and L-G. Bekker. 2019. Organisational best practices towards gender equality in science and medicine. *The Lancet* 393, no. 10171: 587–593. https://doi.org/10.1016/S0140-6736(18)33188-X.

Cortes, L.R., C. D. Cisternas, and N. G. Forger. 2019. Does gender leave an epigenetic imprint on the brain? *Frontiers in Neuroscience* 13: 173. https://doi.org/10.3389/fnins.2019.00173.

COYA Partners. 2020. Surprising facts about women's health. https://www.coyapartners.com/post/surprising-facts-about-women-s-health (accessed March 5, 2021).

Crenshaw, K. 1989. Demarginalizing the intersection of race and sex: A black feminist critique of antidiscrimination doctrine, feminist theory and antiracist politics. *University of Chicago Legal Forum.* https://chicagounbound.uchicago.edu/uclf/vol1989/iss1/8 (accessed December 20, 2021).

Curno, M.J., S. Rossi, I. Hodges-Mameletzis, R. Johnston, M. A. Price, and S. Heidari. 2016. A systematic review of the inclusion (or exclusion) of women in HIV research: From clinical studies of antiretrovirals and vaccines to cure strategies. *Journal of Acquired Immune Deficiency Syndromes* 71, no. 2: 181–188. https://doi.org/10.1097/QAI.0000000000000842.

Day, S., R. Mason, S. Lagosky, and P. A. Rochon. 2016. Integrating and evaluating sex and gender in health research. *Health Research Policy and Systems* 14. https://doi.org/10.1186/s12961-016-0147-7.

De Lange, A-M.G., E. G. Jacobs, and L. A. M. Galea. 2021. The scientific body of knowledge: Whose body does it serve? A spotlight on women's brain health. *Frontiers in Neuroendocrinology* 60: 100898. https://doi.org/10.1016/j.yfrne.2020.100898.

Eindhoven, D.C., A. D. Hilt, T. C. Zwaan, M. J. Schalij, and C. J. W. Borleffs. 2018. Age and gender differences in medical adherence after myocardial infarction: Women do not receive optimal treatment – The Netherlands claims database. *European Journal of Preventive Cardiology* 25, no. 2: 181–189. https://doi.org/10.1177/2047487317744363.

Eisenstein, M. 2020. Closing the gender gap in migraine research. *Nature* 586, no. 7829: S16–S17. https://doi.org/10.1038/d41586-020-02867-4.

Evans, R.A., H. McAuley, E. M. Harrison et al. 2021. Physical, cognitive and mental health impacts of Covid-19 following hospitalisation: A multi-centre prospective cohort study (preprint). *Infectious Diseases (except HIV/AIDS).* https://doi.org/10.1101/2021.03.22.21254057.

Fausto-Sterling, A. 1993. The five sexes. *The Sciences* 33, no. 2: 20–24. https://doi.org/10.1002/j.2326-1951.1993.tb03081.x.

Fausto-Sterling, A. 2000. The five sexes, revisited. *Sciences (New York)* 40, no. 4: 18–23. https://doi.org/10.1002/j.2326-1951.2000.tb03504.x.

Feldman, S., W. Ammar, K. Lo, E. Trepman, M. van Zuylen, and O. Etzioni. 2019. Quantifying sex bias in clinical studies at scale with automated data extraction. *JAMA Network Open* 2, no. 7: e196700. https://doi.org/10.1001/jamanetworkopen.2019.6700.

Flanagan, K. L., A. L. Fink, M. Plebanski, and S. L. Klein. 2017. Sex and gender differences in the outcomes of vaccination over the life course. *Annual Review of Cell and Developmental Biology* 33: 577–599. https://doi.org/10.1146/annurev-cellbio-100616-060718.

Forbes, A. 2013. Mobilizing women at the grassroots to shape health policy: A case study of the Global Campaign for Microbicides. *Reproductive Health Matters* 21, no. 42: 174–183. https://doi.org/10.1016/S0968-8080(13)42735-0.

Garcia, M., S. L. Mulvagh, C. N. Bairey Merz, J. E. Buring, and J.E. Manson. 2016. Cardiovascular disease in women: Clinical perspectives. *Circulation Research* 118, no. 8: 1273–1293. https://doi.org/10.1161/CIRCRESAHA.116.307547.

García-Moreno, C., H. A. F. M. Jansen, M. Ellsberg, L. Heise, and C. Watts. 2005. *WHO multi-country study on women's health and domestic violence against women: Initial results on prevalence, health outcomes and women's responses*. Geneva: World Health Organization.

GBD 2019 Diseases and Injuries Collaborators. 2020. Global burden of 369 diseases and injuries in 204 countries and territories, 1990–2019: A systematic analysis for the Global Burden of Disease Study 2019. *The Lancet* 396, no. 10258: 1204–1222. https://doi.org/10.1016/S0140-6736(20)30925-9.

Geller, S. E., A. R. Koch, P. Roesch, A. Filut, E. Hallgren, and M. Carnes. 2018. The more things change, the more they stay the same: A study to evaluate compliance with inclusion and assessment of women and minorities in randomized controlled trials. *Academic Medicine* 93, no. 4: 630–635. https://doi.org/10.1097/ACM.0000000000002027.

Germain, A. and J. Liljestrand. 2009. Women's groups and professional organizations in advocacy for sexual and reproductive health and rights. *International Journal of Gynecology & Obstetrics*106, no. 2: 185–187. https://doi.org/10.1016/j.ijgo.2009.03.038.

Global Health 50/50. 2021. 2021 Global Health 50/50 Report gender equality: Flying blind in a time of crisis. https://globalhealth5050.org/2021-report/ (accessed April 30, 2021).

GWAnet. 2021. History and theory of feminism. http://www.gender.cawater-info.net/knowledge_base/rubricator/feminism_e.htm (accessed May 3, 2021).

Hamberg, K. 2008. Gender bias in medicine. *Women's Health* 4, no. 3: 237–243. https://doi.org/10.2217/17455057.4.3.237.

Hankivsky, O., C. Reid, R. Cormier et al. 2010. Exploring the promises of intersectionality for advancing women's health research. *International Journal for Equity in Health*9: 5. https://doi.org/10.1186/1475-9276-9-5.

Hankivsky, O., K. W. Springer, and G. Hunting. 2018. Beyond sex and gender difference in funding and reporting of health research. *Research Integrity and Peer Review*3: 6. https://doi.org/10.1186/s41073-018-0050-6.

Hawkes, S. and K. Buse. 2013. Gender and global health: Evidence, policy, and inconvenient truths. *The Lancet* 381, no. 9879: 1783–1787. https://doi.org/10.1016/S0140-6736(13)60253-6.

Heidari, S., T. F. Babor, P. de Castro, S. Tort, and M. Curno. 2016. Sex and gender equity in research: Rationale for the SAGER guidelines and recommended use. *Research Integrity and Peer Review* 1: 2. https://doi.org/10.1186/s41073-016-0007-6.

Heise, L., M. E. Greene, N. Opper et al. 2019. Gender inequality and restrictive gender norms: Framing the challenges to health. *The Lancet* 393, no. 10189: 2440–2454. https://doi.org/10.1016/S0140-6736(19)30652-X.

Holdcroft, A. 2016. Gender bias in research: How does it affect evidence-based medicine? *Journal of the Royal Society of Medicine* 100, no. 1: 2–3. https://doi.org/10.1177/014107680710000102.

Hughes, R. N. 2007. Sex does matter: Comments on the prevalence of male-only investigations of drug effects on rodent behaviour. *Behavioural Pharmacology*18, no. 7: 583–589. https://doi.org/10.1097/FBP.0b013e3282eff0e8.

Institute for Health Metrics and Evaluation. 2018. Findings from the Global Burden of Disease Study 2017. https://www.healthdata.org/policy-report/findings-global-burden-disease-study-2017 (accessed December 20, 2021).

Jones, T. 2018. Intersex studies: A systematic review of international health literature. *SAGE Open* 8, no. 2: 2158244017745577. https://doi.org/10.1177/2158244017745577.

Kalenga, C. Z., J. Parsons Leigh, J. Griffith et al. 2020. Sex and gender considerations in health research: A trainee and allied research personnel perspective. *Humanities and Social Sciences Communications* 7, no. 1: 1–7. https://doi.org/10.1057/s41599-020-00643-3.

Kirwan, P. D., M. Hibbert, M. Kall et al. 2021. HIV prevalence and HIV clinical outcomes of transgender and gender-diverse people in England. *HIV Medicine* 22, no. 2: 131–139. https://doi.org/10.1111/hiv.12987.

Klein, S. L., S. Dhakal, R. L. Ursin, S. Deshpande, K. Sandberg, and F. Mauvais-Jarvis. 2020. Biological sex impacts Covid-19 outcomes. *PLOS Pathogens* 16, no. 6: e1008570. https://doi.org/10.1371/journal.ppat.1008570.

Klein, S.L. and R. Morgan. 2020. The impact of sex and gender on immunotherapy outcomes. *Biology of Sex Differences* 11, no. 1: 24. https://doi.org/10.1186/s13293-020-00301-y.

Klein, S. L. and A. Pekosz. 2014. Sex-based biology and the rational design of influenza vaccination strategies. *Journal of Infectious Diseases* 209, suppl. 3: S114–S119. https://doi.org/10.1093/infdis/jiu066.

Learmonth, C., R. Viloria, C. Lambert, H. Goldhammer, and A. S. Keuroghlian. 2018. Barriers to insurance coverage for transgender patients. *American Journal of Obstetrics and Gynecology* 219, no. 3: 272.e1–272.e4. https://doi.org/10.1016/j.ajog.2018.04.046.

Liu, K. A. and N. A. DiPietro Mager. 2016. Women's involvement in clinical trials: Historical perspective and future implications. *Pharmacy Practice (Granada)* 14, no. 1: 708. https://doi.org/10.18549/PharmPract.2016.01.708.

Maan, A. A., J. Eales, A. Akbarov et al. 2017. The Y chromosome: A blueprint for men's health? *European Journal of Human Genetics* 25, no. 11: 1181–1188. https://doi.org/10.1038/ejhg.2017.128.

Mann, S., M. Davison, L. Logan et al. 2018. *What do women say: Reproductive health is a public health issue.* London: Public Health England.

Mauvais-Jarvis, F., N. Bairey Merz, P. J. Barnes et al. 2020. Sex and gender: Modifiers of health, disease, and medicine. *The Lancet* 396, no. 10250: 565–582. https://doi.org/10.1016/S0140-6736(20)31561-0.

Mazure, C. M. and D. P. Jones. 2015. Twenty years and still counting: Including women as participants and studying sex and gender in biomedical research. *BMC Womens Health* 15: 94. https://doi.org/10.1186/s12905-015-0251-9.

McGregor, A. J., M. Hasnain, K. Sandberg, M. F. Morrison, M. Berlin, and J. Trott. 2016. How to study the impact of sex and gender in medical research: A review of resources. *Biology of Sex Differences* 7, suppl. 1: 46. https://doi.org/10.1186/s13293-016-0099-1.

Miller, I. N. and A. Cronin-Golomb. 2010. Gender differences in Parkinson's disease: Clinical characteristics and cognition. *Movement Disorders* 25, no. 16: 2695–2703. https://doi.org/10.1002/mds.23388.

Nelson, L. H. and J. Nelson. 1996. The feminism question in the philosophy of science. In *Feminism, science, and the philosophy of science*, ed. L. H. Nelson and J. Nelson, 3–15. Dordrecht: Springer. https://doi.org/10.1007/978-94-009-1742-2_1.

Nieuwenhoven, L. and I. Klinge. 2010. Scientific excellence in applying sex- and gender-sensitive methods in biomedical and health research. *Journal of Women's Health* 19, no. 2: 313–321. https://doi.org/10.1089/jwh.2008.1156.

O'Neil, A., A. J. Scovelle, A. J. Milner, and A. Kavanagh. 2018. Gender/sex as a social determinant of cardiovascular risk. *Circulation* 137, no. 8: 854–864. https://doi.org/10.1161/CIRCULATIONAHA.117.028595.

Palmer-Ross, A., P. V. Ovseiko, and S. Heidari. 2021. Inadequate reporting of Covid-19 clinical studies: A renewed rationale for the sex and gender equity in research (SAGER) guidelines. *BMJ Global Health* 6: e004997. https://doi.org/10.1136/bmjgh-2021-004997.

Parker, R., T. Larkin, and J. Cockburn. 2017. A visual analysis of gender bias in contemporary anatomy textbooks. *Social Science & Medicine* 180: 106–113. https://doi.org/10.1016/j.socscimed.2017.03.032.

Pascual, O. M., E. R. Vallejo, and M. L. García. 2021. Challenging gender bias in research. *BMJ Opinions*. https://blogs.bmj.com/bmj/2021/02/05/challenging-gender-bias-in-research/ (accessed April 4, 2021).

Peters, S. A. E., M. Woodward, V. Jha, S. Kennedy, and R. Norton. 2016. Women's health: A new global agenda. *BMJ Global Health* 1: e000080. https://doi.org/10.1136/bmjgh-2016-000080.

Pivonello, R., R. S. Auriemma, C. Pivonello et al. 2020. Sex disparities in Covid-19 severity and outcome: Are men weaker or women stronger? *Neuroendocrinology* 111, no. 11: 1066–1085. https://doi.org/10.1159/000513346.

Ravindran, S. K., Y. Teerawattananon, C. Tannenbaum, and L. Vijayasingham. 2020. Making pharmaceutical research and regulation work for women. *British Medical Journal* 371: m3808. https://doi.org/10.1136/bmj.m3808.

Regensteiner, J. G., A. M. Libby, R. Huxley, and J. A. Clayton. 2019. Integrating sex and gender considerations in research: Educating the scientific workforce. *Lancet Diabetes & Endocrinology* 7, no. 4: 248–250. https://doi.org/10.1016/S2213-8587(19)30038-5.

Reisner, S. L., T. Poteat, J. Keatley et al. 2016. Global health burden and needs of transgender populations: A review. *The Lancet* 388, no. 10042: 412–436. https://doi.org/10.1016/S0140-6736(16)00684-X.

Rochon, P. A., R. Mason, and J. H. Gurwitz. 2020. Increasing the visibility of older women in clinical research. *The Lancet* 395, no. 10236: 1530–1532. https://doi.org/10.1016/S0140-6736(20)30849-7.

Rodney, N. C. and C. J. Mulligan. 2014. A biocultural study of the effects of maternal stress on mother and newborn health in the Democratic Republic of Congo. *American Journal of Physical Anthropology* 155, no. 2: 200–209. https://doi.org/10.1002/ajpa.22568.

Rogers, P. A. W., T. M. D'Hooghe, A. Fazleabas et al. 2009. Priorities for endometriosis research. *Reproductive Sciences*16, no. 4: 335–346. https://doi.org/10.1177/1933719108330568.

Ruiz-Cantero, M. T., C. Vives-Cases, L. Artazcoz, et al. 2007. A framework to analyse gender bias in epidemiological research. *Journal of Epidemiology & Community Health* 61, suppl. 2: ii46–ii53. https://doi.org/10.1136/jech.2007.062034.

Runnels, V., S. Tudiver, M. Doull, and M. Boscoe. 2014. The challenges of including sex/gender analysis in systematic reviews: A qualitative survey. *Systematic Reviews* 3, no. 1: 33. https://doi.org/10.1186/2046-4053-3-33.

Schaaf, M., A. Kapilashrami, A. George et al. 2021. Unmasking power as foundational to research on sexual and reproductive health and rights. *BMJ Global Health* 6: e005482. https://doi.org/10.1136/bmjgh-2021-005482.

Schurz, H., M. Salie, G. Tromp, E. G. Hoal, C. J. Kinnear, and M. Möller. 2019. The X chromosome and sex-specific effects in infectious disease susceptibility. *Human Genomics* 13, no. 1: 2. https://doi.org/10.1186/s40246-018-0185-z.

Shannon, G., M. Jansen, K. Williams et al. 2019. Gender equality in science, medicine, and global health: Where are we at and why does it matter? *The Lancet* 393, no. 10171, 560–569. https://doi.org/10.1016/S0140-6736(18)33135-0.

Shields, K. and A. Lyerly. 2013. Exclusion of pregnant women from industry-sponsored clinical trials. *Obstetrics & Gynecology* 122, no. 5: 1077–1081. https://doi.org/10.1097/AOG.0b013e3182a9ca67.

Shimabukuro, T. 2021. Covid-19 vaccine safety update from CDC Covid-19 Vaccine Task Force. https://www.cdc.gov/vaccines/acip/meetings/downloads/slides-2021-06/03-COVID-Shimabukuro-508.pdf (accessed December 20, 2021).

Sigfrid, L., T. M. Drake, E. Pauley et al. 2021. Long Covid in adults discharged from UK hospitals after Covid-19: A prospective, multicentre cohort study using the ISARIC WHO Clinical Characterisation Protocol. *Lancet Regional Health Europe* 8: 100186. https://doi.org/10.1101/2021.03.18.21253888.

Smolina, K., L. Ball, K. H. Humphries, N. Khan, and S. G. Morgan. 2015. Sex disparities in post-acute myocardial infarction pharmacologic treatment initiation and adherence: Problem for young women. *Circulation: Cardiovascular Quality and Outcomes* 8: 586–592. https://doi.org/10.1161/CIRCOUTCOMES.115.001987.

Stengel, G. 2020. Women's healthcare: A market ripe for disruption lacks investment. *Forbes*. https://www.forbes.com/sites/geristengel/2020/07/08/womens-healthcare-a-market-ripe-for-disruption/ (accessed May 3, 2021).

Sudre, C. H., B. Murray, T. Varsavsky et al. 2021. Attributes and predictors of long Covid. *Nature Medicine* 27: 626–631. https://doi.org/10.1038/s41591-021-01292-y.

Sugimoto, C. R., Y-Y. Ahn, E. Smith, B. Macaluso, and V. Larivière. 2019. Factors affecting sex-related reporting in medical research: A cross-disciplinary bibliometric analysis. *The Lancet* 393, no. 10171: 550–559. https://doi.org/10.1016/S0140-6736(18)32995-7.

Tannenbaum, C. and D. Day. 2017. Age and sex in drug development and testing for adults. *Pharmacological Research* 121: 83–93. https://doi.org/10.1016/j.phrs.2017.04.027.

Taqueti, V. R. and C. N. Bairey Merz. 2017. Sex-specific precision medicine: Targeting CRT-D and other cardiovascular interventions to those most likely to benefit. *European Heart Journal* 38, no. 19: 1495–1497. https://doi.org/10.1093/eurheartj/ehw684.

Taylor, M. M., L. Kobeissi, C. Kim et al. 2020. Inclusion of pregnant women in Covid-19 treatment trials. *Lancet Global Health* 9: e366–e371. http://dx.doi.org/10.1016/S2214-109X(20)30484-8.

Torgrimson, B. N. and C. T. Minson. 2005. Sex and gender: What is the difference? *Journal of Applied Physiology* 99, no. 3: 785–787. https://doi.org/10.1152/japplphysiol.00376.2005.

United Nations. 1995. Beijing Declaration and Platform of Action, adopted by the Fourth World Conference on Women: Action for Equality, Development and Peace. https://www.unwomen.org/sites/default/files/Headquarters/Attachments/Sections/CSW/PFA_E_Final_WEB.pdf (accessed December 20, 2021).

Van Daal, M., M. E. Muntinga, S. Steffens, A. Halsema, and P. Verdonk. 2020. Sex and gender bias in kidney transplantation: 3D bioprinting as a challenge to personalized medicine. *Women's Health Reports* 1, no. 1: 218–223. https://doi.org/10.1089/whr.2020.0047.

Van Hagen, L. J., M. Muntinga, Y. Appelman, and P. Verdonk. 2021. Sex- and gender-sensitive public health research: An analysis of research proposals in a research institute in the Netherlands. *Women & Health* 61, no. 1: 109–119. https://doi.org/10.1080/03630242.2020.1834056.

Verdonk, P., L. J. L. Mans, and A. L. M. Lagro-Janssen. 2005. Integrating gender into a basic medical curriculum. *Medical Education* 39, no. 11: 1118–1125. https://doi.org/10.1111/j.1365-2929.2005.02318.x.

Vijayasingham, L., E. Bischof, and J. Wolfe. 2021. Sex-disaggregated data in Covid-19 vaccine trials. *The Lancet* 397, no. 10278: 966–967. https://doi.org/10.1016/S0140-6736(21)00384-6.

Vitale, C., M. Fini, I. Spoletini, M. Lainscak, P. Seferovic, and G. M. Rosano. 2017. Under-representation of elderly and women in clinical trials. *International Journal of Cardiology* 232: 216–221. https://doi.org/10.1016/j.ijcard.2017.01.018.

Walli-Attaei, M., P. Joseph, A. Rosengren et al. 2020. Variations between women and men in risk factors, treatments, cardiovascular disease incidence, and death in 27 high-income, middle-income, and low-income countries (PURE): A prospective cohort study. *The Lancet* 396, no. 10244: 97–109. https://doi.org/10.1016/S0140-6736(20)30543-2.

Weber, J. 2006. From science and technology to feminist technoscience. In *Handbook of gender and women's studies*, ed. K. Davis, M. Evans, and J. Lorber, 397–414. London: Sage.

Welch, V., M. Doull, M. Yoganathan et al. 2017. Reporting of sex and gender in randomized controlled trials in Canada: A cross-sectional methods study. *Research Integrity and Peer Review* 2: 15. https://doi.org/10.1186/s41073-017-0039-6.

Wolfe, J., B. Safdar, T. E. Madsen et al. 2021. Sex- or gender-specific differences in the clinical presentation, outcome, and treatment of SARS-CoV-2. *Clinical Therapeutics* 43, no. 3: 557–571.e1. https://doi.org/10.1016/j.clinthera.2021.01.015.

World Health Organization. 1999. DALYs and reproductive health: Report of an informal consultation.

World Health Organization. 2007. Integrating gender into the curricula for health professionals. Meeting report. Department of Gender, Women and Health (GWH). https://www.who.int/gender/documents/GWH_curricula_web2.pdf (accessed December 20, 2021).

World Health Organization. 2011. Gender mainstreaming for health managers: A practical approach. Participant's notes.

World Health Organization. 2013. Global and regional estimates of violence against women: Prevalence and health effects of intimate partner violence and non-partner sexual violence. https://www.who.int/publications/i/item/9789241564625 (accessed December 20, 2021).

World Health Organization. 2020. Incorporating intersectional gender analysis into research on infectious diseases of poverty: A toolkit for health researchers. https://www.who.int/tdr/publications/year/2020/tdr-intersectional-gender-toolkit/en/ (accessed December 20, 2021).

Word Health Organization. 2021a. Endometriosis: Fact sheet. https://www.who.int/news-room/fact-sheets/detail/endometriosis (accessed May 3, 2021).

World Health Organization. 2021b. Gender and health. https://www.who.int/news-room/q-a-detail/gender-and-health (accessed July 9, 2021).

World Health Organization. 2021c. Violence against women prevalence estimates, 2018. https://www.who.int/publications/i/item/9789240022256 (accessed December 20, 2021).

World Health Organization and Council for International Organizations of Medical Sciences. 2017. International ethical guidelines for health-related research involving humans. https://cioms.ch/wp-content/uploads/2017/01/WEB-CIOMS-EthicalGuidelines.pdf (accessed December 20, 2021).

World Health Organization and Program for Appropriate Technology in Health (PATH). 2005. Researching violence against women: A practical guide for researchers and activists. https://www.who.int/reproductivehealth/publications/violence/9241546476/en/ (accessed December 20, 2021).

World Health Organization and UNAIDS. 2016. A tool for strengthening gender-sensitive national HIV and sexual and reproductive health (SRH) monitoring and evaluation systems. https://www.who.int/reproductivehealth/publications/gender_rights/hiv-srhr-monitoring-systems/en/ (accessed December 20, 2021).

Yoon, D. Y., N. A. Mansukhani, V. C. Stubbs, I. B. Helenowski, T. K. Woodruff, and M. R. Kibbe. 2014. Sex bias exists in basic science and translational surgical research. *Surgery* 156, no. 3: 508–516. https://doi.org/10.1016/j.surg.2014.07.001.

Zeeman, L. and K. Aranda. 2020. A systematic review of the health and healthcare inequalities for people with intersex variance. *International Journal of Environmental Research and Public Health* 17, no. 18: 6533. https://doi.org/10.3390/ijerph17186533.

Zeiler, K. 2020. Why feminist technoscience and feminist phenomenology should engage with each other: On subjectification/subjectivity. *Feminist Theory* 21, no. 3: 367–390. https://doi.org/10.1177/1464700120920763.

18

GLOBAL HEALTH INDICATORS AND DATA

Communicative signs and sites of contest

Sara L. M. Davis

Introduction

Numerical indicators and data have become increasingly central to decision-making in global health governance.[1] They appear in numerous places, such as on websites and annual reports, as backdrops to speakers at donor-pledging conferences, and on slides in conference rooms and webinars where diverse global and national health actors meet to align on targets, allocate funds, and assess progress (or lack thereof) toward shared objectives. Global health indicators and data, while appearing objective, are also signs that can communicate success or failure, hope or despair, blame or praise. Thus, they are also sites of debate and contestation among diverse social actors, ranging from United Nations (UN) agencies, to bilateral donors, civil society groups, private enterprises, and many other stakeholders, who frequently gather to negotiate over priorities and funding in global health.

As the global experience of Covid-19 has shown, indicators and data relating to health, disease, and death can be politically explosive, and have significant power to shape political futures. For example, we have seen infectious disease modeling move from academic journals and think tank papers to the mass media, and predictive models used to justify lockdowns or their easing; spurring debates over rises in incidence, what they mean, and the appropriate response to them. There has even been pressure on health officials to reclassify mortality data in order to minimize the impact of Covid-19 on countries (Dyer 2020).

Public health has always been a field dominated by quantitative data (for example, epidemiology, demography, economic analysis, and so on). But over the past several decades, there has been a rapid growth in the prominence of data used for purposes of accountability and in communications as well as in the elevation of mathematical models to serve as decision tools at the center of strategic planning processes in the management offices of global health agencies. The growing demand for indicators, modeling, projections, and data represents a rapid expansion of the mechanisms of audit, transparency, and measurement (Riles 2013). Global health is also increasingly digital health; a transformation was underway before Covid-19 and has further accelerated in the pandemic. Digital technologies used in global health are said to offer the hope of better data and the ability to better target resources and interventions with military precision, even down to the level of clinics. The reality, of course, is that no matter how much data in global health grows, there never seems to be enough.

DOI: 10.4324/9781315675411-22

One perspective on this, as Sally Engle Merry aptly noted is "the process of translating the buzzing confusion of social life into neat categories that can be tabulated risks distorting the complexity of social phenomena" (2016: 1). In other words, global health data, while being used to convey authority, objectivity, and precision, is in reality plagued with gaps and risks.

Medical anthropologists and human rights scholars have tended to view the rise of quantitative measurement with a critical eye, pointing out that metrics are abstractions from complex social contexts that oversimplify these settings in order to create the illusion of commensurability (Davis and Kruse 2007; Merry 2011, 2016; Rosga and Satterthwaite 2009). They reduce social phenomena to make them visible and commensurable across diverse contexts (Bartl, Papilloud, and Terracher-Lipinski 2019; Merry and Wood 2015; Winkler, Satterthwaite, and De Albuquerque 2014). To do this, indicators include and exclude data, and aggregate data. They can be constructed in ways that are often distortive and be used to create oversimplified rank-ordering of complex phenomena (Davis et al. 2012: 73–75).

These critics have shown how numerical indicators can take on the status of law in their operations, though the indicators may be ill-suited to the diverse contexts in which they impose these norms: "The production of indicators is itself a political process, shaped by the power to categorize, count, analyze, and promote a system of knowledge that has effects beyond the producers" (Merry, Davis and Kingsbury 2015: 2). Similarly, big data—in fact, any data—is produced by and embedded in institutional, social, political, and economic contexts (Mosco 2015). Vincanne Adams argues that the trend toward metrics in global health has devalued local health specificities and other ways of knowing (Adams 2016). Part of the problematic work done by indicators is the false sense of transparency they create: the information used to shape them and measure progress may be comprehensible to a small group of experts, while remaining incomprehensible to the public (Bradley 2015).

Critics have further pointed out that indicators and data used in global governance reinforce unequal power relationships within and between countries, especially aid donors and recipients (Escobar 1995). Sally Engle Merry and Summer Wood (2015) show how human rights indicators are selected and defined by officials in high-income countries, such as Switzerland, who may fail to grasp how poorly those indicators work in low- or middle-income countries, such as Tanzania, which are nonetheless expected to report on their progress on these inapt metrics to the UN.

This chapter builds on this critique to argue that indicators used in global health governance function as communicative signs, which, while they do contain the somewhat Orwellian traits outlined above, are not always fixed: there can sometimes be a continuing process of contest and critique. This is because indicators used in global health are a form of signification that is constantly emergent through a process of debate and contest among diverse actors: such as scientists, UN agencies, government officials, civil society activists, or private enterprises. Ferdinand de Saussure says that linguistic signs (such as words) that link concepts and sound-images are inherently arbitrary; there is no link between the concept of "sister" and the sound of the word itself (1959: 67). Moreover, forces are constantly shifting the relationship between signified and signifier (1959: 75); signs are inherently mutable and language shifts over time. For Jacques Derrida, shifts in signification are inherently a form of play: discourse is "a system in which the central signified, the original or transcendental signified, is never absolutely present outside a system of differences" (1978: 280). Indicators used for global health governance are similarly arbitrary abstractions of complex phenomena, interpreted through diverse lenses.

In practice, most of the work done by indicators in governance relies more literally on signs—in the sense of visual displays within meetings, workshops, or webinars where diverse actors collaborate or contend over power, funding, and accountability. Both indicators and charts used to report on progress against targets are often displayed as part of collective speech events, such as presentations, and are embedded in verbal narratives as a form of suasion (Bauman 1977). In medieval times, Buddhist monks traveled in Asia, using scrolls and murals to narrate the life of the Buddha and persuade the masses to follow their edicts and principles (Mair 1988). Today, global health officials travel the world with slide presentations which they use to convince others, in particular health officials in low- and middle-income countries, of the merits of aligning with the current global health strategy and of meeting its related targets.

The question then becomes who is in the meeting and who feels empowered to challenge the speaker: whether the presentation is simply an authoritarian handing-down of norms and standards to a passive audience, or a conversation grounded in multivocality that enables different perspectives, even different epistemologies, to enter the meeting and challenge or contribute to the definition of indicators. Either way, through speech events such as presentations and meetings, indicators as signs are further embedded in histories of expression that are constantly remade, in an infinite chain of communication (Bakhtin 1981).

These contests include debates over what quantitative metrics capture and what (or who) they leave out. Given a global landscape of inequalities that shapes access to health services, some data gaps reflect these inequalities; and, in turn, biased data sets in health can amplify inequalities and have other political effects. When priority-setting or rationing decisions are grounded in quantitative analysis, and fail to adequately consider equity, ethics, or human rights dimensions, those decisions may reinforce existing inequalities.

The following three case examples serve to illustrate and elucidate the complex and sensitive power negotiations that can shape indicators, data, and the work of interpretation. These examples include debates linked to the Sustainable Development Goal (SDG) 5.2 on violence against women; the problems linked to data about the needs of marginalized groups in the HIV response, particularly in setting priorities for resource allocations; and finally, the challenge of eligibility criteria that determine which countries can receive global health funding.

Uncounted in the SDG on violence against women

In global health, indicators are frequently used to set targets that help facilitate coordination of work among diverse actors. Indicators are also important signs for public communications, signaling a level of commitment to addressing a given problem, especially for one that requires intensified efforts to make progress. In every case, an objective, linked to an indicator, helps to shine light on a problem. But this can inadvertently obscure adjacent problems that are not included in the indicator; at the same time, the light shone by the indicator may attract critics who disagree with the priorities it highlights, who interpret it in varying ways, or who may differ on the target and reporting methodology.

An example of this is the indicator-related challenges raised by the SDG on violence against women. Establishing a clear target to catalyze greater action on this issue has helped to give this urgent problem greater visibility. But in the process, the indicator creates new questions related to data-gathering and analysis.

Sexual and gender-based violence (SGBV) is widespread across the world and has a profound impact on the physical and mental health of individuals, families, and communities. Nevertheless, despite being widely recognized as a problem, this stigmatized issue is still not included in the healthcare policies of health agendas of many countries (WHO 2013: 10). For many years, gender-based violence has been denied and ignored, minimized, and deprioritized, swallowed up in the "silences in international discourses" (Anholt 2016: 1). Women's rights advocates pushed for years to break this silence, to put the issue on the global agenda, and to catalyze action by the UN agencies and member states.

The advocates' efforts to get a relevant indicator included in the Millennium Development Goals for 2000–2015 were stymied in part because critics said that gender-based violence was too difficult to measure (Anderson 2013; Ellsberg 2006). They questioned the conceptual coherence of gender-based violence and the plausibility of metrics that track the concept. Despite such objections, advocates continued to push for including gender-based violence in the MDGs by organizing high-level summits and lobbying senior diplomats. And when the UN member states approved the SDGs for 2015–2030, they did include an indicator, SDG 5.2, which committed to "eliminate all forms of violence against all women and girls in the public and private spheres, including trafficking and sexual and other types of exploitation" (UN General Assembly 2015).

As Yadlapalli Kusuma and Bontha Babu (2017) note, the setting of an indicator such as SDG 5.2 is a tacit acknowledgment both that violence against girls and women exists, and that it can be prevented through concerted efforts such as mobilizing resources, designing and implementing interventions, and scaling them up. The global indicator thus offers a tool for national-level advocates to use in advocacy and in accountability work: they could use its normative power to push for programming, resourcing, and to demand updates on progress by states.

However, the problems of reporting on and analyzing the violence against women indicator are shaped significantly by politics: especially, by widespread denialism and gender inequalities. As the World Health Organization (WHO) has noted, the available data on cases of SGBV is almost always a small percentage of the actual incidence. The incomplete picture is "an inevitable result of survivors' well-founded anxiety about the potentially harmful social, physical, psychological and/or legal consequences of disclosing their experience of sexual violence" (WHO 2007: 1). To address fears of reporting, WHO recommends health services and others take a series of steps to protect those who disclose SGBV from harm, and to establish the trust needed to elicit disclosure, in order to link survivors to essential health services.

However, this insight into the dynamics that can contribute to hiding a stigmatized group and also result in low reported incidence of SGBV is not widely shared in the general public. Those less familiar with the complex negotiations and trust-earning required in order to elicit disclosure could simply perceive officially reported statistics of gender-based violence not as the tip of the iceberg, but as the full iceberg. Where reports are few, officials who would prefer to minimize, negate, or deny that violence against women is widespread within their domain of responsibility or authority may use those low reports to justify their position.

This points to a second problem created by many indicators like the one created for violence against women: in the absence of contextual information, data reflected in a single indicator can be so abstracted from situational reality that its meaning becomes open to contesting interpretations of the phenomenon being measured.

This is best exemplified by considering the problem of how to understand a change in reported incidence (Davis, Schopper and Epps 2018; Merry 2016): Should we interpret an increase in reported incidence as an indication of an increase in actual violence? Or, more encouragingly, does an increase in incidence suggest that reporting mechanisms are working better, because more girls and women feel more trusting and empowered to report their experience of violence?

Conversely, does a decrease in reported incidence mean that efforts to reduce violence are failing, because fewer women feel safe to report? Or does a drop in cases mean that there is actually less violence? The purpose of an indicator is to abstract away from the contextual information while retaining essential facts about the relevant phenomenon, and to signal the importance of that phenomenon to the public. However, contradictory conclusions can be drawn from a single indicator without contextual information.

If it is decontextualized, an indicator, especially if it is based on reported data of incidence of a stigmatized problem, can subject a communicative sign to political pressures within the larger discourse. That is, those with a stake in reporting positive progress interpret reported data in ways that reinforce their optimism, perhaps even using it as propaganda to promote their progress. Meanwhile, those with reasons to be critical can present the same data to argue that efforts are failing.

For example, in March 2018, the UN tweeted a link to a report showing that the measures it implemented to end sexual exploitation and abuse by UN staff were having a positive effect and resulting in a reduced number of allegations against UN staff from 165 reports to 148. The responses to this on Twitter included an acerbic critique from a women's rights campaigner, Danielle L. Spencer: "Unfortunately, all this shows is a drop in reporting, not a drop in incidents—they know this and this is a PR stunt" (@daniellewas, March, 14, 2018).

In other words, a lone indicator may not tell the whole story. The idea of measuring a complex and politically sensitive phenomenon such as gendered violence through a lone indicator has been widely critiqued by social scientists and legal scholars.

Furthermore, by shining a light on one problem, an indicator may inadvertently reinforce invisibility of related problems. By exclusion from the indicator, other related issues are rendered less important than the particular phenomena measured in the indicator. There is a good example of this. The SDG 5.2 on violence against women, the related public summits, and other high-level efforts have "brought partial sight to some of the previously gender blind, and generated some political discussion and action aimed at preventing such violence," argues Chris Dolan (2014: 486). Nonetheless, Dolan continues: "The range of victims and survivors that are not just recognized but also addressed needs to be more inclusive—most urgently male and lesbian, gay, bisexual, transgender and intersex (LGBTI) victims and survivors." Dolan is among those who have worked to draw attention to the lived experiences as well as lack of services for male survivors of conflict-related sexual violence (Edström et al. 2016).

As Dolan implies, the invisibility or exclusion of male and LGBTI survivors in the SDG indicator on violence against women in effect makes the indicator a sign that discursively constructs cisgender women as a priority. This can reinforce denialism, invisibility, and lack of services for non-female victims of SGBV. Because of stigma and homophobia, including laws criminalizing same-sex sexual behavior in many countries, gathering data on the extent of sexual violence against men and LGBTIQ+ people is even more challenging than doing so on violence against women; these victims are the uncounted among the uncounted.

Thus, while the SDG 5.2 on violence against women is an important step forward in greater recognition of the problem, and toward reducing the stigma and promoting action on this issue, a single indicator monitoring progress on a stigmatized and political problem can open up conceptual challenges and contestations of interpretations. At the same time, it may unintentionally, even in good faith efforts, contribute to rendering adjacent problems invisible, or suggest that they are somehow less urgent or important. The indicator does important work by setting up a flag that gathers diverse actors who can work together to address the problem signaled by the indicator; at the same time, it draws the attention of critics, who may critique the indicator, the methodology, or use the reported data to press for greater progress.

While the actors engaged in addressing SGBV are relatively sparse, the global HIV response has mobilized many different stakeholders to set goals and collaborate to address them, including through redistributing resources among countries. Here, the political forces shaping health indicators and data are more complex, and are frequently critiqued and contested, as discussed in the next section.

Uncounted in the HIV response

Over the past 40 years, the global HIV response has excelled in coordinating diverse actors globally to provide health services and engage in policy advocacy. A critical part of this mobilization has been the development every few years of political declarations on HIV and AIDS by the UN General Assembly. Work following on from these declarations with targets is led by the Joint UN Programme on HIV and AIDS (UNAIDS), which also gathers data from countries to monitor their progress.

The work of priority-setting done by national health officials is closely tied to these targets and to national HIV strategic plans. Health officials collaborate with UNAIDS, WHO, and donors of Development Assistance for Health, such as the Global Fund to Fight AIDS, TB and Malaria ("the Global Fund"), and the US President's Emergency Plan for AIDS Relief (PEPFAR). This work of national health resource allocation is increasingly based on cost-effectiveness principles: given a limited bucket of funds for health in most countries, health policymakers and planners must prioritize investments in those interventions that deliver the greatest impact for the largest number of people.

However, this approach can inadvertently disfavor small or marginalized groups who may otherwise need to be prioritized for both ethical and efficacy reasons. This challenge is especially clear when considering the problem of reaching key populations who are most at risk of HIV: gay men and other men who have sex with men; sex workers; people who use drugs; and transgender people (WHO 2016). As of 2020, over 60% of new HIV infections globally occur among these populations (UNAIDS 2020). However, in contrast to global estimates, many countries lack adequate or current data on the needs of these key populations within their countries, and also lack services that are geared to reach these key populations (Sabin et al. 2016).

A significant body of human rights research has shown that key populations tend to avoid HIV studies and clinics in countries where their behaviors are also criminalized; they fear being publicly exposed or reported to police (Amon and Kasambala 2009; Booth et al. 2013; Global Commission on HIV and the Law 2012, 2018; Schwartz et al. 2015). Like survivors of SGBV, and for similar reasons, criminalized and stigmatized key populations often evade participating in data and data collecting efforts that might identify them and expose them to families, friends, employers, or the police.

This avoidance leads to what Stef Baral and Matt Greenall (2013) call the "data paradox" for key populations: "Decision-makers deny that most affected populations exist [...] so no research gets done on these populations; the lack of data feeds the denial; and so on." The data paradox for key populations is a vicious cycle of invisibility, in which, once again, absence of data is taken as evidence of absence of the issue by officials who may not be willing to acknowledge the existence of key populations, such as men who have sex with men (Narrain and Vance 2018).

This data paradox becomes clear in reviewing size estimates reported by countries to UNAIDS as part of the agency's routine data-gathering process to measure progress toward shared global targets: criminalization of same-sex sexual behavior is statistically associated with reports of implausibly low (or indeed, entirely missing) population size estimates for men who have sex with men. Especially low population size estimates are found in countries that impose the death penalty (Davis et al. 2017). As a result of these low denominators of key population size, some countries then significantly overestimate their rate of success in reaching men who have sex with men, such as with HIV tests. In reality, they are missing an unknown number of uncounted people.

When these biased data sets are fed into algorithms, the results may magnify existing inequalities that created the biases in the first place. To understand how biased data sets that omit uncounted people are used by and shape decision-making, it may be helpful to briefly examine the use of cost-effectiveness analysis software for decision-making processes, particularly in priority-setting or rationing resources.

HIV cost-effectiveness analysis

Since the first UN Political Declaration on HIV, cost-effectiveness as a discourse and frame for prioritization in financing the HIV response has quickly risen to prominence. This has meant that anyone engaged in developing HIV finance plans, whether at the global or the country level, increasingly needs cost-effectiveness data in order to make the case for financing any intervention.

In one type of cost-effectiveness analysis, a health official inputs data about the costs and the typical health outcomes of each service into mathematical models. These models then generate and compare future potential scenarios of disease transmission. This may include an analysis of allocative efficiency: which populations or interventions a health official might invest in, in order to obtain the highest impact for the lowest expense. By inputting available data on HIV transmission among different populations (for instance, men who have sex with men, sex workers and their partners, or the general population), and the cost of programs that meet the specific needs of each group, as well as national targets for the HIV response, health officials can then receive and review projections produced by the software and select the scenario that delivers maximum health impacts within a fixed budget.

These software tools thus offer users an evidence-based visualization to support a frank discussion about how best to allocate or ration limited resources. However, the software tools create an "epistemic object" representing the future by selectively focusing on specific aspects of that future to display visually. That is, the tools edit out the political, legal, and social contexts in which HIV flourishes: in which negation, laws criminalizing HIV transmission, and other contextual issues create a data paradox that warps data sets and leaves key populations uncounted.

While the decision is framed as an evidence-based choice between health interventions, in effect, the final charts produced by cost-effectiveness software visually pit (interventions for) key populations against one another in a competition for limited resources. Interventions for smaller populations are generally more expensive per person, and thus less likely to be cost-effective. For key populations, as shown above, official size estimates are often implausibly low or missing altogether. Because cost-effectiveness software does not explicitly address the ways in which criminalization may distort the data, the scenarios the software generates may lead health planners to inadvertently deprioritize criminalized groups that appear smaller or do not appear at all. Worse, the software in effect disfavors populations for whom there is no data, reinforcing the historical discrimination that rendered them invisible (Davis 2020).

In a context of flatlining development assistance budgets, these forms of cost-effectiveness analysis do offer important benefits: they support the reduction of waste and maximizing of resources for health services. Failure to use economic evaluation in decision-making could itself be considered unethical in conditions of scarcity (Dudley, Silove, and Gale 2012). For example, to uphold the human right to health, states are obligated to dedicate maximum available resources to progressive fulfillment of the right to health (UN CESCR 2000). Cost-effectiveness analysis can help states to fulfill this human rights obligation.

But at the same time, cost-effectiveness analysis always requires "some form of rationing": "Any way you cut it [...] developing a benefits package will produce winners and losers, especially in poor countries with large populations and small budgets for health. Losers in this context are the group of people that inevitably will get less, in terms of benefits or services, than others" (Yazbeck 2002: 7–8).

Considering historical discrimination against some smaller populations, however, those who lose out on health services may be those who have always lost out in the past. The processes in which these tools are used must be informed by the structural factors that shape the patchy and limited data on marginalized groups and should ensure the value of cost-effectiveness is balanced against other values, such as equity and the human right to non-discrimination. This becomes especially crucial in the digital age, as health institutions shift toward machine learning and algorithmic decision-making. Algorithms such as those used in cost-effectiveness analysis may reflect and shape broader patterns of meaning (Seaver 2017) and even reinforce mistaken assumptions and amplify biases (Duclos 2019).

Criminalization, stigma, and discrimination may distort data about marginalized groups; and when these biased forms of data are crucial to decision-making, they can wreak multiple kinds of havoc. Countries may fail to prioritize resources for uncounted or undercounted populations, may overestimate their levels of success in coverage of key services that, in turn, create data (incidence rates, in this case) which further misrepresent reality (Davis et al. 2017). When absence of evidence is used as evidence of absence, uncounted populations may find themselves caught in a cascade of bad decisions about their health.

However, because the HIV response has incorporated civil society and community representation in many levels of decision-making, in some cases, community activists have been empowered to question the data used to make these decisions. African key populations advocates surveyed about their experiences participating in global health governance meetings described challenging the lack of data on transgender people and refusing to accept size estimates that they found implausibly small (Esom et al. 2016). For example, Peter Njane, a gay rights activist in Kenya, described arguing with PEPFAR over a size estimate of 10,000 men who have sex with men in Kenya: "We had disputes over how the data was collected. We questioned where they got their information. Donors were there, we're shown the final product, the money has been used, and the community didn't accept it" (in Esom et al. 2016: 18).

It is fortunate that in some cases activists feel empowered to challenge global health donors and national officials about the biased data sets. Such dialogic processes of defining indicators and data used to make decisions, when they incorporate diverse voices, offer the potential for indicators to be debated, critiqued, and revised.

The stakes for these contests can be high: as discussed in the third example, below, these local gaps in data can shape high-level decision-making that has life and death effects.

Uncounted in health aid eligibility

In 2016, a group of people living with HIV in Venezuela wrote a letter to the Global Fund headquarters in Geneva, Switzerland, to request urgent help. This letter, and the subsequent responses and debates regarding the contents of the letter, revealed cracks in the global health financing architecture—cracks created by a set of apparently objective numerical indicators, and the data that is used to report on progress against them. The letter led to high-level debates over what the indicators failed to capture, and ultimately, some small but significant changes in use of these indicators.

The Venezuelan activists wrote to request urgent shipments of antiretroviral treatment for people living with HIV in a context of rapid economic collapse. As they explained in their letter, Venezuela's national currency had depreciated by 900%, inflation was 700%, and Venezuelans faced long supermarket lines for basics such as rice or milk: "Literally, we are not only suffering hunger, we are also dying, because our health system is totally collapsed" (RVG+ 2016: 2).

At this time, Venezuela's economic collapse was still being widely denied by its political leaders. Venezuela had long been seen as an oil-rich country and one with a robust and flourishing public health system, which had largely eliminated malaria (Griffing, Villegas and Udhayakumar 2014). Venezuela also had never received Global Fund assistance before. The leadership of the Global Fund delayed their reply to the letter for some time, and finally responded negatively, explaining: "The Board is guided by its approved *Eligibility Policy*, which annually determines the countries eligible for Global Fund funding. Eligibility is determined by a country's income level, measured by an appropriate economic indicator of the World Bank, and official disease burden data" (Hauser and Dybul 2017).

Indeed, this was strictly accurate. After many years of debating how best to allocate resources, the Global Fund Board, a vast parliament made up of hundreds of government and civil society representatives, had finally developed and approved an *Eligibility Policy* that outlined that its resources would be disbursed to low-income countries and countries with a high burden of HIV, TB, and malaria (Global Fund 2016). The *Eligibility Policy* aligned with existing overseas development aid criteria used by many bilateral donors that also contribute to the Global Fund and sit on its Board. However, these criteria had not been developed to respond to a situation that was occurring in a country like Venezuela: one in the midst of rapid economic collapse, and in which government leaders were covering up a failing health system.

First and foremost, guided by the World Bank (which has a seat on the Global Fund Board), the Board uses Gross National Income per capita (GNIpc) as the first sorting indicator to identify the countries in greatest economic need. The World Bank classifies all countries as either low-income, lower-middle-income, upper-middle-income, or high-income.

However, the World Bank never intended GNIpc to be used as an indicator to determine eligibility for health financing. GNIpc is calculated once a year and does not capture income and other social inequalities. It only shows the average income that existed in the country the previous year; not how it is taxed, whether it is subject to debt, or how it is allocated (or otherwise) to health services. As such, GNIpc is at best a crude indicator of national economic capacity for health. This was reflected in the Venezuela case.

In 2016, at the time of the initial urgent appeal from Venezuelan activists to the Global Fund, Venezuela was still classified as "high-income" by the World Bank, thus making it ineligible for aid from the Global Fund. By the time the Global Fund leadership finally responded to the appeal with their own letter pointing that their policy, hyperinflation, and plunging oil prices were sending Venezuela's national income into a tailspin. Shortly, thereafter, Venezuela was reclassified by the World Bank as an "upper-middle-income country."

The 2016 Global Fund *Eligibility Policy* did permit the agency to fund HIV, TB, and malaria programs in some "middle-income" countries, provided those countries met other criteria. One of these was "disease burden": the percentage of people living with HIV in the general population, or the percentage living with HIV among key populations.

However, when it came to data on health, Venezuelans had a second problem: the political leadership of the country actively censored health data. Venezuela's president adamantly denied that there was any crisis for people living with HIV and refused overseas assistance of any kind. He forbade publication of any official information that might paint a different picture: when the Ministry of Health published government bulletins showing increases in infant and maternal mortality, the health minister was promptly fired (BBC 2017).

As an international organization with close UN ties, the Global Fund relies on official health data reported by countries to the UN in order to determine eligibility in compliance with its policy. UNAIDS gathers data on HIV from countries on a regular basis, verifies where it can, and normally shares this official data with the Global Fund to use in decision-making. But the most recent data UNAIDS had for Venezuela at the time of the letter was already several years out of date. Thus, without data on disease burden, the second possibility of eligibility was foreclosed, and Venezuela was again deemed to be ineligible for the Global Fund.

While these debates continued in Geneva and elsewhere, Venezuelan physicians formed an informal network to gather and share health data from clinics and hospitals, passing it on to international allies. Journalists managed to record the stark horrors of hospitals lacking basic equipment and supplies (Faiola 2017). A report from Human Rights Watch (2016) drew on these to publish a report on the dire health crisis unfolding in Venezuelan hospitals.

The Global Fund had one final indicator that could make Venezuela eligible: disease burden in key populations. In cases where countries had low general HIV prevalence but had concentrated epidemics of 5% or higher rates of HIV among key populations, the country could be eligible for funding.

Hoping to assist the Venezuelans, experts at UNAIDS found articles by anthropologists and others showing shockingly high rates of HIV and malaria transmission among the indigenous Warao people and shared these with the Global Fund. But Global Fund managers pointed out that indigenous people were not among the key populations affected by HIV that were officially recognized by the WHO and UNAIDS (ICASO and ACCSI 2018: 24).

So, was there data on the officially recognized key populations? Certainly, neighboring countries had high rates of HIV among men who have sex with men and transgender women. If Venezuela had similar data, that would have made Venezuela eligible for the Global Fund. However, due to homophobia and denialism, official national data on men who have sex with men did not exist in Venezuela. When countries had no official data on key populations, the Global Fund's policy in 2016 was to treat that lack of data as a zero.

In sum, a country in the midst of economic and social collapse, in desperate need for HIV and malaria prevention, treatment, and care, could not receive aid from a fund set up specifically for that purpose. The reasons were because of a set of narrowly defined global indicators, and the country's own politically created gaps in data, including data about stigmatized and marginalized groups. In effect, people living with HIV in Venezuela were being swallowed by a crack in the global health architecture—a structure built on what appeared to be robust and rational systems of quantification. But the structure failed to account for political realities shaping data, and how simple indicators designed in an international organization for use in governance might omit or obscure complex realities in another country.

Venezuelan activists, and their allies in international NGOs, UN agencies and on the Board of the Global Fund persisted in their advocacy. In May 2017, consistent with its *Eligibility Policy*, the Board voted down a proposal to send emergency funding to the country. However, it also created a working group to find another solution. In May 2018, nearly two years after the urgent appeal for lifesaving medications was sent to them, the Board approved a new policy on countries in crisis, which then allowed a small amount of emergency funding to go to Venezuela, channeled by UN agencies and civil society groups (The Global Fund 2018b).

At the same time, the Board went through its periodic review and update of the *Eligibility Policy*, and approved a small change to a footnote in the policy.[2] As a result of proposals put forward by civil society constituencies that have permanent seats and votes on the Global Fund Board, the revised 2018 *Eligibility Policy* clarified that in cases where there was no official government HIV-prevalence data for key populations, or if a change in data led to a change in country eligibility, the Secretariat of the Global Fund was authorized to seek other data from UNAIDS to inform their eligibility determination (The Global Fund 2018a). In practice, this data could include data from peer-reviewed studies, civil society reports, or other data that UNAIDS experts felt was sufficiently credible to inform an eligibility determination.

That these debates happened and unfolded the way they did (including this highly contentious but potentially game-changing footnote) shows how diverse actors—government officials, activists, physicians, and UN agencies—can come together to debate and negotiate over numerical indicators and the data reported against them, as well as over the implications of decisions made with this data. As imperfect as this process of responding was, it was only able to happen at all because in the Global Fund's governance structure, civil society activists have a seat at the table as equal peers with government officials, including voting powers. Without their active lobbying for Venezuela's eligibility, it is likely that the appeal would have ended with the original refusal by the Global Fund leadership. Their advocacy further enabled a revision to the footnote that could open up access to aid for more countries, and establish space for more diverse and credible forms of data to be used in decision-making.

Thus, indicators and data can be valuable as sites of contest that sometimes lead to progressive change when they are part of processes that incorporate transparency, accountability, and debate by diverse actors.

Conclusions

All forms of knowledge are partial and emergent. Health indicators and data are signs abstracted from complex realities, and have far-reaching system effects; but as this chapter has attempted to show, they can also be made open to contest. All communicative signs should be understood as abstractions. One indicator, or one text, cannot capture the prismatic and complex contexts in which ill-health flourishes, or do the complex work needed to inform or function as a sophisticated decision-making or accountability tool.

As critics have observed, indicators used in global health governance exercise normative power that shapes decision-making, priority-setting, and financing in ways that may distort local realities and override local expertise. Moreover, biases in data used to set targets or priorities can be produced by social and political inequalities, such as stigma, discrimination, marginalization, and criminalization. If these biases are not explicitly recognized, they may lead to biased decision-making that amplifies inequalities instead of promoting equity.

At the same time, global health indicators create a rallying point for diverse actors, and can open up space for engagement, contestation, and social accountability work that can make them powerful tools in the hands of activists. It is for this reason that advocates for those most marginalized continue to demand that they be used in order to establish commitments and enable independent monitoring of progress. For example, in the aftermath of a 2019 UN High-Level Meeting on Universal Health Coverage, the Global Network of People

Living with HIV (GNP+) issued a statement that criticized the gathering for its failure to set measurable indicators, expressing the view that the commitments at the meeting without indicators meant that they were purely rhetorical (GNP+ 2019). The statement warned that failure to set indicators "will lead to minimal progress and maximum self-congratulation."

The political authority of indicators and data is significant, and so in contexts where diverse actors have the space, the expertise, and the right to challenge authorities, indicators in global health governance do offer some hope for measurable progress.

Notes

1 This chapter draws from an earlier published book (Davis 2020).
2 As a consultant working for the three civil society delegations on the Global Fund Board, the author contributed to developing this footnote.

References

Adams, V., ed. 2016. *Metrics: What counts in global health*. Durham, NC: Duke University Press.

Amon, J. J. and T. Kasambala. 2009. Structural barriers and human rights related to HIV prevention and treatment in Zimbabwe. *Global Public Health* 4, no. 6: 528–545. https://doi.org/10.1080/17441690802128321.

Anderson, L. 2013. Violence against women: The missing Millennium Development Goal. Thomson Reuters Foundation, September 26. http://news.trust.org//item/20130926123955-d58b7/ (accessed May 26, 2019).

Anholt, R. M. 2016. Understanding sexual violence in armed conflict: Cutting ourselves on Occam's razor. *Journal of International Humanitarian Action* 1, no. 6: 237–247. https://doi.org/10.1186/s41018-016-0007-7.

Bakhtin, M. M. 1981. *The dialogic imagination: Four essays*. Ed. Michael Holquist. Austin: University of Texas Press.

Baral S. and M. Greenall. 2013. The data paradox. Blog, Where there is no data, July 5. https://wherethereisnodata.wordpress.com/2013/07/05/the-data-paradox/ (accessed May 10, 2021).

Bartl, W., C. Papilloud, and A. Terracher-Lipinski. 2019. Governing by numbers: Key indicators and the politics of expectations. An introduction. *Historical Social Research* 44, no. 2: 7–43. https://doi.org/10.12759/HSR.44.2019.2.7-43.

Bauman, R. 1977. *Verbal art as performance*. Austin: University of Texas Press.

BBC. 2017. Venezuela health minister fired over mortality stats. May 12. https://www.bbc.com/news/world-latin-america-39896048 (accessed May 10, 2021).

Booth, R. E., S. Dvoryak, M. Sung-Joon et al. 2013. Law enforcement practices associated with HIV infection among injection drug users in Odessa, Ukraine. *AIDS and Behavior* 17, no. 8: 2604–2614. https://doi.org/10.1007/s10461-013-0500-6.

Bradley, C. G. 2015. International organizations and the production of indicators. In *The quiet power of indicators: Measuring governance, corruption and rule of law*, ed. S. E. Merry, K. E. Davis, and B. Kingsbury, 27–74. Cambridge: Cambridge University Press.

Davis, K. E., B. Kingsbury, and S. E. Merry. 2012. Indicators as a technology of global governance. *Law and Society Review* 46, no. 1: 71–104. http://www.jstor.org/stable/41475254 (accessed December 21, 2021).

Davis, K. E. and M. B. Kruse. 2007. Taking the measure of law: The case of the Doing Business Project. *Law & Social Inquiry* 32, no. 4: 1095–1119. https://doi.org/10.1111/j.1747-4469.2007.00088.x

Davis, S. L. M. 2020. *The uncounted: Politics of data in global health*. Cambridge, UK: Cambridge University Press.

Davis, S. L. M., W. C. Goedel, J. Emerson, and B. Skartvedt Guven. 2017. Punitive laws, key population size estimates, and Global AIDS Response Progress Reports: An ecological study of 154 countries. *Journal of the International AIDS Society* 20, no. 1. https://doi.org/10.7448/ias.20.1.21386.

Davis, S. L. M., D. Schopper and J. Epps. 2018. Monitoring interventions to respond to sexual violence in humanitarian contexts. *Global Health Governance* 12, no. 1: 34–46. https://blogs.shu.edu/ghg/2018/03/15/monitoring-interventions-to-respond-to-sexual-violence-in-humanitarian-contexts/ (accessed December 21, 2021).

De Saussure, F. 1959. *Course in general linguistics*. Trans. W. Baskin, ed. P. Meisel and H. Saussy. New York: Columbia University Press.

Derrida, J. 1978. *Writing and difference*. Chicago, IL: University of Chicago Press.

Dolan, C. 2014. Letting go of the gender binary: Charting new pathways for humanitarian interventions on gender-based violence. *International Review of the Red Cross* 96, no. 894: 485–501. https://international-review.icrc.org/articles/letting-go-gender-binary-charting-new-pathways-humanitarian-interventions-gender-based (accessed August 22, 2021).

Duclos, V. 2019. Algorithmic futures. *Medicine Anthropology Theory* 6, no. 3. https://doi.org/10.17157/mat.6.3.660.

Dudley, M., D. Silove, and F. Gale, eds. 2012. *Mental health and human rights: Vision, praxis and courage.* Oxford: Oxford University Press.

Dyer O. 2020. Russia admits to understating deaths by more than two thirds. *BMJ* 371: m4975. https://doi.org/10.1136/bmj.m4975.

Edström, J., C. Dolan, and T. Shahrokh, with O. David. 2016. Therapeutic activism: Men of Hope Refugee Association Uganda breaking the silence over male rape in conflict-related sexual violence. Report. England: Institute of Development Studies. https://opendocs.ids.ac.uk/opendocs/handle/20.500.12413/9995 (accessed August 22, 2021).

Ellsberg, M. 2006. Violence against women and the Millennium Development Goals: Facilitating women's access to support. *International Journal of Gynaecology and Obstetrics* 94, no. 3: 325–332. https://doi.org/10.1016/j.ijgo.2006.04.021.

Escobar, A. 1995. *Encountering development: The making and unmaking of the third world.* Princeton, NJ: Princeton University Press.

Esom, K., C. Mubanda, T. Khositau et al. 2016. African key populations' engagement with global health financing institutions: A rapid review. Report. Johannesburg: African Men for Sexual Health and Rights. https://megontheinternet.files.wordpress.com/2021/09/african-key-populations-engagement-with-global-health-financing-institutions-a-rapid-review.pdf (accessed December 21, 2021).

Faiola, A. 2017. Sickness and HIV drug shortages rise as Venezuela's economy crumbles. *Independent*, September 8. https://www.independent.co.uk/news/world/americas/venezuela-drugs-shortage-food-hunger-healthcare-nicolas-maduro-chavez-socialism-hiv-a7936956.html (accessed May 10, 2021).

Global Commission on HIV and the Law. 2012. *HIV and the law: Risks, rights and health*. July. New York: UNDP, HIV/AIDS Group. https://hivlawcommission.org/report/ (accessed December 21, 2021).

Global Commission on HIV and the Law. 2018. *Risks, rights and health: Supplement*. New York: UNDP. https://hivlawcommission.org/supplement/ (accessed December 21, 2021).

The Global Fund. 2016. *The Global Fund eligibility policy*. GF/B35/06 – Revision 1. Approved by the Global Fund Board under decision point GF/B35/DP07. https://www.theglobalfund.org/media/4227/bm35_06-eligibility_policy_en.pdf (accessed July 2, 2021).

The Global Fund. 2018. *The Global Fund eligibility policy*. GF/B39/DP03, 9 May. https://www.theglobalfund.org/media/7443/core_eligibility_policy_en.pdf?u=636635807340000000 (accessed May 10, 2021).

The Global Fund. 2018a. *Potential engagement with non-eligible countries in crisis*. GF/B39/DP04. May 9. https://www.theglobalfund.org/board-decisions/b39-dp04/ (accessed May 10, 2021).

GNP+ (Global Network of People Living with HIV). 2019. GNP+ Calls for a strong accountability mechanism for UHC. September 24. https://www.plataformalac.org/en/2019/10/gnp-calls-for-a-strong-accountability-mechanism-for-uhc/ (accessed July 2, 2021).

Griffing, S. M., L. Villegas, and V. Udhayakumar. 2014. Malaria control and elimination, Venezuela, 1800s–1970s. *Emerging Infectious Diseases* 20, no. 10: 1691–1696. http://dx.doi.org/10.3201/eid2010.130917.

Hauser, N. and M. Dybul. 2017. Letter to board members of RVG+ Network of Positive People Venezuelan [*sic*]. NH/AK/OBA, January 18. http://icaso.org/wp-content/uploads/2017/10/letter-to-RVG-from-GF-January-2017.pdf (accessed May 10, 2021).

Human Rights Watch. 2016. *Venezuela's humanitarian crisis: Severe medical and food shortages, inadequate and repressive government response*. Report, October 24. https://www.hrw.org/report/2016/10/24/venezuelas-humanitarian-crisis-severe-medical-and-food-shortages-inadequate-and (accessed August 22, 2021).

ICASO (International Council of AIDS Service Organizations) and ACCSI (Accion Ciudadana Contra el SIDA). 2018. *Triple threat: Resurging epidemics, a broken health system, and global indifference to Venezuela's crisis.* Report. http://icaso.org/new-report-details-health-crisis-venezuela/ (accessed May 10, 2021).

Kusuma, Y. S. and B. V. Babu. 2017. Elimination of violence against women and girls as a global action agenda. *Journal of Injury and Violence Research*, July 9, no. 2: 117–121. https://doi.org/10.5249/jivr.v9i2.908.

Mair, V. H. 1988. *Painting and performance: Chinese picture recitation and its Indian genesis.* Honolulu: University of Hawaii Press.

Merry, S. E. 2011. Measuring the world: Indicators, human rights and global governance. *Current Anthropology* 52, no. 3: 583–595. https://doi.org/10.1017/S0272503700034194.

Merry, S. E. 2016. *The seductions of quantification: Measuring human rights, gender violence, and sex trafficking.* Chicago, IL: University of Chicago Press.

Merry, S. E., K. E. Davis, and B. Kingsbury. 2015. *The quiet power of indicators: Measuring governance, corruption, and rule of law.* Cambridge: Cambridge University Press.

Merry, S. E. and S. Wood. 2015. Quantification and the paradox of measurement: Translating children's rights in Tanzania. *Current Anthropology* 56, no. 2: 205–229. https://doi.org/10.1086/680439.

Mosco, V. 2015. *To the cloud: Big data in a turbulent world.* London: Paradigm.

Narrain, A and K Vance, 2018. Negation, acknowledgement and taking forward the struggle for LGBT rights: The third report of the Independent Expert on Sexual Orientation and Gender Identity. ARC International Blog, http://arc-international.net/research-and-publications/new-arc-reports/negation-acknowledgement-and-taking-forward-the-struggle-for-lgbt-rights-the-third-report-of-the-independent-expert-on-sexual-orientation-and-gender-identity/ (accessed May 9, 2021).

Riles, A. 2013. Market collaboration: Finance, culture and ethnography after neoliberalism. *American Anthropologist* 115, no. 4: 555–569. https://doi.org/10.1111/aman.12052.

Rosga, A. and M. L. Satterthwaite. 2009. The trust in indicators: Measuring human rights. *Berkeley Journal of International Law* 27, no. 2: 253–315. https://doi.org/10.15779/Z38G07R.

RVG+ (Red Venezolana de Gente Positiva). 2016. Venezuela needs your urgent help. Open letter to the Global Fund, June 6. http://vps157773.vps.ovh.ca/wp-content/uploads/2017/10/RVG-public-letter-to-board-Global-Fund-2017.pdf (accessed May 10, 2021).

Sabin, K., J. Zhao, J. M. Garcia Calleja et al. 2016. Availability and quality of size estimations of female sex workers, men who have sex with men, people who inject drugs and transgender women in low- and middle-income countries. *PLoS ONE* 11, no. 5. https://doi.org/10.1371/journal.pone.0155150.

Schwartz, S. R., R. G. Nowak, I. Orazulike et al. 2015. The immediate effect of the Same-Sex Marriage Prohibition Act on stigma, discrimination, and engagement on HIV prevention and treatment services in men who have sex with men in Nigeria: Analysis of prospective data from the TRUST Cohort. *The Lancet HIV* 2, no. 7 (July): e299–e306. https://doi.org/10.1016/S2352-3018(15)00078-8.

Seaver, N. 2017. Algorithms as culture: Some tactics for the ethnography of algorithmic systems. *Big Data & Society* 4, no. 2 (December): 205395171773810. https://doi.org/10.1177/2053951717738104.

UNAIDS (Joint UN Programme on HIV and AIDS). 2020. New HIV infections increasingly among key populations. Press Release, September 28. https://www.unaids.org/en/resources/presscentre/featurestories/2020/september/20200928_new-hiv-infections-increasingly-among-key-populations (accessed May 9, 2021).

UN CESCR (United Nations Committee on Economic Social and Cultural Rights). *General Comment No. 14: The right to the highest attainable standard of health* (Art. 12). 2000 Aug. E/C.12/2000/4. https://www.refworld.org/pdfid/4538838d0.pdf (accessed December 21, 2021).

United Nations General Assembly. 2015. Transforming our world: The 2030 agenda for sustainable development. Resolution A/RES/70/1, adopted September 25, 2018. https://sustainabledevelopment.un.org/content/documents/21252030%20Agenda%20for%20Sustainable%20Development%20web.pdf (accessed December 21, 2021).

WHO (World Health Organization). 2007. *WHO ethical and safety recommendations for researching, documenting and monitoring sexual violence in emergencies.* Geneva, CH: World Health Organization. https://www.who.int/reproductivehealth/publications/violence/9789241595681/en/ (accessed May 10, 2021).

WHO (World Health Organization). 2013. *Responding to intimate partner violence and sexual violence against women: WHO clinical and policy guidelines.* Geneva: World Health Organization. https://www. who.int/reproductivehealth/publications/violence/9789241548595/en/ (accessed May 10, 2021).

WHO (World Health Organization). 2016. *Consolidated guidelines HIV prevention, diagnosis treatment and care for key populations.* 2016 update. Geneva: WHO. http://www.who.int/hiv/pub/guidelines/keypopulations/en/ (accessed May 10, 2021).

Winkler, I. T., M. L. Satterthwaite, and C. de Albuquerque. 2014. Measuring what we treasure and treasuring what we measure: Post-2015 monitoring for the promotion of equality in the water, sanitation, and hygiene sector. *Wisconsin International Law Journal* 32 no. 3: 547–594.

Yazbeck, A. S. 2002. *An idiot's guide to prioritization in the health sector.* Washington, DC: The World Bank. http://documents.worldbank.org/curated/en/850011468013195446/pdf/266380Yazbeck-1AnIdiotsGuide1whole.pdf (accessed July 2, 2021).

19

SECURITIZATION AND HEALTH

Jeremy Youde

Introduction

The linking of health and security—and conceptualizing health as an issue of national and international security—has become increasingly common. The end of the Cold War, the emergence of new diseases like HIV and AIDS, and a shift in the thinking of policymakers at all different levels have contributed to the securitization of health and given military and security forces a greater role in responding to disease outbreaks and even enforcing Covid-19 lockdowns in some countries. As time has gone on, though, there has also been resistance to securitizing health, with various scholars arguing that claims of securitizing health have been overblown, that securitizing health harmfully narrows the global health agenda, and that securitization is an inappropriate frame for understanding the importance of global health. This is at the heart of what Christian Enemark calls the "biosecurity dilemma"—the fact that "security-oriented efforts to prevent or respond to disease outbreaks … have the potential to generate harms as well as benefits" (2017: 180).

This chapter aims to provide an overview of the securitization of health and the arguments for and against it as a strategy. It begins by describing what securitization means and the processes by which it occurs. It next looks at the historical evolution of the securitization of health and its close connection with the emergence of HIV/AIDS as a truly global issue. The third section lays out the arguments presented in favor of securitizing health and the benefits it can bring, and the fourth section identifies the most prominent objections to this strategy. Finally, the fifth section describes some of the contemporary debates over the securitization of health and areas for future research.

What is securitization?

International relations has traditionally equated security with war and the military. There is no central hierarchy to keep order in the international arena, and states cannot rely on others to come to their aid. The only way to provide some measure of safety in this environment is to build, develop, and maintain sufficient power to avoid being taken over by another state. Stephen Walt argues, "Organized violence has been a central part of human existence for millennia […] not surprisingly, therefore, preparations for war have preoccupied organized

DOI: 10.4324/9781315675411-23

polities throughout history" (1991: 213). This does not mean that states lack other interests, but this view of security posits that war and the military must take precedence over any other issue because a state can achieve none of its other goals without first ensuring its security.

Instead of solely equating security with war and assuming that security issues are self-evident, securitization presents the idea of security as part of a project whereby political actors frame an issue as a security threat. It does not argue that war and the military are irrelevant to states, but it emphasizes that understanding what a state sees as a security issue is fundamentally a political process. Rather than taking the notion of security as a given and assuming that the same definition applies universally, securitization presents security as "essentially contested," generating "unsolvable debates about [its] meaning and application" (Buzan 1991: 7). These points are key, as they emphasize that describing something as a security issue necessarily arises out of negotiations or social actions. It also means that notions of security can change based on time, space, and context. This does not necessarily mean that the process of securitizing an issue is one that opens up more debate or discussion within society; rather, it means that political elites are framing and reframing an issue as a security threat largely as a tool for bringing more attention and resources to bear on it. It is largely a top-down phenomenon by which governments prioritize certain issues—and the tools to respond to those issues—while deprioritizing others (Rushton 2019). Framing something as a security issue gives it a degree of importance in the political landscape that it might otherwise lack.

Securitization theory, most commonly associated with the Copenhagen School of Security Studies, focuses on *how* and *why* certain issues become security concerns in the first place. A wide range of non-military issues, like HIV/AIDS, environmental degradation, and global warming, *could* conceivably be security issues, but not all will. Securitization theory emphasizes the role of speech acts. Describing something as a security issue gives it a special social quality for policymakers. The designation itself holds certain connotations and implies a certain sort of response. It also affects how other parties view the issue and its place on the political agenda. In essence, the act of securitizing an issue by calling it a security issue effectively forms an agreement among political actors. Ole Waever notes that the security label "does not merely reflect whether a problem *is* a security problem, it is also a political choice" (1995: 65). Designating something as a security issue is thus a political tool to advance particular goals and aims.

The major implication of securitization theory is that there is not some sort of empirical criteria to determine which issues are security issues. Instead, the intersubjective understandings of a particular issue condition whether it holds a place on a nation's security agenda. It is less about any particular qualities of the issue itself, and more about how the issue is discussed, debated, and presented in public as something that poses an existential threat or challenge to national and international society *if* the securitizing effort is successful.

Securitization becomes a political choice on the part of the government. Securitizers choose, for some reason, to elevate a given issue into the realm of security. Barry Buzan, Ole Waever, and Jaap de Wilde caution against securitizing non-military issues, arguing that it represents "a failure to deal with issues as normal politics" (1998: 29). Reaching for extraordinary powers signals a failure by existing political institutions to accommodate this new issue in a timely and beneficial manner. Security issues are treated differently from other issues; debates over tax policy do not come with the same sort of existential considerations as security issues, nor do they provoke the same sense of immediacy.

The securitization process includes four distinct elements. First, there must be a *securitizing agent* or actor. This entity seeks to have an issue to be understood as a security issue.

Second, there must be an identified *existential threat*. Third, there must be a *referent object*, or something being threatened. Finally, there must be an *audience* that needs to be persuaded to accept that the existential threat truly threatens the referent object. That audience will vary depending on the context and political system; it may or may not be oriented toward the public as a whole (Buzan, Waever, and De Wilde 1998: 36). Ultimately, it is up to the audience, not the securitizing agent, to determine whether an issue is securitized (31); if the audience does not accept that a given issue poses an existential threat, or that it requires the resources associated with national and international security to address adequately, then it does not become a security issue.

To see how a health issue might become securitized, let us use the H5N1 influenza (also known as avian flu) outbreak that began in December 2003 as an example. Over the course of ten years, the World Health Organization reported 649 laboratory-confirmed human cases of the disease causing 385 deaths in sixteen countries (Centers for Disease Control and Prevention 2014). During that time, there were significant worries that H5N1 could cause a worldwide pandemic because of its high rates of virulence and death compared to the seasonal flu (Schnirring 2012). As the virus spread internationally, the World Health Organization and national governments began to sound the alarm about the potential effects an outbreak could have and the need to implement aggressive new policies to stop it.

The United States government's response to H5N1 exhibited many signs of securitization. In November 2005, President George W. Bush released his National Strategy for Pandemic Influenza, calling on Congress to allocate $7.1 billion dollars to bolster responses and preparations for a pandemic. Announcing his program, President Bush made the potential existential threat posed by avian flu clear, "By putting in place and exercising pandemic emergency plans across the country, we can help our nation prepare for other dangers, such as a terrorist attack using chemical or biological weapons" (Bush 2005). This statement likened a pandemic influenza outbreak to terrorism, effectively shifting it into the realm of security. Paula Dobriansky, then the Undersecretary of State for Democracy and Global Affairs, noted in an address to a Washington, DC think tank that an avian flu outbreak "could lead to civil unrest and instability." She argued, "If this [human-to-human H5N1 transmission] does begin to occur, in the worst-case scenario, it could kill millions of people, cripple economies, bring international trade to a standstill, and jeopardize political stability" (Dobriansky 2006). When asked about the strategy, Bush himself remarked:

> If we had an outbreak somewhere in the United States, do we not then quarantine that part of the country, and how do you then enforce a quarantine? When—it's one thing to shut down airplanes; it's another thing to prevent people from coming in to get exposed to the avian flu. And who best to be able to effect a quarantine? One option is the use of a military that's able to plan and move.
>
> *(Bush 2005)*

In this case, we can identify all four elements of securitization. First, the United States government is acting as a securitizing agent, taking active steps to try and convince its audiences of the threat. Second, H5N1 is the existential threat. Third, the referent object is political and economic stability. The spread of this existential threat, according to the government, could challenge the political and economic fabric of the United States (and other countries) and require military intervention in day-to-day life. Finally, the audience is the American public and other branches of the government. The Bush administration is trying to convince the general populace about the seriousness of the threat while also sending a message to the rest of the government that this should be a top priority. It is trying to get them on board with its assuming extraordinary powers and roles in order to keep a pandemic at bay. How successfully the government got the general public on board may be questionable (see Kelley 2005), but the response by the government would suggest a shared vision by American policymakers.

Benefits of securitization

Because securitization is a political act and strategy, policymakers deploy it in order to advance specific objectives. This section highlights three key arguments in favor of securitizing health. First, securitization can bring greater attention to issues that would otherwise be neglected or overlooked on the policy agenda. Framing health as a security issue thus allows the issue to cut through the other political debates, and there is clear evidence of policymakers using a security frame for health issues in order to generate public attention. In 2000, the United Nations Security Council devoted a special session to the national and international security challenges that the HIV/AIDS pandemic posed to the global community. This was the first time that the United Nations Security Council had ever devoted attention to a public health issue (David 2001: 560), and it only came about because of the security framing. Richard Holbrooke, the United States' United Nations ambassador, saw "getting AIDS onto the Security Council's agenda [... as] part of a broader strategy to gain high-level political attention and commitment" (Rushton 2019: 60). Along similar lines, Stefan Elbe (2006) argues that securitizing HIV/AIDS helped to convince some of the states with highest prevalence rates to finally take the disease seriously. Governments that had been "unable or unwilling to demonstrate leadership on the issue" now understood just how important the issue was to their populations and their regime's continued survival (Elbe 2006: 131). This can be particularly important, given that, in many (if not most) countries, health ministries possess only modest levels of political clout and resources compared to security organizations and frequently get overlooked in political debates (Altman 2000).

Securitization need not be an all-or-nothing proposition; the fact that policymakers aim to securitize one infectious disease does not necessarily imply that they will seek to securitize all infectious diseases. Jonathan Herington (2010) finds that the Vietnamese government has taken very different approaches to HIV/AIDS and avian influenza, with the former treated as a public health concern and the latter being securitized. The difference, he states, is that avian influenza brings with it other economic, political, and social threats that lead the government to see it as more of an existential threat. In this framing, HIV/AIDS can be addressed through normal channels, but avian influenza challenges the state's core being and therefore needs to be elevated in order to receive the attention it requires.

The security framing for health issues also reflects strategic choices at both the national and international levels. Elsewhere I argue, for instance, that securitizing global health could have been one way to get the Trump administration, which was notoriously skeptical of the importance of global health, to pay the issue more attention—though ultimately Donald Trump showed little inclination to engage on global health issues (except to blame other countries for them) during his term (Youde 2018). At the global level, Jiyong Jin and Joe Thomas Karackattu (2011) posit that the World Health Organization did not really engage with securitization until the twenty-first century with the emergence of disease threats like Severe Acute Respiratory Syndrome (SARS), avian influenza, HIV/AIDS, and the 2001 anthrax attacks. This move, they find, allowed the organization to assert its authority and highlight its authority and expertise.

Second, the securitization of health can bring with it additional resources. If a health issue constitutes an existential threat to the state, then it follows that policymakers need to devote extraordinary resources to addressing it. Debra DeLaet notes, "The successful securitization of a particular illness results in increased funding" (2015: 342). More resources do not automatically mean a better response to a health issue, but they increase the likelihood that health initiatives will have the funding they need. They also represent a tangible commitment on the part of policymakers to combine their rhetoric with increased financial resources.

Nowhere is the relationship between health securitization and increased resources more apparent than in the responses to HIV/AIDS. One analysis found that global funding for all HIV/AIDS initiatives rose from 6% of total global health spending in 1998 to approximately half of all global health funding in 2007 (Shiffman, Berlan, and Hafner 2009: S45). By 2017, $20.2 billion went to address HIV/AIDS initiatives in low- and middle-income countries in a single year (Institute for Health Metrics and Evaluation 2020: 83). In 2003, President George W. Bush unveiled the President's Emergency Plan for AIDS Relief (PEP-FAR). Pledging $15 billion over the next five years to address HIV/AIDS around the globe, it was the largest ever program ever devoted to an infectious disease—and it only continued to grow in its subsequent reauthorizations. Colin McInnes and Simon Rushton highlight that "through the inclusion of the term 'emergency' in the title, [it] carried clear echoes of security arguments" (2011: 123). The program was reauthorized in 2008, 2013, and 2018, and each time it was expanded to include even more money. As of mid-2020, PEPFAR contributed more than $90 billion to HIV/AIDS programs around the world (Kaiser Family Foundation 2020). Similarly, the World Bank estimated that the securitization of pandemic influenza during the first decade of the twenty-first century led governments to pledge $4.3 billion to prevent any future outbreaks, far outstripping the resources that would have other been made available for influenza preparations (Kamradt-Scott 2011). Another study found that governments had pledged $2.7 billion in 2008 for avian influenza pandemic preparedness efforts (Elbe 2010: 479).

Third, securitizing health brings the concept of security more in line with the security threats that people are more likely to experience in their daily lives. Most people do not go about their lives on a daily basis worried about the outbreak of war or whether some country will drop a nuclear bomb on their community. Many people do worry, though, about their ability to keep their families healthy, ensure sufficient food, secure adequate housing, and avoid becoming a victim of crime. This is the core of the idea of *human security*—the idea that people, rather than states, should be the referent objects for security and that this requires political programs that focus on global vulnerabilities. Human security developed out of the post-Cold War era, when many criticized the traditional view of security as outdated for the new international situation. Robert Ostergard (2002) called the old view overly Western-centric and unable to relate to the actual existential concerns of the vast majority of the population, and Andrew Price-Smith (2001) faulted traditional security studies for ignoring pandemic disease and environmental scarcity, which he posited posed far greater challenges to the lives of the vast majority of the population in the long run. The United Nations Development Program, in its seminal report, explicitly recognized ill-health as a threat to human security (United Nations Development Program 1994: 27–28).

At first glance, this relationship between lived experiences and the definition of security may seem irrelevant to the securitization of health. It is vital to remember, though, that securitization is a process between a securitizing agent *and* an audience. Without the audience's acceptance (or at least acquiescence), the securitizing move does not succeed, and the issue is not framed as a security issue. Thierry Balzacq (2005) emphasizes that successful securitization is audience-focused and context-dependent. By talking about security in terms that resonate with the lived experiences and/or the fears that the audience may have about their own health status, or that of their families and friends, the advocates of the securitization of health have found a useful entry point for gaining attention.

This relationship allows for an appeal to self-interested concerns that may override other justifications. Advocates for global health can (and do) frame their appeals in a variety of different frames, such as development and human rights. These frames may resonate with certain audiences, but they do not necessarily generate the same level of attention and resources. A more cosmopolitan framework, for instance, can be difficult to gain purchase with self-interested policymakers. "Where humanitarian development or other more altruistically inclined international initiatives have failed to generate sufficient political will and resources, for those advocating the HIV/AIDS-security nexus, the appeal to the naked self-interest of states is the only strategy left in light of the pressing daily humanitarian implications of the pandemic," writes Elbe (2006: 134).

This is not to say that the securitization of health is inherently selfish. Indeed, it is abundantly clear that widespread disease outbreaks can cause significant and severe economic, political, and social disruptions through a variety of means—the interruption of trade flows, the costs of mounting an effective response, the closure of international borders, and the interruptions presented to daily life (Rushton 2014: 297). Policymakers are likely to want to minimize these costs as much as possible, and calling attention to them may be the most compelling way for an audience to take the threat seriously. Economic estimates after the SARS outbreak of 2003 and 2004 suggested that it cost between $30 and $100 billion to the economies of affected states, or roughly $3–10 million per case (Keogh-Brown and Smith 2008). These figures are so high that they attract immediate attention—and governments want to avoid these costs as much as possible.

Downsides of securitization

The negative elements of securitizing health can be broken down into four main themes. First, securitization can be counterproductive to its ostensible aims. Elbe (2006) draws on Daniel Deudney's (1990) work against securitizing the environment to argue that securitization's threat logic often works against efforts to implement appropriate policies and efforts to reduce stigmatization. Securitization encourages quick action by policymakers, but speed does not necessarily lead to optimal policies. In particular, he notes that securitization tends to rely on an "us vs. them" dichotomization that frequently directly counteracts the sort of solidarity and cosmopolitan actions that are necessary for addressing cross-border health issues.

Securitization implicitly assumes that there is an external enemy that must be fought because it poses an existential threat to the state. Deudney argues, "Fear is the emotion most intimately linked to security" and "the dynamics of fear" condition how states respond (2006: 32). In the case of securitizing health, this frequently gets caught up in Global North–South relations. States in the Global North frame infectious disease as a security threat—an enemy against which we must protect ourselves. In his dire warning about the threats posed by a global influenza pandemic, Michael Osterholm warns, "Border security would be made a priority, especially to protect potential supplies of pandemic-specific vaccines from nearby desperate countries. Military leaders would have to develop strategies to defend the country and also protect against domestic insurgency with armed forces that would likely be compromised by the disease" (Osterholm 2005: 33). This language reinforces an "us-vs.-them" opposition, warning that *they* would try to violate America's borders to get *our* drugs and vaccines. *We* would have to protect ourselves against enemies—both foreign and domestic—because *we* have to be on guard against *them*. David Fidler points out, "Infectious disease measures historically have served as demarcations by which 'we' protect ourselves from the diseases of 'others'" (Fidler 1998: 9). The framework for responding to a pandemic does not suggest that we are all in this together; instead, it suggests that we need to worry about foreigners who could infect us, or bring the disease to our country.

Similarly, securitization brings with it an element of surveillance as highlighted by Michel Foucault's arguments about biopolitics (Dillon 2008; Foucault 1978–1979 [2008]). When disease becomes a security issue, it implies an existential threat to the state, which, in turn, leads the state to engage in surveillance as a protection strategy (Elbe 2005). This surveillance, both domestically and internationally, attempts to keep people in line by disciplining them to perform (or not to perform) certain tasks. At first glance, this may not appear to be a problem; in fact, making sure that people take appropriate steps to protect themselves and others against disease would appear to be a good thing, and the global health governance system and infectious disease responses place a heavy emphasis on the need for robust surveillance capabilities (Davies and Youde 2015). However, it is important to remember the nature of this surveillance. The developed countries are watching over the developing countries, dictating how they structure their public health infrastructures and which issues they prioritize. They adopt a paternalistic role that may or may not reflect the wants, needs, and desires of those countries over whom they watch. By securitizing health, the Global North essentially reprioritizes how states in the Global South should interpret and respond to potential disease outbreaks. It tells states not to conceive of this as a public health issue, but as a security issue. It encourages states to change their responses to match how states in the Global North see the disease. This is even codified in the International Health Regulations, an international legal treaty that defines the obligations of signatories to develop and maintain certain disease surveillance capabilities. Unfortunately, despite setting up a system that requires states to maintain certain disease surveillance capabilities, the International Health Regulations provide no funding for states to do so. That can lead to a situation where states have to deprioritize local needs in order to achieve international compliance (Gostin and Katz 2006).

Second, securitization is closely linked with militarization and using military forces as key tools in addressing health threats (Watterson and Kamradt-Scott 2016), and it is far from clear that the military is the appropriate instrument for addressing these threats. Despite the efforts of the proponents of human security, security generally remains connected to the military and police forces in popular and policy imaginations. More often than not in many situations, the military or the police force is an object of threat to people in their daily lives. To expect people to ignore their past experiences with these organizations and assume that they are acting with good intentions is a step too far (Wenham 2019). For example, foreign militaries played significant and prominent roles in how the United States, the United Kingdom, France, and China responded to the Ebola outbreak in West Africa from 2014 to 2016. Part of the logic behind using military forces was that they had unique logistical and operational capabilities necessary for addressing such a widespread outbreak (Kamradt-Scott et al. 2016). In interviews with local residents and nongovernmental organizations operating in Liberia, though, there was a strong perception that the use of military troops was less about operational readiness and more about tamping down any potential demonstrations. Furthermore, the reliance on the military did little to promote building long-term resiliency within the public health systems that would be needed to address any future outbreaks (Calcagno

2016). Similar concerns about governments using a health securitization frame to restrict movement and public gatherings as a cover for stifling political opposition have emerged during the Covid-19 pandemic, too.

Third, there remain serious and unanswered questions about whose security matters and why particular health issues resonate in a security context. There is almost no relationship between the leading causes of death worldwide and which health issues are securitized (successfully or not) (Youde 2016). Seven of the ten leading causes of death in 2019 were non-communicable diseases like heart disease, stroke, and chronic obstructive pulmonary disease (World Health Organization 2020); yet, there is almost no effort to reframe these as security issues. Even among the leading infectious disease causes of death, like respiratory conditions and diarrheal diseases, the security frame is rarely—if ever—applied. Instead, the health issues that get securitized are those like HIV/AIDS (McInnes and Rushton 2011), Zika (Wenham and Farias 2019), polio (Calain and Sa'Da 2015), and pandemic influenza (Kamradt-Scott and McInnes 2012) that provoke a unique degree of fear—particularly from wealthy states.

This issue about the distortion of the global health agenda due to securitization takes a number of different forms. Jeremy Shiffman (2009) shows that epidemiology alone is insufficient to understand why certain health issues become securitized. Instead, he argues that these processes depend on the interactions between policy communities, ideas, and institutions, reinforcing the fact that securitization is ultimately a political process. As such, he argues that it is better understood as a reflection of power dynamics and the exercise of power (Shiffman 2014). João Nunes (2014) identifies similar themes, arguing that health insecurity is not coterminous with disease. Instead, he argues that it exists as a contested political category that reflects larger underlying global political assumptions. Lorna Weir (2015) describes the securitization of health as an effort by Northern states for their benefit, which, in turn, further marginalizes states in the Global South because it restricts their agency and portrays them solely as the source of health threats. The concerns of states in the Global South are thus dismissed and given little, if any, voice in the debates about securitizing health issue (Aldis 2008).

These debates also raise questions about the underlying focus of health securitization efforts. Rushton (2011) finds that health securitization focuses on containing diseases rather than preventing outbreaks in the first place. Not only does this position securitization as a reactive strategy, but it also raises questions about whose security counts if the international community is doing little to prevent the initial emergence of potential outbreaks. Similarly, McInnes highlights the seeming disconnect between health and security because "the causal relationship between an adverse health effect and international stability is questionable, and/or the empirical evidence to support the claim is suspect or missing" (McInnes 2015: 9).

More recently, scholars are highlighting how the securitization of health has distinct effects on our understanding of the relationships between health, security, and gender. One fundamental flaw in the securitization of health is that health emergencies rarely, if ever, consider women and non-binary individuals (Davies and Bennett 2016). Women are "conspicuously invisible" in the global health policy space (Harman 2016). As a result, when a securitization lens—which often has strongly "masculine" connotations—is applied to health outbreaks, the resulting policy responses rarely consider the formal and informal roles that women play in the provision of care and the dynamics by which an outbreak works its way through a society. None of the key instruments of the securitization of health, including the International Health Regulations, Biological Weapons Convention, or the World Health Organization Blueprint on R&D for Health Emergencies, show any real evidence of taking gender into account or ensuring that the voices of women and non-binary individuals had a place at the proverbial table (Wenham et al. 2020). While the securitization of health should ostensibly boost health outcomes, recent evidence from the Ebola outbreak in West Africa shows that women suffered higher rates of obstetric and postnatal complications because healthcare resources were diverted away from general health facilities and toward Ebola. Thus, the securitization of Ebola actually made women *more* vulnerable to worsening health outcomes (Davies and Wenham 2020: 1245). As Clare Wenham writes about the responses to the Zika outbreak in South America:

> Temporarily destroying vectors does not address the socio-economic conditions that allow mosquitoes to thrive—such as a lack of water and sanitation, poor-quality housing and inadequate civic waste management that all could create breeding grounds for mosquitoes, nor does it challenge the gender inequalities which are mostly ignored in outbreaks.
>
> *(Wenham 2019: 1107)*

Finally, the securitization of health raises serious questions about accountability and agency at both the domestic and international levels. One of the basic tenets of securitization is that it is a process that removes a given issue from the realm of "normal" politics. Regular political processes move too slowly or involve too much cacophonous debate, which makes them incapable of addressing existential threats that security threats pose (McDonald 2008: 567). In other words, extraordinary times call for extraordinary measures. Removing an issue from the normal bounds of political debate, though, also implies a lack of (public) oversight of those actions. If an issue is so serious that normal political processes cannot apply, then it follows that traditional accountability processes would be inappropriate. Indeed, Adam Côté (2016) argues that traditional securitization theory creates audiences without agency— groups that ultimately empower and affirm policymakers to take securitizing actions, but without the ability to engage in oversight or accountability.

In the health realm, these processes raise a host of serious questions. At the domestic level, there is the question of where the accountability for the actions of policymakers lies. Securitizing health may encourage states to introduce quarantine (restricting the movement of persons who might have been exposed to an infectious agent) or isolation (restricting the movement of someone who is infected with a communicable disease) procedures, but few states include processes whereby someone can challenge their confinement (Youde 2012: 91–92). Given the long history of countries justifying illiberal policies and coercive actions against perceived enemies or outsiders on public health grounds, this could be particularly worrisome.

At the international level, issues get even more difficult—and not just because of the well-known democratic deficits within global governance (Glenn 2008). Securitizing health empowers intergovernmental, international, and nongovernmental organizations to take extraordinary actions in the name of protecting global health. Tine Hanrieder and Christian Kreuder-Sonnen argue that securitization "facilitates the emergence of focal and centralized [international organizations] as authoritative actors whose decisions shape how emerging threats are governed"—even in the absence of the power to compel states to take specific actions (2014: 332). Such powers can lead to the introduction of illiberal measures in the name of protecting public health, but with the added complexity of indirect lines of accountability and oversight. Indeed, because groups like the World Health Organization are ultimately dependent on their member-states to provide them with the opportunity to act—and

Western states tend to be the most dominant within global governance organizations—such organizations may be even *more* prone to implement extraordinary measures that lack easily accessible oversight measures (Davies 2008: 296).

Conclusion

As I write this, the world is still in the midst of the Covid-19 pandemic—a disease outbreak that has profoundly altered life in nearly every country in the world. It is also generating debates about the appropriateness of framing this outbreak as a security threat (see, for example, Gaudino 2020; Liu and Bennett 2020; Nunes 2020; Sears 2020). Nigeria, South Africa, Uganda, and Kenya, for example, have come under criticism for relying heavily on police and military officials to enforce Covid-related curfews and lockdowns and for the brutality those security forces have employed in enforcing these restrictions (Mugabi 2020), while South Korea, New Zealand, and Taiwan have largely relied on more traditional public health techniques of contact tracing, testing, and quarantining (Bremmer 2021). The variation in responses to Covid-19 and whether states that have taken a more securitized approach have handled the pandemic better will present a great deal of opportunities for future research. This ongoing debate follows many of the same contours explained throughout this chapter, and there is no single "right" answer about securitizing any particular health concern. Instead, it is incumbent upon all of us to consider the trade-offs—both philosophically and in terms of policy outcomes—that come with the decisions about whether or not to securitize health.

References

Aldis, W. 2008. Health security as a public health concept: A critical analysis. *Health Policy and Planning* 23, no. 6: 369–375. https://doi.org/10.1093/heapol/czn030.

Altman, D. 2000. Understanding HIV/AIDS as a global security issue. In *Health impacts of globalization: Towards global governance*, ed. K. Lee, 33–43. New York: Palgrave Macmillan.

Balzacq, T. 2005. The three faces of securitization: Political agency, audience, and context. *European Journal of International Relations* 11, no. 2: 171–201. https://doi.org/10.1177/1354066105052960.

Bremmer, I. 2021. The best global responses to the COVID-19 pandemic, 1 year later. *Time*, 23 February. https://time.com/5851633/best-global-responses-covid-19/ (accessed June 15, 2021).

Bush, G. 2005. President outlines pandemic influenza preparations and response. Speech at National Institutes of Health, Bethesda, MD, 1 November. https://georgewbush-whitehouse.archives.gov/news/releases/2005/11/20051101-1.html (accessed January 18, 2021).

Buzan, B. 1991. *People, states, and fear: An agenda for international studies in the post-Cold War Era.* 2nd edition. Boulder, CO: Lynne Rienner.

Buzan, B., O. Waever, and J. de Wilde. 1998. *Security: A new framework for analysis.* Boulder, CO: Lynne Rienner.

Calain, P. and C. Abu Sa'Da. 2015. Coincident polio and Ebola crises expose similar fault lines in the current global health regime. *Conflict and Health* 9: 29. https://doi.org/10.1186/s13031-015-0058-1.

Calcagno, D. 2016. Killing Ebola: The militarization of US aid in Liberia. *Journal of African Studies and Development* 8, no. 7: 88–97. https://doi.org/10.5897/JASD2016.0415.

Centers for Disease Control and Prevention. 2014. Highly pathogenic avian influenza (H5N1) human cases and deaths since 2003. https://www.cdc.gov/flu/pdf/avianflu/avian-flu-human-world-summary.pdf (accessed January 18, 2021).

Côté, A. 2016. Agents without agency: Assessing the role of the audience in securitization theory. *Security Dialogue* 47, no. 6: 541–558. https://doi.org/10.1177/0967010616672150.

David, M. 2001. Rubber helmets: The certain pitfalls of marshaling Security Council resources to combat AIDS in Africa. *Human Rights Quarterly* 23, no. 3: 560–582. https://doi.org/10.1353/hrq.2001.0033.

Davies, S. 2008. Securitizing infectious disease. *International Affairs* 84, no. 2: 295–313. https://doi.org/10.1111/j.1468-2346.2008.00704.x.

Davies, S. and B. Bennett. 2016. A gendered human rights analysis of Ebola and Zika: Locating gender in global health emergencies. *International Affairs* 92, no. 5: 1041–1060. https://doi.org/10.1111/1468-2346.12704.

Davies, S. and C. Wenham. 2020. Why the COVID-19 response needs international relations. *International Affairs* 96, no. 5: 1227–1251. https://doi.org/10.1093/ia/iiaa135.

Davies, S. and J. Youde, eds. 2015. *The politics of surveillance and response to disease outbreaks: The new frontier for states and non-state actors*. London: Routledge.

DeLaet, D. 2015. Whose interests is the securitization of health serving? In *Routledge handbook of global health security*, ed. S. Rushton and J. Youde, 339–348. London: Routledge.

Deudney, D. 1990. The case against linking environmental degradation and national security. *Millennium* 19, no. 3: 461–476. https://doi.org/10.1177/03058298900190031001

Deudney, D. 2006. *Bounding power: Republican security theory from the polis to the global village*. Princeton, NJ: Princeton University Press.

Dillon, M. 2008. Underwriting security. *Security Dialogue* 39, no. 2–3: 309–332. https://doi.org/10.1177/0967010608088780.

Dobriansky, P. 2006. Social, economic, and security implications of avian influenza. Speech at Nixon Center, Washington, DC, June 26. https://2001-2009.state.gov/g/rls/rm/68811.htm (accessed January 18, 2021).

Elbe, S. 2005. AIDS, security, biopolitics. *International Relations* 19, no. 4: 403–419. https://doi.org/10.1177/0047117805058532.

Elbe, S. 2006. Should HIV/AIDS be securitized? The ethical dilemmas of linking HIV/AIDS and security. *International Studies Quarterly* 50, no. 1: 119–144. https://doi.org/10.1111/j.1468-2748.2006.00395.x.

Elbe, S. 2010. Haggling over viruses: The downside risks of securitizing infectious disease. *Health Policy and Planning* 25, no. 6: 476–485. https://doi.org/10.193/heapol/czq050.

Enemark, C. 2017. *Biosecurity dilemmas: Dreaded diseases, ethical responses, and the health of nations*. Washington, DC: Georgetown University Press.

Fidler, D. 1998. Microbialpolitik: Infectious diseases and international relations. *American University International Law Journal* 14, no. 1: 1–53. https://digitalcommons.wcl.american.edu/auilr/vol14/iss1/1/ (accessed December 21, 2021).

Foucault, M. 1978–1979 [2008]. *The birth of biopolitics: Lectures at the College de France, 1978–1979*. Ed. Graham Burchell. New York: Palgrave Macmillan.

Gaudino, U. 2020. The ideological securitization of COVID-19: Perspectives from the right and the left. *E-International Relations*, 28 July. https://www.e-ir.info/2020/07/28/the-ideological-securitization-of-covid-19-perspectives-from-the-right-and-the-left/ (accessed February 1, 2021).

Glenn, J. 2008. Global governance and the democratic deficit: Stifling the voice of the South. *Third World Quarterly* 29, no. 2: 217–238. https://doi.org/10.1080/01436590701806798.

Gostin, L. and R. Katz. 2006. The International Health Regulations: The governing framework for global health security. *Milbank Quarterly* 94, no. 2: 264–313. https://doi.org/10.1111/1468-0009.12186.

Hanrieder, T. and C. Kreuder-Sonnen. 2014. WHO decides on the exception? Securitization and emergency governance in global health. *Security Dialogue* 45, no. 4: 331–348. https://doi.org/10.1177/0967010614535833.

Harman, S. 2016. Ebola, gender, and conspicuously invisible women in global health governance. *Third World Quarterly* 37, no. 3: 524–541. https://doi.org/10.1080/01436597.2015.1108827.

Herington, J. 2010. The securitization of infectious diseases in Vietnam: The cases of HIV and avian influenza. *Health Policy and Planning* 25, no. 6: 467–475. https://doi.org/10.1093/heapol/czq052.

Institute for Health Metrics and Evaluation. 2020. *Financing global health 2019: Tracking health spending in a time of crisis*. Seattle: Institute for Health Metrics and Evaluation. https://www.healthdata.org/policy-report/financing-global-health-2019-tracking-health-spending-time-crisis (accessed December 21, 2021).

Jin, J. and J.T. Karackattu. 2011. Infectious diseases and securitization: WHO's dilemma. *Biosecurity and Bioterrorism: Biodefense Strategy, Practice, and Science* 9, no. 2: 181–187. https://doi.org/10.1089/bsp.2010.0045.

Kaiser Family Foundation. 2020. The U.S. President's Emergency Plan for AIDS Relief (PEPFAR). 27 May. https://www.kff.org/global-health-policy/fact-sheet/the-u-s-presidents-emergency-plan-for-aids-relief-pepfar/ (accessed February 1, 2021).

Kamradt-Scott, A. 2011. Changing perceptions of pandemic influenza and public health responses. *American Journal of Public Health* 102, no. 1: 90–98. https://doi.org/10.2105/AJPH.2011.300330.

Kamradt-Scott, A., S. Harman, C. Wenham, and F. Smith III. 2016. Civil-military cooperation in Ebola and beyond. *The Lancet* 387, no. 10014: 104–105. https://doi.org/10.1016/S0140-6736(15) 01128-9.

Kamradt-Scott, A. and C. McInnes. 2012. The securitization of pandemic influenza: Framing, security, and public policy. *Global Public Health* 7, suppl. 2: S95–S110. https://doi.org.10.1080/1744169 2.2012.725752.

Kelley, L. 2005. Is H5N1 the one? Avian flu facts and fiction. *Health Policy Outlook*, November–December. https://www.aei.org/wp-content/uploads/2011/10/20051130_19303HPONov_ Dec_g.pdf?x88519 (accessed January 18, 2021).

Keogh-Brown, M. and R. Smith. 2008. The economic impact of SARS: How does the reality match the predictions? *Health Policy* 88, no. 1: 110–120. https://doi.org/10.1016/j.healthpol.2008.03.003.

Liu, X. and M. Bennett. 2020. Viral borders: COVID-19's effects on securitization, surveillance, and identity in Mainland China and Hong Kong. *Dialogues in Human Geography* 10, no. 2: 158–163. https://doi.org/10.1177/2043820620933828.

McDonald, M. 2008. Securitization and the construction of security. *European Journal of International Relations* 14, no. 4: 563–587. https://doi.org/10.1177/1354066108097553.

McInnes, C. 2015. The many meanings of health security. In *Routledge handbook of global health security*, ed. S. Rushton and J. Youde, 7–17. London: Routledge.

McInnes, C. and S. Rushton. 2011. HIV/AIDS and securitization theory. *European Journal of International Relations* 19, no. 1: 115–138. https://doi.org/10.1177/1354066111425258.

Mugabi, I. 2020. COVID-19: Security forces in Africa brutalizing civilians under lockdown. *DW*, 20 April. https://www.dw.com/en/covid-19-security-forces-in-africa-brutalizing-civilians-under-lockdown/a-53192163 (accessed June 15, 2021).

Nunes, J. 2014. *Security, emancipation, and the politics of health: A new theoretical perspective*. London: Routledge.

Nunes, J. 2020. The COVID-19 pandemic: Securitization, neoliberal crisis, and global vulnerablization. *Cadernos de Saude Publica* 36, no. 5: e00063120. https://doi.org/10.1590/0102-311x00063120.

Ostergard, R. 2002. Politics in the hot zone: AIDS and national security in Africa. *Third World Quarterly* 23, no. 2: 333–350. https://doi.org/10.1080/01436590220126676.

Osterholm, M. 2005. Preparing for the next pandemic. *Foreign Affairs* 84, no. 4: 24–37. https://doi.org/10.2307/20034418.

Price-Smith, A. 2001. *The health of nations: Infectious disease, environmental change, and their impact on national and international security*. Cambridge, MA: MIT Press.

Rushton, S. 2011. Global health security: Security for whom? Security from what? *Political Studies* 59, no. 4: 779–796. https://doi.org/10.1111/j./1467-9248.2011.00919.x.

Rushton, S. 2014. Arguments for securitizing global health priorities. In *Handbook of global health policy*, ed. G. Brown, G. Yamey, and S. Wamala, 289–304. Malden, MA: Wiley Blackwell.

Rushton, S. 2019. *Security and public health*. Cambridge: Polity Press.

Schnirring, L. 2012. Debate on H5N1 death rate and missed cases continues. *CIDRAP*, 24 February. https://www.cidrap.umn.edu/news-perspective/2012/02/debate-h5n1-death-rate-and-missed-cases-continues (accessed January 18, 2021).

Sears, N. 2020. The securitization of COVID-19: Three political dilemmas. *Global Policy*, 25 March. https://www.globalpolicyjournal.com/blog/25/03/2020/securitization-covid-19-three-political-dilemmas (accessed February 1, 2021).

Shiffman, J. 2009. A social explanation for the rise and fall of global health issues. *Bulletin of the World Health Organization* 87, no. 8: 608–613. https://doi.org/10.2471/BLT.08.060749.

Shiffman, J. 2014. Knowledge, moral claims, and the exercise of power in global health. *International Journal of Health Policy and Management* 3, no. 6: 297–299. https://doi.org/10.15171/ijhpm.2014.120.

Shiffman, J., D. Berlan, and T. Hafner. 2009. Has aid for AIDS lifted all funding boats? *Journal of Acquired Immune Deficiency Syndromes* 52, suppl. 1: S45–S48. https://doi.org/10.1097/QAI.0b013e 3181bbcb45.

United Nations Development Program. 1994. *Human development report 1994*. New York: Oxford University Press.

Waever, O. 1995. Securitization and desecuritization. In *On security*, ed. R. Lipschutz, 46–86. New York: Columbia University Press.

Walt, S. 1991. The renaissance of security studies. *International Studies Quarterly* 35, no. 2: 211–239. https://doi.org/10.2307/2600471.

Watterson, C. and A. Kamradt-Scott. 2016. Fighting flu: Securitization and the military role in combating influenza. *Armed Forces and Society* 42, no. 1: 145–168. https://doi.org/10.1177/0095327X14567364.

Weir, L. 2015. Inventing global health security, 1994–2005. In *Routledge handbook of global health security*, ed. S. Rushton and J. Youde, 18–31. London: Routledge.

Wenham, C. 2019. The oversecuritization of global health: Changing the terms of debate. *International Affairs* 95, no. 5: 1093–1110. https://doi.org/10.1093/ia/iiz170.

Wenham, C. and D. Farias. 2019. Securitizing Zika: The case of Brazil. *Security Dialogue* 50, no. 5: 398–415. https://doi.org/10.1177/0967010619856458.

Wenham, C., J. Smith, S. Davies et al. 2020. Women are most affected by pandemics: Lessons from past outbreaks. *Nature* 583, no. 7815: 194–198. https://doi.org/10.1038/d41586-020-02006-z.

World Health Organization. 2020. The top 10 causes of death. https://www.who.int/news-room/fact-sheets/detail/the-top-10-causes-of-death (accessed January 31, 2021).

Youde, J. 2012. Biosurveillance, human rights, and the zombie plague. *Global Change, Peace, and Security* 24, no. 1: 83–93. https://doi.org/10.1080/14781158.2012.641278.

Youde, J. 2016. High politics, low politics, and global health. *Journal of Global Security Studies* 1, no. 2: 157–170. https://doi.org/10.1093/jogss/ogw001.

Youde, J. 2018. The securitization of health in the Trump era. *Australian Journal of International Affairs* 72, no. 6: 535–550. https://doi.org/10.1080/10357718.20188.1534936.

20

HEALTH, PLACE, AND JUSTICE

A philosophical appraisal of promoting equity in Covid-19 through disadvantage indices

Samantha Fritz, Tuhina Srivastava, Emily Sadecki, and Harald Schmidt

Introduction

In Spring 2020, when Covid-19 first began to affect the United States, distributive justice questions quickly came into focus. For example, allocative decisions needed to be made regarding the limited supply of personal protective equipment such as masks, and ventilators. One year in, the focus shifted to the distribution of vaccines. How should hospitals or the government in the United States handle the shortfall of supply relative to demand? Should the fact that certain populations are more vulnerable to Covid-19 effects due to prior societal inequities play a role in allocation frameworks? If so, practically, how should such considerations be incorporated? The case of vaccine allocation in the United States with an unprecedented recognition of the need to address existing disparities offers a case study with plausible relevance much beyond vaccines and pandemic scarcity.

The aim of this chapter is to describe a novel approach toward equitable allocation by combining phased vaccine rationing systems with disadvantage indices. This approach was rapidly and widely adopted in the United States in the critical period between November 2020 and March 2021. This was the time period when allocation plans were first established, and the extent of scarcity was the most severe. The chapter will proceed as follows: in the first section, we describe why and how *disadvantage indices* came to be included in rationing frameworks to reduce inequity affecting vulnerable communities, and how they actually were used in practice. In the second section, we compare the way that disadvantage is conceptualized under what came to be the dominant model—the Centers for Disease Control and Prevention's (CDC's) Social Vulnerability Index (SVI) and related measures—relative to a leading philosophical conception of disadvantage as articulated by Jonathan Wolff and Avner de-Shalit. We close the chapter with an outline of possible broader applications of place-based measures of disadvantage to other areas of public health policy.

Disadvantage in the United States

As in other countries, not everyone in the United States has felt the effects of Covid-19 equally. More economically disadvantaged groups have been hit harder. And impact in terms of unemployment, infections, hospitalizations, and deaths has also varied significantly across

DOI: 10.4324/9781315675411-24

racial and ethnic groups (Karmakar, Lantz, and Tipirneni 2021). The reasons for these differences are not genetic, but due to structural racism and systemic disadvantage (Flood et al. 2020; Venkatapuram 2021; Yearby and Mohapatra 2020). For example, larger proportions of more disadvantaged people of color (DPOC) are represented among essential workers; such workers are more likely to get infected and also further spread the infections (CDC 2021a). DPOC are also more likely than non-Hispanic White people to live in crowded housing, and their worse healthcare access is well documented, and reflected in their limited access to Covid-19 testing sites (CDC 2020a).

These group-level inequalities have been evident since the start of the pandemic. Chicago's African-American community is a prime example. Black Chicagoans make up about 30% of the city's population. But as of April 2020, just one month into the pandemic, they made up over 50% of infection cases and nearly 70% of Covid-19 deaths. The immediate and disproportionate impact of the new health threat is not because African Americans are genetically more vulnerable. Due to systemic racism and poverty, many American people of color are more likely to have underlying health conditions and less likely to have access to healthcare, which likely contributed to the severity of infections (Jane Addams College of Social Work 2020). Justice in healthcare requires us to acknowledge that communities of color have been hit harder by Covid because they account for a disproportionate number of the people who are disadvantaged. This is due to society's structure, which reduces their economic mobility and their odds of leading a long and healthy life (O'Brien et al. 2020).

In the United States, guidance on vaccine allocation in pandemic and other emergency situations is provided by the CDC's Advisory Committee on Immunization Practices (ACIP). In recognizing from early Spring 2020 that the pandemic was compounding existing social and health inequities, and that the development of any Covid-19 vaccine allocation framework needed to be particularly sensitive to this trend, the heads of the National Institute of Health (NIH) and the CDC requested the National Academies of Science, Engineering, and Medicine (NASEM) to produce guidance on equitable Covid-19 vaccine allocation.

NASEM's final report was published in October 2020, and it reviewed general resource allocation frameworks, those focused on pandemic and Covid-19-related resources, and those focused on vaccines, more specifically (NASEM 2020). In full continuity or alignment with many of these frameworks, the overall focus of the report was on maximizing benefits "by reducing morbidity and mortality caused by transmission of the novel coronavirus" (NASEM 2020). At the same time, the framework expressly noted that "the vaccine allocation criteria should mitigate the negative effects of existing health inequities" (NASEM 2020). This emphasis was in direct contrast to an influential framework that conceptualized worse-off groups as either younger or sicker, and it called for their prioritization only in a secondary and instrumental way, namely, insofar as doing so aligned with maximizing benefits (Emanuel et al. 2020).

Concretely, NASEM's framework integrated social equity considerations in two main ways. First, through the sequence of priority population groups that are grouped in four sequential phases over time. Second, while within phases there is equal priority among the included population groups, within each population group, access should be prioritized by social vulnerability; see Figure 20.1.

The implication for equity of sequential prioritization *across* phases and of priority groups is readily appreciated. NASEM's proposal to prioritize *within* each phase, which amplified a more basic earlier proposal from the academic literature that suggested to prioritize by disadvantage in allocating vaccines to the general population (Schmidt 2020), is perhaps less obvious. What this approach is getting at is that there are such close links between health

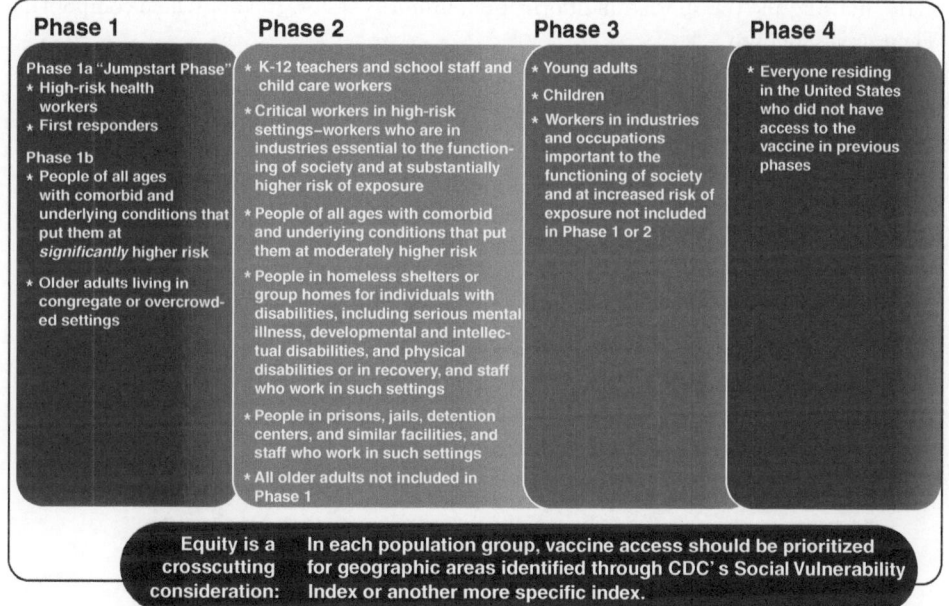

Figure 20.1 A phased approach to vaccine allocation for Covid-19. Republished with permission of The National Academies Press from NASEM, and Health and Medicine Division; Board on Population Health and Public Health Practice; Board on Health Sciences Policy; Committee on Equitable Allocation of Vaccine for the Novel Coronavirus. *A Framework for Equitable Allocation of COVID-19 Vaccine. Framework for Equitable Allocation of COVID-19 Vaccine* (Washington, DC: The National Academies Press, 2020)

(disease/illness), place, and social status that socioeconomically worse-off groups are more at risk of getting and spreading the virus than better-off ones, typically because of worse baseline health and living circumstances. For example, two elderly couples living at different locations in the same city are both at a heightened risk of death due to their biological vulnerability or frailty. But the older couple in the affluent suburban area is less likely to have underlying health conditions while also being more able to social distance. This is compared with, say an elderly couple who are both people of color, living in the inner city, and living at the poverty threshold. Due to the consequences of structural racism, people living in the inner city, and living in poverty, are more likely to be people of color. These communities of color, moreover, are less likely to live as long as their counterpart White residents (City Health Dashboard 2015; Gourevitch 2021). As such, a disadvantage index such as the SVI, combined with sequentially phased allocation frameworks, is well suited to contribute "to effectively control the epidemic, but with significant attention to equity because the deaths and suffering are socially caused" (Venkatapuram 2021).

The SVI was not developed for Covid-19 specifically, but for largely natural disaster situations such as earthquakes, hurricanes, or flooding (Flanagan et al. 2011; Srivastava et al. 2021). It is a statistical measure tied to a geographic area and captures the average of the relative advantage and disadvantage of people living there (Kind and Buckingham 2018). The SVI includes fifteen equally weighted variables collected from census data and applied to geographic regions (known as census tracts), comprising between 1,200 and 8,000 people (Flanagan et al. 2018). The fifteen variables are grouped into four categories: socioeconomic status, housing and transportation information, minority status, and household composition. These are as follows:

1   Socioeconomic status

    a   Whether a person is below the poverty line
    b   If a person is unemployed
    c   What a person's income is
    d   Whether a person has a high school diploma

2   Household composition and disability

    a   Whether there are people 65+ in the home
    b   Whether there are people <17 in the home
    c   Whether there are people 5+ with a disability in the home
    d   Whether it is a single-parent home

3   Minority status and language

    a   Whether a person is a minority
    b   Whether a person speaks language less than well

4   Housing and transportation

    a   Whether a person lives in a multiunit structure
    b   Whether a person lives in a mobile home
    c   Whether there is crowding in the home
    d   Whether a person has a vehicle
    e   Whether a person lives in group quarters (Flanagan et al. 2018).

In integrating these variables into an index, and despite its pragmatic construction, the SVI recognizes that disadvantage can take many different forms; different combinations of the fifteen variables can produce the same high scores. The SVI computes an overall score for each census tract, which then enables one to compare its rank on two different rank-orderings, that is, relative to all census tracts within a state or across the entire country.

Used in the pandemic vaccine context, an index like the SVI can capture population groups for whom the protection offered by vaccines is both more necessary in health terms (with individual- and population-level health benefits) and more valuable, given the reduced ability of more disadvantaged populations to absorb the pandemic's economic shock. The groups captured by the SVI are typically more dependent on regular income (little savings), less able to socially distance, and more likely to contract and spread the infection and die from it (Dasgupta et al. 2020; NASEM 2020; Schmidt 2020). In addition to increasing the epidemiological benefit of vaccines (containment), disadvantage indices also address health inequities (Schmidt 2020). Expressly, NASEM notes that an index such as SVI incorporates "the variables that the committee believes are most linked to the disproportionate impact of COVID-19 on people of color and other vulnerable populations" (NASEM 2020). In practical terms, NASEM recommends that each time a new batch of vaccines is distributed (typically in weekly intervals), 10% of federally available vaccines should be set aside for vulnerable communities (identified via an index such as SVI and defined as the 25% most disadvantaged people). These additional allocations should then be added to the shares of vaccines that would otherwise be offered proportionately to population (NASEM 2020).

While 10% would not be sufficient to provide vaccines to all people falling under the most disadvantaged quartile, the extra allocations will reduce the severity of scarcity that these populations face and have the consequence that larger shares of vaccines are offered to people of color (Schmidt et al. 2020). Furthermore, the CDC's administrative units are asked to "ensure that special efforts are made to deliver vaccine to residents of high-vulnerability areas (defined as the twenty-five percent highest in the state)," for example, through targeted outreach (NASEM 2020).

In the January 2021 national Covid-19 strategy published by the Biden-Harris Administration, states and other administrative units were instructed to "update their pandemic plans to describe how they have or will provide equitable access […] using [SVI] or other indices" (Office of the President 2021). And, in response to CDC data demonstrating the disproportionately lower vaccine uptake by people of color after the first month of the vaccine roll-out, the CDC recognized the index's utility. Officials stated that "monitoring coverage by [SVI] will be useful to ensure equity and to identify communities where focused immunization efforts might be required" (Painter, Ussery, and Patel 2021). Aside from public health goals, assessing coverage rates by SVI deciles, for example, can also support a disparate impact monitoring, a legal concept focused on determining whether policies negatively affect a protected group, even if they do not have that express intention and do not directly use information about that group. The point is that should allocation trends have the consequence that, for example, more disadvantaged minority populations have a lesser chance at receiving a vaccine, such data can motivate policy responses to redress this outcome (Foster, Cannon, and Bloche 2020; Kakani et al. 2020).

Practical applications of place-based measure of disadvantage to improve equitable vaccine allocation

While ACIP emphasized the need to reduce social inequities in vaccine allocation, the committee chose to accomplish this mainly through the sequence of priority groups. ACIP members did not embrace NASEM's proposal to integrate within-population group prioritization in its phased system (Bell, Romero, and Lee 2020; McClung et al. 2020). By contrast, adopting a measure such as the SVI had clear appeal to the CDC's 64 jurisdictions (50 states, the District of Columbia, 5 cities, and 8 territories), each of which had to determine their own binding allocation frameworks. When jurisdictions first published their plans, 17 jurisdictions indicated the intention to use an index, and by the end of January, this had increased to 30. By the end of March, this increased to 37, including the majority of states (34) (Schmidt et al. 2021). Below, we will outline these specific uses and then discuss ways in which the CDC's SVI and other indices compare to a prominent model on disadvantage in the philosophical literature.[1]

The 37 CDC jurisdictions that used different vulnerability indices applied them at five different points spanning the vaccine allocation process: (1) prioritizing disadvantaged groups through providing them with larger proportion of vaccines or vaccination appointments, (2) defining priority groups or areas in the phased systems, (3) planning tailored outreach and communication, (4) planning the location of vaccine-dispensing sites, and (5) monitoring uptake (Schmidt et al. 2021). We set aside differences in the design of types of indices used and outline these purposes in more detail below (Srivastava et al. 2021). It should be noted that, aside from using vulnerability indices, fourteen jurisdictions (three cities and eleven states) describe postal ZIP-code-based prioritizations, that combine the United States Postal Office geographic zone structure with other proxies for disadvantage, and in several cases, combine several such proxies. The three most frequent combinations were measures of Covid-incidence ($n=5$); vaccine uptake rates ($n=4$), and Covid-associated mortality ($n=3$) per ZIP code (Schmidt et al. 2021). One implication of using ZIP codes in combination with such metrics is that the justificatory burden falls on the jurisdiction-level planner. In contrast, from a pragmatic perspective, using the CDC's SVI—which has the implicit authority of being an index by a governmental agency—can sidestep needing to explain the choice of metric to governors, relevant sections of state governments, or the public. For a more focused discussion, we concentrate on disadvantage indices, but note that much of the description also applies to states and cities that used ZIP-code-based equity weights, instead of indices.

The most frequent use of indices, adopted by 24 jurisdictions, took the form of direct adaptation of NASEM's recommendations by increasing either vaccine allocations or appointments for high vulnerability areas. SVI weights can be added to the allocation formulas such that more disadvantaged areas receive larger amounts of doses. California had one of the more robust state plans, where 40% of vaccinations were reserved for communities in the first quartile of the Healthy Places Index (HPI). Other states—including New Hampshire, Massachusetts, and Connecticut—similarly pledged specific percentages of their total allocation to be distributed based on vulnerability (ranging from additional 5% to 30%). North Carolina provided guidance to its vaccine providers to promote equity, and specifically suggested that a certain number of vaccination slots could be reserved for historically marginalized populations in the state. Cities like Houston in Texas and Philadelphia in Pennsylvania disproportionately invited individuals from vulnerable ZIP codes to receive vaccination (Schmidt et al. 2021).

The different national jurisdictions also used a vulnerability index to help promote access to vaccines such as through planning locations of dispensing sites (eleven jurisdictions) or targeted outreach or communication strategies (fifteen jurisdictions). This use of SVI recognizes that setting aside larger shares of vaccines alone can be meaningless for reducing inequity. Reserving vaccines arriving in warehouses have to be matched with genuine and proactive efforts to reduce the barriers from there until the injections get into people's arms. Vaccine dispensaries being conveniently located and in trusted settings is one such effort. Some strategies used by jurisdictions to increase vaccines in vulnerable communities include deploying mobile vaccine clinics, enrolling more providers in underserved areas, utilizing community health workers, planning vaccination events, and extending site hours. Robust, appropriate, and relevant communication campaigns can both provide information about where to get vaccinations and help to build trust in the vaccinations and public health system. It is precisely the lack of trust in the healthcare system, in the government behind the public health efforts, and ongoing experiences of structural racism in healthcare and beyond that are powerful and substantive barriers to vaccine uptake (Bunch 2021). What is particularly notable is that North Carolina developed a robust communications plan specifically for outreach to historically marginalized communities. As all the above illustrates, vulnerability indices allow states to first identify the most vulnerable communities, and then subsequently develop creative strategies to reach those groups.

Finally, monitoring uptake is a key component to all the above-mentioned strategies, as recognized expressly by nine jurisdictions. If planners can quickly identify areas of increased need, they can use tools like increased allocation, targeted outreach, and placement of dispensing sites to course correct in real time. Targets such as Michigan's Zero Disparity goal (aimed at no disparity in vaccination rates across racial and ethnic groups or by SVI) provide critical orientation (Schmidt et al. 2021). Such goals succinctly articulate a central notion of health equity that aims to allocate resources not just per capita alone, but also in ways that address avoidable and unfair differences in health outcomes. Real-time monitoring contributes to achieving these types of goals. Such monitoring also gains particular importance after the initial time of scarcity in ensuring ongoing equity in vaccinations upon opening to the whole public. For this, as well as all other purposes, it is not always straightforward to disentangle whether public health goals (such as limiting the spread of the infection, or the impact of the pandemic on health system capacity) or social justice goals (such as prioritizing historically or otherwise marginalized communities) were primary, or were pursued in parallel. However, it is noteworthy that 25 jurisdictions use language in their allocation plans that makes it clear that a place-based measure not only has public health relevance, but can also be used for promoting equity. Traditionally, such rationales would not be found in technocratic allocation plans (and are, for example, entirely absent from pandemic flu planning guidance, which focuses on professional and health groups exclusively) (CDC 2020b; Schmidt et al. 2021).

Disadvantage and vulnerability

Philosophical account of disadvantage

We now transition to discuss the philosophical framework at issue. In the book *Disadvantage*, Jonathan Wolff and Avner de-Shalit explore a method of measuring disadvantage. To do this, the authors started with the work on well-being and social justice by Amartya Sen, Martha Nussbaum, and John Rawls. Specifically, they draw on both Sen's and Nussbaum's interpretations of the capabilities approach and Rawls's notion of reflective equilibrium (Wolff and de-Shalit 2013: 37–41). The capabilities approach, in general terms, and in articulations focused on the health context (Venkatapuram 2013), looks at advantage and disadvantage in terms of what a person is practically capable of achieving. For example, two people with equal resources may not have equal capabilities because one might have a disability and requires more resources to achieve the same capability level. And, in the space of capabilities, the able-bodied person is advantaged (that is, is capable), and the disabled person is disadvantaged (Sen 1979: 215). Capabilities, in other words, are the real abilities of a person to achieve what they want to do. Nussbaum expanded on Sen's capabilities approach and developed ten central categories that would constitute a minimally decent human life.[2] (For a list of these ten basic capabilities, see below.) Methodologically, Wolff and de-Shalit complement Sen's and Nussbaum's conceptual approach with the Rawlsian notion of reflective equilibrium— going back and forth between philosopher's intuitions and the public's intuitions until equilibrium is reached (Wolff and de-Shalit 2013: 42). They proceed in finding equilibrium by initially coming up with a list of capabilities functionings, interviewing members of the public to check the philosopher's intuitions, and then revising the philosophical principles until the two become one (Wolff and de-Shalit 2013: 187).

Wolff and de-Shalit began this process with Nussbaum's ten categories (see 1–10 below). Their initial public consultations led them to add three additional functionings (see 12–14 below) and one "independence" functioning to ensure engaged participation among participants (see 11 below) (Wolff and de-Shalit 2013: 47). Once they confirmed these fourteen functionings, they conducted a total of 98 interviews in the United Kingdom and Israel to engage the public more broadly with these functionings (Wolff and de-Shalit 2013: 49).[3] The thirteen genuine functionings were all received positively, and some people also thought positively about the control functioning. Wolff and de-Shalit ultimately left out the control from their final list of functionings. However, for our discussion purposes here, we include it, for two reasons. First, among the group interviewed, two interviewees pointed out how important independence is for elderly people and people with disabilities (Wolff and de-Shalit 2013: 58). Second, as will become apparent in our comparison to the indices used in the various United States allocation frameworks, notions of independence also surface prominently there, which makes the discussion of the "independence" functioning relevant for our purposes, even if it was not relevant for Wolff and de-Shalit's purposes.

With the exception of number 11, the control independence functioning, genuine opportunity to satisfy these functionings would be considered a non-disadvantaged life (Wolff and de-Shalit 2013: 87). While not a perfect measurement, roughly, the less a person is able to realize one or more of these functionings, the more disadvantaged they are. The fourteen functionings are as follows:

1 **Life**: Being able to live to the end of a human life of normal length.
2 **Bodily health**: Being able to have good health, including reproductive health; to be adequately nourished; to have adequate shelter.
3 **Bodily integrity**: Being able to move freely from place to place; being secure against assault, including sexual assault, child sexual abuse, and domestic violence; having opportunities for sexual satisfaction and for choice in matters of reproduction.
4 **Sense, imagination, and thought**: Being able to use the senses, to imagine, think, and reason—and to do these things in a way informed and cultivated by an adequate education. Freedom of expression, speech, and religion.
5 **Emotions**: Being able to have attachments to things and people outside ourselves; to love those who love and care for us.
6 **Practical reason**: Being able to engage in critical reflection about the planning of one's life.
7 **Affiliation**: Being able to live with and toward others, to recognize and show concern for other human beings, to engage in various forms of social interaction. Having the social bases of self-respect and non-humiliation. Not being discriminated against on the bases of gender, religion, race, ethnicity, and the like.
8 **Other species**: Being able to live with concern for and in relation to animals, plants, and the world of nature.
9 **Play**: Being able to laugh, to play, to enjoy recreational activities.
10 **Control over one's environment:** Being able to participate effectively in political choices that govern one's life. Being able to have real opportunity to hold property. Having the right to seek employment on an equal basis with others.
11 **Complete independence**: Being able to do exactly as you wish without relying on the help of others.
12 **Doing good to others**: Being able to care for others as part of expressing your humanity. Being able to show gratitude.
13 **Living in a law-abiding fashion**: The possibility of being able to live within the law; not to be forced to break the law, cheat, or deceive other people or institutions.
14 **Understanding the law**: Having a general comprehension of the law, its demands, and the opportunities it offers to individuals. Not standing perplexed before the legal system
(Wolff and de-Shalit 2013: 51–59).

One novel contribution Wolff and de-Shalit made to the theory of capabilities is that they provide an account of fertile functionings and corrosive disadvantage. Fertile functionings are specific functionings that tend to positively impact other functions; corrosive disadvantage occurs when the lack of a specific functioning tends to negatively impact other functionings (Wolff and de-Shalit 2013: 133–134). To use their example, the lack of bodily integrity would be corrosive as it would inhibit a person's ability to play, interact with other species, affiliate with others, and so forth (Wolff and de-Shalit 2013: 134). When a person does not have control over their own body or lives in fear of physical assault, other functionings are severely restricted. On the other side, having full bodily integrity positively enables a person to live within the law or do good to others. These illustrations all serve to point out that functionings are often interrelated, and the absence or presence of certain functionings can snowball into more or less disadvantage.

SVI and disadvantage

We now turn to how key indices compare with the philosophical framework. In the period between November 2020 and March 2021, when vaccine scarcity was the most acute, the majority of CDC jurisdictions that used a disadvantage index for prioritizing worse-off groups used the SVI (28 states, 1 city). The SVI is not driven by a larger theoretical framework that would seek to reduce a particular notion of disadvantage, but it is pragmatically constructed by integrating readily available census data deemed relevant and sufficiently robust for disaster planning (Srivastava et al. 2021). The relative weights of its fifteen constituent elements are generally thought of as being equal in that the numeric scores are produced by scoring a census tract on each of the fourteen variables, and then sum-totaling all the scores.

Nine states and two cities referred to or used seven other established or internally developed indices: the Community Vulnerability Index (CCVI, $n=5$), the Area Deprivation Index (ADI, $n=2$), two newly developed indices (Covid Vulnerability Index and HPI), and two indices, both referred to as Covid Vulnerability Index but distinct. Five states used more than one index. Among the twenty jurisdictions with the largest numbers of disadvantaged people (where more than 25% of the local population are among the nationwide most disadvantaged group, as measured by SVI), fourteen reported using an index (Schmidt et al. 2021).[4] Table 20.1 provides an overview of the indices for which documentation about their design is publicly available. All data integrated into these indices are usually CDC or census data (see Srivastava et al. 2021 for further details).

As the table conveys, there is considerable overlap between the dimensions of disadvantage captured in the functionings, and the variables in the indices, respectively. In the following, we discuss the extent of overlap and discrepancies in the sequence of the functionings. Further to the description of how NASEM intended the SVI to be used, we describe below their concrete uses. For now, it is sufficient to note that incorporating a particular variable such as disability, for example, means that the disadvantage that is associated with the variable will be recognized in such a way that increases the chances of receiving a vaccine for those people living in an area where, on average, there are disproportionately higher rates of that variable.

We set aside here the exact arithmetic importance of each variable relative to others included under an index. For example, as noted, in the SVI, each variable is counted equally, so would be weighed at one-fourteenth if planners used all fourteen variables, whereas the ADI specifies differential weights for each of its seventeen variables (Srivastava et al. 2021). The focus is on the conceptual relationship between the type of disadvantage that is articulated under the functionings, and indices' domains or variables, respectively. We also set aside the normative justification of disadvantage underlying Wolff and de-Shalit's project, and we provide concrete examples of how disadvantage articulated under each of the functionings

Table 20.1 Alignment of Wolff and de-Shalit's functionings with dimensions of disadvantage used to promote equity in Covid-19 vaccine rationing (Wolff and de-Shalit 2013: 51–59 and Srivastava et al. 2021)

Wolff and de-Shalit's functionings	SVI	ADI	CCVI	HPI
Total domains	4	4	7	8
Total variables	15	17	40	24
Life	Household composition and disability (age)		Socioeconomic status (age)	
Bodily health	Household composition and disability (disability status) Socioeconomic status (access to insurance, poverty, income) Housing type and transportation (housing type, housing quality)	Income (poverty, health) Housing quality (housing quality, housing type)	Socioeconomic status (income, poverty) Housing type, transportation, household, composition and disability (disability status, housing quality, housing type) Epidemiological factors (rates of disease) Healthcare system factors (insurance access, healthcare access)	Economy (income) Healthcare access (insurance access, healthcare access) Neighborhoods (supermarket access) Housing (housing quality, housing type)
Bodily integrity	Housing type and transportation (vehicle access)	Housing quality (vehicle access)	Housing type, transportation, household, composition and disability (vehicle access) Healthcare system factors (access to PCP, cost of medical care) Long-term care	Transportation (vehicle access, non-vehicle commuting)
Sense, imagination, and thought Emotions	Socioeconomic status (education status)	Education	Socioeconomic status (education status)	Education
Practical reason	Socioeconomic status (education status)	Education	Socioeconomic status (education status)	Education
Affiliation	Housing type and transportation (vehicle access) Minority status and language (minority status, speaks English) Population	Housing quality (vehicle access, telephone access)	Housing type, transportation, household, composition and disability (vehicle access) Minority status and language (minority status, speaks English) Population density	Transportation (vehicle access, non-vehicle commuting) Social environment (index of dissimilarity)

Domain				
Other species				Clean environment Neighborhoods (access to nature)
Play				Clean environment Neighborhoods (access to nature) Social environment (access to alcohol sales, access to retail, entertainment, and education)
Control over one's environment	Socioeconomic status (employment status) Housing type and transportation (housing quality) Population	Employment (employment status, employment type) Housing quality (housing quality, housing type, housing costs)	Socioeconomic status (employment status) Housing type, transportation, household, composition and disability (housing quality, housing type) High risk environments (prison population)	Housing (housing quality, housing type) Economy (employment status, employment type)
Complete independence	Housing type and transportation (vehicle access) Minority status and language (speaks English) Household composition and disability (disability status, single-parent households)	Housing quality (vehicle access, telephone access, single-parent households)	Housing type, transportation, household, composition and disability (vehicle access) Minority status and language (speaks English) Housing type, transportation, household, composition and disability (disability status, single-parent households)	Transportation (vehicle access)
Doing good to others				
Living in a law-abiding fashion				
Understanding the law				

This table shows the broad domain categories that each of the indices uses and, in the parenthetical, we added the relevant variables that are applicable to the domain and functioning. There is some overlap among the functionings and variables found within the indices. For the purposes here, rather than assigning each variable to one functioning only, we felt that it was more useful to list variables where there was a plausible overlap.

mattered in the context of Covid-19 vaccine allocation (and, where applicable, was addressed through concrete policies). The purpose is to understand how the notions of vulnerability map onto the notions of disadvantage and to understand how indices developed under the constraints of realpolitik of public health policy relate to more normative frameworks. As will become clear, equitable vaccine allocation requires that policy incorporates the notions of disadvantage and/or vulnerability.

Turning to the analysis, first, we have the functioning of life (no. 1). This is relevant to the way age and premature death are integrated in indices as they seek to realize the capability of living a full length of life. The SVI and other indices take age into account by prioritizing areas with larger shares of both older populations, who are more at risk, and younger ones, who have not yet lived a full lifespan.

Bodily health (no. 2), as conceptualized by Nussbaum/Wolff and de-Shalit, finds direct correspondence in many indices' recognition that disability status, access to insurance, poverty, income, housing type and quality, rates of disease, and access to healthy and affordable food affect disadvantage. While variation exists in the variable across the indices, two things are clear. First, all are relevant to promoting bodily health, and second, geographical areas scoring lower are likely to be more disadvantaged and individuals living there are vulnerable to getting, spreading, and dying from Covid-19. Bodily health's ability to negatively affect so many aspects of a person's life likely points to this being a corrosive functioning: where absence of the functioning negatively spills over into other areas.

Regarding bodily integrity (no. 3), four of the five indices take into account vehicle access (understood as vehicles available for household use) in ways that correspond to this functioning's conceptualization. Such access matters for a person's ability to have freedom of movement, which increases in importance when vaccination sites are not in walking distance. One factor of bodily integrity that the various indices do not take into account is freedom from abuse and control. This affects over 10 million people in the United States every year (National Coalition Against Domestic Violence).[5] And this likely impacts vaccine uptake. For example, a woman in an abusive relationship with little to no freedom over her own body and health will face additional barriers in accessing vaccines. Even if the mobile vaccine clinic is parked down the road, someone experiencing domestic violence has more hurdles to overcome to get vaccinated. So it is surprising that that data was not included.

We can discuss the functioning of sense, imagination, and thought (no. 4) and that of practical reason (no. 6) together. Both functionings are related to education, which four of the five indices expressly take into account. A person needs to have access to adequate education in order to develop these functionings. Lack of education can undermine one's ability to independently appraise information on vaccines, which, given the politicization of the vaccine development and roll-out, can have major implications on the decision to receive a vaccine. Education, along with social status, also directly affects vaccine access as more educated groups are typically more able to navigate often complex healthcare systems, including vaccination registration procedures, and prioritizing less-educated groups can therefore help blunt such tendencies.

Next we move to affiliation (no. 7). In Wolff and de-Shalit's functioning, the more affiliation you have, the better off you are. Affiliation also matters in the indices, albeit with a different valence. Certain affiliations, like being part of a certain racial group, mean that you are *more* disadvantaged according to the indices. Capturing racial and ethnic status is meaningful as a recognition of structural racism, which, as noted, also manifests in the disproportionate impact of Covid-19 on communities of color. This sort of inverse relationship does not hold for all of the variables, though. When people are able to speak the dominant language, they are typically better able to navigate health systems (even if, for example, the CDC recognized this form of disadvantage from the outset, in issuing its "vaccinate with confidence" information materials initially in, ultimately, over 30 languages [CDC 2021b]). The relationship between the functioning and the variables for this domain is more complicated than some of the other relationships.

The functioning of other species and play (no. 8 and 9, respectively) can also be grouped together in terms of the reflection they find in the indices. People, including those who are severely disadvantaged, turn to developing relationships with other species. Homeless people often develop close relationships with dogs despite not having access to other necessities (Wolff and de-Shalit 2013: 56). Access to parks or beaches is often one of the few ways that people can have access to nature and other species. While we do not see very obviously how relationships with other species directly correspond to any of the variables that are part of various indices, there is an indirect relationship between a person's access to nature and whether they are more disadvantaged. For example, poor air quality from living in an urban environment is related to poor health such as experiencing asthma symptoms (AAFA 2015). And there is large body of evidence about the importance of access to nature for both mental and physical health; this became more widely understood when social lockdowns were put into place (Mell and Whitten 2021).

The functioning of control over one's environment (no. 10) is reflected in the indices' recognition of such variables as employment status, housing quality, and prison population. By definition, prisoners have almost no control over their environment. While, as shown in Figure 20.1, NASEM expressly listed prisoners as a discrete priority population, ACIP declined to do so (Bell, Romero, and Lee 2020; McClung et al. 2020), and numerous CDC jurisdictions followed suit (Strodel et al. 2021). Where prisons are not included expressly in a particular phase, an index such as SVI can still help reduce scarcity in prisons as they are typically located in more disadvantaged areas. Housing quality, which includes crowding, also increases disadvantage because people in crowded housing are at a higher risk of getting and transmitting Covid. When a person has less control over their living environment, they typically are less able to mitigate risks posed by Covid. Equity aside, prioritizing crowded areas also makes good epidemiological sense, as it can help achieve meaningful herd immunity more quickly (Azuma et al. 2020).

The last relevant functioning is complete independence, which, as a reminder, was Wolff and de-Shalit's additional "control" functioning (no. 11). They included a control functioning in order to ensure that the participants were actively engaging in the discussion of the other thirteen functionings. Being independent is related to speaking English, vehicle access, telephone access, disability status, and single-parent households. When a person cannot speak English, they have trouble communicating on their own and would typically require help. They are more disadvantaged. When a person does not have access to a vehicle or telephone, they cannot make their own appointments and could struggle to travel to their own appointments, including their vaccination appointments. Single parents have more trouble taking time off of work or having time away from their children to go to vaccination appointments. Lack of complete independence makes a person more disadvantaged because they are not as able to make or access vaccine appointments.

Stepping back, it is noteworthy that Wolff and de-Shalit's philosophical framework does not expressly integrate quantifiable measurements of people's socioeconomic status. The indices capture this in assigning weights for, in particular, education, employment status, poverty level, and income. The exclusion of quantifiable measures of socioeconomic status is intentional from the philosophical framework's perspective because those measures often fail to capture what people are actually capable of achieving, and thus, according to the capabilities theorist, it is preferable to look to other measures. The indices, however, directly account for these dimensions of disadvantage.

On the side of the indices, it is noteworthy that they fail to include the more personal aspects of measuring disability. They fail to include things like an ability to express care for others and emotions. These are the more interpersonal aspects of advantage or disadvantage. A person who is unable to express care for others is likely to be disadvantaged. A person who does not have an ability to develop emotions for other people is likely very lonely, unhappy, and disadvantaged. The factors that influence personal development are not included in any way in the indices.

The takeaway from this section is this: while there are some differences, there is also substantial overlap between the philosophical framework and the far more pragmatically developed examples of disadvantage indices that were used for vaccine allocation.

Conclusion

From spring 2020, Covid-19 began to tear the social fabric of the United States and the rest of the world, exposing with cruel clarity prior social and health inequities. In an equally unprecedented turn, Covid-19 vaccine policy guidance shifted from a narrow focus on maximizing overall benefits and promoting equity through the phased sequence of priority populations alone to addressing equity within each phase/priority group, by capturing different levels of disadvantage though place-based indices. On April 19, 2021, when the federal government opened vaccine eligibility for all residents of the United States, an analysis by the *New York Times,* drawing on SVI and CDC data, found that the difference in vaccination uptake at this point between the most and least disadvantaged groups was around 5% (around 22.5% of the most disadvantaged had been fully vaccinated, compared to 27% of the most advantaged) (New York Times 2020). Given the historical disparities in healthcare access in the United States, it would have been reasonable to expect this margin to be much larger. With the majority of CDC jurisdictions, and the majority of states having adopted a disadvantage index for the above noted purposes, it is plausible to conclude that the disadvantage indices contributed to the difference not being larger. Furthermore, it is also worth noting that despite some variance, the pragmatically designed indices find considerable backing in the philosophical model of disadvantage we used as a comparison. Our analysis hopefully further contributes to the reflective equilibrium approach used in its development, and could be of use to others working toward theories of disadvantage.

We also hope that the analysis will be of use to those more directly focused on public health policy. We have noted that calls to integrate epidemiology and social justice need not remain abstract but, along with other interventions focused on the social determinants of health (Venkatapuram and Marmot 2009), can find direct translation in vaccine allocation and beyond through disadvantage indices and other place-based measures. As one outlook, California's HPI exemplifies policymaker's interest in this area, and illuminates possible broader uses.

Initially developed in 2015 (Rudolph et al. 2013), the HPI was used during the pandemic to guide the state's reopening (State of California 2021a) and vaccine allocating strategy (State of California 2021b), as noted above. The HPI has been used by numerous state and local groups to write grants, make investment decisions, plan for programs, and conduct community health needs assessments. One example is a partnership between the state health department and Los Angeles hospitals, where the HPI was used to develop a Community

Birth Plan addressing pre-term births among African-American women (California Healthy Places Index 2021). Additionally, eight different policy areas are identified to help communities address areas of disadvantage in the HPI, including economic, social, education, transportation, neighborhood, housing, clean environment, healthcare access, and climate change. The policy examples include things both within the realm of things typically associated with health (supporting expanded insurance coverage, access to healthy foods, and safe drinking water) and in other sectors (supporting universal preschool, livable wages, and affordable housing) (Delaney et al. 2021) that are directly related to addressing the social determinants of health and social justice (Venkatapuram and Marmot 2009).

The HPI is also offered as a resource to a wide range of community groups (businesses, community organizations, and so on) for consideration in organizational programming and policy development (California Healthy Places Index 2021). Similarly, prior to the Covid pandemic, other community- and hospital-based teams across the United States were exploring ways to use vulnerability indices to target resources and improve outcomes. At the governmental public health level, SVI has been used to identify areas in need of community-based interventions to prevent teen pregnancy (Yee, Cunningham, and Ickovics 2019). Within hospitals, the SVI has been used to identify patients who may need additional support following surgical intervention (Carmichael et al. 2020; Diaz et al. 2020; Hyer et al. 2021).

We also note that broader exploration of indices requires an assessment of the relative strengths and weaknesses of different types of indices (Srivastava et al. 2021). Beyond this, in July 2021, the Department of Health and Human Services announced that the CDC and Office of Minority Health had launched a new index, the Minority Health Social Vulnerability Index, to capture and target the systemic inequalities we have discussed throughout this chapter (US Department of Health and Human Services 2021). Among the uses that are highlighted are planning targeted programs and services to address chronic disease disparities, and planning community-level efforts to address systemic factors related to the social determinants of health (CDC 2021c). Looking outside the United States, other countries use similar methods and data collection to measure poverty, so the implications are relevant beyond health policy, too (Dirksen 2020; WHO 2008). This further demonstrates the importance of this project.

Health in all policies has long been an interest to planners—the idea that health considerations should be taken into account when developing policy even outside of health sectors because of the implications that decisions in other sectors (transportation, criminal justice, energy, and so on) have in addressing social determinants of health (Rudolph et al. 2013; WHO 2008). Vulnerability indices provide a concrete and complementary way to incorporate disadvantage considerations, and avoid policies becoming complicit in sustaining health disparities, even if unintentionally. Incorporating disadvantage indices can help mitigate the consequences of past, and in many ways still ongoing, wrongs, and, as we sought to show here, connects well with important philosophical accounts of social and individual disadvantage.

Notes

1 For other methods of approaching disadvantage, see Florencia Luna, Michael Otsuka, and Sridhar Venkatapuram.
2 There is disagreement over whether to use the term "capabilities" or rather "functionings" here, but to remain consistent with Wolff and de-Shalit and Nussbaum, we use "functionings."
3 Wolff and de-Shalit interviewed 38 adults total in Israel and England in the first round of interviews, and 60 total in a second round of interviews. They interviewed both providers and

recipients of welfare services. They brought in the notion of reflective equilibrium through an ongoing conversation with the interviewees. For a more in-depth discussion, see Wolff and de-Shalit (2013, Appendix I).

4 Note that thirteen jurisdictions (four cities and ten states) describe ZIP-code-based prioritizations combining the United States Postal Office geographic structure with different proxies for disadvantage. In several cases, more than one proxy was mentioned. By frequency, ZIP code in combination with Covid-incidence (n=5) was the most frequent, followed by vaccine uptake rates (n=4); Covid-associated mortality (n=3); bespoke algorithms developed by the respective health department (n=2); economic data (n=2); general health data (n=2); hospitalization rates (n=1); and social data (n=1). In five cases, the metric applied to the ZIP code was unclear. The dominance of disadvantage indices over ZIP-code approaches is likely explained by NASEM's recommendation to use the SVI or a similar index, and by the fact that combining ZIP codes with proxy measures for disadvantage incurs a justificatory burden for the metric chosen. To focus the discussion, we set the ZIP-code-based approach aside here. For more context, see Schmidt et al. (2021).

5 See https://ncadv.org/STATISTICS (accessed May 2, 2021).

References

AAFA (Asthma and Allergy Foundation of America). 2015. Air pollution and asthma. https://www.aafa.org/air-pollution-smog-asthma/ (accessed December 21, 2021).

Azuma, K., U. Yanagi, N. Kagi et al. 2020. Environmental factors involved in SARS-CoV-2 transmission: Effect and role of indoor environmental quality in the strategy for COVID-19 infection control. *Environmental Health and Preventive Medicine* 25, no. 66. https://doi.org/10.1186/s12199-020-00904-2.

Bell, B., J. Romero, and G. Lee. 2020. Scientific and ethical principles underlying recommendations from the advisory committee on immunization practices for COVID-19 vaccination implementation. *JAMA* 324, no. 20: 2025. https://doi.org/10.1001/jama.2020.20847.

Bunch, L. 2021. A tale of two crises: Addressing Covid-19 vaccine hesitancy as promoting racial justice. *HEC Forum* 33, no. 1–2: 143–154. https://doi.org/10.1007/s10730-021-09440-0.

California Healthy Places Index. 2021. https://healthyplacesindex.org/ (accessed May 2, 2021).

Carmichael, H., A. Moore, L. Steward, and C. Velopulos. 2020. Disparities in emergency versus elective surgery: Comparing measures of neighborhood social vulnerability. *Journal of Surgical Research* 256: 397–403. https://doi.org/10.1016/j.jss.2020.07.002.

CDC (Centers for Disease Control and Prevention). 2020a. COVID-19 Racial and ethnic health disparities. https://www.cdc.gov/coronavirus/2019-ncov/community/health-equity/racial-ethnic-disparities/increased-risk-exposure.html#ref7 (accessed December 21, 2021).

CDC (Centers for Disease Control and Prevention). 2020b. Interim updated planning guidance on allocating and targeting pandemic influenza vaccine during an influenza pandemic. https://www.cdc.gov/flu/pandemic-resources/national-strategy/planning-guidance/index.html?web=1&wdLOR=cF03500B8-2110-BB4A-8AB6-568AFFF8D109 (accessed December 21, 2021).

CDC (Centers for Disease Control and Prevention). 2021a. Health equity considerations and racial and ethnic minority groups. https://www.cdc.gov/coronavirus/2019-ncov/community/health-equity/race-ethnicity.html (accessed April 19, 2021).

CDC (Centers for Disease Control and Prevention). 2021b. Information for limited-English-proficient populations. https://www.cdc.gov/coronavirus/2019-ncov/need-extra-precautions/communication-toolkit.html (accessed December 21, 2021).

CDC (Centers for Disease Control and Prevention). 2021c. Minority health social vulnerability index fact sheet. https://www.minorityhealth.hhs.gov/Assets/PDF/MH%20SVI%20Fact%20Sheet_7.15.2021.pdf?utm_medium=email&utm_source=govdelivery. (accessed July 22, 2021).

CityHealthDashboard.2015.https://www.cityhealthdashboard.com/il/chicago/metric-detail?metric=837&metricYearRange=2010-2015%2C%2B6%2BYear%2BModeled%2BEstimate&dataRange=city (accessed December 21, 2021).

Dasgupta, S., V. Bowen, A. Leidner et al. 2020. Association between social vulnerability and a county's risk for becoming a COVID-19 hotspot—United States, June 1–July 25, 2020. Centers for Disease Control and Prevention. https://www.cdc.gov/mmwr/volumes/69/wr/mm6942a3.htm (accessed December 21, 2021).

Delaney, T., W. Dominie, H. Dowling, and N. Maizlish. 2021. Healthy Places Index (HPI 2.0). https://healthyplacesindex.org/wp-content/uploads/2021/04/HPI2Documentation2018-02-20-FINALrev2021-04-22.pdf (accessed April 22, 2021).

Diaz, A., J. Madison Hyer, Elizabeth Barmash et al. 2020. County-level social vulnerability is associated with worse surgical outcomes especially among minority patients. *Annals of Surgery.* Publish ahead of print. https://doi.org/10.1097/sla.0000000000004691.

Dirksen, J. 2020. Which are the dimensions and indicators most commonly used to measure multidimensional poverty around the world? *Dimensions.* https://mppn.org/national-mpi-dimensions-and-indicators/ (accessed December 21, 2021).

Emanuel, E. J., G. Persad, R. Upshur et al. 2020. Fair allocation of scarce medical resources in the time of Covid-19. *New England Journal of Medicine* 382, no. 21: 2049–2055. https://doi.org/10.1056/nejmsb2005114.

Flanagan, B. E., E. W. Gregory, E. J. Hallisey, J. L. Heitgerd, and B. Lewis. 2011. A social vulnerability index for disaster management. *Journal of Homeland Security and Emergency Management* 8, no. 1. https://doi.org/10.2202/1547-7355.1792.

Flanagan, B., E. Hallisey, E. Adams, and A. Lavery. 2018. Measuring community vulnerability to natural and anthropogenic hazards: The Centers for Disease Control and Prevention's Social Vulnerability Index. *Journal of Environmental Health* 80, no. 10: 34–36. https://svi.cdc.gov/Documents/Publications/CDC_ATSDR_SVI_Materials/JEH2018.pdf (accessed December 21, 2021).

Flood, C., V. MacDonnell, T. Sophie, S. Venkatapuram, and Jane Philpott. 2020. *Vulnerable: The law, policy and ethics of COVID-19.* Ottawa: University of Ottawa Press.

Foster, S., Y. Cannon, and G. Bloche. 2020. Health justice is racial justice: A legal action agenda for health disparities. *Health Affairs Blog.* https://doi.org/10.1377/hblog20200701.242395

Gourevitch, M. 2021. The power of local data in action. Robert Wood Johnson Foundation. https://www.rwjf.org/en/blog/2019/08/the-power-of-local-data-in-action.html (accessed April 13, 2021).

Hyer, M., D. Tsilimigras, A. Diaz et al. 2021. High social vulnerability and "textbook outcomes" after cancer operation. *Journal of the American College of Surgeons* 232, no. 4: 351–359. https://doi.org/10.1016/j.jamcollsurg.2020.11.024.

Jane Addams College of Social Work. 2020. COVID-19: The disproportionate impact on marginalized populations. https://socialwork.uic.edu/news-stories/covid-19-disproportionate-impact-marginalized-populations/ (accessed April 29, 2020).

Kakani, P., A. Chandra, S. Mullainathan, and Z. Obermeyer. 2020. Allocation of COVID-19 relief funding to disproportionately black counties. *JAMA* 324: 1000–1003. https://doi.org/10.1001/jama.2020.14978.

Karmakar, M., P. Lantz, and R. Tipirneni. 2021. Association of social and demographic factors with COVID-19 incidence and death rates in the US. *JAMA Network Open* 4, no. 1. https://doi.org/10.1001/jamanetworkopen.2020.36462.

Kind, A. and W. Buckingham. 2018. Making neighborhood-disadvantage metrics accessible—The neighborhood atlas. *New England Journal of Medicine* 378, no. 26: 2456–2458. https://doi.org/10.1056/nejmp1802313.

Luna, F. 2009. Elucidating the concept of vulnerability: Layers not labels. *International Journal of Feminist Approaches to Bioethics* 2, no. 1: 121–139. http://www.jstor.org/stable/40339200 (accessed August 20, 2021).

McClung, N., M. Chamberland, K. Kinlaw et al. 2020. The Advisory Committee on Immunization Practices' ethical principles for allocating initial supplies of COVID-19 vaccine—United States, 2020. *Morbidity and Mortality Weekly Report* 69, no. 47: 1782–1786. https://doi.org/10.15585/mmwr.mm6947e3.

Mell, I. and M. Whitten. 2021. Access to nature in a post Covid-19 world: Opportunities for green infrastructure financing, distribution and equitability in urban planning. *International Journal of Environmental Research and Public Health* 18, no. 4: 1527. https://doi.org/10.3390/ijerph18041527.

NASEM (National Academies of Sciences, Engineering, and Medicine), and Health and Medicine Division; Board on Population Health and Public Health Practice; Board on Health Sciences Policy; Committee on Equitable Allocation of Vaccine for the Novel Coronavirus. 2020. *A framework for equitable allocation of COVID-19 vaccine.* Washington, DC: The National Academies Press. https://www.ncbi.nlm.nih.gov/books/NBK564091/.

New York Times. 2020. See how the vaccine rollout is going in your county and state. *The New York Times.* https://www.nytimes.com/interactive/2020/us/covid-19-vaccine-doses.html?action=-click&module=Top+Stories&pgtype=Homepage (accessed December 21, 2021).

O'Brien, R., T. Neman, N. Seltzer, L. Evans, and A. Venkataramani. 2020. Structural racism, economic opportunity and racial health disparities: Evidence from U.S. counties. *SSM - Population Health* 11: 100564. https://doi.org/10.1016/j.ssmph.2020.100564.

Office of the President. 2021. National strategy for the COVID-19 response and pandemic preparedness. https://www.whitehouse.gov/wp-content/uploads/2021/01/National-Strategy-for-the-COVID-19-Response-and-Pandemic-Preparedness.pdf (accessed December 21, 2021).

Otsuka, M. 2003. *Libertarianism without inequality.* Oxford: Oxford University Press. https://doi.org/10.1093/0199243956.001.0001.

Painter, E., E. Ussery, and A. Patel. 2021. Demographic characteristics of persons vaccinated during the first month of the COVID-19 vaccination program—United States, December 14, 2020–January 14, 2021. *Morbidity and Mortality Weekly Report* 70, no. 5: 174–177. http://dx.doi.org/10.15585/mmwr.mm7005e1external icon.

Rudolph, L., J. Caplan, K. Ben-Moshe, and L. Dillon. 2013. *Health in all policies: A guide for state and local governments.* Washington, DC and Oakland, CA: American Public Health Association and Public Health Institute.

Schmidt, H. 2020. Vaccine rationing and the urgency of social justice in the Covid-19 response. *Hastings Center Report* 50, no. 3: 46–49. https://doi.org/10.1002/hast.1113.

Schmidt, H., P. Pathak, T. Sönmez, and M. Ünver. 2020. Covid-19: How to prioritize worse-off populations in allocating safe and effective vaccines. *BMJ* 371: m3795. https://doi.org/10.1136/bmj.m3795.

Schmidt, H., R. Weintraub, M. Williams et al. 2021. Equitable allocation of COVID-19 vaccines in the United States. *Nature Medicine* 27: 1298–1307. https://doi.org/10.1038/s41591-021-01379-6.

Sen, A. 1979. Equality of what. In *Tanner lectures on human values,* ed. S. M McMurrin, 197–220. Cambridge: Cambridge University Press.

Srivastava, T., H. Schmidt, E. Sadecki, and M. Kornides. 2021. Social vulnerability, disadvantage, and COVID-19 vaccine rationing: A review characterizing the construction of disadvantage indices deployed to promote equitable allocation of resources in the United States. https://ssrn.com/abstract= (accessed July 8, 2021).

State of California. 2021a. Blueprint for a safer economy. Coronavirus COVID-19 response, April 27. https://covid19.ca.gov/safer-economy/ (accessed December 21, 2021).

State of California. 2021b. California's commitment to health equity. Coronavirus COVID-19 response, April 28, 2021. https://covid19.ca.gov/equity/ (accessed December 21, 2021).

Strodel, R, L. Dayton, H. Garrison-Desany et al. 2021. COVID-19 vaccine prioritization of incarcerated people relative to other vulnerable groups: An analysis of state plans. *PLoS ONE* 16, no. 6: e0253208. https://doi.org/10.1371/journal.pone.0253208.

US Department of Health and Human Services. 2021. CDC and OMH partner to launch minority health Social Vulnerability Index (SVI). Office of Minority Health, July 15. https://content.govdelivery.com/accounts/USOPHSOMH/bulletins/2e62d06 (accessed December 21, 2021).

Venkatapuram, S. 2013. *Health justice: An argument from the capabilities approach.* Oxford: Wiley.

Venkatapuram, S. 2021 An attention to equity must guide our pandemic responses. *Policy Options.* https://policyoptions.irpp.org/magazines/september-2020/an-attention-to-equity-must-guide-our-pandemic-responses/ (accessed December 21, 2021).

Venkatapuram, S. and M. Marmot. 2009. Epidemiology and social justice in light of social determinants of health research. *Bioethics* 23, no. 2: 79–89. https://doi.org/10.1111/j.1467-8519.2008.00714.x.

WHO Regional Office for Southeast Asia. 2008. Social determinants of health: Report of a regional consultation Colombo, Sri Lanka, 2–4 October 2007. https://apps.who.int/iris/bitstream/handle/10665/206363/B3357.pdf (accessed December 21, 2021).

Wolff, J. and A. de-Shalit. 2013. *Disadvantage.* Oxford: Oxford University Press.

Yearby, R. and S. Mohapatra. 2020. Law, structural racism, and the COVID-19 pandemic. *Journal of Law and the Biosciences* 7, no. 1. https://doi.org/10.1093/jlb/lsaa036.

Yee, C., S. Cunningham, and J. Ickovics. 2019. Application of the Social Vulnerability Index for identifying teen pregnancy intervention need in the United States. *Maternal and Child Health Journal* 23, no. 11: 1516–1524. https://doi.org/10.1007/s10995-019-02792-7.

PART 4

Rights and duties

21

SOCIAL JUSTICE AND PUBLIC HEALTH

Maxwell J. Smith

Introduction

Social justice is central to the vocabulary of public health. In fact, it is often described as the "foundation of public health" (Beauchamp 1976; Krieger and Birn 1998; Levy and Sidel 2006; Powers and Faden 2006; Tod and Hirst 2014). Social justice—so the argument typically goes—affects the way people live, their chance of illness, and risk of premature death (Commission on Social Determinants of Health 2008). Injustice, then, is considered to be responsible for profound differences in health between populations (Wilkinson and Pickett 2010). An oft-cited example of this is the correlation between socioeconomic position and the social gradient in health; those occupying lower socioeconomic positions will tend to have worse health than those occupying higher socioeconomic positions, and the steepness of this gradient affects the population's health overall (Marmot 2005). Hence, social justice is affirmed as a "fundamental condition for health" in the Ottawa Charter for Health Promotion (World Health Organization 1986), and links between persistent health inequalities and unjust social conditions served as the motivation for forming the World Health Organization's Commission on Social Determinants of Health (2008).

Yet, despite the ubiquity and stature of social justice as a declared value in public health, it is unclear or remains unsettled what public health's "commitment to social justice" actually requires for social action (National Collaborating Centre for Determinants of Health 2020; Smith 2015; Smith, Thompson and Upshur 2018; Smith, Thompson and Upshur 2019). A sufficiently robust conception of social justice should be capable of providing analytic and/or action-guiding insight into the major controversies and situational challenges that are often confronted in public health and enable the interrogation of the content, scope, and justification of public health policy recommendations (Gostin and Powers 2006; Venkatapuram 2009). It may also be able to help supply policy imperatives regarding future public health action (Krieger and Birn 1998). Conceptual underdevelopment or muddiness will therefore render such a normative framework either barren or disordered, which increases the likelihood that the ideals and aims of social justice, whatever they may be, will not be realized.

Without a sophisticated understanding of what social justice requires when it is invoked in public health, myriad conflicting views will be accommodated, and disagreements will be

DOI: 10.4324/9781315675411-26

concealed. This is problematic insofar as these sorts of tacit disagreements are likely to confuse policy deliberation (Giacomini et al. 2004), stymie progress on important public health initiatives, or because they may simply lead to muddy and imprecise policies. However, there are even more insidious implications. Varied and potentially conflicting views about what social justice requires, even if they remain tacit, directly impact the public's health. In the worst case, this may contribute to the creation or exacerbation of social injustice—the very outcome against which the value is intended to militate.

Fortunately, an emerging body of philosophical scholarship cutting across public health ethics and political philosophy has supplied plausible theories that interrogate what justice requires in this context. This chapter explores these philosophical treatments and foundations of social justice in public health.

Justice and ethics

Despite the centrality of social justice to public health, it is important to note at the outset that ethical issues and obligations in public health can be thought of in ways according to criteria other than what can be called "just-making," including other "right-making" criteria or justifications (for example, beneficence, efficiency, and so on) (see Sridhar Venkatapuram's chapter in this volume). In other words, just-making considerations are only one species of right-making considerations (Mill 1962 [1861]; Nozick 1974; Rawls 1999). While this may appear to be uncontroversial, some (for example, Plato) construe justice as closer to the whole of morality (Buchanan and Mathieu 1986). Others, like William Frankena, argue that "this seems to be distributing justice a little thin" (1966: 3). The latter view—that justice is a large part but not all of morality/ethics, particularly social ethics—is adopted in this chapter.

So, what does it then mean to invoke social justice in public health? An example may be helpful. The mere fact that some are in poor health ought to be considered morally concerning, which provides moral force to claims made against the state to have such poor health remediated. The fact that we might also consider the poor health of some to be *unjust* can provide additional moral force to those claims. Identifying an injustice related to poor health may indicate a particular type, or perhaps a special type, of wrongness that requires remediation. It implies that a right exists that can be claimed against society or the state, which the latter has a duty to fulfill (Frankena 1962; Mill 1962 [1861]). The pertinent task is to specify the just-making criteria that should be used to identify the nature of such moral claims and duties in public health.

Theoretical foundations of social justice

Justice as an idea has benefited from numerous intellectual, political, social, and religious traditions. Given the scope of this volume, the following focuses on the contributions that philosophy has made to understanding the nature, scope, and architecture of justice, and does so in a way that is necessarily brief.

At its core, justice is said to consist of the apportionment of benefits and burdens to individuals in accordance with that to which they have a moral claim. In other words, justice exists when individuals are rendered what is due to them (Cohen 1986; Miller 2001; Sandel 2009). Yet, people do not necessarily have equal moral claims. Some may have stronger claims, and others may have no claim at all. This is formalized in what is commonly referred to as the formal logic of justice: "Treat equals equally and unequals unequally in proportion to relevant similarities and differences" (Frankena 1962; Perelman 1963; Sidgwick 1907).

People are alike and unalike in a number of important ways, and so a pertinent task is to identify those similarities and differences relevant for justice.

Conceptions of justice tend to be understood in distributive, relational, and/or procedural terms. As the name suggests, *distributive* justice concerns itself with how and why benefits and burdens are distributed among members of society. Accounts of distributive justice commonly answer two questions: (1) Distribution of what? (that is, the valuable goods or "currency" of justice, sometimes referred to as the "distribuendum" or "distribuans"); and (2) distribution according to what rule or pattern?

Currencies of justice are the goods that individuals are thought to be "due" as a matter of justice (Miller 2001). Common currencies of justice include welfare (for example, satisfaction of preferences or health status); opportunities (for example, educational or vocational); capabilities (for example, to be healthy or to be able to participate in political life); and resources (for example, income or healthcare resources). Specifying the currency or currencies relevant to justice is a normative task, requiring one to establish the moral relevance and importance of that good (and its distribution) to justice. Drawing the boundaries between relevant and irrelevant currencies of justice depends, in part, on the capacities of social institutions to influence the distribution of such goods and the degree of consensus in society about their value (Miller 2001). Insofar as accounts of justice and social justice might be distinguished, the currency or currencies relevant to the latter could plausibly be construed as the goods that are created through social cooperation (and, in terms of the distribution of burdens, may be construed as the burdens whose remediation requires social cooperation).

The pattern or basis of distribution corresponds to the varying criteria used to determine how to distribute the currency of justice. Of particular significance to theories of justice in public health are distributive principles of maximization, equality, priority, and sufficiency. The principle of maximization requires that the currency of justice be maximized irrespective of how it is distributed within or between groups. Maximization is a key component of utilitarianism—a set of theories that propose the right course of action is that which tends to maximize the greatest utility for the greatest number of people (Sinnott-Armstrong 2015). Utilitarianism is the paradigm example of consequentialism, where *outcomes* of actions are considered to be the only factor of moral relevance. Which outcomes are valued (for example, pleasure, happiness, preference satisfaction, health status, or life expectancy) distinguishes many forms of utilitarianism (Bellefleur and Keeling 2016; Lyons 1965). In its most basic form, utilitarianism as a conception of justice establishes that individuals have claims of justice based on (rule) utilitarian grounds (Harsanyi 1985). As such, a society (or social institutions) may be considered just when it is arranged so as to achieve the greatest net balance of utility for all individuals (Mill 1962 [1861]). John Stuart Mill, a prominent figure in utilitarian philosophy, argues that utility (in his theory of utilitarianism) is "the highest abstract standard of social and distributive justice" (Mill 1962: 318).

In contrast to utilitarians, egalitarians distinguish themselves insofar as they value equality, and value it in itself; they believe "it is bad in itself that some people are worse off than others" (Parfit 1998: 3). Instances of inequality are therefore morally urgent for the egalitarian. Egalitarians now tend to depart from what could be considered "strict" equality (that is, everybody gets equal things or treatment). This is due to the formidable objection that equality for its own sake can become absurd if it requires depriving people of some good, even if everyone has sufficient amounts of that good, simply in order for equality to obtain—imagine blinding people in order that everyone is equally sighted. Non-egalitarians of different types, however, do not consider equality to be of intrinsic value (though it may be considered instrumentally valuable). The central concern for sufficientarians is whether individuals have *enough* of a given valuable social good to satisfy justice, not whether every-one has an equal amount. As Harry Frankfurt argues, "If everyone had enough, it would be of no moral consequence whether some had more than others" (1987: 21). Finally, pri-oritarians argue that the most important job of justice is benefiting the worse off, where the relative position of the worse off to others is of no moral significance (as it is for the egalitar-ian). Rather, as Derek Parfit argues, "Benefits to the worse off matter more, but that is only because these people are at a lower absolute level. It is irrelevant that these people are worse off than others" (1998: 13).

Clearly, different views regarding the relative importance of different currencies and dis-tributive principles of justice result in multiple combinations for how distributive justice might be conceptualized and defended, both in terms of how we ought to measure injustice (for example, inequalities in access to health services; shortfalls below a sufficient level of health status) and in terms of the objectives of interventions (for example, equal access to health services; everyone achieving a level of sufficient health). A non-exhaustive illustration of different possible combinations is found in Table 21.1.

Relational justice falls outside this distributive paradigm by focusing the concerns of justice on social interactions (Anderson 1999; Young 1990). Justice, on a relational account, requires a disposition to treat individuals in accordance with principles expressing just relations, like social equality. Relational justice also situates justice in its social and historical context, shifting the focus from which goods and how they are merely distributed toward the recog-nition and critical investigation of social phenomena such as power, privilege, oppression, discrimination, subordination, exploitation, and marginalization (Bies and Moag 1986; Jost and Kay 2010; Miller 2001; Young 1990). In so doing, the relational justice paradigm focuses attention on *social group* differences (for example, race or socioeconomic status), including the ways in which social identities intersect to create overlapping systems of discrimination and disadvantage, and the pernicious effects of phenomena such as racism, sexism, classism, and colonialism.

Finally, *procedural* justice involves the application of just-making criteria to decision-making processes rather than directly to distributions, outcomes, or relations. Proponents of procedural justice argue that injustice can exist even where distributions of the currency of justice align with desired distributive principles (Miller 2001). For example, the fact that some have the power to unilaterally make decisions that profoundly impact the health of a population might suggest that a certain procedural injustice exists irrespective of distributive circumstances. Moreover, in finding that there are many possible distributive rules (maximi-zation, need, benefit, and so on) that could be valid, some theorists focus on fair procedures for guiding reasoning and justifying outcomes. Many factors or principles have been con-sidered of relevance to procedural justice, chief among them being neutrality, consistency, transparency, reasonableness, revisability, timeliness, and inclusiveness (Daniels and Sabin 2002; Jost and Kay 2010; Leventhal, Karuza and Fry 1979).

Social justice and public health

As Nancy Krieger and Anne-Emanuelle Birn (1998) note, the idea that "social justice is the foundation of public health" emerged over 170 years ago during the emergence of modern public health and important social and political movements of the mid-nineteenth century. Yet, perhaps the earliest, well-known philosophical treatment of the intersection of social justice and public health was made by Dan Beauchamp in his article, "Public Health as So-cial Justice" (Beauchamp 1976). In this seminal article, Beauchamp acknowledges that there

Table 21.1 A partial mapping of common currencies and principles of justice

Currency of justice ➡ / Distributive principle of justice ⬇	Resources	Opportunities	Capabilities	Health
Maximization	*"Maximize the resources important for health"* Objective: the greatest increase in overall resources important for health	*"Maximize opportunities to be healthy"* Objective: the greatest increase in overall opportunities	*"Maximize opportunities to be healthy"* Objective: the greatest increase in overall capabilities to be healthy	*"Maximize health outcomes"* Objective: the greatest increase in overall health outcomes
Equality	*"Equality of resources"* Objective: equal resources important in bringing about health	*"Equality of opportunity"* Objective: equal opportunities to be healthy	*"Equality of capabilities"* Objective: equal capabilities to be healthy	*"Equality of health"* Objective: equal health outcomes
Sufficiency	*"Sufficiency of resources"* Objective: improve everyone's share of the resources important in bringing about health to a threshold, beyond which differences in those resources are of no ethical importance to address	*"Sufficiency of opportunity"* Objective: improve everyone's opportunity to be healthy to a threshold, beyond which differences in those opportunities are of no ethical importance to address	*"Sufficiency of capabilities"* Objective: improve everyone's capabilities to be healthy to a threshold, beyond which differences in those capabilities are of no ethical importance to address	*"Sufficiency of health"* Objective: improve everyone's health to a threshold, beyond which differences in health are of no ethical importance to address
Priority to the worst off	*"Priority to those with the fewest resources"* Objective: improve resources for those with the worst level of resources	*"Priority to those with the fewest opportunities to be healthy"* Objective: improve opportunity for those with the fewest opportunities to be healthy	*"Priority to those with the fewest capabilities to be healthy"* Objective: improve capabilities for those with the fewest capabilities to be healthy	*"Priority to those with the worst health"* Objective: improve the health of those with the worst health

are competing just-making criteria (namely: merit, equality, or need), but argues that all individuals are equally entitled to key ends, like health protection or minimum standards of income. Consequently, all individuals ought to equally share the costs of collective action required to achieve this goal, except where unequal burdens result in increased protection of everyone's health, and especially potential victims of preventable death and disability.

With that said, it has only been since the dawn of the present millennium that health has begun to figure meaningfully in the philosophical treatment of social justice. John Rawls, in many ways the standard bearer of contemporary thinking about justice, framed health as a "natural good." This meant health did not fall within the scope of social justice, given that it was not a good that can be directly or significantly socially produced (Rawls 1999). This has prompted many, including Norman Daniels (2007), Amartya Sen (2002, 2009), Martha Nussbaum (2000), and Sridhar Venkatapuram (2011), for example, to disagree with Rawls and argue for the significance, if not centrality, of health to social justice, citing, among other things, the influence of social arrangements on health and the importance of health in securing opportunities and capabilities that are central to social justice.

With the emergence of the field of public health ethics in the late 1990s and early 2000s, there has been a surge in theoretical interest and examination of social justice and its role in public health. The first scholarship exploring and, indeed, constructing the field of public health ethics identified social justice as a key value or ethical consideration in public health (Callahan and Jennings 2002; Childress et al. 2002; Gostin 2003; Kass 2001, 2004; Thompson, Robertson and Upshur 2003). For instance, in her seminal article introducing an ethics framework for public health, Nancy Kass proposes that one should ask whether public health programs are "implemented fairly," a question she says corresponds to "the ethics principle of distributive justice, requiring the fair distribution of benefits and burdens" (2001: 1780). James Childress and colleagues, as another example, suggest that two of the general moral considerations in public health involve "distributing benefits and burdens fairly (distributive justice)" and "the participation of affected parties (procedural justice)" (2002: 171–172).

In addition to the "fair" distribution of benefits and burdens from public health activities, both Kass and Childress et al. locate at least part of the scope of social justice in addressing the social conditions that determine or impact health, a feature that has remained a hallmark of thinking around justice in public health. Childress and colleagues argue that "social injustices expressed in poverty, racism, and sexism have long been implicated in conditions of poor health" (2002: 177), which are considered to be public health's responsibility to remediate as a matter of justice. And Kass argues that it is appropriate, if not obligatory, for public health to reduce poverty, substandard housing conditions, and threats to a meaningful education. In a similar vein, Daniel Callahan and Bruce Jennings assert that "much of the research and expertise in public health throughout its history has shown how social deprivation, inequality, poverty, and powerlessness are directly linked to poor health and the burden of disease," and that this corresponds to public health's "strong orientation toward equality and social justice" (2002: 172).

Nuala Kenny, Susan Sherwin, and Françoise Baylis (2010) more explicitly situate their account of social justice in the relational justice paradigm. They argue that what is of primary significance is fair access to social goods such as rights, opportunities, power, and self-respect, which are produced through social relations. The authors indicate that this relational account of justice attunes attention to the context in which political and social policies and structures are maintained and how they create inequalities in access and opportunity. Ultimately, Kenny and colleagues argue that relational social justice "enjoins us to correct patterns of systemic injustice among different groups, seeking to improve rather than worsen systematic disadvantages in society," and "requires attention to the needs of the most disadvantaged" (2010: 10).

It is worth acknowledging the prominence that the concept of "health equity" enjoys within public health, and its relationship to justice. Health inequities are commonly understood as being inequalities in health (that is, differences in health) that are considered to be unjust (Smith 2015; Wilson 2011). Consequently, the identification of health inequities and the pursuit of health equity are predicated on an account that specifies which health inequalities ought to be identified as just and unjust. As Paula Braveman and colleagues (2011) so succinctly argue, the issue is justice. Yet, there is reason to believe that, in practice, given the lack of explicit connection to concerns of social justice, health equity is perceived as operating in a manner that is value neutral and largely divorced from the normative concern of injustice (Smith, Thompson and Upshur 2018).

Since the emergence of the field of public health ethics, several important theories at the intersection of social justice and public health have been proffered. Daniels's (2007) theory of justice, for instance, can be said to operate in the theoretical space of equal opportunity theories of justice insofar as it argues that we have obligations to protect and promote health, given the special contribution health makes to the range of opportunities available to each of us—opportunities we have obligations to protect. Shlomi Segall (2009) operates in this egalitarian space as well, though he advances an account of "luck" egalitarianism that rejects the idea that health is a special good. Instead, he insists the job of justice is to compensate for, if not rectify, negative impacts on equal opportunities resulting from any factors over which individuals have no control ("bad brute luck"). For luck egalitarians such as Segall, the claim on society by the individual who is responsible for their own disadvantage must be separated from, and is weaker than, the claim of the person whose disadvantage is a consequence of factors over which they have no control.

By contrast, theoretical contributions made by Sridhar Venkatapuram (2011) and Jennifer Prah Ruger (2010) are informed by the capabilities approach first developed by Martha Nussbaum and Amartya Sen. The capabilities approach to health advances the understanding and role of health as a capability, to which we have moral entitlements as a matter of justice. For both theorists, the capability to be healthy—the real, practical capabilities, rather than mere formal opportunities, to achieve one's potential "doings" and "beings"—is placed as the focal point for assessing justice. What so starkly sets Ruger apart from Venkatapuram's health capability theory, as well as most other prominent theories in this area, is that her theory is confined to healthcare policy as well as her argument that "it is unwise to attempt to improve health with broad non-health policies, such as completely flattening socio-economic inequalities," as doing so tends to "cloud rather than clarify the means and ends of health policy and our ability to evaluate the impact of public policy on health" (Ruger 2010: 6). Ruger, adopting here what is called a "separate spheres" view of justice, does not necessarily dispute the influence of many policy domains on health, but instead favors avoiding this complexity rather than addressing it directly. For instance, in citing her reasoning for embracing the separate spheres view, Ruger asserts that "we are far from understanding the precise societal mechanisms that influence health or how to weight different social objectives" (2010: 6). Yet, in addition to arguably downplaying the contributions of social epidemiology in understanding these societal mechanisms, it is not clear whether uncertainty or conflicting views in these areas should altogether preclude their consideration in a conception of social justice for public health, nor whether doing so might actually work to exacerbate injustice.

Finally, Madison Powers and Ruth Faden's (2006) "Twin Aim" theory of justice takes an explicit focus on well-being. The authors argue that the object of justice is successful "functioning" in six dimensions of well-being and not simply someone's "opportunity" or "capability" to achieve functionings, as is argued (variably) by Daniels, Segall, Venkatapuram, and Ruger. While the capabilities approach interprets capabilities in terms of what individuals are able "to do and be," Powers and Faden's theory concerns itself with the achievement of states of "being" well-nourished, "being" educated, "being" healthy, or "doing" certain activities, such as voting in elections; that is, in contrast to the capabilities approach, which focuses on the practical opportunities or freedoms to achieve, Powers and Faden focus on outcomes, and they fix on a minimum set of domains of well-being.

The first aim of justice for Powers and Faden, which they call the "Basic Well-being Aim" (Powers and Faden 2019), requires social arrangements to secure six core elements of well-being characteristic of a decent human life. These include health, cognition, personal security, personal attachment, respect of others, and self-determination. According to this aim, well-being is a condition or state of affairs that is good for someone to be in; a deprivation in well-being exists when one is outside the range of what is required for a decent human life. Consequently, justice demands that everyone receive a sufficient amount of each of the essential dimensions of well-being, including health. This positive aim is outcome-oriented and can be considered to be in the theoretical space of sufficientarianism.

Their second aim of justice, which Powers and Faden call the "Structural Fairness Aim," requires that social arrangements combat serious forms of systematic disadvantage that act as social impediments to the realization of a minimum level of well-being. This second aim can be considered to be in the theoretical space of equal opportunity theories of justice. Thus, while the Basic Well-being Aim seeks to combat deprivations in each element of well-being, the Structural Fairness Aim seeks to locate injustice in the structural unfairness of social arrangements that distribute advantages and disadvantages in certain ways.

The foregoing discussion does not do "justice" to the full breadth of carefully crafted theoretical treatments of social justice in public health, and as a result, is not intended to comprehensively represent these and other theories. It should also be appreciated that the theories briefly discussed here, as well as much of the theory discussed in this chapter, largely reflect contributions to justice from the Anglo-American/European liberal tradition. It is possible that these commitments run counter to widely held principles of justice based on, for example, concepts of moral desert (Buchanan 2008), the injunction to maximize collective health outcomes (Faden and Shebaya 2015), or libertarian ideals (Beauchamp 1976). And it should be appreciated that appeals to a multitude of different values or theoretical commitments exist in public health, including communitarian values (Ataguba and Mooney 2011; Jennings 2009), liberal values (Powers, Faden and Saghai 2012; Radoilska 2009), and human rights (Mann 1997; Nixon and Forman 2008; Powers and Faden 2019; VanderPlaat and Teles 2005), to name just a few examples. Thus, despite an apparent degree of consensus regarding public health's "commitment to social justice," it is unclear whether this actually reflects the "reality" or "goings-on" of public health, and it remains contested as to exactly which normative considerations these ought to entail, particularly outside the Anglo-American/European liberal tradition.

Utilitarianism and public health

Utilitarianism has been described as "the main competitor among theoretical alternatives discussed among public health theorists" (Faden and Powers 2008: 151). For instance, it is common for authors in this literature to suggest that "public health has strong roots in utilitarianism because of its fundamental focus on collective health" (Nixon and Forman 2008: 2), "public health has long been associated with the utilitarian school of moral philosophy" (Buchanan 2008: 17), "the utilitarian analysis of consequences has, and will continue to have, a central role in public health practice" (Roberts and Reich 2002: 1056), or that "utilitarianism is very much alive in the real world, and nowhere more kicking than in public health and health policy" (Venkatapuram 2011: 26). Some suggest the moral justification for public health is predominantly utilitarian, or at least consequentialist, in nature, due to its concern with the health outcomes of the public as the primary source of measuring success (Childress et al. 2002; Nixon et al. 2005).

While not referencing utilitarianism directly by name, Nancy Edwards and Colleen Davison argue that "some distancing from public health's social justice values" (2008: 102) occurred following a mid-twentieth-century shift toward reductionist thinking and an increased demand for empirical evidence to support public health interventions. For some, the use (and, often, reliance) on cost-effectiveness analyses and expert-determined indices of health status in public health, such as quality-adjusted life years (QALYs) and disability-adjusted life years (DALYs), represents a utilitarian approach to producing the greatest amount of health for the greatest number of people (Jonsen 1986; Kotalik 2006). Indeed, some consider utilitarianism to be one of the leading frameworks for contemporary health policy and welfare economics (Ruger 2010; Weinstein 1990; Weinstein and Stason 1977). Though, despite the ubiquity of utilitarianism in public health discourse, it is worth noting that it is far less common to find an unabashed defense or justification of a commitment to utilitarianism in philosophical treatments of public health in contrast to what as is found with non-utilitarian commitments to social justice.

Justice in a global (health) context

While present space does not permit a full discussion of justice in a global (health) context, it is important to acknowledge that public health and our obligations of justice cannot, and arguably should not, be divorced from the broader global context within which they exist, particularly given the global economic and political forces that so often privilege the wealthy at the expense of the poor (Powers and Faden 2019).

Moreover, it is also worth acknowledging that theories of justice developed in the context of global health remain anthropocentric insofar as they neglect the justice-relevant relationships between humans, the environment, and nonhuman animals. Missing from most, if not all, accounts are analyses of the duties that exist to promote the flourishing of the environment and nonhuman animals either in-and-of-themselves or given their instrumental role in advancing human health and well-being. An account of justice that considers the distribution of benefits and burdens between species (that is, interspecific justice) is crucial for global actors to develop common interests like shared health threats (for example, pandemics) and vulnerabilities that emerge as a result of humans' relationship with the environment (for example, deforestation, habitat encroachment, and anthropogenic climate change) and nonhuman animals (for example, wet markets), which can create conditions for poor health and injustice on a grand scale. It is also critical that such an account considers trade-offs that must be reconciled between different spatial scales (for example, between local, national, and global contexts and actors) and temporal scales (for example, intergenerational justice) (Buse, Smith and Silva 2018).

Complexity arises in the moral calculus required to consider and justify trade-offs between intergenerational, interspecies, and environmental conditions across multiple spatial scales that is (by comparison) attenuated in leading accounts of justice in public health and global health. Moreover, as accounts of justice strive to promote just health outcomes at a global scale, many other determinants of health and associated interventions ought to be weighed carefully against ecosystem values, recognizing that environmental change precipitates social and health impacts that influence global health security (Buse, Cole and Parkes 2020). This complexity warrants explicit analytic focus if we are to succeed in coordinating actors and actions, bring coherence, clarity, and legitimacy to formerly chaotic conditions, and generate and limit authority with the aim of preventing and responding to threats like pandemics and climate change in a manner that is just.

From theory to practice

"Social justice is the foundation of public health": a decades-old idea, now the beneficiary of focused and sustained philosophical attention. Between these important theoretical contributions and intrepid advocacy for social justice in practice, the optimist might conclude that we have arrived at an important juncture where meaningful reform and action for social justice is more possible than ever. Yet, it is presently unclear how this body of philosophical scholarship might interact with, let alone inform, the interpretation and pursuit of social justice in "real-world" public health policy and practice. One might be inclined to interpret this as a mere issue of knowledge translation, requiring one to simply select a theory from this literature and translate it to the public health policy and practice context. But which theory should be selected? Which would be most capable of supplying a satisfactory framework for policy and practice? As a distinct philosophical project, this may involve "reasoning out" which account of social justice we should prefer and then asking public health professionals to conform their actions to it (Wilson 2009).

While the philosophical project is no doubt an important one, we might be skeptical as to whether normative theory developed from philosophical investigation *alone* can meaningfully inform or guide public health policy and practice without further empirical insights. This is because the philosophical project, at it currently stands, largely does not directly engage with practical, messy matters of public policy (Buyx, Killar and Laukötter 2016), nor the lived experiences of those who experience forms of disadvantage and injustice (Wolff and de-Shalit 2007). This means that no matter the degree of coherence, elegance, or soundness of philosophical theory, that theory may be unworkable in the "real" world. The philosopher may be unfazed by this. G.A. Cohen, for instance, believed that justice is not primarily about what we ought to do, but rather what we ought to think (Cohen 2003). On this view, the practical import of theories of social justice may be of little consequence to their value (Valentini 2011). To be fair, this is not true of all theories or theorists; many philosophers do in fact believe that a sound theory of justice ought to be action-guiding (Valentini 2009). Nevertheless, if our goal is to understand how social justice ought to be conceived in order for it to be successfully pursued in policy and practice—in other words, for social justice to have the capacity to *operate* as a value in public health—then information about this messy context is crucial.

In contrast to the philosophical project, this pragmatic aim embraces the practical nature of ethics as an inquiry directed at "what to do" rather than a mere theoretical inquiry directed toward "what is the case" or "what we ought to think" (Finlay 2007). It acknowledges that the task of specifying and clarifying the values that form the basis for policy decisions and actions in public health is both a theoretical and practical endeavor. Pursuing this goal necessitates engagement with the "realities" of the context of public health policy and practice. It requires non-ideal theory and meaningful engagement with the injustices that are uniquely experienced by individuals and populations.

Moreover, philosophy's general neglect of the practical matters of public health policy and practice means that important moral information about social justice itself may be overlooked. As Jonathan Ives and Heather Draper argue, there is "something lacking in an approach that appeals solely to abstract theoretical principles and rationality when the problems addressed are experienced in a particular context" (2009: 250). The problems addressed are also experienced in myriad ways by different populations. The theoretical literature has paid insufficient attention to the social context in which public health is practiced—the context in which the value of social justice is actually interpreted, negotiated, ignored, experienced, and pursued (Smith, Thompson and Upshur 2018, 2019). A robust understanding of this context, including the considerations that shape or constrain what is perceived by those practicing in public health to be desirable or possible, may contribute to an understanding of the value's pragmatic features and role (Musschenga 2005), which is crucial for the actual achievement of justice. As Sen argues,

> there is clearly a strong case for not leaving out the perspectives and reasonings presented by anyone whose assessments are relevant, either because their interests are involved, or because their ways of thinking about these issues throw light on particular judgements—a light that might be missed in the absence of giving those perspectives an opportunity to be aired.
>
> *(2009: 44)*

Indeed, an understanding of these perspectives can help us to recognize which moral principles or considerations are most at stake in this context (Solomon 2005), and what policy and practice solutions would be best poised to make meaningful progress on addressing this world's injustices.

References

Anderson, E. 1999. What is the point of equality? *Ethics* 109, no. 2: 287–337. http://dx.doi.org/10.1086/233897.

Ataguba, J. E. and G. Mooney. 2011. A communitarian approach to public health. *Health Care Analysis* 19, no. 2: 154–164. https://doi.org/10.1007/s10728-010-0147-7.

Beauchamp, D. E. 1976. Public health as social justice. *Inquiry* 13, no. 1: 3–14. https://www.jstor.org/stable/29770972 (accessed December 22, 2021).

Bellefleur, O. and M. Keeling. 2016. Utilitarianism in public health. National Collaborating Centre for Healthy Public Policy. http://www.ncchpp.ca/docs/2016_Ethics_Utilitarianism_En.pdf (accessed December 22, 2021).

Bies, R. J. and J. Moag. 1986. Interactional justice: Communication criteria of fairness. In *Research on negotiation in organizations*, ed. B. Sheppard, 43–55. Greenwich, CT: JAI Press.

Braveman, P., S. Kumanyika, J. Fielding et al. 2011. Health disparities and health equity: The issue is justice. *American Journal of Public Health* 101, suppl. 1: S149–S155. https://dx.doi.org/10.2105%2FAJPH.2010.300062.

Buchanan, A. and D. Mathieu. 1986. Philosophy and justice. In *Justice: Views from the social sciences*, ed. R. Cohen, 11–43. New York: Plenum Press.

Buchanan, D. R. 2008. Autonomy, paternalism, and justice: Ethical priorities in public health. *American Journal of Public Health* 98, no. 1: 15–21. https://doi.org/10.2105/ajph.2007.110361.

Buse, C. G., D. C. Cole, and M. Parkes. 2020. Health security in the context of social-ecological change. In *Human security in world affairs: Problems and opportunities*, ed. A. Lautensach and S. Lautensach. https://opentextbc.ca/humansecurity/chapter/social-ecological-change/ (accessed December 22, 2021).

Buse, C. G., M. J. Smith, and D. S. Silva. 2018. Attending to scalar ethical issues in emerging approaches to environmental health research and practice. *Monash Bioethics Review* 37, no. 1–2: 4–21. https://doi.org/10.1007/s40592-018-0080-3.

Buyx, A., E. Killar, and S. Laukötter. 2016. Sridhar Venkatapuram's *Health justice:* A collection of critical essays and a response from the author. *Bioethics* 30, no. 1: ii–iv. https://doi.org/10.1111/bioe.12220.

Callahan, D. and B. Jennings. 2002. Ethics and public health: Forging a strong relationship. *American Journal of Public Health* 92, no. 2: 169–176. https://doi.org/10.2105/ajph.92.2.169.

Childress, J. F., R. R. Faden, R. D. Gaare et al. 2002. Public health ethics: Mapping the terrain. *Journal of Law, Medicine, & Ethics* 30, no. 2: 170–178. https://doi.org/10.1111/j.1748-720x.2002.tb00384.x.

Cohen, G. A. 2003. Facts and principles. *Philosophy and Public Affairs* 31, no. 3: 211–245. https://doi.org/10.1111/j.1088-4963.2003.00211.x.

Cohen, R. L. 1986. Introduction. In *Justice: Views from the social sciences*, ed. R. Cohen, 1–10. New York: Plenum Press.

Commission on Social Determinants of Health. 2008. *Closing the gap in a generation: Health equity through action on the social determinants of health. Final report of the commission on social determinants of health.* Geneva: World Health Organization.

Daniels, N. 2007. *Just health: Meeting health needs fairly.* New York: Cambridge University Press. https://doi.org/10.1017/CBO9780511809514.

Daniels, N. and J. Sabin. 2002. *Setting limits fairly: Can we learn to share medical resources?* Oxford: Oxford University Press. https://doi.org/10.1093/acprof:oso/9780195149364.001.0001.

Edwards, N. E. and C. M. Davison. 2008. Social justice and core competencies for public health: Improving the fit. *Canadian Journal of Public health* 99, no. 2: 130–132. https://doi.org/10.1007/BF03405460.

Faden, R. and M. Powers. 2008. Health inequities and social justice: The moral foundations of public health. *Bundesgesundheitsblatt Gesundheitsforschung Gesundheitsschutz* 51, no. 2: 151–157. https://doi.org/10.1007/s00103-008-0443-7.

Faden, R. and S. Shebaya. 2015. Public health ethics. In *The Stanford encyclopedia of philosophy*, ed. E. N. Zalta. https://stanford.library.sydney.edu.au/archives/spr2015/entries/publichealth-ethics/ (accessed December 22, 2021).

Finlay, S. 2007. Four faces of moral realism. *Philosophy Compass* 2, no. 6: 820–849. https://doi.org/10.1111/j.1747-9991.2007.00100.x.

Frankena, W. K. 1962. The concept of social justice. In *Social justice*, ed. R. B. Brandt, 1–29. Englewood Cliffs, NJ: Prentice-Hall.

Frankena, W. K. 1966. Some beliefs about justice. The Lindley Lecture, Department of Philosophy, University of Kansas. http://hdl.handle.net/1808/12382 (accessed December 22, 2021).

Frankfurt, H. 1987. Equality as a moral ideal. *Ethics* 98, no. 1: 21–43. https://doi.org/10.1086/292913.

Giacomini, M., J. Hurley, I. Gold, P. Smith and J. Abelson. 2004. The policy analysis of "values talk": Lessons from Canadian health reform. *Health Policy* 67, no. 1: 15–24. https://doi.org/10.1016/s0168-8510(03)00100-3.

Gostin, L. O. 2003. Public health ethics: Traditions, profession, and values. *Acta Bioethica* 9, no. 2: 177–188. https://doi.org/10.4067/S1726-569X2003000200004.

Gostin, L. O. and M. Powers. 2006. What does social justice require for the public's health? Public health ethics and policy imperatives. *Health Affairs* 25, no. 4: 1053–1060. https://doi.org/10.1377/hlthaff.25.4.1053.

Harsanyi, J. C. 1985. Rule utilitarianism, equality, and justice. *Social Philosophy and Policy* 2, no. 2: 115–127. https://doi.org/10.1017/S026505250000323X.

Ives, J. and H. Draper. 2009. Appropriate methodologies for empirical bioethics: It's all relative. *Bioethics* 23, no. 4: 249–258. https://doi.org/10.1111/j.1467-8519.2009.01715.x.

Jennings, B. 2009. Public health and liberty: Beyond the millian paradigm. *Public Health Ethics* 2, no. 2: 123–134. https://doi.org/10.1093/phe/php009.

Jonsen, A. R. 1986. Bentham in a box: Technology assessment and health care allocation. *Law, Medicine & Health Care* 14, no. 3–4: 172–174. https://doi.org/10.1111/j.1748-720x.1986.tb00974.x.

Jost, J. T. and A. C. Kay. 2010. Social justice: History, theory, and research. In *Handbook of social psychology*, ed. S. Fiske, D. Gilbert, and G. Lindzey, 1122–1165. 2nd edition. Hoboken, NJ: John Wiley & Sons.

Kass, N. E. 2001. An ethics framework for public health. *American Journal of Public Health* 91, no. 11: 1776–1782. https://doi.org/10.2105/ajph.91.11.1776.

Kass, N. E. 2004. Public health ethics: From foundations and frameworks to justice and global public health. *Journal of Law, Medicine, & Ethics* 32, no. 2: 232–242. https://doi.org/10.1111/j.1748-720x.2004.tb00470.x.

Kenny, N. P., S. B. Sherwin, and F. E. Baylis. 2010. Re-visioning public health ethics: A relational perspective. *Canadian Journal of Public Health* 101, no. 1: 9–11. https://doi.org/10.1007/BF03405552.

Kotalik, J. 2006. Ethics of planning for and responding to pandemic influenza: Literature review. Swiss National Advisory Commission on Biomedical Ethics. https://www.nek-cne.admin.ch/inhalte/Externe_Gutachten/gutachten_kotalik_en.pdf (accessed December 22, 2021).

Krieger, N. and A-E. Birn. 1998. A vision of social justice as the foundation of public health: Commemorating 150 years of the spirit of 1848. *American Journal of Public Health* 88, no. 11: 1603–1606. https://doi.org/10.2105/ajph.88.11.1603.

Leventhal, G., J. Karuza, and W. R. Fry. 1979. Beyond fairness: A theory of allocation preferences. In *Justice and social interaction*, ed. G. Mikula, 167–218. New York: Springer.

Levy, B. S. and V. W. Sidel. 2006. *Social injustice and public health*. New York: Oxford University Press. https://doi.org/10.1093/med/9780199939220.001.0001.

Lyons, D. 1965. *Forms and limits of utilitarianism*. London: Oxford University Press. https://doi.org/10.1093/acprof:oso/9780198241973.001.0001.

Mann, J. M. 1997. Medicine and public health, ethics and human rights. *Hastings Center Report* 27, no. 3: 6–13. https://doi.org/10.2307/3528660.

Marmot, M. 2005. Social determinants of health inequalities. *The Lancet* 365, no. 9464: 1099–1104. https://doi.org/10.1016/S0140-6736(05)71146-6.

Mill, J. S. 1962 [1861]. *Utilitarianism, on liberty, and essay on Bentham*. New York: Penguin Books.

Miller, D. 2001. *Principles of social justice*. Cambridge, MA: Harvard University Press.

Musschenga, A. W. 2005. Empirical ethics, context-sensitivity, and contextualism. *Journal of Medicine and Philosophy* 30, no. 5: 467–490. https://doi.org/10.1080/03605310500253030.

National Collaborating Centre for Determinants of Health. 2020. *Let's talk: Ethical foundations of health equity*. National Collaborating Centre for Determinants of Health, St. Francis Xavier University. https://nccdh.ca/resources/entry/lets-talk-ethical-foundations-of-health-equity (accessed December 22, 2021).

Nixon, S. and L. Forman. 2008. Exploring synergies between human rights and public health ethics: A whole greater than the sum of its parts. *BMC International Health and Human Rights* 8, no. 2: 140–149. https://doi.org/10.1186/1472-698X-8-2.

Nixon, S., R. E. Upshur, A. Robertson, S. R. Benatar, A. K. Thompson, and A. S. Daar. 2005. Public health ethics. In *Public health law & policy in Canada*, ed. N. M. Ries, T. Bailey, and T. Caulfield. Markham: LexisNexis Canada.

Nozick, R. 1974. *Anarchy, state, and utopia*. New York: Basic Books.

Nussbaum, M. 2000. *Women and human development: The capabilities approach*. Cambridge: Cambridge University Press. https://doi.org/10.1017/CBO9780511841286.

Parfit, D. 1998. Equality and priority. In *Ideals of equality*, ed. A. Mason, 1–20. Oxford: Wiley-Blackwell.

Perelman, C. 1963. *The idea of justice and the problem of argument*. New York: Humanities Press. https://doi.org/10.1093/ajj/9.1.186.

Powers, M. and R. Faden. 2006. *Social justice: The moral foundations of public health and health policy*. New York: Oxford University Press.

Powers, M. and R. Faden. 2019. *Structural injustice: Power, advantage, and human rights*. New York: Oxford University Press.

Powers, M., R. Faden, and Y. Saghai. 2012. Liberty, Mill and the framework of public health ethics. *Public Health Ethics* 5, no. 1: 6–15. https://doi.org/10.1093/phe/phs002.

Radoilska, L. 2009. Public health ethics and liberalism. *Public Health Ethics* 2, no. 2: 135–145. https://doi.org/10.1093/phe/php010.

Rawls, J. 1999. *A theory of justice*. Cambridge, MA: Harvard University Press.

Roberts, M. J. and M. R. Reich. 2002. Ethical analysis in public health. *The Lancet* 359, no. 9311: 1055–1059. https://doi.org/10.1016/S0140-6736(02)08097-2.

Ruger, J. P. 2010. *Health and social justice*. New York: Oxford University Press.

Sandel, M. J. 2009. *Justice: What's the right thing to do?* New York: Farrar, Straus and Giroux.

Segall, S. 2009. *Health, luck, and justice*. Princeton, NJ: Princeton University Press.

Sen, A. 2002. Why health equity? *Health Economics* 11, no. 8: 659–666. https://doi.org/10.1002/hec.762.

Sen, A. 2009. *The idea of justice*. Cambridge, MA: Belknap Press of Harvard University.

Sidgwick, H. 1907. *The methods of ethics*. Indianapolis, IN: Hackett Publishing Company.

Sinnott-Armstrong, W. 2015. Consequentialism. In *The Stanford encyclopedia of philosophy*, ed. E. N. Zalta. https://plato.stanford.edu/entries/consequentialism/ (accessed December 22, 2021).

Smith, M. J. 2015. Health equity in public health: Clarifying our commitment. *Public Health Ethics* 8, no. 2: 173–184. https://doi.org/10.1093/phe/phu042.

Smith, M. J., A. Thompson, and R. E. G. Upshur. 2018. Is "health equity" bad for our health? A qualitative empirical ethics study of public health policy-makers' perspectives. *Canadian Journal of Public Health* 109, no. 5–6: 633–642. https://doi.org/10.17269/s41997-018-0128-4.

Smith, M. J., A. Thompson, and R. E. G. Upshur. 2019. Public health as social justice? A qualitative study of public health policy-makers' perspectives. *Social Justice Research* 32, no. 3: 384–402. https://doi.org/10.1007/s11211-019-00327-7.

Solomon, M. Z. 2005. Realizing bioethics' goals in practice: Ten ways ""is" can help "ought." *Hastings Center Report* 35, no. 4: 40–47. https://doi.org/10.2307/3528827.

Thompson, A., A. Robertson, and R. Upshur. 2003. Public health ethics: Towards a research agenda. *Acta Bioethica* 9, no. 2: 157–163. https://doi.org/10.4067/S1726-569X2003000200002.

Tod, A. M. and J. Hirst. 2014. Public health for a fairer society. In *Health and inequality: Applying public health research to policy and practice*, ed. A. M. Tod and J. Hirst, 1–14. London: Routledge.

Valentini, L. 2009. On the apparent paradox of ideal theory. *Journal of Political Philosophy* 17, no. 3: 332–355. https://doi.org/10.1111/j.1467-9760.2008.00317.x.

Valentini, L. 2011. Paradigm shift in theorizing about justice? A critique of Sen. *Economics and Philosophy* 27, no. 3: 297–315. https://doi.org/10.1017/S0266267111000228.

VanderPlaat, M. and N. Teles. 2005. Mainstreaming social justice: Human rights and public health. *Canadian Journal of Public Health* 96, no. 1: 34–36. https://doi.org/10.1007/BF03404011.

Venkatapuram, S. 2009. A bird's eye view: Two topics at the intersection of social determinants of health and social justice philosophy. *Public Health Ethics* 2, no. 3: 224–234. https://doi.org/10.1093/phe/php031.

Venkatapuram, S. 2011. *Health justice: An argument from the capabilities approach*. Cambridge: Polity Press.

Weinstein, M. C. 1990. Principles of cost-effective resource allocation in health care organizations. *International Journal of Technology Assessment in Health Care* 6, no. 1: 93–103. https://doi.org/10.1017/S0266462300008953.

Weinstein, M. C. and W. B. Stason. 1977. Foundations of cost-effectiveness analysis for health and medical practices. *New England Journal of Medicine* 296, no. 13: 716–721. https://doi.org/10.1056/NEJM197703312961304.

Wilkinson, R. G. and K. E. Pickett. 2010. *The spirit level: Why equality is better for everyone*. London: Penguin Books.

Wilson, J. 2009. Towards a normative framework for public health ethics and policy. *Public Health Ethics* 2, no. 2: 184–194. https://doi.org/10.1093/phe/php012.

Wilson, J. 2011. Health inequities. In *Public health ethics: Key concepts and issues in policy and practice*, ed. A. Dawson, 211–230. New York: Cambridge University Press.

Wolff, J. and A. de-Shalit. 2007. *Disadvantage*. Oxford: Oxford University Press. https://doi.org/10.1093/acprof:oso/9780199278268.001.0001.

World Health Organization. 1986. *Ottawa charter for health promotion*. Geneva: World Health Organization.

Young, I. M. 1990. *Justice and the politics of difference*. Princeton, NJ: Princeton University Press.

22

HEALTH, HEALTHCARE, AND PUBLIC HEALTH AS OBJECTS OF (HUMAN) RIGHTS

Michael Da Silva

Introduction

Advocates for rights to health, healthcare, or public health (health rights) claim special moral entitlements to various health-related goods.[1] They further hold that certain entities possess duties that are correlative with such rights. These duties require taking actions to at least ensure reasonable access to the objects of these rights and that duty-bearing entities wrong the rights-holders when they fail to take relevant actions. Claims such as "I have a right to health" are taken to entail "You wrong me when you fail to secure my access to goods necessary for health." At a minimum, that wrong then further entails "You owe me an explanation for this failure."

Health rights claims play important roles in health policy discourse. Many advocates believe that making health, healthcare, or public health into objects of rights (that is, recognizing rights thereto) is an appropriate way to highlight their moral importance and protect them against appeals to other values and rights that are at play in shaping health policy or its neglect. Justified rights to healthcare or public health could, for instance, protect against liberty-based arguments being used against single-payer healthcare programs or public health initiatives with proven health efficacy (for example, vaccine mandates). Often, domestic national governments are posited as health rights' primary duty-bearers.[2] Within and across countries, legal health rights aim to protect key health-related interests through legal institutions (Rosevear et al. 2019; United Nations 1966).

Health rights claims nonetheless face various challenges. Some reject *any* positive obligations or duties to provide health-related goods to others (for example, Goodman 2005). Others recognize possible positive obligations but argue that no plausible *rights* trigger duties to provide health-related goods. These arguments note that not all morally important things are necessarily the proper objects of rights. Even if governments should secure my access to insulin, for example, it need not necessarily mean that I have a right to health or to insulin, or that my government owes me a unique, personal explanation when I do not receive it. Rights claims are, moreover, often considered even less pressing or demanding regarding public health programs. Critics (for example, Sreenivasan 2012) suggest that no one has a unique individual right to pure public goods, such as sanitation.[3] That is, if we are all wronged by governmental failures or neglect in providing such services, it is hard to see why *I* can say that *I* was individually wronged and am owed a personal explanation.

DOI: 10.4324/9781315675411-27

These challenges raise questions about which health-related goods, if any, are proper objects of rights. Broad rights to health or public health face greater challenges meeting the philosophical standards for recognition as rights than a narrower right to healthcare (RTHC). That is, unique individual claims to insulin or acetaminophen are easier to explain than claims to large-scale sanitation, let alone health *simpliciter*. At the same time, values that may justify RTHCs (basic health, capabilities, dignity, and so on) may also serve to prioritize public health programs and policies over providing individuals healthcare. Recognizing a RTHC for individuals may actually distort health policymaking and expenditures. For example, realizing a RTHC would require prioritizing individual healthcare-related goods in contexts where resources are limited (as they are in most places), and could force a trade-off in funding and delivering healthcare versus public health initiatives.[4]

These considerations raise a puzzle: Can plausible health rights claims meet necessary philosophical strictures, rather than just serve rhetorical utility, *and* adequately recognize the moral importance of population-level public health? This theoretical puzzle has immediate and practical import. Extant legal health rights frame the policymaking of many states and directly impact individual and population health outcomes.[5] Whether the rights are fully coherent and justified depends partly on whether they adequately solve our puzzle. This chapter accordingly motivates and outlines possible solutions to the puzzle. In the process, it introduces related issues at the intersection of rights theory and health policy that warrant independent scrutiny.

Background

While "rights" is a contested term in philosophy, there is broad agreement that rights protect important moral goods and impose duties on others. A rights-holder has a special moral status that permits them to make unique claims on corresponding duty-bearers and provides a "privileged basis for complaint" (Wilson 2016: 370) when the correlative duties are unfulfilled. Most also agree that rights trigger second-order duties of (at least) explanation and (most likely and most often) redress, where first-order duties to provide the goods are unfulfilled. One may use the term "rights" to refer to other phenomena, but most philosophers accept that rights at least have these basic features.[6] Any right properly-so-called should explain why duty-bearers owe rights-holders some entitlement(s) and why not receiving the entitlement triggers special second-order duties of explanation, if not compensation.[7]

Rights also come in moral and legal forms. On standard accounts, moral rights provide special grounds for complaint (and perhaps compensation) where the correlative duties are unfulfilled. Legal rights are, in turn, those recognized in in a given legal system whose nonfulfillment triggers legal censure or sanction according to a legal system's rules. Whether domestic or international legal rights must reflect or be grounded in corresponding moral rights remains contested.[8] Health rights claims are deployed and contested in both moral and legal domains.

Health rights are considered positive, socioeconomic rights, which entail correlative duties to perform certain acts, most often the provision of goods/services. Positive rights are most often contrasted with negative rights, which correlate with duties not to interfere with right-holders' pursuit of certain ends.[9] Positive socioeconomic rights require positive action to provide basic social goods. It should be noted that health rights advocates do not claim rights to everything that is health-related. For instance, most right to health advocates do not claim a right to total well-being come what may. Instead, they posit a right to some social determinants of health needed to secure a certain level of well-being ("health") consistent with natural mortality. Yet, there is still great debate regarding the particular health-related goods to which one can plausibly make claims, and what the duty-bearers must provide.

Formal conditions for health rights

Plausible arguments for health rights should meet certain basic conditions if the rights are to have more than just rhetorical value. To meet the formal schema for rights, health rights theorists should establish:

> *Correlativity:* Rights-holder A has right X which triggers duty-bearer B's duty Y, and B's second-order duties Z where Y remains unfulfilled.

As part of action-guiding theories, health rights theorists must further specify the content of X and Y in enough detail for A and B to understand their respective moral powers, requiring:

> *Determinacy:* A and B can be reasonably expected to know the act or sets of acts required that comprise duty Y and are accordingly necessary to fulfill right X and avoid triggering second-order duties Z.

Health rights advocates may not need to identify the precise actions Y needed to fulfill X but must identify at least *some* goods X duty-bearers must guarantee. For example, B should be able to know whether A's claims to insulin and to Botox both fall under A's right to X, and the relative strength of the claim to each.[10]

If a claim is to be normatively compelling, health rights theorists must further establish:

> *Justification:* There are a set of strong moral reasons that could not be reasonably rejected tying AX to BYZ.

In health rights cases, this requires explaining why duty-bearers must provide access to health-related goods. Such justification does not necessarily require that Y always has to be fulfilled but it must explain why Z is triggered upon Y's nonfulfillment. Recall that "rights" denote a concern of high moral import, so the reasons provided in the justification must be tied to weighty values. A theory seeking to ground health rights in a concern with dignity, for example, should explain how dignity grounds health rights; the entitlements inherent in dignity-based rights; and whether, why, and when they trigger specified duties to be carried out by certain duty-holders.

Action-guiding rights should also be realizable in pluralist societies, supporting:

> *Practicality:* Fulfilling Y must further health-related moral values without substantially undermining B's ability to further other moral values/rights/social goals.[11]

Health rights cannot be so broad so as to be practically unrealizable, or only realizable at unacceptable (and perhaps unlimited) cost, as when they would require spending to the point where one cannot fund other goods like education programs. At the same time, health rights also cannot be so specific or so narrow as to make them rights to particular goods, like lorazepam or a specific vaccine.[12] Such rights not only lack "vision" (Gostin 2001: 123). They are also better described as rights *to those goods* alone. Existing health rights theories and practices are often critiqued for failing to correctly balance the need for a distinct, circumscribed set of entitlements that health rights should entail and the need to create entitlements that can produce real change (Cohen 2020 (also discussing other rights)).

Health rights must also avoid a type of "imperialism" whereby all policy/political decisions must be addressed through a single analytical lens (Prah Ruger 2006).[13] That is, health is not the only concern of pluralist societies or of individuals. Health rights should not turn all governmental issues into health issues, obscuring distinctions between diverse social concerns and obfuscating their relative contributions to health. At the same time, rights-based approaches need not hold that *only* rights matter. Stating that rights provide a special kind of protection to some interest need not entail that those interests are of primary moral importance in all conflicts. Other moral phenomena may matter. Indeed, broad approaches to health rights could challenge the possibility of a distinct rights-based approach to health justice. If rights are to be distinct moral phenomena, they should add something distinctive to our moral ontology. This distinctiveness is meant to come from how they change rights-holders and duty-bearers' moral powers and create unique moral relationships between them. However, broad social rights collapse into general theories of social justice if they create entitlements to a just social order.[14] If health rights require ideal allocations of the social determinants of health, they seemingly require achieving health justice. Even if this were practicable, rights-based approaches to health justice would no longer appear distinct where "I have a right to health" is ultimately equivalent to "You must achieve health justice."

The puzzle

Even if one grants health rights' general plausibility, meeting some of the conditions above fits uneasily with prioritizing population-level health. Other conditions, however, seemingly require exactly such prioritization. This is our puzzle.

Correlativity, determinacy, and practicality arguably motivate a form of rights minimalism that is more amenable to healthcare-focused theories.[15] A RTHC appears most likely to establish concrete health-related duties governments can, and plausibly should, fulfill, and thus maintain rights-based theories' distinct characteristics. While healthcare is multifarious, a circumscribed list of preventative, diagnostic, and curative procedures fit under the category. Individuals can plausibly assert distinct rights claims to such concrete goods. These accounts are also more practicable: providing the healthcare goods needed for a set level of well-being seems a lot easier than providing various social determinants of health. That is, funding some essential medicines can be expensive but is less so than funding all health-relevant programs. Countries are thus more likely to be able to realize a RTHC than broader health rights. RTHCs will be *more* practical if the level of well-being in question is sufficiently low. But one should not underestimate even a narrower or minimal RTHC's transformative potential. A right that secures wide access to insulin, acetaminophen, lorazepam, and some other essential goods, such as childhood vaccines, is important even if lacking the kind of vision desired by some health rights advocates.

A RTHC also keeps health rights distinct from other moral considerations and permits weighing health rights against those considerations, possibly including population-level interests. This blunts practicality objections and provides a framework for responses that fulfill second-order duties upon nonfulfillment. Saying that someone has a right to insulin need not entail that they receive it, come what may. It entails that they are owed a duty of explanation when relevant duty-holders such as their own governments choose to fund other health or social goods instead. If, for example, a RTHC is justified only when it contributes to basic species-typical functioning, we can examine the extent to which a good contributes to that end before deciding whether to fulfill a claim thereto. We can also weigh that claim against those to other goods, including public health, when deciding which rights to fulfill. A public health initiative's relative contribution to basic species-typical function or realizing another good, like some subpopulation's self-determination rights, can then be part of explanations provided to rights-holders whose rights are unfulfilled.

However, the interests that justify a RTHC seem to also justify broader health rights even more. And the empirical record on RTHCs' ability to improve access to healthcare, let alone improve population-level health through public health measures, is at best mixed.[16] Access to healthcare alone is insufficient to protect the values commonly invoked to justify health rights, such as basic species-typical functioning (Daniels 1985), dignity (Da Silva 2018: Gilabert 2018 (on human rights generally with a social rights focus)), and capabilities (Prah Ruger 2006; Venkatapuram 2011). Healthcare alone may not even contribute to the justificatory values as well as other health-related entitlements can. In this light, the case for a RTHC could collapse into preferences for healthcare-centered health policy. Such preferences may themselves prove problematic. For instance, Lawrence Gostin (2014: xv, 420) suggests that people behind a Rawlsian veil of ignorance would much prefer "an environment with healthy living conditions" produced by public health initiatives over "access to medical care" when sick. As a result, RTHC advocates owe an explanation for why recognizing a RTHC does not reflect mere idiosyncratic preferences for healthcare.

Existing legal health rights provide special protections for healthcare, through explicit recognition of a RTHC, or a right to health focused on healthcare entitlements. This can distort health policy priorities. For instance, it seems that many constitutional health rights in different countries result in largely middle-class citizens securing access to expensive healthcare goods at the cost of public health programs that greatly protect the worst-off in society (Flood and Gross 2014; Gauri and Brinks 2010; King 2012; Yamin 2019; Yamin and Gloppen 2011). Even many RTHC advocates consider such situations unjust. Consequently, one should note that RTHCs could undermine health justice, rather than offer distinct, rights-based approaches to it.

To avoid such unjust outcomes, theorists emphasizing rights to healthcare entitlements must better address public health- and population-level concerns. Yet, capturing public health's moral value or priority while also meeting the requirements identified above is remarkably difficult in both theory and practice. Recent philosophical accounts that discuss RTHCs (for example, Hessler and Buchanan 2002; Powers 2015) or that emphasize healthcare-related components of the right to health (for example, Hassoun 2020a) are better able to address concerns about the philosophical requirements of rights. Yet, many also make public health concerns less central. This is especially odd given that even traditional advocates of healthcare justice are now calling for attending to broader health concerns, beyond healthcare (for example, Daniels 2008).

The continuing puzzle, then, is to specify a health right that can meet requirements favoring minimalist health rights, and also account for public health's apparent moral priority. Arguments for rights to health or public health present possible solutions and unique challenges. I will now outline some of these solutions and their drawbacks before exploring how a different account of a RTHC may offer a better, if still incomplete, solution to the puzzle than even these broader health rights.

Rights to health

Numerous moral goods could ground a right to health. Many plausibly argue that at least some minimal level of well-being is necessary to enjoy other rights or values. Health is of basic importance in many theories, including those interested in protecting basic species-typical functioning (Daniels 1985) and capabilities (Prah Ruger 2006; Venkatapuram 2011). Several such theories suggest that all persons have a basic right to at least a minimal level of well-being and the basic entitlements necessary to reach it or sustain it. This can be understood as a moral right to health. The international legal human right to health (United Nations 1966), in turn, purports to reflect a basic concern with dignity. This legal right could be justified by the way in which the international legal right promotes state and third-party improvements in health justice even absent a corresponding moral right (though the justification would rely on legal rights being independently justifiable outside morality and shown through analysis of empirical data).[17]

A moral right to health can plausibly recognize the moral importance of population-level concerns and public health initiatives. The international legal right includes public health entitlements, including constitutive sub-rights to many social determinants of health, and requires attending to health distributions or inequalities across populations (Da Silva 2018; Nixon and Forman 2008; Tobin 2012; Wolff 2012). Its operation in international law arguably provides some determinative content that does not unduly favor healthcare. Moreover, where rights are supposed to protect important moral interests, a direct right to the interest (for example, health) can be preferable to rights to goods instrumental to producing it (for example, healthcare). This is especially true where claimed instrumental goods may not best realize that interest. A right-to-health framework, then, permits focus on the goods, whatever they might be in the specific context, that actually promote health. If public health initiatives are strong contributors to individual and collective health outcomes, in certain places or times, such a framework can even prioritize public health entitlements over other entitlements that are part of the right.

A right to health that also meets other requirements could resolve our puzzle. But rights to health face correlativity, determinacy, and practicality issues. It is simply very hard to identify who must do what to fulfill a moral right to health. For instance, Gopal Sreenivasan (2012) argues that no account of such rights clearly articulates their correlativity relationships in a normative defensible, non-ad hoc fashion that can further health rights advocates' desired ends. Even if governments are duty-bound to provide some health-related goods to their citizens, no *individual* holds unique rights to broad social programs necessary for health. It is, again, hard to see why I have a *special* complaint when a government fails to provide basic sanitation if the government's duty applies equally to everyone. A plausible right to health should connect to concrete goods to which individuals could have distinct entitlements, such as access to particular immunizations or clean water in one's home. One is then likely better off recognizing rights to those goods, not health. If, in turn, one could identify specific health entitlements to which an individual plausibly should have a right, the same values that could justify such entitlements may also justify entitlements to other goods, raising demandingness concerns. Attempts to funds only a narrow set of goods may prove ad hoc and again provide fewer entitlements than what advocates desire.

One way around these objections may be to argue for collective rights to health. But this too presents issues. Collective rights make every member of a polity or group into rights-holders who can make claims on a duty-bearer. Right X belongs to collective A who can be represented by members from $A^\star$ to A^n. However, collective rights raise questions about which collectives are relevant or legitimate, how collective interests interact with the individual interests of their members, and how collective rights relate to individual rights. An account of collective rights that answers those questions would need to explain why and when member $A^\star$ in particular can make a claim to $X^\star$. So, the collective suffers the same challenges as that of an individual making rights claims. Moreover, any collective right to health raises questions about competing health-related interests within the collective. A collective is unlikely to have only one health-related interest. Pursuing a collective right to health in order to categorically favor public health initiatives could collapse the right to health into a right to public health (RTPH). This raises further issues discussed below and seems like an ad hoc way to resolve conflicts.

Indeed, right-to-health frameworks' difficulties making trade-offs cut against their potential solution of our puzzle. Operationalizing a right to health requires setting priorities within it. Yet, placing all priority setting within a single analytical framework itself distorts moral calculi. Mere appeals to collective rights or the moral priority of public health cannot resolve related rights imperialism concerns or explain how to resolve health-health trade-offs (Sunstein 1996). If health includes all its causal contributors, a right to health is not only vague but seemingly all-encompassing (Morales 2018; Prah Ruger 2006; Weinstock 2015a, 2015b). This is not merely an over-demandingness problem. It makes health amorphous and a right thereto difficult to parse, undermining understandings of health and related, otherwise independent concepts. More pressing still, such a broad right would not permit weighing relevant values against each other or explain how each causal contributor is relevant to the present task (Weinstock 2018). This could result in worse policy distortions than those produced from healthcare-emphasizing rights.

Appealing to international law may not resolve this issue. International law avoids over-demandingness charges by only making states responsible for initially providing a minimum core of health entitlements, and then achieving other health-related goods as funds permit through a progressive realization process (Nixon and Forman 2008; Tobin 2012). Many core right to health entitlements are healthcare-related; other entitlements form parts of other, non-health rights (Da Silva 2018). If the international right to health is practically realizable, then, it may also (at least initially) be not sufficiently broad enough to produce entitlements to expensive public health programs that are not part of other rights. Our puzzle would largely remain in place.

Rights to public health

RTPHs are narrower than rights to health, helping blunt some specificity/practicality issues, and reflect public health's moral import. Those comfortable with collective responses to correlativity charges may thus view a collective RTPH as a useful middle ground (Coggon and Gostin 2015; Gostin 2014; Meier 2007; Meier et al. 2018). Proponents claim that these public health rights supersede any individual healthcare-focused equivalents.[18] If the moral goods justifying health rights always instrumentally prioritize public health, recognizing a RTPH could also help address lingering justifiability concerns.

A RTPH could also help justify public health interventions despite its impact on other rights. For example, public health is often challenged for violating individual liberty rights. Per James Wilson (2016: 374), if there is a RTPH, interfering with other rights in order to fulfill RTPH is legitimate; "anything that is morally legitimate is either not paternalistic at all, or paternalistic but not morally wrong. Therefore, paternalism cannot be a valid objection to proportionate action in the name of the right to health." If nothing else, then, a RTPH could help justify public health policies. This seemingly gets our moral priorities correct from a health promotion standpoint. The case for recognizing this right to resolve our puzzle is thus initially compelling.

Yet, RTPHs raise the same correlativity issues as the right to health, and do not blunt specificity or practicability concerns as much as desired. RTPHs raise aforementioned concerns about rights to pure public goods (Sreenivasan 2012). Specifying the particular, concrete goods to which those with a RTPH should be entitled to in a way that avoids even just the most common criticisms of health rights is exceedingly difficult. Why I should be able to make a *distinct individual* claim to public sanitation or anti-obesity measures when these goods can only be enjoyed collectively (again) remains hard to parse.[19] Notably, the leading RTPH advocate, Wilson, eschews specifying his RTPH's content. He recognizes "risk reduction measures" as core content but otherwise leaves specification up to a procedural framework (2016: 372–373). How a non-redundant RTPH can meet the desiderata above and ground feasible practices is unclear.

Extant accounts of RTPHs raise specificity and practicality concerns. For instance, RTPH advocate Benjamin Mason Meier's (2007: 547) "expanded" definition of public health grounds a right that "protects and promotes the health of entire societies by employing multi-disciplinary, multi-agency interventions to address the collective causes of health and disease." This approach faces over-demandingness and imperialism charges. While RTPH proponent Lawrence Gostin (2001: 123) admirably warns against "limitless" conceptions of public health, his characterization of basic public health shift throughout his text, with nutrition and education sometimes appearing as public health and also sometimes as social determinants of health. Indeed, RTPH advocates' disagreements on what qualifies as public health suggests that expanded understandings of the category have made it too amorphous to determinatively and plausibly set a RTPH's content.

Wilson's, Meier's, and Gostin's respective accounts of what counts as public health, basic or otherwise, could also collapse distinctions between healthcare, public health, and underlying social determinants of health. The most obviously distinct public health goods also raise democracy concerns and cannot ground plausible rights. For instance, Gostin's (2014: 426) right would require graphic cigarette warnings, tobacco taxes, and clean air laws. Wilson (2016: 372) promotes bans on alcohol advertising and alcohol and tobacco taxes as public health "best buys" that a RTPH must include. Requiring such substantive policies challenges the pluralism that should operate in the relevant spheres. This is particularly worrisome where each measure's contribution to health is contested. Still other candidate RTPH components can be fulfilled through other rights. For example, S. Matthew Liao (2019)'s public health-emphasizing right to health is restricted to basic nutrition, healthcare, and nutrition education. Yet there are already legal rights to nutrition, healthcare, and education that can guarantee these goods in many jurisdictions. If there is a right to anti-obesity measures (2018: 54), that right can be fulfilled through good healthcare and education programs as part of a RTHC and a right to education. A distinct RTPH is unnecessary.

RTPHs also threaten our ability to attend to different moral considerations that should play prominent roles in health policymaking. For instance, Wilson's (2016) RTPH-inspired very strong weighting of public health concerns in moral analyses can obscure other relevant interests. His RTPH also seems to come at the expense of our best understanding of public health's relationship to other goods. Making public health the object of a right makes all conflicts between promoting public health and human rights into conflicts between *rights*. Wilson views this positively but comes dangerously close to suggesting that nothing is wrongful about restricting rights in paternalism cases. That could help justify public health measures and ease the move toward conciliation between health and human rights but only at the cost of attending to real trade-offs between public health and human rights that pluralists should recognize.

These costs may not be worth it where RTPHs may also be unnecessary. Holding that states *should* promote health for good governance could also highlight public health's relative value.[20] For instance, countries should prioritize scientifically sound health promotion programs, set indicators for success, collect data on the same, and so on, as Meier (2007) seeks, absent RTPHs. As I will now explain, a RTHC may also require some of these actions. Moreover, public health and (other) population-level goods could justify not realizing a narrower RTHC where one must choose between healthcare and public health funding even in the absence of a moral or legal RTPH. The difference here is that any conflicts would not be conflicts between *rights*.

A path forward?

Attempts to specify health rights will find it hard to solve our puzzle. One may thus conclude that no health right can meet all the relevant criteria. Non-rights-based approaches to health justice could then be preferable, especially given existing legal health rights' distorting effects. Alternatively, the above discussion could suggest that rights-based approaches to health justice should emphasize and examine the relative contribution of other rights and their importance to the realization of health justice. One can consider rights to health, healthcare, and public health problematic and still remain committed to examining and strengthening relationships between health and other moral and legal rights. This may render specific health rights redundant but would vindicate ongoing health and human rights research and rights-based policymaking.[21]

The idea of health rights is, however, still compelling to many. Moreover, Wilson's call to recognize such rights to protect health interests against competing concerns that are already objects of rights is important. So, seeking to solve our puzzle remains a good project.

My preferred approach is to adopt a modified RTHC that attends to at least some population-level interests and that can be limited by overriding population-level concerns, including the need for public health measures. I can only provide an outline of this approach and even what I contend is the most promising route admittedly may only partially solve the puzzle at hand. However, the view has some benefits over competitors and even attending to its limitations (and potential problems) will deepen understanding of the puzzle and possible solutions.

In brief, I believe that a defensible "complex" RTHC that includes substantive, procedural, and systemic content will improve public health and offers specific opportunities to attend to population-level health concerns. Such a right is unlikely to fully account for the moral importance of public health established by any plausible principle that will ground a complex RTHC. However, I do not take this as evidence that one must recognize broader health rights. Simply recognizing public health as important enough to sometimes constrain the pursuit of complex RTHCs permits one to recognize a right that meets necessary formal criteria and will likely fulfill some population-level goods while also recognizing the relative moral importance of public health. Indeed, this approach permits one to recognize that the very principles justifying the right might also provide reason to limit the right to pursue other, population-level goods. This addresses the tension at our puzzle's core (if not related empirical concerns about "distortion").

As discussed above, a RTHC with minimalist content appears most likely to address traditional challenges to health rights. A modified RTHC also provides opportunities to address at least some population-level concerns. Elsewhere (for example, Da Silva 2020, 2021), I argue that any plausible RTHC is inherently complex in that it requires procedural guarantees to set its content beyond an uncontroversial core (for example, the essential medicines, basic maternal and infant care, and vaccines guaranteed in international law that are plausibly necessary for dignity) and a functioning healthcare system instrumental to securing the core content and procedural justice. Purely substantive RTHC conceptions focused on particular goods are incomplete: principles for selecting substantive goods admit borderline cases, and content must change over time. Procedural fairness guarantees are needed to resolve borderline conflicts and update coverage. Yet, purely procedural conceptions focused on ensuring fair processes in healthcare decision-making are redundant where other rights to fair decisions already exist. Identifying *some* substantive content is necessary. Systemic features of functioning political and healthcare systems are then instrumentally required to guarantee substantive and procedural content.

The complex version of the RTHC that I envision would produce (at least governmental) duties to provide a *de minimus* list of goods required to fulfill some basic value. I prefer a dignity-based approach, but other sufficientiarian values, such as basic health, may also help identify a circumscribed set of goods that governments could plausibly be justifiably required and practically able to realize. If the principle is suitably circumscribed, procedural guarantees can be indexed to countries' specific needs, permitting a path between overly narrow and over-demanding rights. Several candidate principles mentioned above can plausibly justify correlative rights/duties relationships that require the provision of basic health entitlement. The list in question is, in turn, not terribly demanding economically, blunting demandingness objections. The costs for many such goods, such as insulin, may not be too high for most governments to fulfill, avoiding over-demandingness charges (Da Silva 2018). They are at least less than the costs of broader rights. A plausible complex RTHC would also include procedural fairness guarantees whereby other health policy decisions, including funding decisions, would need to fulfill basic justificatory requirements, such as the provision of acceptable reasons for policy decisions and opportunities to challenge those decisions.[22] Formally requiring explanations for why healthcare entitlements are not fulfilled would establish mechanisms for ensuring second-order duties are fulfilled when first-order duties are unfulfilled. Functioning healthcare and legal systems will then guarantee the complex RTHC's other elements. Adequate hospitals, administrative review bodies, and so on may then also improve population-level health. Establishing each of these factors would require the kind of data collection Meier desires.

Adopting a complex RTHC alone provides a partial solution to the puzzle at hand by taking the path offered by a RTHC that addresses correlativity- and determinacy-based challenges lodged against many accounts of health rights while also providing at least some of the goods intended by a RTPH. A complex RTHC in particular also offers means of securing some of the goods desired by RTPH and opportunities to specifically attend to population-level concerns.

Many principles for selecting substantive content likely require ensuring that the basic goods are evenly distributed across populations. Some theorists (for example, Hassoun 2020a) and international legal standards (Da Silva 2018) thus call for attending to vulnerable and marginalized groups in rights analyses. A right prioritizing goods needed for basic health, rather than luxury goods, may not solve all inequities but should not produce further ones. Raising all persons to, for example, that basic health level should have a salutary impact on population health and address *some* inequities.[23] Yet if better access to healthcare does not improve or adequately raise population-level health procedural and systemic content, it will still likely have population-level effects by securing political systems that correlate with better health outcomes. A functioning healthcare system that makes evidence-based rationing decisions and provides basic care to everyone in a jurisdiction should improve population-level health. Even if one thinks that providing the goods necessary for dignity is unambitious, then, claims that RTHCs are too narrow become even less compelling where they necessarily require systemic content. Indeed, a complex RTHC allows one to anchor rights to systems in concrete entitlements to specific goods, helping avoid charges that there are no rights to pure public goods.

A complex RTHC also offers specific opportunities to address population-level considerations. To wit, fulfilling the procedural and systemic requirements requires opportunities for public deliberations on how health policy is set. That discourse should plausibly address public health considerations where the procedural right too is justified by a concern with dignity, basic health, or some other good that would seem to prioritize public health and where reasonable people disagree on what values (individual, population-level, and so on) *should* guide health policy. Decisions on which goods to provide in a procedurally just system should be transparent and address relevant interests in ways those subject to the decisions could accept (Daniels and Sabin 2002). If decisions are made that are completely insensitive to their population-level effects, the reasons for those decisions are plausibly incomplete and unlikely to be fair. If the reasons are to be compelling, in turn, they too will require the kind of data collection RTPH advocates desire.

Viewing the right as defeasible and permitting it to be limited by other considerations helps further address some concerns with this approach. Adopting a complex RTHC along with a form of moral pluralism whereby rights do not always trump other moral considerations provides another way to recognize the moral importance of public health while only recognizing a RTHC. Any principle one may use to establish a complex RTHC's basic substantive content may still prioritize public health. Yet, only recognizing *rights* to some goods that fulfill a value is non-ad hoc where the purported right to other goods cannot meet formal requirements for recognition. Basic health, for example, may prioritize public health, but this is not determinative of whether we should recognize a RTPH thereto given other conceptual issues with RTPH recognition.

This approach too may only provide a partial solution to our puzzle. Specifying a plausible RTHC that serves a unique moral role and how and when it can be limited by public health considerations remains theoretically difficult.[24] It may be harder still in practice. Whether recognizing public health as an important value that can justify not fulfilling a RTHC will secure access to public health goods or avoid the distortions motivating our puzzle remains unclear. While one may contest whether a RTHC or RTPH will provide better outcomes in reality or the reasons why some RTHC are problematic in practice, appealing to a RTHC does lead to prioritizing healthcare over health goods in at least some cases.[25] Whether and when a RTHC will distort priorities is an empirical question. Such distortion is not inevitable. Yet much more needs to be said to specify how a complex RTHC could work in practice and when it can be justifiably constrained in the name of public health to fully address our puzzle's underlying concern. I suspect that a complex RTHC nonetheless provides the best path forward in this debate.[26] Yet if my outline alone is uncompelling, I hope that attending to its strengths and limits further deepens our understanding of the puzzle and related issues in rights theory and public health ethics.

Notes

1 Many internationally recognized human rights are relevant to health (Mann et al. 1994). Consider rights to nondiscrimination in healthcare provision, information about sexual health, or free association with fellow patient advocates. Yet, distinct "health rights" should not merely describe how other rights impact health systems.

2 Some view international bodies, corporations, and so on as duty-bearers, albeit often in subsidiarity cases where domestic governments do not fulfill their primary duties (for example, Hassoun 2020a).

3   Sreenivasan nonetheless thinks that a *legal* right can be independently justified (Buchanan and Sreenivasan 2018). He can make this move via his position in debates discussed in note 8. Empirical distortion worries may still arise.

4   See representative accounts in Meier (2007) and Easterly (2009) and related claims in Meier et al. (2018) and Cohen (2020).

5   See, for example, Langford (2008); Tobin (2012); Gauri and Brinks (2010); Yamin and Gloppen (2011); King (2012); and Flood and Gross (2014). See also general works on social rights like Langford et al. (2017) or Young (2019).

6   Any definition of rights will be controversial. This account is agnostic on most debates about right summarized by Wenar (2020). Yet, it broadly follows the classic structure of claim rights in Hohfeld (1913) and captures key features in several contemporary works on health rights (for example, Wilson 2016) and rights generally (for example, Etinson 2018).

7   I follow the leading exponent of the right to public health, Wilson (2016), in bracketing debates about the precise second-order duties required. Questions about which first-order duties that could trigger them remain central.

8   Etinson (2018) summarizes these debates. See also Pavel (2019)'s argument that healthcare can be an object of a conventional, rather than human, right.

9   Many criticize the positive/negative rights distinction. Critics suggest that realizing negative rights requires positive actions. See, for example, Holmes and Sunstein (1999).

10 This language follows Simpson (2021), though his definition of the term closely links it to correlativity. His alternative criteria are feasibility, which speaks to my practicality concern, and pluralistic adequacy, which requires that any justificatory requirements apply in many settings and which I do not explicitly adopt here.

11 I take a minimalist approach to specifying the conditions here. For more detailed conditions, see Gilabert (2018).

12 For good overviews of these and related debates, see Powers (2015), Rumbold (2017), and Hassoun (2020b).

13 This imperialism is distinct from related concerns about Western values being imposed elsewhere. It refers to a single concept subsuming others within its ambit and overriding them.

14 See Beitz (2013: 39) on social rights generally (and more details in Beitz 2011).

15 Minimalism admits many forms (Cohen 2004; Simpson 2021). Minimalism here concerns content (in Powers 2015's sense).

16 For the mixed record, see, for example, sources in note 5. Per Sreenivasan (2016), any narrow health rights that address most conceptual issues are unlikely to fulfill advocates' aims. Health rights might be valuable without securing direct access to goods. They can, for example, inspire and support other forms of advocacy (Hassoun 2020ab). Whether narrow rights further even these ends is debatable. See also Cohen (2004) (on rights generally).

17 Third-party influence is the kind of benefit in the previous note. On legal/moral rights, recall note 8.

18 Per Meier (2007), medical rights are only justifiable if they achieve overlapping public health goals.

19 Granted, an individual's lack of access to a specific concrete good, like a nutrition class, could more easily provide grounds for complaint. Yet focusing on these discrete rights raises other challenges discussed in this section.

20 One reading of Gostin (2014) could support this claim. More broadly, the standard view on which all rights must have corresponding duties does not entail that all duties have corresponding rights.

21 The kind of work discussed in note 1 would remain compelling on this approach.

22 Daniels and Sabin (2002) inspire this element.

23 Recall the mixed record on legal rights discussed above (and in note 5 sources). Gostin (2014) and Hassoun (2020a) read the literature positively. Yet, Gauri and Brinks (2010) notwithstanding, the comparative law texts above provide more complex, less sanguine accounts.

24 Another reason one might challenge the proposal is that appealing to a defeasible RTHC but granting that other considerations, like public health, can overwhelm it does not maintain a distinctive role for rights. The way in which these rights change moral powers appears distinctive to me. However, this account does rely on a form of pluralism and a recognition that rights can be overwhelmed that I lack space to adequately defend here.

25 Again, see the empirical sources discussed above (focusing especially on Latin American cases). Yamin (2019) is especially compelling on this point.

26 I thank audiences at the Carnegie Mellon University Workshop on Political Philosophy in Bioethics, the London School of Economics and Political Science and UK Faculty of Public Health Paternalism and Public Health Workshop, and the Universidad Austral de Chile International Seminar on Law and Health for feedback on these issues. I also thank Sridhar Venkatapuram and Alison Lockhart for careful editing and assistance.

References

Beitz, C. R. 2011. *The idea of human rights.* Oxford: Oxford University Press. https://doi.org/10.1093/acprof:oso/9780199572458.001.0001.

Beitz, C. R. 2013. What human rights mean. *Daedalus* 132, no. 2: 36–46.

Buchanan, A. and G. Sreenivasan. 2018. Taking international legality seriously: A methodology for human rights. In *Human rights: Moral or legal?*, ed. A. Etison, 211–229. Oxford: Oxford University Press. https://doi.org/10.1093/oso/9780198713258.003.0013.

Coggon, J. and L. O. Gostin. 2015. Beyond medicine, patients, and the law: Policy and governance in 21st century health law. In *Pioneering healthcare law: Essays in honor of Margaret Brazier*, ed. C. Stanton, S. Devaney, A. Farrell, and A. Mullock, 78–88. New York: Routledge.

Cohen, J. 2004. Minimalism about human rights: The most we can hope for? *Journal of Political Philosophy* 12, no. 2: 190–213. https://doi.org/10.1111/j.1467-9760.2004.00197.x.

Cohen, J. 2020. Paradigm under threat: Human rights today. *Health and Human Rights Journal* 22, no. 2: 309–312. https://www.hhrjournal.org/2020/09/paradigm-under-threat-health-and-human-rights-today/ (accessed December 22, 2021).

Da Silva, M. 2018. The international right to health care. *Michigan Journal of International Law* 39, no. 3: 343–384. https://repository.law.umich.edu/mjil/vol39/iss3/3/ (accessed December 22, 2021).

Da Silva, M. 2020. The complex structure of health rights. *Public Health Ethics* 13, no. 1: 99–110. https://doi.org/10.1093/phe/phaa001.

Da Silva, M. 2021. *The Pluralist Right to Health Care: A Framework and Case Study.* Toronto: University of Toronto Press.

Daniels, N. 1985. *Just health care.* Cambridge: Cambridge University Press. https://doi.org/10.1017/CBO9780511624971.

Daniels, N. 2008. *Just health: Meeting health needs fairly.* Cambridge: Cambridge University Press. https://doi.org/10.1017/CBO9780511809514.

Daniels, N. and J. E. Sabin. 2002. *Setting limits fairly: Can we learn to share medical resources?* Oxford: Oxford University Press. https://doi.org/10.1093/acprof:oso/9780195149364.001.0001.

Easterly, W. 2009. Human rights are the wrong basis for healthcare. *Financial Times.* https://www.ft.com/content/89bbbda2-b763-11de-9812-00144feab49a (accessed December 22, 2021).

Etinson, A., ed. 2018. *Human rights: Moral or political?* Oxford: Oxford University Press. https://doi.org/10.1093/oso/9780198713258.001.0001.

Flood C. M. and A. Gross, eds. 2014. *The right to health at the public–private divide: A global comparative study.* Cambridge: Cambridge University Press. https://doi.org/10.1017/CBO9781139814768.

Gauri, V. and D. M. Brinks, eds. 2010. *Courting social justice: Judicial enforcement of social and economic rights in the developing world.* Cambridge: Cambridge University Press. https://doi.org/10.1017/CBO9780511511240.

Gilabert, P. 2018. *Human dignity and human rights.* Oxford: Oxford University Press. https://doi.org/10.1093/oso/9780198827221.001.0001.

Goodman T. 2005. Is there a right to health? *Journal of Medicine and Philosophy* 30, no. 6: 643–662. https://doi.org/10.1080/03605310500421413.

Gostin, L. O. 2001. Public health, ethics, and human rights: A tribute to the late Jonathan Mann. *Journal of Law, Medicine & Ethics* 29, no. 2: 121–130. https://doi.org/10.1111/j.1748-720x.2001.tb00330.x.

Gostin, L. O. 2014. *Global health law.* Cambridge, MA: Harvard University Press.

Hassoun, N. 2020a. *Global health impact: Extending access to essential medicines.* Oxford: Oxford University Press. https://doi.org/10.1093/oso/9780197514993.001.0001.

Hassoun, N. 2020b. The human right to health: A defense. *Journal of Social Philosophy* 51, no. 2: 158–179. https://doi.org/10.1111/josp.12298.

Hessler, K. and A. Buchanan. 2002. Specifying the content of the human right to health care. In *Medicine and social justice: Essays on the distribution of health care*, ed. R. Rhodes, M. Battin, and A. Silvers, 84–101. Oxford: Oxford University Press.

Hohfeld, W. N. 1913. Some fundamental legal conceptions as applied in judicial reasoning. *Yale Law Journal* 23, no. 1: 16–59. https://doi.org/10.2307/785533.

Holmes, S. and C. Sunstein. 1999. *The costs of rights: Why liberty depends on taxes.* New York: W. W. Norton.

King, J. 2012. *Judging social rights.* Cambridge: Cambridge University Press. https://doi.org/10.1017/CBO9781139051750.

Langford, M., ed. 2008. *Social rights jurisprudence: Emerging trends in international and comparative law.* Cambridge: Cambridge University Press. https://doi.org/10.1017/CBO9780511815485.

Langford, M., C. Rodríguez-Garavito, and J. Rossi, eds. 2017. *Social rights judgments and the politics of compliance: Making it stick.* Cambridge: Cambridge University Press. https://doi.org/10.1017/9781316673058.

Liao, S. M. 2019. Human rights and public health ethics. In *The Oxford handbook of public health ethics,* ed. A. C. Mastroianni, J. P. Kahn, and N. E. Kass, 47–56. Oxford: Oxford University Press.

Mann, J., L. Gostin, S. Gruskin, T. Brennan, Z. Lazzarini, and H. V. Fineberg. 1994. Health and human rights. *Health and Human Rights Journal* 1, no. 1: 6–23. https://cdn1.sph.harvard.edu/wp-content/uploads/sites/2469/2014/03/4-Mann.pdf (accessed December 22, 2021).

Meier, B. M. 2007. Advancing health rights in a globalized world: Responding to globalization through a collective human right to health. *Journal of Law, Medicine, and Ethics* 35, no. 4: 545–555. https://doi.org/10.1111/j.1748-720X.2007.00179.x.

Meier, B. M., D. P. Evans, M. M. Kavanagh, J. M. Keralis, and G. Armas-Cardona. 2018. Human rights in public health: Deepening engagement at a critical time. *Health and Human Rights Journal* 20, no. 2: 85–91. https://www.hhrjournal.org/2018/12/perspective-human-rights-in-public-health-deepening-engagement-at-a-critical-time/ (accessed December 22, 2021).

Morales, L. 2018. The discontent of social and economic rights. *Res Publica* 24, no. 2: 257–272. https://doi.org/10.1007/s11158-017-9353-6.

Nixon, S. and L. Forman. 2008. Exploring synergies between human rights and public health ethics: A whole greater than the sum of its parts. *BMC International Health and Human Rights* 8: 2. https://doi.org/10.1186/1472-698X-8-2.

Pavel, C. E. 2019. Healthcare: Between a human and a conventional right. *Economics and Philosophy* 35, no. 3: 499–520. https://doi.org/10.1017/S0266267118000366.

Powers, M. 2015. Health care as human right. *Jurisprudence* 6, no. 1: 138–143. https://doi.org/10.5235/20403313.6.1.138.

Prah Ruger, J. 2006. Toward a theory of a right to health: Capability and incompletely theorized agreements. *Yale Journal of Law & the Humanities* 18, no. 2: 273–326. https://openyls.law.yale.edu/handle/20.500.13051/7382

Rosevear E., R. Hirschl, and C. Jung. 2019. Justiciable and aspirational economic and social rights in national constitutions." In *The future of economic and social rights,* ed. K. G. Young, 37–65. Cambridge: Cambridge University Press. https://doi.org/10.1017/9781108284653.003.

Rumbold, B. E. 2017. The moral right to health: A survey of available conceptions. *Critical Review of International Social and Political Philosophy* 20, no. 4: 508–528. https://doi.org/10.1080/13698230.2014.995505.

Simpson, R. M. 2021. Minimalism, determinancy, and human rights. *Canadian Journal of Law and Jurisprudence* 34, no. 1: 149–169. https://doi.org/10.1017/cjlj.2020.25.

Sreenivasan, G. 2012. A human right to health? Some inconclusive scepticism. *Proceedings of the Aristotelian Society Supplementary Volumes* 86, no. 1: 239–265. https://doi.org/10.1111/j.1467-8349.2012.00216.x.

Sreenivasan, G. 2016. Health care and human rights: Against the split duty gambit. *Theoretical Medicine and Bioethics* 37, no. 4: 343–364. https://doi.org/10.1007/s11017-016-9375-7.

Sunstein, C. R. 1996. Health–health tradeoffs. *University of Chicago Law Review* 63, no. 4: 1533–1571. https://doi.org/10.2307/1600280.

Tobin, J. 2012. *The right to health in international law.* Oxford: Oxford University Press. https://doi.org/10.1093/acprof:oso/9780199603299.001.0001.

United Nations. 1966. *International convention on economic, social, and cultural rights. United Nations Treaty Series* 993: 3.

Venkatapuram, S. 2011. *Health justice: An argument from the capabilities approach.* Cambridge: Polity.

Weinstock, D. 2015a. Health justice after the social determinants of health revolution. *Social Theory & Health* 12, no. 3–4: 437–453. https://doi.org/10.1057/sth.2015.11.

Weinstock, D. 2015b. Integrating intermediate goods to theories of distributive justice. *Res Publica* 21, no. 2: 171–183. https://doi.org/10.1007/s11158-015-9274-1.

Weinstock, D. 2018. Les déterminants sociaux de la santé. *Éthique Publique* 20, no. 2. http://journals.openedition.org/ethiquepublique/4173. DOI: 10.4000/ethiquepublique.4173 (accessed December 22, 2021).

Wenar, L. 2020. Rights. In *The Stanford encyclopedia of philosophy*, ed. E. N. Zalta. https://plato.stanford.edu/entries/rights/ (accessed December 22, 2021).

Wilson, J. 2016. The right to public health. *Journal of Medical Ethics* 42, no. 6: 367–375. https://doi.org/10.1136/medethics-2015-103263.

Wolff, J. 2012. *The human right to health.* New York: W. W. Norton.

Yamin, A. E. 2019. The right to health in Latin America: The challenges of constructing fair limits. *University of Pennsylvania Journal of International Law* 40, no. 3: 695–734. https://scholarship.law.upenn.edu/cgi/viewcontent.cgi?article=1986&context=jil (accessed December 22, 2021).

Yamin A. E. and S. Gloppen, eds. 2011. *Litigating health rights: Can courts bring more justice to health?* Cambridge, MA: Harvard University Press.

Young, K. ed. 2019. *The future of social and economic rights.* Cambridge: Cambridge University Press. https://doi.org/10.1017/9781108284653.

23

DISABILITY JUSTICE AND PUBLIC HEALTH

Agnès Berthelot-Raffard

Introduction

Although impairments, developmental disabilities, chronic diseases, mental illness, and severe injuries are all part of the human condition, one of public health's missions remains to prevent them. Counterintuitively, it can be argued that the goals of reducing mortality, morbidity, and disability have encouraged discrimination, harmful stereotypes, and abuse toward people with disabilities in the healthcare system. This can be made visible if we see that the Industrial Revolution both motivated public health and played a significant role in the mistreatments and coercive institutionalization of people living with disabilities influenced by their relation to "productive labor." In the 1960s, many ethical, political, and epistemological debates emerged about the treatments, stigma, and injustices toward people with disabilities in the healthcare system. These debates emerged alongside the disability rights movements and challenged the views that people living with a temporary or permanent disability are "abnormal," "dysfunctional," or "deviant," "to be fixed" as well as being viewed as "costly" in terms of healthcare resources. Such stereotypes and assumptions highlight the difficult relationship between the disabled and their advocates on the one side, and the public health community, on the other. The relationship was contentious despite both communities sharing the same central concern regarding the promotion of health equity, including realizing equal access to healthcare services. Decades later, even where they have access to healthcare and public health amenities, disabled individuals are still subject to epistemic injustices and stigma (Goldberg 2020). According to the disability rights movement, the meaning of disability, its ontology, phenomenology, and culture do not seem to be accurately understood when it comes to implementing new public health policy, law, and interventions.

This chapter discusses the relationship between public health and disability. Through an examination of the two main models of disability, the social and the medical, the first part of the chapter sets out to define disability and underlines how different meanings of disability represent a significant challenge for public health. The second part presents an analysis of the ethical stakes at the heart of the concept of normal functioning and its relationship with health. And from a disability justice perspective, the last part of this chapter examines how public health should promote health equity to properly center on disability justice. Inspired

DOI: 10.4324/9781315675411-28

by the principle of universal design that promotes equal access for all, the disability justice framework leads to more equal opportunity (Swenor 2021) and distributive justice in public health, irrespective of the abilities or disabilities of those who have access to it (Möller 2015).

Conceptualizing disability

Fifteen percent of the global population is currently living with an impairment—some form of chronic physical or a mental illness that affects their capacity to perform certain social roles. Disabilities are extremely diverse in nature and various situations can create disability. Birth defects (for example, Down syndrome, cerebral palsy, or fetal alcohol syndrome) and developmental conditions affecting children and adolescents lead to substantial functional limitations over their lifespan such as cognitive impairments. And severe injuries (for example, traumatic brain injury) or a chronic disease limiting the capacity to work or live without the support of a caregiver are conditions affecting the lives of many adults around the world.

Prima facie, from the public health perspective, disability is most often assumed to emerge from a specific disease or impairment. Physical incapacities due to a mental illness, chronic ill-health, or intellectual or sensory impairment create limits across a lifespan. Many conditions can exist on a long-term basis, and disability can become permanent. However, many people with disabilities only experience inability on a temporary basis. Indeed, some symptoms of disorders or illness (for example, symptoms of mental illness and fibromyalgia) are not ongoing. Consequently, due to the diversity of conditions, and the fact that each condition does not affect all people in the same way, the term disability does not refer to a static condition. All these disabilities do not have the same impacts on people in their everyday life, on their capacity to perform in a workplace, to receive an education, how they can spend their leisure time, and so forth. The experience of disability is on a continuum experienced by people in multiple social and cultural environments, and with diverse identities shaped by their age, race, ethnicity, gender, sexual orientation, spirituality, and so forth.

In terms of public health, disability is often understood as a condition that affects the capacity to perform basic life activities such as taking a bath, getting dressed, going to the toilets, preparing meals without the support of another person, et cetera. Disability is defined in a negative way—as a limitation that is the direct result of biomedical conditions that prevents a person from being or remaining autonomous in daily life. This kind of understanding of disability leads to measurement of individual or bodily ability/inability to perform daily self-care tasks. And, consequently, the individual is assessed whether they are functional enough to be considered autonomous.

Since the 1950s, healthcare professionals have used measurements such as the Activity of Daily Living (ADL) or the Instrumental Activities of Daily Living (IADL) in the provision of care to people with disabilities. These measurements also serve to evaluate the autonomy of older people in long-term care. Nevertheless, for the disability rights community, such measurements do not necessarily acknowledge the fact that people's ability or inability should also take into account the social environment of the person subjected to such evaluation, and the ways in which a person understands her own autonomy. Moreover, perceptions of function level are dependent on a local culture, and on particular conceptions of autonomy grounded in liberal philosophy. So this approach, for example, does not take relational autonomy (Sherwin 1998) into consideration, which deconstructs the concept of autonomy/independence by highlighting the existing interdependencies among human beings.

The debates between public health and disability studies, in particular, identify the limits of a biomedical definition of limitations. Limitations, and consequently disability experienced by individuals, are not just physiological and psychological as highlighted by biomedical model. Disability also limits people in a broad range of social contexts: the incapacity to work; pay bills or debts; use public transportation; or walk without the assistance of someone else or medical devices such as a stroller or a wheelchair. In North American universities, disability also encompasses the difficulty for some students to complete exams without additional time due to specific conditions (for example, mental illness, brain injury, neurodiversity, chronic illness, and so on). Such a social functioning conception of limitation is shared widely by disability scholars and activists. According to them, disability is not necessarily or only a condition diminishes the health state of a person. Disability is much more—something that is linked with the social environment that impedes the capacity of a person to perform a social role, such as studying or working, or the ability to function in a specific environment because of social barriers.

This social model of disability is not robustly or even minimally incorporated into public health research, policy, law, and interventions. The contrasts between biomedical and social views on disability at the heart of the two different disability models (Wasserman et al. 2016) reflect the complexity public health organizations face when they try to promote interventions and policy addressing the needs of people with disabilities (Lollar and Crews 2003). Promoting interventions in public health requires a balance between the medical and social views of disability. This balance between both views creates a significant challenge for promoting a public health system that includes a disability justice framework as claimed by the disabled's movement.

"Nothing about us without us"

Everywhere in the world people with impairments have always been part of every human society. Historically, despite their loss of capacity to perform movements, sensory limitations due to physical, cognitive, or mental conditions, they may not have necessarily been excluded from their families and communities. This is not to say that disabled individuals have not been treated poorly throughout history. However, the start of the Industrial Revolution in the United Kingdom in the late eighteenth century seems to be pivotal regarding the place of the disabled in societies. The establishment of capitalist production norms created a new imperative of production. Before the Industrial Revolution, labor production was in the hands of the family/village under the aegis of the private patriarchy. Capitalism displaced the line of family labor production and established the state's public patriarchy. A boundary was also created between the public and private spheres, which influenced the separation between the labor market and reproductive/care labor performed by families for sustaining the needs of the most vulnerable. Caregivers taking care of people with disabilities also began to be socially devalued and subjected to "discrimination by association" in the labor market (Berthelot-Raffard 2015a, 2015b).

Since then, the capitalist system has been intertwined with ableism, not least by creating expectations of having the necessary abilities for reaching the labor market's standards of performance. People living with disability began to be seen as socially undesirable because of their inability to perform labor roles in the new capitalist system. From then onward, any sign of weakness, idiosyncrasy, or physical dysfunction began to be regarded as a marker of disorder and disruption from the norms for the able body. Impairments were perceived through notions such as abnormality, pathology, or deviance from this norm. Seen as a deviance from the normal functioning of humanhood, the presence of people with impairments began to motivate implementing specific controls against them in order to exclude bodies that did not follow what was being established as the biostatistical norm of health (Ouellette 2011; Satz 2020).

For the sake of economic and social progress, protecting the "normal" from the "abnormal" became a broad medical and social imperative. This political aspect of modern nation-building led to coercive and violent actions and state policies separating people according to who holds the right to function as a full citizen from those who are not desirable due to their "abnormal" functioning linked to their genes, intellectual or physical capacities, or phenotypes. We should note here that this devaluation of humanhood was also deployed against racialized people, such as indigenous and Black people in North America and Caribbean islands. Black, indigenous people, and people living with impairments were all the targets of a growing eugenics perspective. This perspective aimed for populations with "good" genetic stock and contributed to the implementation of coercive interventions to protect the "normal" from the "abnormal." Until the early twentieth century, people living with mental and cognitive disabilities were segregated from the rest of the population, interned in medical and residential institutions where they received very poor medical treatment and even objectified and used for unethical research, such as the Willowbrook experiment (1956–1970) (Savulescu and Hope 2010). The eugenic perspective also led to the sterilization of many girls and women with intellectual disabilities (Tilley et al. 2012).

During the nineteenth and twentieth centuries, at least in Europe and the United States, the lives of people with severe disabilities were restricted to hospices or rehabilitation facilities where they were subjected to pity, patronization, objectification, or even fetishization. Given the conception of disability as a defect, as a failure of the bodily system that is inherently abnormal and pathological, and a personal tragedy that inflicts damage upon minds and bodies, the related mission of public health became the search for treatments, rehabilitation, or the possibility of cure. For a long time, this conception of disability was embedded in the public health system, and justified medical treatments and other interventions to prevent biological or genetic conditions that could impede the capacity to pursue an ordinary life course. The medical model became hegemonic, encouraging us to frame disability in a very particular way when considering issues such as assisted suicide, euthanasia, and antenatal termination. Even today, professionals in public health still may view disabilities as an individual problem that requires medical as well as legal interventions, as evidenced by the unprecedented case of the young Ashley X (Edwards 2011; Gunther and Dickema 2006; Ouellette 2008; Sobsey 2009).

According to critical disability studies, it was only in the middle of the twentieth century that the conception of disability and lives of people with disabilities began to meaningfully change. With the advancements of women's liberation, Black civil rights issues, and many other struggles, disabled people's movements also emerged leading to a new conceptualization of disability as something social, rather than medical. Diverse people, from those using wheelchairs to those with intellectual disabilities living in residential institutions, created community organizations worldwide to promote disability rights, equal citizenship, and independent living. In the 1960s, the most prominent cause of disability advocates was the deprivations of people with disabilities incarcerated within residential homes. At a time when charity organizations were most often speaking on behalf of people with impairments, people living with disabilities advocating for themselves was itself revolutionary. In September 1972, Paul Hunt, a disability activist living in a residential home, wrote a letter published in the *Guardian* newspaper inviting other disabled individuals to write to him:

> Severely physically handicapped people find themselves in isolated unsuitable institutions where their views are ignored, and they are subject to authoritarian and often cruel regimes. I am proposing the formation of a consumer group to put forward nationally the views of actual and potential residents of these successors of the Workhouse.

Hunt subsequently became a major figure in the United Kingdom, and his self-help approach contributed to understanding of disability as social oppression. Many people living with disabilities responded to his letter, and led to the formation of the Union of the Physically Impaired against Segregation (UPIAS), a forum to debate disability issues for and by disabled people. UPIAS rejected prevailing concepts and norms of disability rights being advocated by people who were not themselves disabled, and yet were allowed to speak and advocate for people living with disabilities. UPIAS went on to significantly challenge general practices and ethics of how people from the medical professions and charities engaged with and treated/controlled disabled people in a paternalistic way.

During the 1980s, across the United Kingdom and internationally, disability studies emerged as a transdisciplinary academic discipline. Notable contributors to research and teaching include Mike Oliver (1945–2019), who proposed a new perspective on disability. Oliver shifted the discourses of statistics, medicine, and law since the nineteenth century that presented impairments as "deviance," "abnormality," or "disorder" (Oliver 1990). His research and analysis illustrated why disability should be understood as a form of social oppression, rather than a physical or functional problem that arises from physical deficits.

The theorization of the social model of disability then further helped to identify systemic barriers, derogatory attitudes, and intentional and inadvertent social exclusions toward disabled people. While rejecting the biomedical model of disability, the social model also calls for equity, social justice, and human rights. Furthermore, as Jane Campbell highlights in her conference presentation titled "Fighting for a Slice, or for a Bigger Cake?": "the social model of disability [...] became the hallmark of [disabled people's] struggle" (Campbell 2008). It began changing the way in which people living with disabilities were seen by non-disabled people, and demonstrated that they were and should be able to participate as equal citizens like the non-disabled.

In the United Kingdom, this shifting paradigm motivated new legislation such as the Disability Discrimination Act in 1995. This Act and other legislation served to extend the moral and functional autonomy of people living with physical or cognitive disability, mental illnesses, hearing and vision impairments, infectious diseases, or other long-term health conditions. This Act acknowledges that people living with disabilities can participate in the labor market and should be granted better access to employment, and education, public transportation and all public services, by removing the barriers that limit or impede their access. The 1990s was also when HIV/AIDS was spreading, and due to the awful ways patients were being treated in medical institutions, the media, and general social life, AIDS and gay rights activists fought for the inclusion of aspects of living with infectious diseases in the definition of disability. Consistent gains such as within the United Kingdom and elsewhere contributed to beginning of eradication of social barriers faced by disabled people—barriers that were economic, political, cultural, relational, or psychological. Unfortunately, change within the public health system regarding disability remains limited partly due the primacy of the conception of normal biological functioning across research, interventions, policies, laws, et cetera.

The normal function and health performance model

Worldwide, disability rights activists and scholars have been promoting inclusion, equal citizenship, and independent living, de-institutionalization, and de-stigmatization of people with disabilities. However, public health as a profession and discipline, largely continues to promote the medical model of disability. The persistence of this model is due to a particular and prominent definition of health. Indeed, as it shall be demonstrated below, disability and health are often conceived of as being opposites. This antinomy is illustrated in the biostatistical concept of normal functioning that conveys a naturalistic conception of health.

As discussed below, a conception of disability was embedded in the medical model, which defined what is normal and what is pathological. This conception was illuminated and theorized by the French philosophers Georges Canguilhem and Michel Foucault (Tremain 2015). The distinction between the normal and the pathological is at the heart of controversial discussions about the validity of the concept of normal functioning as well as the definitions of health.

Health as normal functions

Developed by Christopher Boorse in the 1970s, the concept of health as normal functioning defines in statistical terms the biological functions human beings need to live, survive, and reproduce (Barnes 2020). Boorse argues that physiologically and psychologically, the human organism is anatomically organized to reach or achieve these goals. Normal is defined statistically in terms of the most frequent level of functioning of organisms of same age and sex. Consequently, if an organism's organ or sub-part is not functioning in the statistically normal range for the age and sex group, the organism is seen as abnormal or pathological because of its non-normal functioning.

The concept of normal species functioning does not illuminate the conceptual differences between disability and impairments. The problem with this concept is that pathologies and abnormal functions are seen as mutually overlapping. However, all impairments are not pathological. For example, deafness and blindness may be biostatistically infrequent, but they are not pathologies and do not necessarily need to be treated (Shakespeare 2014). Moreover, all human beings have physical or mental variations that become a source of vulnerability or disadvantage in some settings even though they are not necessarily impaired. In addition, impairments are not static. There are continuous variations of impairments among people and several people who have the same impairment may not function in the same way. Consequently, if people with disabilities have trouble functioning, or if they have poor health outcomes, it is not necessarily because they are impaired. Indeed, depending on their way of life, their job occupation, their mode of leisure, the support they have from their families, caregivers, or social services, all people do not experience what is supposed to be an abnormal function in the same way (Barnes 2020).

As a result, incorporating the notion of normal function in public health leads to thinking that abnormal functions as pathology and not as something influenced by the environment of a person who lives with an impairment. The concept of normal function can be considered to be "ableist" as when it is applied to people's capacities and their performance of some social role is compared to their fellow citizens who are non-disabled. The action that a person is supposed to perform is "biomedically typical of the human species (suitability relativized to age and perhaps sex)" (Amundson 1992: 108). Such a definition puts emphasis on the fact that having an impairment impedes the capacity of a human being to function normally.

A naturalistic view of human being

For an advocate of disability rights, normal function is problematic as it equates health exclusively with the physiological ability to perform an activity or social role. First of all, for critical disability theorists, the problem with this statistical norm is that it tends to be used to define health in terms of a naturalistic view (Barnes 2020). This is considered a problem even if public health needs to measure normal function to explain and regulate mortality, morbidity, and disability. In this view of normal function, health is not a normative concept. It is a naturalistic concept since health is seen as the capacity associated with the norms of human lives. A person can have a normal lifespan when she is without dysfunctions that could prevent her from living normally. Consequently, the concept of normal species functioning connects health with a condition which depends on the capacity to perform something specific (holding something, working, social interactions, et cetera). Moreover, this concept also implicitly promotes an ideal of the good life in a Rawlsian sense. Indeed, an individual with an impairment would be reduced to being a holder of lower function, which renders the person unable to reach the same aspirations as someone who fits within a normal level of abilities.[1] The notion of normal species functioning expresses an ideal of social performance that seems to have little relationship with health but rather society's understanding of the social role based on sex and age. Indeed, the physiological ability to perform an activity or a particular social role, such as having a professional occupation, does not take into account how people with disabilities (as well as elderly people) value their personal activities, even if they do not fit in with existing social standards of functioning (Lanoix 2021). Living with a disability or being elderly does not mean not healthy. Unfortunately, the notion of normal function carries an ableist view. Moreover, the ways in which people with disabilities adapt to their environments are not always considered. Since the concept of normal species functioning is limited to an evaluation of capacities and inabilities, it does not offer the healthcare professionals a deeper understanding of the disabled and the elderly's needs. It also does not offer an understanding of the disability culture.

Furthermore, as the concept of normal function refers to pathology that impedes the normal lifespan, philosophers of public health, such as Norman Daniels with his "prudential lifespan" account, make use of the idea of normal function in their arguments for fair healthcare distribution (Daniels 2007). According to Daniels, healthcare should be a social good, and his account promotes a way to allocate healthcare resources based on health needs. Under a critical disability lens, this concept of needs is limited. The health needs of someone are defined by an estimation of what is normal for people of same age and sex. However, this measurement does not pay enough attention to the social determinants of health. It is not accurate just to base the healthcare needs on the physiological and psychological normal functioning of people in groups of same age and sex. For example, the health determinants of a woman in her sixties who is socially active, working in an office and who has been living in an urban area all her life are different from the health determinants of a woman in same age group who has been living in a rural community and working in professional areas such as agriculture or mining. Both women do not have the same health outcomes, health determinants, and needs, despite being of the same age and sex. This shows how the concept of normal function does not provide an effective method for measuring health and health needs. Furthermore, this concept does not seem consistent with the idea of health equity at the heart of the new public health, and progress being made in our society regarding disability rights.

Eradicating or fixing disability: the mission of public health?

The public health mission is about reducing mortality, morbidity, and disability. In this view, impairments and other conditions under the umbrella of disability are perceived as a problem to be addressed or failure of the public health system. Consequently, public health laws, organizations, and practices could be understood as being rooted in the ableist assumption that disabled people require being cured and controlled under prevention campaigns dedicated to reducing the number of birth defects, injuries, and chronic diseases such as cancer and HIV. Indeed, the mission of public health emphasizes the prevention or eradication of physical or mental impairment due to intellectual or sensory dysfunctions, chronic health conditions, and mental illness (Lollar and Crews 2003). So how can public health pursue its mission while doing justice to those who are disabled? Considering that disability impacts people's capacity to live and perform in society without barriers, the public health's mission should be founded on a universal design which complies with a disability justice framework for promoting health equity.

Public health orients interventions and campaigns to empower people in order to guide them in the development of their abilities, especially so that they can take control of their own physical and mental well-being. This mission promotes a positive vision of health as something of a resource that helps people to participate socially, maintain a good life balance, and live in harmony with their values. And health campaigns promoting the importance of well-being help to sustain the effort toward reaching these valuable goals. Nevertheless, this positive definition of health presupposes that people for whom these campaigns are developed have the capacities to live and function normally in society. Consequently, having an impairment or a particular health condition (for example, a mental health issue) could be seen as something that would prevent self-care.

A contrasting view is that disability is not a failure or a condition that inherently impedes the goals of health promotion. For disability activists and scholars, positive and anti-ableist descriptions of health must drive public health initiatives and programs to strengthen abilities of all people to take control of their own well-being. In this positive description, all people and all dis/abilities are included (Möller 2015). When public health tries to eradicate or to "fix" disability, the field can be seen as failing. Moreover, public health reproduces distinct classifications of people living with disabilities and those who are non-disabled. The public mission geared toward the non-disabled embeds an ableist view that typical or most frequent abilities are superior. Ableism, in public health's organization, laws, and practices is grounded in the primacy of the biomedical model, which stems from a negative description of health (the "absence of disease") and, at the same time, a biostatistical representation of normal functioning.

Also, despite the fact that the disability rights and public health community members share central concerns about health promotion, access and participation, and health equity policies, these communities do not have the same way of defining and applying a disability justice framework (Gaventa, Stahl, and McDonald 2020).

Toward disability justice in public health

Perceptions of what is normal human functioning are exactly what have long been used to restrict the rights of people with disabilities, including their rights to access public health resources. The history of treatment of people with disabilities in the public health system has been shaped by the public beliefs of their deficiency. Implicitly, disability is considered as an antonym of health. As claimed by Wendy Lu, an American disability activist, "disabled people don't need to be fixed."[2] Disability does not need a cure. Furthermore, public health organizations tend to follow official or legal definitions of disability. Some of them are subtly ableist despite them being accepted by government bureaucracies and social service agencies. Many of these official definitions are often based on an ideal view of human abilities (Wendell 1996). Take, for example, the definition of disability proposed by the World Health Organization's *International Classifications of Impairment, Disability and Handicaps* (ICIDH) (WHO 1980). Although it separates impairment and disability, it is limited to the effects of disability and does not include the discrimination faced by people with disabilities. According to this definition, impairments describe any loss or abnormality of a psychological, physiological, or anatomical structure or function and disability defines any restriction or lack of (resulting from an impairment) of ability to perform an activity in the manner of or within the range considered normal for a human being. And, the concept of handicap is defined as the disadvantage that a person with disabilities experiences in his or her environment. Although disability is conceived as a personal limitation arising from the functional impairments that are part of a person's physical constitution—whether those impairments are congenital or acquired—the full consequences of impairment and disability are not well enough reflected in such a definition of handicap.

The notion of social barriers such as due to architecture, the governments' regulations, or professional attitudes are not reflected in the ICIDH. This lack of understanding of the social environmental role in disability has enormous consequences when used to promote an institutional design that is not all-inclusive of people with disability. In contrast, the United Nations' definition of disability handicap seems more inclusive as it highlights the consequences of impairments and disability. In this definition:

> Handicap is, therefore, a function of the relationship between disabled persons and their environment. It occurs when they encounter cultural, physical, or social barriers which prevent their access to the various systems of society that are available to other citizens. Thus, a handicap is the loss of opportunities for taking part in the life of the community on an equal level with others.
>
> *(United Nations 1982)*

Consequently, a new understanding of the notion of handicap was reflected in the revision of the ICIDH in 1993. The new document, *International Classification of Functioning, Disability and Health* (ICF), acknowledges environmental barriers and how they impede the capacity of people with disabilities to participate in society (Lollar and Crews 2003).

At the same time, public health ethicists constantly work to develop ethical guidelines to resist or prevent the mistreatment of individuals, particularly those considered vulnerable by researchers and healthcare providers. In order to promote a disability justice framework, people with disabilities must be included in the decision-making process. Unfortunately, even if we are living in an apparently more inclusive society, people with disabilities are still at the margins when it comes to making decisions about their needs within the public health system. They are still excluded from this public health debate. As expressed in the Convention of the Rights of Persons with Disabilities (CRDP): "Persons with disabilities have the right to the enjoyment of the highest attainable standard of health without discrimination on the basis of disability" (United Nations 2006).

Disability rights activists and scholars go beyond a negative or a positive description of health. They offer a different and more proper understanding of what disability means. Indeed, the disability rights community and the public health community share the same concern regarding the access for all individuals in the healthcare system and their equal treatment. And, they share a central interest in the protection of the most vulnerable communities. Nevertheless, disability advocates have pushed for "supported decision-making," which brings people living with disabilities to the decision-making table. Many public health policies and programs reflect stigma associated with disability and the misinformation regarding the capacities of people with disabilities to have a good quality of life. The disability community considers that the real tragedy is not due to the fact of disability itself but rather because of the failure of social support, and the lack of intervention that reflects that lives of people with disability are equally valued.

As activists and scholars, the disability rights community, which is diverse, shares the aim of deconstructing the idea of disability as a curse or a personal tragedy. Emphasizing the social oppression of people with disabilities, the disability rights community promotes the protection of people with disabilities as a group. They struggle against the subtle exclusion of people with disabilities from society. In particular, they have fought against the systematic exclusion of persons with disabilities from employment and education. They have also used personal narratives to counter the systematic devaluation of people with disabilities in popular culture. And they have taken part in discourses that resist the ableist public health view of disability.

The tension between the fields of public health professionals and researchers and the disability scholars and activists can be partly explained by the different levels of awareness or knowledge regarding the lived experience of being disabled. It can be said that people with disabilities share a common "moral knowledge" (Scully 2008, cited by Garland-Thompson 2017: 329) regarding their common experience of social oppression. This knowledge is not accessible for those who are not currently disabled, or are not family members or caregivers of someone with disabilities. When the two communities talk about disability, they often do not have the same understanding of what its meaning and experience. In medical and legal settings, disability can often only be seen as impairments that involve pain and suffering, or as being incompatible with a good life. Disability can also be narrowly understood as a severe condition that prevents independent living. In response, the disability rights community pleads for a different kind of epistemic ethics and understanding regarding their experiences, their realities, and their needs.

The difference between public health and disability rights communities can also be explained through an analysis of moral psychology—an investigation of human actions in moral contexts. A conflict exists between the public health and the disability rights communities when it comes to an understanding of the real-life experience of disability. Due to a lack of knowledge on the phenomenology of disability, public health professionals and researchers, bioethicists and legal scholars do not have the epistemic resources to understand the norms and culture of the disability communities. As a result, they do not easily recognize or acknowledge the social context of oppression within which a person with disabilities can make a supposed choice or exercise autonomy. They also do not understand how the conditions created by this context compromise the authenticity of the individual's choice.

Public health originates from a position of privilege and reflects the social power of those who are non-disabled. It reflects the norms and values of the majority and their moral perception of people with disabilities. Public health also follows an ethical reasoning framework that does not pay attention to human interdependency, and the fact that people who are not currently disabled could become disabled in the future, or at least vulnerable. Following the principles of feminist ethics of care, a disability perspective in public health would center the discussion on the subjective experience of vulnerability, on the necessity to develop a relational conception of autonomy to encompass this fact of human life, and allows people with disabilities to explain their own experiences without being patronized by those who do not experience disability. This requirement for the abled also motivates disability activists and scholars to also think about their realities through ethical principles and arguments. There is much that both communities can learn from each other.

As a feminist disability philosopher, I agree with Rosemarie Garland-Thompson that public health ethicists and disability scholars and human rights activists really need to learn from each other. In my view, the divide between public health professions and people who live with disabilities is grounded in what Miranda Fricker calls "testimonial injustices" (Fricker 2007: 27). In this regard, public health needs to develop an anti-oppressive praxis that promotes epistemic justice toward the experience of people living with disabilities. Garland-Thompson advocates for the development of disability bioethics to guide public health fields. Centered on the disability experience and epistemology, this would allow articulating knowledge and informing knowledge produced in the social sciences, humanities, social services, and public policy. Garland-Thompson writes, "Disability bioethics is to strengthen the cultural, political, institutional, and material environment in which people with disabilities can most effectively flourish" (2017: 330). Epistemic justice is the key to reaching this flourishment.

According to Garland-Thompson, disability is an "essential characteristic of being human" (2017: 328). Ontologically vulnerable, all human beings need care and assistance to live. But, in our society, vulnerability is not valued enough. Nobody seems to pay attention to the knowledge that arises from the experience of living with a disabled body. As with other marginalized groups, people with disabilities hold knowledge of their own realities. They have an "embodied cognition" meaning a moral knowledge or a politicized consciousness within which they construct an independent self-definition (Hill Collins 2009: 111) coming from their experience of navigating a society that is not created for their flourishing. Through its theoretical and descriptive dimensions, disability bioethics can allow theorizing this experience while facilitating the construction of a material environment that improves the quality of the lives of those with disabilities. A disability bioethics should propose a tool to better understand and integrate the people with disabilities' lives: a "disability cultural competence," which "involves five interconnected elements: 1) biomedical decision-making 2) disability culture and history 3) accessible technology and design 4) disability legislation and social justice and 5) disability cultural competence research" (Garland-Thompson 2017: 335).

Taking the experiences of people living with disabilities seriously may have important implications for health policy. Disabled people are not frequently included in many public health policy discussions. Health professionals tend to see their conditions as far worse than what is reported by the disabled community itself. The idea of disability cultural competence promotes a better understanding of how the social and cultural structure shapes the health outcome. This tool also opens the conversation on disability, and to participate in disability literacy. Even if someone is non-disabled today, this person cannot be sure that she will never be disabled. Garland-Thompson mentions that even when someone becomes disabled due to an injury or from an illness, due to a lack of disability cultural competency (Garland-Thompson 2017: 331), this individual is not equipped with the necessary information in order to effectively live with her new disability. In other words, a disability cultural competency answers these questions: What is a disability? What is the experience of people with disabilities? How to live with a disability? How to include the experience of people living with disabilities in our institutions?

Public health ethics must include a disability curriculum that takes into consideration the history, the culture—including the disability narratives—and the theories of the disability movements. Moreover, a disability culture that goes beyond the experience of people with disabilities to include their families and caregivers should be promoted. In addition, this disability culture should also promote disability pride and participate in developing a positive identity for those who are disabled. And, a disability cultural competency would focus on tools for flourishing and reaching a high quality of life. That also means the promotion of the acceptance of people with disabilities where they are. They should be supported in learning how to be disabled rather than trying to push themselves to reach the standards of a non-disabled society.

I postulate that the relationship between the disability rights field and the public health field does not only related to the way in which disability and health have been theorized and constructed. The differences between the two areas are more an expression of our performance-based society and the way it interferes with health management. Instead of being based on a feminist ethic of care that recognizes the interdependence between individuals and the vulnerability of each, the healthcare system distinguishes between two categories of human beings. On the one hand, there are those who are able-bodied, and consequently meet the standards of good health defined by health promotion and, on the other hand, those who are vulnerable because of their different level of functioning. The presence of these two categories of people express, in fact, the way in which the performance society we are all living in does not allow people to be vulnerable. The tragic history of people with disabilities within the healthcare system demonstrates the interconnection between the standards of a capitalist society and the creation and subjugation by the norms of able bodies. Nevertheless, a feminist ethics of care promotes the recognition of those who are vulnerable, and those who take care of them, and acknowledges our mutual dependency and challenges the politics behind the ideal of our performance society whereby being vulnerable or disabled, or taking care of people who are in these situations are viewed as limiting the development of the capitalist production.

Conclusion

Following the initial claim that public health and disability rights share a difficult relationship, this chapter has briefly reviewed the conceptualization of disability and its interconnection with the definition of health through the notion of normal function. There are four basic points to remember. First, historically, the disability community has been active in challenging the ways in which people living with disabilities have been subjected to mistreatments, harmful stereotypes, and injustices. Disability activists and scholars make the case that disability should be understood as a form of social oppression, rather than only as a physical or functional problem that arises from physical impairments. Second, the concept of normal function within an ideal of social performance of roles has no relationship with health. In fact, normal function limits the understanding of differences in human capacities for performing a social role. Third, with regard to positive and negative descriptions of health, I have demonstrated that the health promotion mission has understood health as something to be performed. The conception of health in which health promotion is embedded separates bodies who can perform with good health. Fourth, through disability cultural competence, we are able to have a better understanding of how social and cultural structures can shape health outcomes. The values of capitalism bear a particular view about what health is, and about the standards of normal functioning. The implementation of the disability cultural competence would sustain society where everybody vulnerable will not to be pushed to perform according to standards that are derived from capitalism and ableism/capacitism. Promoting a new framework would help to shift the moral reasoning on disability. At the same time, the disability justice framework would promote a new vision about the lives of all human beings and the worth of their social contributions. The implementation of the disability cultural competence would work toward the eradication of what I have coined "capacitalism,"[3] which represents the interconnection between the ability and economic performance standards imposed by capitalism.

Notes

1 For more discussion of this issue, please refer to the debates on the "marginal case" in animal ethics in which Eva Fedder Kittay (2009) opposes Jeff McMahan's arguments.

2 Wendy Lu's narrative statement has been published on the blog *Everyday Feminism,* on May 21, 2018. The disability activist spoke up about the way in which people tend to think that disability can be cured. She suggests curing ableism instead.

3 It should be noted that in French the word *ableism* is translated as *capacitisme* in relation to capacities. This word being close to the word *capitalism,* I propose the term *capacitalism* to describe how the ability standards are interlocked in the standard of economic performance imposed by capitalism, a society that claims that people should be capable to constantly overcome themselves.

References

Barnes, E. 2020, Disability, health and normal function. In *Disability, health law and bioethics*, ed. I. G. Cohen, C. Shachar, A. Silvers, and M. A. Stein, 5–19. Cambridge: Cambridge University Press. https://doi.org/10.1017/9781108622851.

Berthelot-Raffard, A. 2015a. La discrimination par association: Une expression du *care* dominé. *La Revue des Sciences Sociales* 52: 102–109. https://doi.org/10.4000/revss.3236.

Berthelot-Raffard, A. 2015b. Penser le *care* comme cœur de la justice: Un outil pour analyser une des institutions de la vie ordinaire. In *Le care: Éthique féministe actuelle*, ed. S. Bourgeaut and J. Perreault, 117–132. Montréal: Les Éditions du Remue-Ménage.

Campbell, J. 2008. Fighting for a slice, or for a bigger cake? Sixth annual disability lecture, St John's College, University of Cambridge. https://disability-studies.leeds.ac.uk/wp-content/uploads/sites/40/library/Campbell-Fighting-for-a-slice-of-the-cake-FINAL-FINAL-29-04-08.pdf (accessed December 23, 2021).

Daniels, N. 2007. *Just health: Meeting health needs fairly.* Cambridge: Cambridge University Press. https://doi.org/10.1017/CBO9780511809514.

Edwards, S. D. 2011. The case of Ashley X. *Clinical Ethics* 6, no. 1: 39–44. https://doi.org/10.1258%2Fce.2011.011007.

Fricker, M. 2007. *Epistemic injustice: Power & the ethics of knowing.* New York: Oxford University Press.

Garland-Thompson, R. 2017. Disability bioethics: From theory to practice. *Kennedy Institute of Ethics Journal* 27, no. 2: 323–339. https://doi.org/10.1353/ken.2017.0020.

Gaventa, B., D. Stahl, and K. McDonald. 2020. Public health ethics and disability: Centering disability justice. In *Public health perspectives on disability: Science, social justice, ethics and beyond*, ed. D. J. Lollar, W. Horner-Johnson, and K. Froehlich-Grobe, 129–148. New York: Springer.

Goldberg, D. 2020. Epistemic injustice, disability stigma and public health law. In *Disability, health law and bioethics*, ed. I. G. Cohen, C. Shachar, A. Silvers, and M. A. Stein, 33–46. Cambridge: Cambridge University Press. https://doi.org/10.1017/9781108622851.

Gunther, D. and D. Dickema. 2006. Attenuating growth in children with profound developmental disability. *Archives of Pediatrics and Adolescence Medicine* 160, no. 10: 1013–1017. https://doi.org/10.1001/archpedi.160.10.1013.

Hill Collins, P. 2009. *Black feminist thought: Knowledge, consciousness and the politics of empowerment.* New York: Routledge.

Kittay, E. 2009. The personal is philosophical is political: A philosopher and mother of a cognitively disabled person sends notes from the battlefield. *Metaphilosophy* 40, no. 3–4: 606–627. https://doi.org/10.1111/j.1467-9973.2009.01600.x.

Lanoix, M. 2021. Aging and the prudential lifespan account. *Medicine, Health Care and Philosophy* 24, no. 3: 351–366. https://doi.org/10.1007/s11019-021-10009-4.

Lollar, D. and J. Crews. 2003. Redefining the role of public health in disability. *Annual Review of Public Health* 24: 195–208. https://doi.org/10.1146/annurev.publhealth.24.100901.14084.

Möller, A. 2015. Disability from a public health perspective. *Scandinavian Journal of Public Health* 43, suppl.16: 81–84. https://doi.org/10.1177/1403494814568601.

Oliver, M. 1990. *The politics of disablement.* London: Macmillan.

Ouellette, A. 2008. Growth attenuation, parental choice, and the rights of disabled children: Lessons from the Ashley X case. *Houston Journal of Health & Policy* 8: 207–244. https://www.law.uh.edu/hjhlp/volumes/Vol_8_2/Ouellette.pdf (accessed December 23, 2021).

Ouellette, A. 2011. *Bioethics and disability: Towards a disability conscious bioethics.* Cambridge: Cambridge University Press.

Satz, A. B. 2020. Healthcare as eugenics. In *Disability, health law and bioethics*, ed. I. G. Cohen, C. Shachar, A. Silvers, and M. A. Stein, 20–32. Cambridge: Cambridge University Press. https://doi.org/10.1017/9781108622851.

Savulescu, J. and T. Hope. 2010. The ethics of research. In *The Routledge companion to ethics*, ed. S. Skorupski, 781–795. London: Routledge.

Shakespeare, T. 2014. *Disability rights and wrongs revisited.* 2nd edition. London: Routledge.

Sherwin, S. 1998. A relational approach to autonomy in health care. In *Health care ethics in Canada*, ed. F. Baylis, B. Hoffmaster, S. Sherwin, and K. Borgerson, 242–258. Toronto: Nelson Education.

Sobsey, D. 2009. Cutting-edge treatment: Pain and surgery in the Ashley X case. *Development Disabilities Bulletin* 37, no. 1: 63–90. https://eric.ed.gov/?id=EJ920690 (accessed December 23, 2021).

Swenor, B. K. 2021. Including disability in all health equity efforts: An urgent call to action. *The Lancet Public Health* 6, no. 6: e359–e360. https://doi.org/10.1016/s2468-2667(21)00115-8.

Tilley, E. J. Walmsley, S. Earle, and D. Atkinson. 2012. "The silence is roaring": Sterilization, reproductive rights and women with intellectual disability. *Disability and Society* 27, no. 3: 413–426. https://doi.org/10.1080/09687599.2012.654991.

Tremain, S., ed. 2015. *Foucault and the government of disability.* Ann-Arbor: University of Michigan. https://doi.org/10.3998/mpub.8265343.

United Nations. 1982. World programme of action concerning disabled persons. https://www.un-.org/development/desa/disabilities/resources/world-programme-of-action-concerning-disabled-persons.html (accessed December 23, 2021).

United Nations. 2006. United Nations convention on the rights of persons with disabilities. https://www.un.org/disabilities/documents/convention/convention_accessible_pdf.pdf (accessed December 23, 2021).

Wasserman, D., A. Ash, J. Blustein, and D. Putman. 2016. Disability: Definitions, models, experience. In *The Stanford encyclopedia of philosophy*, ed. E. N. Zalta. https://plato.stanford.edu/entries/disability/ (accessed December 23, 2021).

Wendell, S. 1996. *The rejected body: Feminist philosophical reflections on disability.* New York: Routledge.

WHO (World Health Organization). 1980. *International classification of impairments, disabilities and handicaps.* Geneva: WHO. https://apps.who.int/iris/bitstream/handle/10665/41003/9241541261_eng.pdf;jsessionid (accessed December 23, 2021).

24

AGEING AND JUSTICE IN HEALTH

A conceptual map toward a unified view

Kebadu Mekonnen Gebremariam and Ritu Sadana

Introduction

Global population projections indicate that the number of older persons aged 60 or over is expected to more than double between 2020 and 2050, which would be a rise from just over 1 billion to 2.1 billion (UN 2019). The demographic transition occurring in many societies, and in the world as a whole, in terms of population aging due to increasing longevity and declining fertility is well known and has some key, projected, and predicable milestones. For example, in 2020, for the first time in recorded history, there were more people aged 65 and over living in the world than children under five years. Moreover, these population ageing dynamics are not limited to high-income countries where life expectancy is the highest; two-thirds of older people live in middle-income countries.

Although there is no typical older person, on average, with increasing age, many people experience higher rates of disease and disability, including chronic conditions or multiple morbidities. Older people also experience declines in physical and cognitive capacities. However, there is tremendous variability within and across countries regarding both (WHO 2015). In response, the United Nations (UN) policy frameworks, including the Sustainable Development Goal on health (in Agenda 2030) assert that, at each age, people should have access to health promotion – these can be across many sectors; services to prevent ill health including screening; treatment for ill health; rehabilitation services; palliative care – this is end of life but not limited to older adults as needed, whether these are provided in health facilities, in community settings, or at home (UN 1948, 2015). Moreover, optimizing people's functioning and well-being in their current environments, at whichever level of physical or cognitive capacity, is the goal of "healthy ageing," a concept endorsed by the World Health Organization (WHO) in 2016 and within the UN Decade of Healthy Ageing 2021–2030. This requires that the immediate environments where people live should offer equitable access to health-promoting opportunities, strive to eliminate negative environmental exposures (for example, air pollution), as well as mitigate decline in individual capacities, such as through improved household and community design, including appropriate transportation options that enable older people to get where they need and want to go (WHO 2015, 2020).

Concerning health and social care services, older persons might require more frequent visits to health facilities, or at home visits by health and social care providers. On average,

DOI: 10.4324/9781315675411-29

where services are available, per capita costs for health services for older people can be higher than for younger people. This has far-reaching consequences for wider concerns of social equity and justice. Older persons with the greatest health needs tend to also be those with the least access to institutional, social, and financial resources. This is particularly the case for older persons who live alone or only with other older people aged 60 and over (WHO 2020). For many older people with longer-term care needs, most of the care is provided by families—overwhelmingly by female relatives. This is a consistent finding across high-, middle-, and low-income countries. It means that neglecting the legitimate care needs of older persons can set off a series of unjust outcomes, starting with the older person and much beyond. All of the above shows that societies currently do not consistently value and invest in maintaining the capacities of older people, or foster their abilities essential for well-being, as they should.

More broadly, there are age-related inequalities in the coverage of health services and in the environments that are health-promoting. Some are justifiable, while others are not. For example, bestowing equal moral concern to people in terms of health may mean inequality in the provision of health services, such as increased investment in early life and at older age than other ages. Yet, in some societies, there is a presumption or prevailing view that providing adequate and affordable health services for older persons is too costly to societies, or futile or wasteful. However, research indicates that it can be affordable and of great overall social benefit across high-, middle-, and low-income countries. This is due to an overestimation of the costs of services for older persons (Williams et al. 2019), and the often overlooked but critically important benefits to society, including social capital created by older adults experiencing healthy ageing (a phenomenon referred to as "the third demographic dividend") (Fried 2016).

Poor health at older age is, for the most part, inappropriately explained away by invoking biological factors, or a "natural" process, and as a consequence identifying poor health and old age with a fatalistic air of inevitability. Some may see poor health in later life as due to poor luck or a tragedy. However, our chances in life, including healthy life expectancy, are greatly determined by social, economic, and other structural factors, and their interaction with our individual traits and behaviors. The overwhelming importance of social determinants of health (SDOH), which are outside a person's control and yet not random brute luck, cannot but be central to assess justice and health (Ben-Shlomo and Kuh 2002; Kuh et al. 2014; Sadana et al. 2016). This includes the extent to which older people experience healthy ageing. Furthermore, inequalities in brute luck often translate into health inequalities through social determinants. In sum, there is no natural reason that functioning (understood as an individual's internal physical and mental capacities interacting with their surrounding environment) should significantly decline with increasing age, if the background institutions of society and environments are supportive.

For every individual, social determinants influence, on the one hand, the extent to which capacities are built up and maintained. And on the other hand, they determine the onset of morbidities and rate of decline in capacities. Moreover, social determinants do not only mean national factors. Trajectories of health are influenced by local and global events (also shaped by policy choices). This is demonstrated by two events at the start of this decade: the COVID-19 pandemic that has predominantly resulted in deaths of older people (as of late 2021) (WHO 2021a, 2022), and the opportunity for global action driven by the UN Sustainable Development Goals (Agenda 2030) and the UN declaration of a Decade of Healthy Ageing (2021–2030) (UN 2020). That being the case, which policy choices will be resourced and implemented over the next decade by national governments and global institutions, and what kind of measurable impact that will have on the lives of older people, remains to be seen.

Our aim in this chapter is three-fold. First is to provide a conceptual map of the problem of distributive justice in health across age groups by utilizing the two approaches of conceptualizing the ageing process: the life course and life stages approaches. Second is to show how three different conceptions of justice can provide insight into the general debate about the requirements of social justice, and we use that insight to highlight the specific problems of justice that relate to population ageing. Our third aim is to explore the practical policy implications of the two ageing process approaches for addressing age-related inequalities in health. This includes exploring three future scenarios regarding inequalities (deterioration, stagnation, and improvement) in light of the commitments made in the UN Decade for Healthy Ageing and its policy implications. The argumentative thrust of this chapter is that older persons are owed, as a matter of justice, the social provision of conditions to create sufficient functional abilities that are essential to leading a dignified life.

Healthy ageing through the prism of life course and life stages approaches

From a population science perspective, healthy ageing in later ages is influenced by multiple factors throughout the life course. These factors include cumulative impacts that start from before we are born and through to factors at each age or stage of the life course. There are also certain "programming mechanisms and exposures" that may occur at sensitive time periods during the life course, and sort people into different and dynamic life course trajectories. From a justice perspective, these events taken together reflect and shape one's opportunities in life. Policies and actions must, therefore, consider what we can do across the entire life course to enhance reserves of people's capacities, delay declines in capacities, and when declines occur, to modify, or slow the rate of decline (Kuh et al. 2014).

Life course perspective

A life course perspective asserts that, first, a person's intrinsic capacity during early development and during critical stages or periods of life can be influenced by a diverse range of factors (biological, socioeconomic, and environmental) (WHO 2020). This, in turn, influences the age of attainment of peak functioning and the potential onset and rate of declines. This means that health and other interventions targeting pregnancy, infancy, childhood, and adolescence, aimed at enhancing intrinsic capacity in the first half of life, can also help individuals to attain their full health potential, and thereby promote fair access to the attendant age-relative ranges of opportunities for pursuing life plans. Moreover, healthy lifestyles and enabling environments during adulthood help to maintain intrinsic capacities even after peak capacity is obtained (Figure 24.1). These factors minimize the risk of early declines in physical and mental capacities. Examples include reducing the incidence of noncommunicable diseases (NCDs) such as cardiovascular and chronic lung disease, diabetes, and some forms of cancer, associated with accelerated declines in capacities at older ages. Enabling environments can also mitigate declines in capacities by supporting individuals to maintain their abilities to be and do what they value, such as through better design of homes, public transport for people of all ages, lifelong learning opportunities, flexible working conditions,

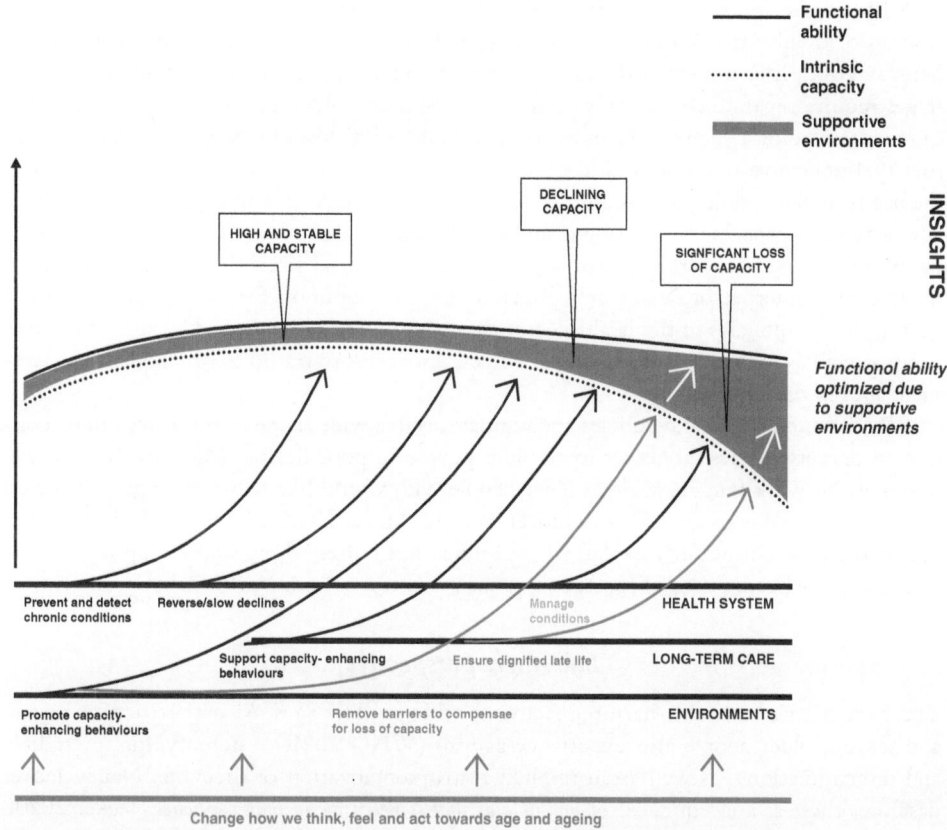

Figure 24.1 Trajectories of healthy ageing: optimizing functional ability (WHO 2020)

intergenerational social networks, and social care and support for those with significant loss of capacities (Figure 24.1).

Second, SDOH literature adds further insight into the cumulative health impact of social and economic disadvantages or, indeed, privilege that sorts people into different life course trajectories. These trajectories shape opportunities and vulnerabilities as people age and contribute to people's functional abilities. Furthermore, intergenerational transmission of social disadvantages (or privileges), where effects of advantage or disadvantage become embedded in genetic material and passed on, can alter healthy ageing trajectories from birth.

Third, almost all of these underlying social and structural determinants are amenable to change through public policy. Results from an analysis of longitudinal cohort studies (that track the same people over time) report the positive impacts that higher levels of education, wealth, and physical activity have on trajectories that lead to better health at older ages (Moreno-Agostino et al. 2020; Wu et al. 2020). A combination of structural changes that improve socioeconomic conditions for vulnerable social groups, healthy lifestyles, coverage of health and long-term care services, and enabling environments during adulthood can improve the trajectories of both intrinsic capacity and functional ability for each person, or for a group of people (Figure 24.1).

A life course approach can help map out the interdependence of socioeconomic opportunities or disadvantages and health status at earlier stages in life, with health status at the latter stages in life. Importantly, however, health-determining factors specific to older life stages require separate consideration. In many countries, older age coincides with the end of remunerated or valued work, and with that comes some loss of power and social status in society. Public investment in health, education, and economic security often tends to neglect the needs of older adults, which, in turn, contributes to the decline in capacities and abilities at older age. A probable loss of power and social standing can occur due to one or a combination of factors: not working, care dependency, or financial stress that is amplified due to institutional, interpersonal, and self-directed ageism. Common forms of institutionalized ageism include policies in the health sector that allow care to be rationed by age rather than need, as well as discriminatory hiring practices, less access to training, or mandatory retirement ages in the labor sector.

When combined, public policies and regulations in a wide range of countries can be considered perverse—these together force older people in poor health, with limited financial resources, to work longer, whereas older people who would like to work longer are forced to stop working due to a mandatory retirement age (Madero-Cabib et al. 2020). These types of situations cannot be fully explained, and much less redressed, by solely adopting the life course approach: adopting a life stages approach is also required.

Life stages perspective

There are particular health-harming factors specific to older ages. As with structural racism and sexism, older people also experience ageism (WHO 2021c)—stereotyping, prejudice, and discrimination—as well as an implicit instrumentalization of their life. Nancy Jecker describes these as consequences of *midlife bias that is pervasive in many societies* (Jecker 2020). Midlife bias involves applying the values that are central to midlife, such as the capacity for autonomy, to all life stages. It figures as an underlying attitude about human values, choices, and behavior that privileges a particular life stage, particularly midlife in which human beings are generally considered to be at the peak of their cognitive and physical capacities, and are valued for specific economic or reproductive roles. Such bias is also reflected, for example, in the attitude toward the education of children; their education is often deemed valuable, instrumentally, for the cultivation of their capacity for autonomy later as adults (Buchanan et al. 2000; Feinberg 1980).

We ought to care about the autonomy of older persons for interconnected reasons. One reason is that it is an indispensable component of respect for persons. Another reason relates to the special responsibility we have to our fellow citizens to treat them as free and equal members of the political community. But this does not imply that autonomy ought to be the singular, or overriding, value at older life stages. Increased risk for chronic disease and disabilities may justify making the value of respecting and preserving human dignity more central. Taking autonomy at midlife as the epitome of one's true self, on the one hand, results in thinking of older life in purely instrumental terms—as a means for preserving the autonomy had or gained at midlife. And, on the other hand, it entrenches the view that equates ageing with decline and loss. One way of avoiding the midlife bias is to conceive of autonomy as both diachronic and relational, in the sense that autonomy is exercised over time for which social relations are indispensable (Baumann 2008; Christman 2007). While avoiding the midlife bias is indispensable, other reasons may still require that societies should do their best to maintain or increase individual functioning despite decline in intrinsic capacities older age may bring.

The available data on ageing and health also shows that age-relative inequalities are so pervasive that they prima facie raise concerns of social (in)justice. As part of efforts to establish a global baseline, in 2020 the WHO collated and analyzed comparable and nationally representative data on the ability of older people to meet their basic needs. The data was primarily from high-income countries and some middle- and low-income countries. According to the data collected from more than 127,000 people aged 60 and over from 37 countries, the majority of older people (86%) scored in the highest score band of 80–100. However, our attention should focus on the remaining 14% of older people who are unable to meet some of the basic needs necessary for a life of meaning and dignity. This 14% represents some 71 million older people across the 37 countries studied (WHO 2020). Extrapolating the results from the 37 countries to the world, a key finding is that at least 142 million older persons are unable to meet at least some of their basic needs. This finding provides only a snapshot and is probably an underestimation of the global context, given the selected range of countries with data. Moreover, these data were collated and analyzed prior to the start of the COVID-19 pandemic.

That there is a great spectrum in intrinsic capacities (WHO 2020) underlines the assertion that there is no typical older person, and that declines in capacities are neither automatic nor symmetrical to age. The evidence of a wide spread in functioning also highlights a policy imperative. Policies should consider ways to shift the entire distribution, and not only to improve an average. Improving population averages, although a worthy goal, will not necessarily solve distributive injustice, a pressing problem especially regarding something that can legitimately be claimed as a right. Improving averages may also lead to neglect of the worst-off. Furthermore, one of the main challenges in developing policy choices regarding older people is that despite such great variation in functioning, all people who are 60 and older are often lumped into one single age demographic category. Policies and programs need to be informed by disaggregated data, by age groups above 60. This would better document and reveal the lived experiences of individuals and age groups often erased by the 60 and older category.

Unsurprisingly, the richest countries in the world have the highest life expectancies. And there is currently a maximum difference of 33 years for life expectancy at birth between rich countries and the rest, where most older people live. Among those who reach the age of 60 worldwide, those who live in rich countries can expect to live up to twelve more healthy years than their contemporaries from other countries (WHO 2021a). At the same time, care needs are far higher for older people living in sub-Saharan Africa than for people of similar ages in higher-income countries. That is, just as some in the 90+ age group can be healthier than people twenty years younger, a significant proportion of older people in one country can be much healthier than many of the youngest of the older people in other countries. In Ghana, for instance, more than 50% of people between the ages of 65 and 75 required assistance with daily activities, while the percentage jumps to 65% for those 75 years and older. As a comparison, in Switzerland, for the same age groups, the percentages are less than 5% and 20%, respectively (WHO 2017).

Globally, the proportion of time spent in ill-health has slightly increased at birth and at age 60 (WHO 2021a). Despite the variation within and across countries, the fact that the time spent in ill-health has increased with age makes older persons vulnerable to experiencing structural adversities—to the very same social determinants that are partly responsible for producing ill-health in the first place.

All of this research from the baseline study and others raises the question what is, if anything, distinctive about age-related inequalities in health that can or do generate obligations to societies? What weight should societies give to this age-related health inequalities? And how should they determine responsibility in responding to the inequalities in health that are caused by brute bad luck such as hereditary older-age-onset syndromes? We would argue that answering these questions requires identifying those inequalities between age groups that are distinctively salient for considerations of justice. In addition, we need to establish what are the things that older people have reason to value, and the normative weight we ought to give their interests in contrast to the interests and values of younger age groups. This is precisely what it means to adopt a life stages approach to healthy ageing.

The assertion that there are distinct life stages does not, however, mean that life stages represent a natural and enduring distinction. For example, in many societies, individuals are granted full autonomy rights at age eighteen, although we know that biologically the brain's prefrontal cortex is not fully developed until age twenty-five or so, with biological differences between women and men. And the traditional association of life stages with socially structured stages in life, such as education, work, reproduction, and retirement are shifting with changing ways of life, including longer lives. However, the stratification of life stages as it is currently embedded in our social structures fundamentally determines our opportunities in life and thus has a practical relevance.

The life stages approach is indispensable for articulating the institutional and social manifestations of the midlife bias, more specifically giving an account for how ageism figures in health services rationing in both normal and emergency settings. Moreover, it helps in articulating these structural problems from the standpoint of age-relativity of values and provides a groundwork for the following claims: older people have rights to lead a healthy and dignified life, regardless of their place in the social distribution of income or social status. With respect to basic entitlements that they are owed, older persons should not be disadvantaged on the basis of their perceived economic value to society, a practice that is neither accurate nor ethical.

Age groups and birth cohorts: an integrated approach

Not all problems of justice for health relating to the fair treatment of older persons can be modeled on fairness between age groups. One reason being that, since we all age, age group distinction can be a synchronic but not a diachronic basis of comparison. The institutions that currently disfavor an older person are usually the same ones from which the person may have unfairly benefited at earlier age. Moreover, it is difficult to adequately capture interpersonal injustices across time on the basis of age group distinction in the same way as unjust treatment of people on the basis of gender and skin color that invariably operates across the life course. Where there is social progress with respect to inequalities between genders and that of racialized groups, such progress is more tractable by looking at how it improves the lives of different birth cohorts within these groups. Similarly, Norman Daniels asserts that "we should distinguish age groups, which do not age, from birth cohorts, which do, and provide an integrated solution to the distinct problems of distributive justice that arise from each" (Daniels 2008: 476).

To illustrate the problem of justice between birth cohorts, take the baby boomer generation in the United States and Western Europe—the demographic cohort born between the end of World War II and the mid-1960s. They are currently between 57 and 75 years old, and comprise the largest birth cohort among older adults, namely, the 65–75 age group; they are double the size of the 75–85 age group (US Dept. of Health 2020). In the United States and Western Europe, most members of this cohort grew up during booming economies coupled with higher marginal tax rates and generous provision of public goods such as education and health services. It was an era in which societies were more egalitarian than previously and the flow of inheritance was virtually stamped out as evidenced by the fact that "bequest and gifts accounted for just a few points of national income" (Piketty 2014: 480). For this cohort, what they own is largely due to effort and savings accumulated over their lifetime within this enabling environment. In contrast, for those born in the 1970s and 1980s, inheritance (which accounts for roughly 15% of the national income in the United States and Western Europe) has a profound effect on their life chances. This effectively sorts people at birth into designated socioeconomic status, which, in turn, exacerbates the wealth gap while reducing the rate of social mobility (Hout 1988, 2018; Marsden et al. 2020). This is relevant for the present discussion as studies show the link between hierarchies of social advantage and health across the life course (Braveman et al. 2010; McMaughan et al. 2020). Inequalities in inheritance—and therefore the wealth gap—are still expanding and will translate into future inequalities in opportunities and health status when this cohort reaches older age.

For birth cohorts such as the baby boomer generation, inequalities between birth cohorts have more salience and are central to considerations of justice. But when there are gross inequalities within a birth cohort, one must evaluate and identify the possible injustice of such inequalities before venturing to examine what justice demands in distribution across birth cohorts.

More than 60% of the world's working population are in the informal economy, ranging from less than 20% in some countries to 90+% in other countries (ILO 2018). For older birth cohorts living in low- and middle-income countries, where many of them worked in the informal sectors with little or no access to pensions if they ever retire, and with wider inequalities within cohorts than their US or European counterparts, the cumulative experience over time is expected to be exacerbated by the effects of socioeconomic disadvantages at older age. When social injustices compound over the life course, older ages then become acute periods of unfairness, and that matters for distributive justice (Corna 2013; Ferraro, Shippee, and Schafer 2009; Graham 2002). The socioeconomic inequalities within these birth cohorts are ultimately fundamental drivers of significant differences in health status in later life. Hence, the healthy ageing policies that are designed to address objectionable within age group inequalities must also respond to prior injustices that are compounded over the life course.

These concerns above show that our thinking about what is fair between age groups must complement, but not supplant, our thinking about fairness between and within birth cohorts. Having discussed the difference between adopting the life course approach and that of life stages approach for ageing and health justice, we now turn to insights we can draw from some mainstream conceptions or approaches to justice.

Theories of distributive justice and health

We would argue that age-related concerns of justice in health can be framed along three philosophical approaches to distributive justice—two egalitarian and one sufficientarian. The two egalitarian views draw on luck egalitarianism (LE) and from social/relational egalitarianism (SE). We discuss each, in turn, below, and then sufficientarianism.

Luck egalitarianism

LE begins with the observation that some life disadvantages or inequalities are generated by individual choices (option luck) while others are due to unchosen factors, termed brute luck. Luck egalitarians argue that choice-sensitive inequalities are outside the scope of justice; the goal of justice being "to eliminate the impact of brute luck in human affairs" (Anderson 1999: 288). One's brute luck includes being born into a certain family—which determines their draw in the genetic lottery as well as their social class—or the place where they were born, which may determine their nationality. The basic intuition of LE is that factors such as age, sex, gender, race, or the particular social circumstances into which a person is born are neutral from the moral point of view. Consequently, LE asserts that no one should be disadvantaged because of these and other such factors beyond the person's control—inequalities are fair or just only if they are responsibility-sensitive in the sense that inequalities must be side outcomes of a series of choices freely undertaken by the individuals.

Consequently, individuals are responsible for the bad (health) outcomes resulting from the risks that they deliberately undertake or that were within their effective control to avoid (Dworkin 2000). The claim that choice-sensitive social inequalities are permissible also commits luck egalitarians to the principle of compensation for brute/bad luck (Arneson 1989; Cohen 1989; Lippert-Rasmussen 2015, 2018). According to this principle, society should step in to reduce or eliminate bad (health) outcomes that people suffer as a result of brute bad luck.

Ageing and luck egalitarianism

It is plausible to think that declines in sensory capacities (hearing or vision) and cognition (including dementia), would fall under consequences of brute bad luck, whereas diseases largely caused by lifestyle choices, such as smoking and alcoholism, are within the remit of option luck. However intuitively appealing this distinction may seem, in reality, the complexity of life defies separation of causal factors neatly into either one of the two choice/brute luck categories. This makes LE impractical and error prone. LE is limited for two other reasons. One, it imposes a narrow criterion for assigning responsibility for health outcomes. Responsibility aptness of an action requires more than meeting the formal conditions for agency, namely, mental capacity and absence of obstacles for exercising one's will. Individuals must, in addition, possess the capacity and resources effectively to exercise their will (Van-Parijs 1997). A person lacks real freedom to choose when, for example, long working hours with meager pay in a dilapidated environment means that the practical set of available lifestyle choices are all likely to result in ill-health.

Second, critics accuse LE of being too harsh on individuals suffering from ill-health and for disregarding care as an important aspect of morality. In response, it has been argued that individuals' basic needs must be secured before activating responsibility-sensitive requirements to regulate the health services (Robinson 2011; Segall 2009). As stated earlier, globally at least 14% of older adults do not have their basic needs met. So, applying LE would require that this group of older persons make healthy choices which could amount to asking them to pull themselves up by their own bootstraps. In sum, LE does not adequately account for multifactorial and multilayered causes of ill-health at older age, and the diverse reasons for social responsibility (not only or largely personal responsibility) in addressing them.

Social/relational egalitarianism

SE holds that the point of equality is "not to eliminate the impact of brute luck from human affairs, but to end oppression, which by definition is socially imposed" (Anderson 1999: 288). SE is what might be called a gateway theory. In such a view, anyone residing within a gateway (by virtue of being a member of, say, the moral community, or a society conceived as a cooperative entity) ought to stand in relation of equality with one other. What sort of treatment is owed to persons in their relations as equals depends on which version of SE one adopts. Equal standing is defined in terms of equality of authority, power, status, or standing (Anderson 1999, 2010, 2012; Scheffler 2010, 2015; Schemmel 2011, 2012). However, barring paradigmatic cases of abuse that clearly imply unequal standing for the abused, the requirement of standing in relation of equality seems to be oddly compatible with remarkably low but equal standing between age groups.

Age-related inequality in health is unjustified from SE point of view to the extent that it prevents people from standing in equal social relations with their fellow citizens. As a gateway theory, it is unclear to what extent SE's commitment to standing in relation of equality can guide our judgments about what older persons are minimally owed as a matter of public health policy. Imagine two free and democratic societies, where one has the misfortune of living under severe resource scarcity while the other lives in abundance. Both would equally satisfy the requirements of SE as long as their residents stand in relation of equality with their respective fellow citizens, whatever equal standing means. SE is not a principle of ranking and cannot tell us what each society ought to prioritize. Moreover, a commitment to SE cannot guide us on how low the equal standing threshold can be allowed to go.

SE also seems to build on implausible explanations of why persons have entitlements to health services that are grounded in justice. Intuitively, we think that people have health services entitlements for reasons that do not necessarily follow from their standing in egalitarian social relationships with others with whom they share a social space. In addition, SE does not tell us about the distributive pattern or set of entitlements that reflect, or are deemed constitutive of, egalitarian social relations (Barkey 2018; Kelleher 2016; Voigt and Wester 2015). We would argue that the ideal of equal standing ought, therefore, to be supplemented with sufficiency conditions that independently stipulate the threshold of decent life prospects that every society has an obligation to secure for everyone (Frankfurt 1987, 2000; Miller 1995; Nussbaum 1990, 2000; Walzer 1983).

Sufficientarianism

All sufficientarian views share a positive thesis that justice requires everyone has enough and not that everyone is equally well off (Rid 2016). Each person is owed a threshold level of valuable goods/benefits, where the currency of sufficientarian justice is defined either in terms of welfare (Powers and Faden 2006), capabilities (Nussbaum 1988; Ram-Tiktin 2009; Sen 1999; Venkatapuram 2011), or other things. Once everyone has enough, one of two alternatives can be defended (Timmer 2021): either a negative thesis that no further distributive criteria can be asserted as a demand of justice (Casal 2007), or a *shift thesis* that our reasons for providing further social benefits shifts (Shields 2012, 2016). A common objection holds that it is hard to draw a sufficiency threshold such that equal distribution is required just below the threshold, and yet equality is not that important just above the threhold line (Arneson 2005; Casal 2007).

Ageing and justice: toward a unified view

The two egalitarian and the sufficientarian accounts of justice under consideration are, in different ways, pertinent to conferring normative content to the two schemes at conceptualizing ageing and health justice, namely, the life stages and life course approaches.

For LE, ageing-dependent impairments either due to genetic predisposition or social circumstances are a matter of brute luck, and society, therefore, has the obligation to reduce their negative effect on the lives of older people. A responsibility-sensitive approach such as LE can also capture the SDOH within the remit of brute luck; that is, poor health caused by social determinants are objectionable from the point of view of justice. Brute bad luck can affect individuals, age groups, and birth cohorts in specific ways.

Similar to LE, which seeks to eliminate default inequality in health that is not a result of individual choice, SE considers as unjust the SDOH in so far as they generate relations of inequality between age groups. The sufficientarian view provides an adequate account of why societies ought to take seriously the health of older persons. Endorsing the sufficientarian view does not carry the troubling implications manifested by LE's negative thesis, which holds that ill-health would have little concern with justice, unless it is invariably linked to misfortune of birth or social circumstances. It also has the advantage of being compatible with the fact that specific needs, intrinsic capacities, and functional abilities could vary at different stages of life, due to critical periods, that may justify unequal investment in the provision of social goods at different stages. Sufficientarianism permits, for example, deriving a principle of justice in health for older adults that converges the capabilities approach to health, as first developed by Amartya Sen and Martha Nussbaum, and currently defended by Sridhar Venkatapuram, with Nancy Jecker's notion of age-relativity of values. According to this combined theory, as found in Efrat Ram-Tiktin's blended approach, justice requires that the institutions of society guarantee older persons the sufficient functional abilities essential for them to live dignified lives (Ram-Tiktin 2012: 342). In achieving that, the life stages approach informs age-based structural injustices, while the life course approach addresses the problem of justice between birth cohorts.

The dynamic within and between birth cohorts is more tractable for policy design should we focus our analysis on whether people have enough, and on the presence and extent of social oppression, rather than attempting to define and measure the effects of brute luck on people's health. Hence, distributive approaches to justice such as LE and sufficientarianism "should be complemented by a concern for relational equality" (Barkey 2018).

Policy implications: the future of healthy ageing

What policy inputs are needed for realizing the United Nations' Decade of Healthy Ageing in a manner that is commensurate with the requirements of distributive justice?

In developing the Decade of Healthy Ageing, member states of the UN have endorsed the importance of healthy aging as a policy response to population ageing—and identified four pathways to improve functional ability, intrinsic capacity, and environments. This includes combatting ageism, ensuring communities foster the functional abilities of older people, delivering person-centered integrated care to older persons, and ensuring access to long-term care for older people who need it. Together, these actions should foster healthy ageing and improve the well-being of older people.

Three possible global scenarios regarding quality of life of older people—deterioration, stagnation, and improvement (Table 24.1)—are envisioned from 2021 to 2030. On the one hand, these scenarios are anchored to the key finding that at least 142 million older people globally do not have the ability to meet some of their basic needs, prior to the COVID-19 pandemic. On the other hand, these scenarios recognize that the COVID-19 pandemic has had concentrated impacts on the lives and livelihoods of older people and their families.

As of December 2021, there are signs of deterioration being predominant due to the fact that the initial pandemic response has not been inclusive of older people in all countries, and that services for older people are being cut back, including pension benefits, and that the

Table 24.1 Scenarios toward healthy ageing

Scenario 1 Deterioration	Scenario 2 Stagnation	Scenario 3 Improvement
The situation relative to the baseline increases significantly the number of older people who cannot meet their basic needs—especially those who have few opportunities whether by age, gender, location, or other markers of inclusion or exclusion.	The situation remains largely unchanged with some deterioration. Unequal pace of global progress remains.	Significant improvement reflecting the ability of older people to meet their basic needs relative to the baseline, a rebound after the pandemic, and improved access to services.

• Health and social services for older people are cut back	• Out-of-pocket expenditures are maintained	• Person-centered integrated care and long-term care for older people developed and provided as part of UHC
• Out-of-pocket payments for health and social services increase	• Pension benefits remain unchanged, without flexibility for those who wish to work longer	• Attitudes toward older people change positively
• A greater proportion of households suffer from catastrophic payments for health services	• No improvements in coverage of quality affordable services for older people	• Faster recovery and inclusive response, mitigating the pandemic's disruptions
• Pension benefits decrease	• Legislation to address age-based discrimination neither introduced nor enforced	• Accelerated improvements in the meaningful and inclusive engagement of older people
• Pandemic response and recovery is not inclusive of older people	• Attitudes toward older people remain unchanged	• Governments, civil society, and the private sector work together to optimize functional ability
• Unequal pace of global progress	• Delayed recovery and unequal inclusion of older people in pandemic response	• Better distribution of global investments and progress
	• Policymaking remains in silos for most countries	

unequal pace of global progress continues. Significant cuts on development aid for health, and even for global health research such as by the United Kingdom government, are a telling indicator and predictor of deterioration.

Regarding the baseline situation (stagnation), if the decline of resource allocation within countries and through the status quo emitting rules of financial institutions and development assistance for health is allowed to persist, it will perpetuate the current grotesque injustices faced by older persons. For instance, WHO documented in 2020 and again in 2021 the knock-on effects of COVID-19 that caused wide disruptions of other health services across high-, middle-, and low-income countries, including those for noncommunicable disease management, and home and social care—services that are vital for the health of older adults (WHO 2021b). That adds to the fact that most of the deaths due to COVID-19 are among older people, whether recorded or estimated (WHO 2021a, 2022). Although the risk of death due to COVID-19 is documented to increase with age, recent research shows that the most powerful factor for variation in deaths across communities is income inequality (Wildman 2021). Despite the reality that in many countries pandemic responses have been nothing short of disastrous, the accelerated changes since 2020 to adapt to pandemic conditions and drive the development of COVID-19 vaccines indicate that rapid change and innovation are possible.

However, globally, the scenario unfolding is one of deterioration. Due to the fact that only ten countries have administered more than 75% of COVID-19 vaccines, as of August

2021, the WHO Director-General alarmingly wrote: "Low income countries have received just over 1%—nowhere near enough to fully vaccinate their health workers, older populations and others at highest risk of severe disease and death" (Ghebreyesus 2021).

Yet, of the three, the Improvement scenario is what the stakeholders have committed to in the UN Decade. This would require global cooperation focused on improvement, and would result in the ability of all older people to meet their basic needs. It would also require that attitudes toward older people change positively. Social responsibility with regard to enabling older persons to meet their basic needs can be justified on grounds of sufficientarian reason, which has it that justice requires that everyone has enough. The same requirement may also be defended on social egalitarian grounds due to the fact that older people whose basic needs are unmet are vulnerable to oppressive social relations. Ageism undercuts social equality in two senses: ageist norms and practices are direct expressions of social oppression, and they impair older persons' sense of their self-worth.

The commitments to the Improvement scenario are framed in generic terms for which further elucidation is necessary. There is a requirement to ensure a fair distribution of global investments between countries and communities, on the one hand, and between age groups and birth cohorts, on the other. One area of comparison involves tracking the structure of development assistance for health (DAH). DAH does benefit older people but in contrast to global burden of disease, it targets younger more than older age groups (Figure 24.2). As things stand, this disparity is projected to increase further between 2030 and 2040 (Dieleman et al. 2020). The mismatch should be viewed within the broader context of ensuring each country invests in areas that promote better health across the life course and ensure older people get a fair share. This requires national commitments to invest in older people and not only reliance on the flow of international development assistance for health.

Country-specific information on the disease burden and interventions that can be effectively implemented at scale across age groups will help to identify what can be done. General conclusions can, however, be drawn using available information. For instance, a sufficientarian approach to health justice can guide our judgment about fair allocation of resources between age groups, and between birth cohorts, necessary for ensuring that everyone has enough. The particular form that the evaluation of fairness must adopt depends on the country-specific structure

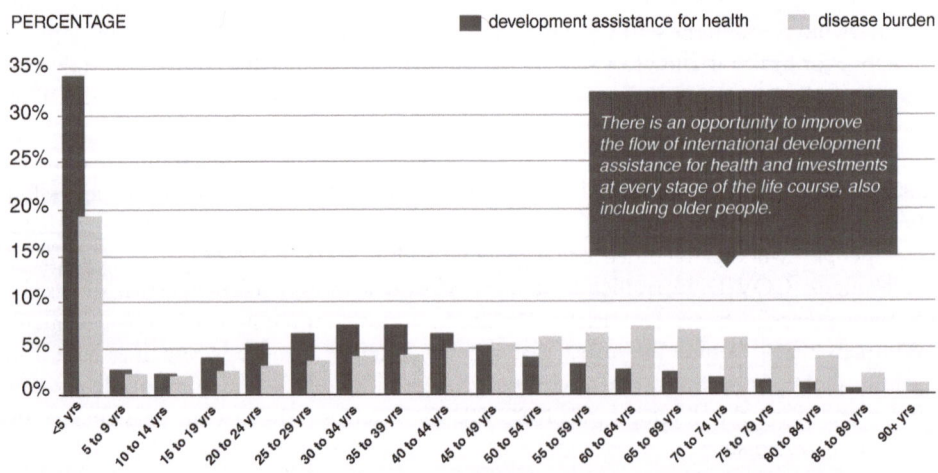

Figure 24.2 Development assistance for health and disease burden in 2017, by age groups (WHO 2020)

of inequalities between age groups, and where applicable, between birth cohorts. Health investments with respect to, for instance, an internally egalitarian birth cohort can be uniform and focused on health inequalities vis-à-vis other birth cohorts. Such shift in focus can be defended on LE as well as SE grounds. Considering the repugnance of existing inequalities in health, both globally and within countries, a vastly increased global investment that privileges individual wellbeing across all ages, rather than the current paradigm of economic growth (tracked by GDP), is required to have a decent chance of meeting a threshold status of health for all.

Conclusion

The current state of health decline at older age is neither inescapable nor morally neutral. Health declines occur at older age; however, the distribution can be improved and the rate can be delayed and decreased for many. As research in health and social sciences has attested, opportunities for healthy ageing across the life course is largely a consequence of the SDOH. In this chapter we have attempted to formulate a unified model of normative diagnosis by drawing from LE, SE, and sufficientarian conceptions of justice to show that the current state of healthy ageing is not merely regrettable but unjust. One key policy implication is that governments bear the primary responsibility, which is grounded in justice, to ensure that older persons secure sufficient functional abilities indispensable for leading a dignified life and to shape the conditions in which other actors operate. Moreover, the community of nations ought to take responsibility under the auspices of the UN Decade of Healthy Ageing, to exponentially increase investments in health and other sectors with specific benefits to older persons, also engaging older persons.

Three mainstream conceptions of justice have been deployed in this chapter to understand and frame the dynamic interplay between synchronic concerns of justice between life stages and the diachronic concern of justice between (and within) birth cohorts. While distributive approaches to justice, namely— LE and sufficientarianism—help to estimate the amount of goods (such as health and social services) to be distributed, SE encompasses values such as dignity and autonomy that cannot be quantified in terms of the provision of goods but are liable to be violated by the institutions of society. Public policymakers, including those in the health sector, ought, therefore, to consider not only a just allocation of resources for health and social services and ensuring an enabling environment, but also the non-distributive entitlements of older persons that their health status must be commensurate with, namely, a life of dignity.

Acknowledgments

This chapter partially draws on sections 1 and 3 of the WHO *Decade of Healthy Ageing Baseline Report,* of which Ritu Sadana was the lead author. The three scenarios were developed with civil society inputs, particularly benefiting from Prakash Tyagi, Executive Director, Gramin Vikas Vigyan Samiti (GRAVIS), Jodhpur, India. We would like to thank Sridhar Venkatapuram and Alison Lockhart for their invaluable comments and suggestions on earlier versions of this chapter.

Ritu Sadana is a staff member of the World Health Organization. All listed authors alone are responsible for the views expressed in this publication, and they do not necessarily represent the decisions, policy, or views of the World Health Organization. WHO acknowledges financial support from the Velux Stiftung to conduct research, including preparation of the WHO's baseline report for the UN Decade of Healthy Ageing 2021–2030 (https://apps.who.int/iris/handle/10665/338677).

References

Anderson, E. 1999. What is the point of equality? *Ethics* 109, no. 2: 287–337. https://doi.org/10.1086/233897.

Anderson, E. 2010. The fundamental disagreement between luck egalitarians and relational egalitarians. *Canadian Journal of Philosophy Supplementary Volume* 36: 1–23. https://doi.org/10.1080/00455091.2010.10717652.

Anderson, E. 2012. Equality. In *The Oxford handbook of political philosophy*, ed. D. Estlund, 40–57. Oxford: Oxford University Press.

Arneson, R. 1989. Equality of opportunity for welfare. *Philosophical Studies* 56, no. 1: 77–93. https://doi.org/10.1007/BF00646210.

Arneson, R. 2005. Distributive justice and basic capability equality: "Good enough" is not good enough. In *Capabilities equality: Basic issues and problems*, ed. A. Kaufman, 17–43. London: Routledge.

Barkey, B. 2018. Relational egalitarianism and the grounds of entitlements to healthcare. *Les atheliers de l'ethique* 13, no. 3: 85–104. https://doi.org/10.7202/1061220ar.

Baumann, H. 2008. Reconsidering relational autonomy: Personal autonomy for socially embedded and temporally extended selves. *Analyse & Kritik* 30: 445–468. https://doi.org/10.1515/auk-2008-0206.

Ben-Shlomo, Y. and D. Kuh. 2002. A life course approach to chronic disease epidemiology: Conceptual models, empirical challenges and interdisciplinary perspectives. *International Journal of Epidemiology* 31, no.2: 285–293. https://doi.org/10.1093/ije/31.2.285.

Braveman, P. A., C. Cubbin, S. Egerter, D. R. Williams, and E. Pamuk. 2010. Socioeconomic disparities in health in the United States: What the patterns tell us. *American Journal of Public Health* 100, suppl. 1: S186–S196. https://doi.org/10.2105/AJPH.2009.166082.

Buchanan, A., D. W. Brock, N. Daniels, and D. Wikler. 2000. *From chance to choice: Genetics and justice.* Cambridge: Cambridge University Press.

Casal, P. 2007. Why sufficiency is not enough. *Ethics* 117, no. 2: 296–326. https://doi.org/10.1086/510692.

Christman, J. 2007. Autonomy, history, and the subject of justice. *Social Theory and Practice* 33, no. 1: 1–26. https://doi.org/10.5840/soctheorpract200733133.

Cohen, G. A. 1989. On the currency of egalitarian justice. *Ethics* 99, no. 4: 906–944. https://doi.org/10.1086/293126.

Corna, L. M. 2013. A life course perspective on socioeconomic inequalities in health: A critical review of conceptual frameworks. *Advances in Life Course Research* 18, no. 2: 150–159. https://doi.org/10.1016/j.alcr.2013.01.002.

Daniels, N. 2008. Justice between adjacent generations: Further thoughts. *Journal of Political Philosophy* 16, no. 4: 475–494. https://doi.org/10.1111/j.1467-9760.2008.00320.x.

Dieleman, J. L., E. Maddison, R. Sadana, and A. Micah. 2020. An aging world requires more support for health systems: Development assistance should reflect this need. *Think Global Health.* https://www.thinkglobalhealth.org/article/aging-world-requires-moresupport-health-systems (accessed December 23, 2021).

Dworkin, R. 2000. *Sovereign virtue.* Cambridge, MA: Harvard University Press.

Feinberg, J. 1980. The child's right to an open future. In *Whose child?*, ed. W. Aiken and H. LaFollette, 124–153. Totowa, NJ: Rowman & Littlefield.

Ferraro, K. F., T. P. Shippee, and M. H. Schafer. 2009. Cumulative inequality theory for research on aging and the life course. In *Handbook of theories of aging*, ed. V. L. Bengston, D. Gans, N. M. Pulney, and M. Silverstein, 413–433. New York: Springer.

Frankfurt, H. 1987. Equality as a moral ideal. *Ethics* 98, no. 1: 21–42. https://doi.org/10.1086/292913.

Frankfurt, H. 2000. The moral irrelevance of equality. *Public Affairs Quarterly* 14, no. 2: 87–103. https://www.jstor.org/stable/40441279 (accessed December 23, 2021).

Fried, L. P. 2016. Investing in health to create a third demographic dividend. *The Gerontologist* 56, suppl. 2: S167–S177. https://doi.org/10.1093/geront/gnw035.

Ghebreyesus, T. A. 2021. Why there should be a moratorium on COVID-19 booster shots until low-income countries get vaccinated. *TIME,* August 12. https://time.com/6089974/who-moratorium-covid-19-vaccine-boosters/ (accessed December 23, 2021).

Graham, H. 2002. Building an inter-disciplinary science of health inequalities: The example of life-course research. *Social Science & Medicine* 55, no. 11: 2005–2016. https://doi.org/10.1016/s0277-9536(01)00343-4.

Hout, M. 1988. More universalism, less structural mobility: The American occupational structure in the 1980s. *American Journal of Sociology* 93, no. 6: 1358–1400. https://doi.org/10.1086/228904.

Hout, M. 2018. Americans' occupational status reflects the status of both of their parents. *PNAS* 115, no. 38: 9527–9532. https://doi.org/10.1073/pnas.1802508115.

ILO (International Labour Organization). 2018. *Women and men in the informal economy: A statistical picture*. 3rd edition. Geneva: International Labour Organization.

Jecker, N. 2020. *Ending midlife bias: New values for old age*. New York: Oxford University Press.

Kelleher, J. 2016. Health inequalities and relational egalitarianism. In *Understanding health inequalities and justice: New conversations across the disciplines*, ed. R. L. Walker, M. Buchbinder, and M. Rivkin-Fish, 88–111. Chapel Hill: University of North Carolina Press.

Kuh, D., R. Cooper, R. Hardy, M. Richards, and Y. Ben-Shlomo. 2014. *A life course approach to healthy ageing*. Oxford: Oxford University Press.

Lippert-Rasmussen, K. 2015. *Luck egalitarianism*. London: Bloomsbury.

Lippert-Rasmussen, K. 2018. Precis of luck egalitarianism. *Critical Review of International Social and Political Philosophy* 22, no. 3: 245–252. https://doi.org/10.1080/13698230.2018.1438783.

Madero-Cabib, I., L. Corna, and I. Baumann. 2020. Aging in different welfare contexts: A comparative perspective on later-life employment and health. *Journals of Gerontology - Series B Psychological Sciences and Social Sciences* 75, no. 7: 1515–1526. https://doi.org/10.1093/geronb/gbz037.

Marsden, P., T. Smith, and M. Hout. 2020. Tracking U.S. social change over a half century: The GSS at fifty. *Annual Review of Sociology* 46: 109–134. https://doi.org/10.1146/annurev-soc-121919-054838.

McMaughan, D. J., O. Oloruntoba, and M. L. Smith. 2020. Socioeconomic status and access to health: Interrelated drivers for healthy ageing. *Frontiers in Public Health* 8: 231. https://doi.org/10.3389/fpubh.2020.00231.

Miller, D. 1995. *On nationality*. Oxford: Oxford University Press.

Moreno-Agostino, D., C. Daskalopoulou, Y-T. Wu et al. 2020. The impact of physical activity on healthy ageing trajectories: Evidence from eight cohort studies. *International Journal of Behavioral Nutrition and Physical Activity* 17: 92. https://doi.org/10.1186/s12966-020-00995-8.

Nussbaum, M. 1988. Nature, Function, and Capability: Aristotle on Political Distribution. In *Oxford Studies in Ancient Philosophy*: Supplementary Volume, ed. J. Annas and R.H. Grimm, 145-184. Oxford: Clarendon Press.

Nussbaum, M. 1990. Aristotelian social democracy. In *Liberalism and the good*, ed. R. B. Douglas, G. M. Mara, and H. Richardson, 203–252. New York: Routledge.

Nussbaum, M. 2000. Aristotle, politics, and human capabilities: A response to Antony, Arneson, Charlesworth, and Mulgan. *Ethics* 111, no. 1: 102–140. https://doi.org/10.1086/233421.

Piketty, T. 2014. *Capital in the twenty-first century*. Cambridge, MA: Harvard University Press.

Powers, M. and R. Faden. 2006. *Social justice: The moral foundation of public health and health policy*. New York: Oxford University Press.

Ram-Tiktin, E. 2009. Distributive justice in health care. PhD diss., Bar-Ilan University.

Ram-Tiktin, E. 2012. The right to health care as a right to basic human functional capabilities. *Ethical Theory and Moral Practice* 15: 337–351. https://doi.org/10.1007/s10677-011-9322-7.

Rid, A. 2016. Sufficiency, health, and health care justice: the state of the debate. In *What is enough? Sufficiency, justice, and health*, ed. C. Fourie and A. Rid. Oxford: Oxford University Press.

Robinson, F. 2011. *The ethics of care: A feminist approach to human security*. Philadelphia, PA: Temple University Press.

Sadana, R., E. Blas, S. Budhwani, T. Koller, and G. Paraje. 2016. Healthy ageing: Raising awareness of inequalities, determinants, and what could be done to improve health equity. *Gerontologist* 56, suppl. 2: S178–S93. https://doi.org/10.1093/geront/gnw034.

Scheffler, S. 2010. *Equality and tradition: Questions of value in moral and political theory*. Oxford: Oxford University Press.

Scheffler, S. 2015. The practice of equality. In *Social equality: On what it means to be equals*, ed. C. Fourie, F. Schuppert, and I. Walliman-Helmer. Oxford: Oxford University Press.

Schemmel, C. 2011. Why relational egalitarians should care about distribution. *Social Theory and Practice* 37, no. 3: 365–390. https://doi.org/10.5840/soctheorpract201137323.

Schemmel, C. 2012. Distributive and relational equality. *Politics, Philosophy, and Economics* 1, no. 2: 123–148. https://doi.org/10.1177/1470594X11416774.

Segall, S. 2009. *Health, luck, and justice*. Princeton, NJ: Princeton University Press.

Sen, A. 1985. *Commodities and capabilities*. Amsterdam: Elsevier (North-Holland Publishing Co.).

Sen, A. 1999. *Development as freedom*. New York: Alfred Knopf.

Shields, L. 2012. The prospects for sufficientarianism. *Utilitas* 24, no. 1: 101–117. https://doi.org/10.1017/S0953820811000392.

Shields, L. 2016. *Just enough: Sufficiency as a demand of justice*. Edinburgh: Edinburgh University Press.

Timmer, D. 2021. Justice, thresholds, and the three claims of sufficientarianism. *Journal of Political Philosophy*. Early view. https://doi.org/10.1111/jopp.12258.

UN (United Nations). 1948. *The universal declaration of human rights*. New York: United Nations.

UN (United Nations). 2015. *United Nations sustainable development goals*. New York: United Nations.

UN (United Nations). 2020. United Nations decade of healthy ageing (2021–2030). In United Nations, *General assembly seventy-fifth session, agenda item 131: Global health and foreign policy*. New York: United Nations.

U.S. Dept. of Health and Human Services 2020. 2019 profile of older Americans. https://acl.gov/sites/default/files/Aging%20and%20Disability%20in%20America/2019ProfileOlderAmericans508.pdf (accessed December 23, 2021).

Van-Parijs, P. 1997. *Real freedom for all: What (if anything) can justify capitalism?* Oxford: Oxford University Press.

Venkatapuram, S. 2011. *Health justice: An argument from the capabilities approach*. Cambridge: Polity.

Voigt, K. and G. Wester. 2015. Relational equality and health. *Social Philosophy and Policy* 31, no 2: 204–229. http://dx.doi.org/10.1017/S0265052514000326.

Walzer, M. 1983. *Spheres of justice: A defense of pluralism and equality*. New York: Basic Books.

WHO (World Health Organization). 2015. *World report on ageing and health*. Geneva: WHO.

WHO (World Health Organization). 2017. Towards long-term care systems in sub-Saharan Africa. https://www.who.int/publications/i/item/9789241513388 (accessed December 23, 2021).

WHO (World Health Organization). 2020. *Decade of healthy ageing baseline report*. Geneva: WHO. https://apps.who.int/iris/handle/10665/338677 (accessed December 23, 2021).

WHO (World Health Organization). 2021a. *World health statistics 2021: Monitoring health for the SDGs, sustainable development goals*. Geneva: WHO.

WHO (World Health Organization). 2021b. *Second round of the national pulse survey on continuity of essential health services during the COVID-19 pandemic*. Geneva: WHO.

WHO (World Health Organization). 2021c. *Global report on ageism*. Geneva: WHO.

WHO (World Health Organization). 2022. *Global excess deaths associated with COVID-19, January 2020 – December 2021* (who.int). Geneva: WHO.

Wildman, J. 2021. Covid-19 and income inequality in OECD countries. *European Journal of Health Economics* 22: 455–462. https://doi.org/10.1007/s10198-021-01266-4.

Williams, G. A., J. Cylus, T. Roubla, P. Ong, and S. L. Barber. 2019. *The economics of health and active ageing: Sustainable health financing with an ageing population—will population ageing lead to uncontrolled expenditure growth?* Copenhagen: European Observatory on Health Systems and Policies.

Wu, Y-T., C. Daskalopoulou, G. Muniz Terrera et al. 2020. Education and wealth inequalities in healthy ageing in eight harmonised cohorts in the ATHLOS consortium: A population-based study. *Lancet Public Health* 5, no. 7: e386–e394. https://doi.org/10.1016/s2468-2667(20)30077-3.

25

PHILOSOPHICAL ISSUES IN CANCER AND PUBLIC HEALTH

Anya Plutynski

Introduction: two questions

Cancer is one of the leading causes of mortality in the world and some estimate that cancer mortality worldwide will triple by 2050 (Pilleron et al. 2021). Moreover, there are significant disparities in both cancer incidence and mortality in different groups, and in different nations. In the United States, while overall rates of mortality have fallen (Hashim et al. 2016), rates in racial minorities are almost double that of other groups,[1] and these mortality rates tend to covary with socioeconomic status (SES) (Zavala et al. 2021). In low- and middle-income countries, cancer incidence and mortality are starting to surpass higher-income countries; over half of new breast cancer cases, for instance, and 62% of all deaths, occur in low- and middle-income countries (DeSantis et al. 2015; Torre et al. 2015).

Yet, many causes of cancer are in principle controllable. Colditz et al. (2012) argue that with smoking-cessation programs, vaccination efforts,[2] improvements in diet, reduced alcohol consumption, improved environmental quality, and workplace safety, cancer incidence in the United States could be reduced as much as 54%. Worldwide, incidence and mortality might be significantly reduced with greater efforts made toward the reduction of smoking, control of AIDS (and thus, Karposi sarcoma), as well as hepatitis and human papillomavirus (HPV), and greater access to screening and treatment options. If this is true, then why has more not been done?

This question invites two further questions.

- First, what do scientists *know* about how public health interventions affect cancer incidence and mortality? Is such knowledge *warranted*?
- Second, what *obligations* do we have as *individuals, and as a society,* to ameliorate cancer risk?

First, how exactly do we *know* that such interventions would reduce cancer incidence by 54%? Why not 80% or 20%? What exactly are the relative contributions of smoking,[3] genetics, or workplace safety? Can we predict how interventions on these factors will change outcomes, especially given that these factors interact in such complicated ways?

DOI: 10.4324/9781315675411-30

The question of how to define and measure causation has raised an array of methodological and conceptual questions in epidemiology and public health, discussed further below. Such debates are profoundly political, insofar as they may have very different implications for whether we ought to judge these disparities unjust. In other words, answers to the first question inform and are in turn informed by competing views about how best to answer the second question. Reducing worldwide cancer incidence and mortality could require massive social reform, economic investment, and political will, as well as changes in behavior at the individual level. How such reforms should take place hinges not only on one's views of the roles and responsibilities of the state, but on whether, or how (if at all!), cancer's causes can be identified and disambiguated.

In what follows, these intertwined questions are brought into focus by considering debates over racial disparities in cancer mortality. This is only one of many potential case studies, which illustrate the overlapping epistemic and normative disputes concerning standards of evidence for assignment of causal, legal, and moral responsibility.

Health disparities along racial and other lines are of course not limited to cancer, and the study of cancer causation faces some of the same methodological challenges as many other chronic, multifactorial diseases. So, what is distinctive about cancer?

Arguably, cancer is distinctive in both the suffering and expense it causes,[4] and insofar as cancer causation has been a focal point for debates among public health scientists over standards of evidence and conceptualization of causation for decades, going back as far as the 1950s. Cancer research has also been a focal point around wider debates—not only among scientists, but also within funding agencies, government bodies, and the wider public—over how best to invest in research, whether "basic" or "applied." Such debates (implicitly or explicitly) invoke broad questions over the goals of science, methodological ideals for scientific inquiry (for example, "experimental" versus "observational"), and the appropriate institutional organization and reward system for science. For instance, our current institutional reward system tends to favor speed or frequency of publication; arguably, this carries a bias against public health science at the outset, given that genomic data-mining efforts could produce a paper in a month, whereas epidemiological cohort studies can require decades. Cancer research has also been promoted as a vivid example of the great potential of both "precision" and "big data" science. Molecular biomarkers and genomic research on cancer have yielded important insights about prognosis and treatment. This makes cancer as a subject of research in public health particularly fraught. There are both intrinsic methodological challenges facing public health efforts at prediction and explanation, and there are ethical challenges, given that such debates take place on the public stage, in the shadow of widely acclaimed (and generously funded) research efforts in molecular medicine.

Cancer causation and causal inference: the DAG-wagging controversy

Cancer causation is complex,[5] in the following senses: there are many remote causes, which act and interact with proximate causes. The relative contributions of these causes are not additive, and their effects can be highly context-sensitive. Thus, cancers' causes are not easy to discriminate from one another, or to generalize about. Whether from one patient population to another, or from one cancer to another, heterogeneity in both causes and effects makes extrapolation profoundly difficult. Carcinogenicity of various exposures, for instance, can be significantly different for individuals at different ages, in different sexes, and in light of differences in heritable features, or life history, such as parity (number of children). Environmental causes are mediated by multiple factors and may have intergenerational effects. While dramatic one-time environmental exposures can provide strong evidence of causation, these cases are rare, and their implications for conditions of lower exposure often subject to dispute, particularly with respect to multigenerational effects (Cranor 2011; Elliott 2011; Proctor 1994).

For instance, the diethylstilboestrol (DES) "daughters"—daughters of women who took DES during pregnancy—had fertility problems, and significantly elevated rates of cancers of the reproductive tract (Verloop et al. 2017). The mechanistic bases for these cancers are by now relatively well understood. Sex hormones like endocrine often play a very important role during certain stages of development; thus, endocrine disruptors like DES can disrupt sexual development and lead to higher rates of various cancers of the reproductive system. Most cancers of the reproductive system are "hormone sensitive," that is, many tend to grow in the presence of estrogen, progesterone (ER- or PR-positive breast cancer), or testosterone (in the case of prostate cancer). Hormone-blocking drugs such as tamoxifen or the aromatase inhibitors in women, or "chemical castration" in men with prostate cancer, reduce risk of recurrence, or can act as a prophylactic in high-risk populations. Populations exposed to extreme levels of endocrine disruptors such as DES daughters show significantly elevated rates of cancer in the breast, testes, and ovaries. Similarly, an explosion in Seveso in Italy in 1976 exposed residents to the highest levels of 2,3,7,8-Tetrachlorodibenzo-para-dioxin (TCDD) ever in a human population (Warner et al. 2011), leading to an epidemic of cancers of the reproductive organs (among other conditions affecting fertility). Yet these cases of clear links between environmental exposure and elevated cancer risk are rare and extreme; most cases of environmental exposure are much less significant, and the effects are difficult to detect. Moreover, epidemiologists have competing views about whether and how we can extrapolate from such extreme cases to estimates of risk of lower levels of exposure to endocrine disruptors. Challenges facing how best to infer from extreme cases of environmental exposures to more moderate cases are one of several vivid examples in public health science of what philosophers of science call "evidential underdetermination."

Evidential underdetermination has been used as a "wedge" to undermine arguments on behalf of restrictive regulatory law or more proactive, precautionary policies aimed at ameliorating health risks, across the board (Broadbent 2011; Oreskes and Conway 2011; Shrader-Frechette 2007, 2008, 2010, 2012). This wedge strategy has in some cases delayed and, in others, undermined public health and legal efforts in service of regulating potential carcinogens (Cranor 2005, 2017). The debate among epidemiologists regarding the concept of causation, or what count as legitimate causal variables, and methodological standards for causal inference is best understood against the background of these politically charged conversations around regulation and responsibility.

For instance, starting as early as the 1950s, Richard Doll and Austin Bradford Hill (1950) and Ernest Wynder and Evarts Graham (1950) did their first epidemiological studies of the link between smoking and lung cancer. Critics, such as Ronald Fisher (1958), argued that such studies lacked the methodological rigor of randomized, controlled trials. It was in principle possible (and, he argued, plausible) that hereditary factors explained the link between smoking and lung cancer. In a famous presidential address to the Section of Occupational Medicine of the Royal Society of Medicine in 1965, Hill defended his research on smoking and lung cancer, and offered a set of general, qualitative, "viewpoints" (often referred to as "Hill's criteria") that the medical community should consider in assessing claims about environmental causes of disease: strength of association, consistency across different times and places, in different populations, specificity of association (or, how common a particular outcome is associated with a specific type of exposure), temporal priority of exposure to the outcome, dose-response relationship (or, higher rates of incidence given higher exposure), biological plausibility (based on our best current understanding of the mechanistic basis of the disease etiology), coherence with our best current science, experiment (if possible), and analogical reasoning with similar exposures and disease pairings (Hill 1965).

Hill insisted these "viewpoints" do not provide anything like a test for causation. Hill was emphatic on this point: no one of these factors was necessary or sufficient to establish that a given environmental factor caused disease. The best way to interpret these "viewpoints" is perhaps as a set of guidelines for better or worse inferences to the best explanation, and as a pragmatic guide to setting standards of evidence for appropriate intervention (Broadbent 2015; Reiss 2015). However, Hill's lesson has never really sunk in. Unfortunately, the way statistics is typically taught reinforces a notion that randomization and experimental tests are necessary and sufficient for establishing causation—as if the applications of Neyman-Pearson tests of significance are essential to establishing causal relationships.

During the latter half of the twentieth century, with rapid advances in biomedicine and discoveries of precise clinical interventions on disease, such as insulin, vaccines, and antibiotics (Greene 2007), randomized clinical trials gradually become the "gold standard" against which all other research methods in medicine and public health were to be compared. This became solidified in the "evidence-based medicine" movement of the 1990s (Guyatt et al. 1992). In the late 1990s and early 2000s, a new approach to causal modeling gained ever wider popularity, canonized by Judea Pearl's (2009) classic book, *Causality,* first published in 2000. Pearl's book provides a thorough, clear defense of the value of structural equations, or DAGs (directed acyclic graphs) for modeling causation and avoiding problems of confounding. For many epidemiologists in the early 2000s, this seemed to be a solution to the ever-widening gap between the methodological ideals promoted by mainstream medicine and epidemiology. As Pearl himself explains, "The rise of Fisher's RCT to the 'gold standard' of experimental science further entrenched manipulability as a prerequisite for causation. In some communities, this entrenchment has turned into a dogma, cast for example in the mantra 'no causation without manipulations'" (Pearl 2018: 1).

Defenders of DAGs in epidemiology argue that this approach provides a precise set of methodological standards for causal inference. In this view, causal claims are to be understood as counterfactual claims: "Precise predictions about contrary-to-fact scenarios that would be brought about by some intervention or manipulation" (Vandenbroucke, Broadbent and Pearce 2016: 1778). Causation in this view is closely tied to prediction and, in particular, prediction about interventions. Nancy Krieger and George Davey Smith elaborate: "The ability to discern (and quantify) 'causal effects' hinges on positing counterfactuals that involve 'manipulable' exposures which could, in principle, be randomized [...] if an exposure cannot be 'manipulated' [...] it cannot produce 'causal effects'" (2016: 1788). These criteria, however, are often interpreted in restrictive terms. What can be manipulated? Are all and only manipulable variables causal? According to some advocates of this approach, race cannot be said to cause health disparities, since direct manipulation of race per se is impossible (cf. Krieger and Davy Smith 2016).

In the 2000s, the debate over this formal tool became a focal point around which epidemiologists debated not only this particular methodology, but also competing views about standards of evidence for making claims about causation. If all and only variables that can be "well-defined" and "precisely" manipulated are causes, we may be limited in what we can legitimately claim about social inequalities as causes of ill-health. Yet, identifying such social determinants of ill-health seems in principle a worthy pursuit. For instance, Michael Marmot and colleagues demonstrated that the "social gradient"—the extent of the divide between rich and poor, privileged and materially deprived—was a positive predictor of higher mortality and worse health outcomes (Marmot et al. 1978). While one cannot (directly) manipulate such a gradient, Marmot's research suggested that policies that (directly or indirectly) widened economic inequality promoted worse health, an important insight that could shift one's views about the justice of such policies.

Social determinants of health (SDOH) refer to causes of better and worse health, such as lack of safe and secure employment, poor housing conditions, discrimination, lack of self-respect, poor personal relationships, low community cohesion, and income inequality. These social determinants, insofar as they shape individual biology, behaviors, and proximate exposures to harmful agents are—some argue—essential to investigate, if we wish to pursue the larger goal of improving overall public health (Valles 2018). Though, here is where the debate becomes contentious: some epidemiologists have argued that since these determinants are often remote, and deeply intertwined with other less remote causes, efforts at measuring their precise effects are inevitably flawed. We should rather measure causes that one can directly intervene upon, and avoid the many confounding and intermediate causal factors intersecting with the social determinants of health.[6]

The attraction of structural models was that they seemed to promise a means of bypassing exactly these problems of confounding causal variables. Some defenders of what is called the "restricted potential outcomes approach" (RPOA) to causal reasoning in epidemiology (Hernán, Hernández-Díaz, and Robins 2004; Hernán and Taubman 2008; Robins, Hernán, and Brumback 2000; VanderWeele 2012, 2015) argue that this approach provides a way to mark off which causal factors are "well defined": namely, "when interventions are well specified" or how intervening on causal variables would change outcome variables. The goal of this account is to strive to make causal inference in epidemiology as close as possible to the model of randomized controlled trials, where intervention on one, precise variable can be shown to directly influence outcomes of interest.

The problem from the perspective of critics of the RPOA approach, however, is that such restrictions seemed to set to one side decades of work on the complex, indirect, structural, institutional, and economic factors contributing to health disparities, insofar as such factors could not be "well specified." As Krieger and Davey Smith have argued: "The stakes, after all, are high: riding on the findings of epidemiological research are not only scientific credibility but also accountability and agency: who and what is shaping population distributions of health, disease and well-being, within and across societies, and at what cost—and what benefit—to whom?" (20161788)

Let's turn to an example and see exactly how this divide informs competing answers to questions about cancer causation.

Case study: race and breast cancer mortality

In the United States, Black women have much higher mortality from breast cancer than White women. More precisely, "Black women in the United States are twice as likely as Whites to die from breast cancer developed before menopause" (McClintock et al. 2005: 33). In part, this may be because Black women experience much higher rates of estrogen-receptor negative (or ER) breast cancer. ER status is of relevance because those whose breast tumors are ER-positive (ER+) can be treated with antiestrogenic drugs (for example, tamoxifen and raloxifene), and hence have better long-term survival. Thus, ER-negative status is a predictor of higher rates of mortality, and so called "triple negative" cancers (estrogen, progesterone, and Her2neu negative) cancers are associated with highest mortality, overall. Black women have higher incidence of these latter cancers. Moreover, there is a striking age dynamic of cancer mortality for Black women in the United States when compared with White women, "with young Black women experiencing a sharp increase between 30 and 44 years of age and then a relatively low rate thereafter that is relatively independent of age. In sharp contrast, breast cancer incidence in White women increases exponentially with age, with the greatest age-dependent frequency occurring after menopause" (McClintock et al. 2005: 33).

What causes these differences in patterns of incidence and mortality? Explanations are overlapping and contested. Disparities in mortality have been associated with many, complex, overlapping causes: age at first menarche, parity, breastfeeding, SES, lifetime exposure to environmental carcinogens, sleep-wake cycles, and much else. According to Martha McClintock et al., however: "This striking health disparity likely arises from the reciprocal interplay of culture and biology that *defines ethnicity and race*" (McClintock et al. 2005: 33).

How does the "DAG-wagging" controversy come into play in this debate? Krieger and colleagues have done decades of epidemiological detective work to demonstrate how patterns of Jim Crow legislation and red lining[7] in the United States have shaped disparities in health overall (Krieger et al. 2005), and cancer incidence and mortality, in particular (Krieger et al. 2020). They argue that the evidence from their research strongly supports the view that social and socioeconomic factors—racism, inequality—are the primary drivers of these disparities in mortality (not, as some argue, "endogenous" or "intrinsic" difference in racial groups) (Krieger, Chen, and Waterman 2011). Their reasoning was as follows.

ER+ tumors are associated with early age at menarche, delayed age at first birth, low parity (that is, fewer children), postmenopausal obesity, and use of hormone therapy (estrogen plus progestin). In contrast, ER-negative and PR-negative (progesterone-negative) tumors are associated with early ages at first birth, higher parity, and race. That is, there is higher incidence of ER-negative/PR-negative breast cancer in African American women, and this incidence occurs at relatively young ages. For decades, it was more or less assumed that this difference was due primarily to "endogenous" (that is, strictly genetic, inherited) differences. If they were, then these relative patterns of incidence should remain consistent in Black women relative to White, regardless of such women's environment or circumstances, and should not change over time, as changes in environment or social determinants of health change. However, Nancy Krieger, Jacquelyn Jahn, and Pamela Waterman (2017) documented change in incidence by age of ER-negative cancers in Black women, in relation to Jim Crow birthplace (birth in a state that is subject to segregation), showing that women who had been subject to lifelong racist institutions had higher rates of ER-negative cancers. In their own words:

> Changes according to biological generation were greater among black women than among white women, and among black women, they were greatest among those born in Jim Crow (versus non–Jim Crow) states […] Our study's analytical

approach and findings underscore the need to consider history and societal context when analyzing ER status among breast cancer patients and racial/ethnic inequities in its distribution.

(2017: 960)

The strength of the study comes from looking at changes in birth cohorts over time, and the key finding was that Jim Crow birthplace was importantly predictive of excess risk of ER-negative breast cancer for Black women (and not White women). The impact was greatest for the earliest birth cohorts—that is, those exposed to Jim Crow policies for the longest time, during the course of their development. This challenges hereditarian explanations of excess risk. In other words, this study provides suggestive evidence in favor of the relationship between racist institutions and ER-negative status, in that the change in the proportion of Black women with this variant was traceable to living under Jim Crow versus not.

What is the causal pathway by which this lifetime exposure yields higher rates of cancer? To be sure, this is a matter that is still open to debate, but one hypothesis is what is sometimes called the "weathering" hypothesis, summarized briefly here by Arline Geronimus et al.:

> The weathering hypothesis [...] emphasizes health as an emergent capacity of human beings that dynamically develops over the life course in response to repeated or chronic and *structurally rooted material, psychosocial, or environmental stressors*. Weathering theory recognizes health as dynamic across the full life course as biopsychosocial mechanisms link fundamental social causes (Link and Phelan 1995) to population distributions of health, disease, and longevity. Mechanistically, advances in stress physiology, human stress genomics, epigenetics, and the mechanisms of telomere attrition confer biological plausibility on and suggest pathways for causal links between high-effort coping with chronic stress exposure and disease [...] This feedback system prepares the body for responses to stressful situations.

(Geronimus et al. 2019: 224)

Linnenbringer et al. (2017), among others, have drawn upon the weathering hypothesis to explain the disproportionate mortality in Black women. They argue that weathering provides a mechanistic link between life stressors and elevated cancer risk, and in particular risk of HR− (hormone receptor negative) breast cancers in Black women. While access to (or utilization of) healthcare resources (such as breast cancer screening) may influence higher rates of mortality, it cannot explain the significant differences in HR− status. Moreover, while HR− status is more common in women with inheritable risk factors (such as BRCA I and II mutations), there is no evidence of higher population prevalence of these mutations in Black women. Thus, they eliminate at least two potentially confounding upstream causes of health disparities, leaving stress, anxiety, and its effects on bodily health—via a variety of mechanistic pathways. According to Linnenbringer et al. (2017) stress leads to increased cortisol secretion, and "dysregulation of glucocorticosteriods, neurotransmitters, and inflammatory cytokines" (544). Over time, persistent activation of this system can lead to both dysregulation and acceleration of normal cellular aging process, or weathering and age-patterns of allostatic load, such as changes to epigenetic regulation of cell division, such as DNA methylation patterns, and changes to telomere length in Black women (Geronimus et al. 2010, 2015). In other words, there is a direct mechanistic link from stress, through molecular and epigenetic as well as genomic changes, to cancer risk.

However, Krieger's group disagrees that the "weathering hypothesis" is sufficient to explain the results observed. The "weathering hypothesis" focuses overwhelmingly on biological responses to *psychosocial* stress. However, they claim that *psychosocial* stress (alone) is unlikely to be sufficient to explain the trends observed. They argue that "biological pathways that could potentially link these social changes to breast cancer ER status include social adversity starting in early life, affecting *nutrition, body build, and reproductive history* (including age at menarche, age at first birth, parity, and breastfeeding)" (Krieger et al. 2018: 981, italics added). That is, impacts of *material* deprivation, and especially the high levels of impoverishment and lack of adequate nutrition early in life, likely matter enormously to ER status. This disagreement may seem to be minor, but the underlying mechanisms linking psychosocial stress to cancer are far more controversial than those linking *material* factors such as nutrition, body build, age at first menarche, parity, and breast feeding, to cancer. That is, Krieger's group emphasizes the role of material deprivation due to Jim Crow laws over the course of the lifespan, which occurs well before an infant would understand and have a psychosocial response to racism. Further evidence for this is that ER-negative tumors are found more frequent in materially deprived populations, such as those from the Great Famine in China (Alimujiang et al. 2016).

Whatever the causal pathways between Jim Crow and ER-negative breast cancer, there is an alternative explanation: some have identified heritable biomarkers of higher risk of some such cancers in Black women (Huo et al. 2016; Park, Cheng, and Haiman 2018). Dezhong Huo's group found a novel susceptibility locus for ER-negative breast cancer to be more prevalent in women of African descent. However, Africa is an enormously diverse, heterogeneous continent. Indeed, though Huo claimed (on the basis of a single study of 500 some patients in 2009 (Huo et al 2009)) that ER-negative status was more common in indigenous Africans, according to a more recent meta-analysis of 54 studies from North Africa involving 12,284 women with breast cancer (mainly living in Egypt or Tunisia) and 26 studies from sub-Saharan Africa involving 4,737 women with breast cancer (mainly living in Nigeria or South Africa) to calculate the proportions of ER+, PR+, and HER2+ tumors across indigenous populations in Africa (Eng, McCormack, and Dos-Santos-Silva 2014), the distribution of receptor-defined subtypes of breast cancer in Africa is not dramatically different from that found in Western populations. That is, the evidence so far suggests that the population distribution of (and social inequalities in) breast cancer ER status in the United States are likely historically contingent, in at least two (possible) senses: a product of a particular subpopulation of West Africans being the majority in the United States (who may have particularly high rates of this genetic marker), or simply because Black women in the United States have been disproportionately subject to excess material deprivation and psychosocial stress. They are perhaps more likely products of the distinct time and place in which they occur, rather than traceable to hereditary factors distinctive of all (or most) women of African descent.

Moreover, the study by Huo et al. of the biomarker for ER-negative status was based on mining data from genome wide association studies in the United States and established only a statistical association between an SNP (single nucleotide polymorphism) and elevated risk of ER-negative cancer. Little is known about the functional role of this genetic factor, or, for that matter, the etiology of ER-negative cancer. Disentangling these heritable factors from the extragenomic factors is, of course, difficult. Both may indeed play an important causal role, but focus on inherited genetic (as opposed to epigenetic) causes, (some fear) may direct focus away from interventions on extrahereditary factors. In any case, one can acknowledge that there may well be a genetic factor without necessarily undermining the case for extrahereditary factors also playing a role, historically, and currently. Calls for social action, in any case, do not require that there are no genetic components to inequitable distributions in health.

Social imbalances in health are often due to a complex of economic, environmental, structural, and psychosocial factors: poverty, inequitable access to education and opportunity, patterns of gender, racial, or ethnic segregation, poor physical conditions, lack of access to fresh food, open spaces, or basic medical care. It is enormously difficult to parse the relative causal contribution of each to cancer incidence and mortality, let alone directly manipulate the complex factors associated with such factors to improve health outcomes. Arguably, the controversy discussed above over relative significance of causal variables is not (or not merely) a methodological debate about what causal variables should or can be measured, but also a debate over the larger goals of epidemiological research and matters of justice. Historical redlining (as opposed to contemporary illegal racial discrimination) cannot be "manipulated" because from a policy standpoint it is no longer operative. However, it is another question entirely as to whether it is possible to (a) discern their continued impact on population health (necessary for understanding who and what is driving health inequities), and (b) allocate resources to redress and repair the documented harms (and thus, potentially prevent future harms).

Conclusions

The hope standing behind the RPOA was that if we can pin down more precisely which causes, and which interventions, will make a difference to outcomes, we can more effectively intervene. As such, it seems an attractive view. As Jan Vandenbroucke, Alex Broadbent, and Neil Pearce (2016: 1778) point out "It identifies an advantage [...] namely prediction under hypothetical scenarios; and it advocates restricting our attention to causal claims that clearly specify such hypothetical scenarios. It further restricts the hypothetical scenarios to those we can humanly bring about, again apparently because of a motivation of pragmatism." While identification of causes we can intervene upon is a good thing, the RPOA unduly limits the scope of causal inference and thus legitimate questions of interest to epidemiologists, and to the public at large.

Defenders of "fundamental cause" theory have argued that SES and systematic racism are "fundamental causes" of inequities in health and mortality. Fundamental causes comprised:

a set of flexible resources, and a superior set of resources generates superior results on some outcome. The level of resources varies between social groups, and groups with superior resources are advantaged on the outcome. The flexibility of the resources allows them to influence the outcome under a wide range of circumstances and through multiple pathways.

(Phelan and Link 2015: 315)

The problem—according to critics of this "fundamental causes" approach—is that this approach either neglects biology, or that SES is a poorly defined, or vague category of cause; it could be measured in multiple ways, not all of which are systematically related: income, wealth, education level, social status, and so on. Claiming that SES is a "fundamental cause," according to defenders of RPOA, ultimately provides us with no or very little precise information about how, or exactly what, to intervene upon, if we wish to change outcomes in a systematic way. (For more discussion see Goldberg, this volume.)

Likewise, there are many ways to measure and define systemic racism, which in fact feed into and are fed by the very same factors contributing to SES: access to positions in government and commercial institutions; financial resources, knowledge, power, prestige, and beneficial social connections; and social psychological advantages, such as expectations for success. Since such causal variables cannot be separated or measured with precision, some argue, we ought to stop pretending we can measure their relative effects. However, as the case study above attests, there are creative and instructive ways to identify patterns, and thus processes, yielding cancer disparities, demonstrating lasting effects of race and racism in health. Demanding particular formal ways of representing and measuring causal factors runs the risk of ignoring such factors, and thus discovering how and why such factors shape our long-term health outcomes.

Defenders of more permissive approaches to causal reasoning in public health argue that the more appropriate standard of evidence in such contexts is inference to the best explanation. That is, one ought in such cases to limit one's consideration to plausible alternatives and infer to that cause with the highest plausibility (or, perhaps, loveliness and likeliness), given the total evidence (Broadbent 2013; Lipton 2003): "Causal inference remains a judgment based on integration of diverse types of evidence" (Vandenbroucke, Broadbent, and Pearce 2016: 1785). Epidemiologists can use "(ii) diverse strategies to assess causality by ruling out alternatives, such as triangulation, negative controls and interlocking evidence from other types of science; (iii) the elements of all types of epidemiological study designs, inclusive of those types of design that do not match the ideal counterfactual situation."[8] As Broadbent has argued (2015), restricting causes to all and only "manipulable" variables is both vague and unduly restrictive.

Arguably, this debate is not only about matters of what counts as a cause, but about which causes we can and should invest in shifting. Institutional and economic changes associated with lifelong stress and chronic disease—of the sort typically found in Black women and men in the United States—are much more difficult to change than targeted interventions on specific variables.[9]

It is enormously difficult not only to identify and measure the causal contributions to cancer incidence and mortality, but also to translate this into action. Such sentiments may be behind much of the skepticism of preventive public health science; the question is not just whether we can measure the relevant risks, but how we can change complex institutional causes of disparity. In addition, the siloed nature of research leads to disagreements about not only method, but also effective translation of epidemiological evidence into policy. Efforts are consciously underway to change this state of affairs, however (on "translational" epidemiology, see Neta et al. 2015).

Notes

1 For the sake of this chapter, I treat these ethnic/racial categories as unproblematic, following much of the epidemiological literature. Of course, self-reported race may or may not coincide with ancestry, and whether ancestry is a meaningful indicator of biological difference is itself highly contested. For a detailed discussion of how these questions are far from resolved, see, for example, Burchard et al. (2003); Kaplan (2010); Roberts (2011); Valles (2012); Spencer (2016, 2018); Yudell et al. (2016); and Glasgow et al. (2019). I will also use upper case "Black" and "White" to signify that I am referring to a person who is taken to fall this category, rather than a color.

2 HPV and HBV are two of several infectious agents, chronic infection with which is associated with cancer (in these cases, cancers of the cervix and liver). So, vaccination can reduce rates of infection and thus cancer risk.

3 Talk of how much different causes "contribute" to risk of cancer is complicated by the problem of interaction. As I discuss below, it is a mistake to try to sum the different causes to 100%, as some epidemiologists still do, in service of making comparative judgments about relative contribution of risk factors. (For further discussion of this problem, see Krieger 2017.)

4 With respect to suffering: in parts of the world without access to the latest diagnostic tools or therapies, many patients and their families struggle with access to drugs and suffer long processes of decline (Livingston 2012). Cancer treatments can be enormously expensive (Mailankody and Prasad 2015; Prasad 2020), and end-stage cancer can be a long and painful process that many struggle to endure. Indeed, cancer is the most common diagnosis among those who choose to end their life, in those parts of the world where this option is available. As many as 70% of patients who opt for euthanasia, or physician-assisted death, are suffering from end-stage cancer (Al Rabadi et al. 2019).

5 Of course, the very use of the term "complex" is varied; it is applied and interpreted in various ways by cancer scientists, philosophers, and the general public. For an overview of the senses in which cancer is spoken of as "complex," see Plutynski (2021).

6 The question of whether SDOH can be directly manipulated depends on who is doing the manipulating. Public health/health professionals by themselves cannot enact economic policies that increase taxes on the wealthy, direct more funds to reinvest in communities shortchanged by economic and racial injustice, and reduce impoverishment, but they can inform the debates over the impacts doing so would have on population health. However, that health professionals per se cannot by themselves "manipulate" SDOH does not mean that these SDOH cannot be "manipulated" by others.

7 Jim Crow legislation were laws that enforced racial segregation in the American South beginning in the 1890s, mandating segregation of schools, parks, libraries, drinking fountains, restrooms, buses, trains, and restaurants.

   Red lining refers to both official and unofficial segregated patterns in access to property in many major cities in the United States, shaping access to housing, schooling, and public resources in the Black community.

8 Perhaps needless to say, there is a large and complex literature on inference to the best explanation in science; questions about the form of the inference, and warrant, are still widely disputed. For an overview of this literature, see Plutynski (2011).

9 As Vandenbroucke, Broadbent, and Pearce (2016) point out, there are many perfectly legitimate "causes that are not (or do not correspond to) feasible human interventions. Moving tectonic plates cause earthquakes; heat waves cause deaths; mutations cause drug resistance" (1781).

References

Alimujiang, A., M. Mo, Y. Liu et al. 2016. The association between China's Great Famine and risk of breast cancer according to hormone receptor status: A hospital-based study. *Breast Cancer Research and Treatment* 160, no. 2: 361–369. https://doi.org/10.1007/s10549-016-3994-6.

Al Rabadi, L., M. LeBlanc, T. Bucy et al. 2019. Trends in medical aid in dying in Oregon and Washington. *JAMA Network Open* 2, no. 8: e198648-e198648. https://dx.doi.org/10.1001%2Fjamanetworkopen.2019.8648.

Broadbent, A. 2011. Epidemiological evidence in proof of specific causation. *LEG* 17, no. 4: 237–278. http://dx.doi.org/10.1017/S1352325211000206.

Broadbent, A. 2013. *Philosophy of epidemiology*. London: Palgrave Macmillan.

Broadbent, A. 2015. Causation and prediction in epidemiology: A guide to the "Methodological Revolution." *Studies in History and Philosophy of Science Part C: Studies in History and Philosophy of Biological and Biomedical Sciences* 54: 72–80. https://doi.org/10.1016/j.shpsc.2015.06.004.

Burchard, E. G., E. Ziv, N. Coyle et al. 2003. The importance of race and ethnic background in biomedical research and clinical practice. *New England Journal of Medicine* 348, no. 12: 1170–1175. https://doi.org/10.1056/NEJMsb025007.

Colditz, G. A., K. Y. Wolin, and S. Gehlert. 2012. Applying what we know to accelerate cancer prevention. *Science Translational Medicine* 4, no. 127: 127rv4–127rv4. https://doi.org/10.1126/scitranslmed.3003218.

Cranor, C. 2005. Scientific inferences in the laboratory and the law. *American Journal of Public Health* 95, no. 1: S121–S128. https://doi.org/10.2105/AJPH.2004.044735.

Cranor, C. 2011. *Legally poisoned: How the law puts us at risk from toxicants*. Boston, MA: Harvard University Press.

Cranor, C. F. 2017. *Tragic failures: How and why we are harmed by toxic chemicals*. New York: Oxford University Press.

DeSantis, C. E., F. Bray, J. Ferlay, J. Lortet-Tieulent, B. O. Anderson, and A. Jemal. 2015. International variation in female breast cancer incidence and mortality rates. *Cancer Epidemiology, Biomarkers & Prevention* 24: 1495–1506. https://doi.org/10.1158/1055-9965.EPI-15-0535.

Doll, R. and A. B. Hill. 1950. Smoking and carcinoma of the lung. *British Medical Journal* 2, no. 4682: 739. https://doi.org/10.1136/bmj.2.4682.739.

Elliott, K. C. 2011. *Is a little pollution good for you? Incorporating societal values in environmental research*. New York: Oxford University Press.

Eng, A., V. McCormack, and I. dos-Santos-Silva. 2014. Receptor-defined subtypes of breast cancer in indigenous populations in Africa: A systematic review and meta-analysis. *PLOS Medicine* 11: e1001720. https://doi.org/10.1371/journal.pmed.1001720.

Fisher, R. A. 1958. Lung cancer and cigarettes? *Nature* 182, no. 4628: 108. https://doi.org/10.1038/182108a0.

Geronimus, A. T., J. Bound, T. A. Waidmann, J. M. Rodriguez, and B. Timpe 2019. Weathering, drugs, and whack-a-mole: Fundamental and proximate causes of widening educational inequity in U.S. life expectancy by sex and race, 1990–2015. *Journal of Health and Social Behavior* 60, no. 2: 222–239. https://doi.org/10.1177/0022146519849932.

Geronimus, A. T., M. T. Hicken, J. A. Pearson et al. 2010. Do US black women experience stress-related accelerated biological aging? A novel theory and first population-based test of black-white differences in telomere length. *Human Nature* 21, no. 1: 9–38. https://doi.org/10.1007/s12110-010-9078-0.

Geronimus, A. T., A. Jay, E. L. Pearson et al. 2015. Race-ethnicity, poverty, urban stressors, and telomere length in a Detroit community-based sample. *Journal of Health and Social Behavior* 56, no. 2: 199–224. https://doi.org/10.1177/0022146515582100.

Glasgow, J., S. Haslanger, C. Jeffers, and Q. Spencer. 2019. *What is race? Four philosophical views*. New York: Oxford University Press.

Greene, J. A. 2007. *Prescribing by numbers: Drugs and the definition of disease*. Baltimore, MD: Johns Hopkins University Press.

Guyatt, G., J. Cairns, D. Churchill et al. 1992. Evidence-based medicine: A new approach to teaching the practice of medicine. *Journal of the American Medical Association* 268, no. 17: 2420–2425. https://doi.org/10.1001/jama.1992.03490170092032.

Hashim, D., P. Boffetta, C. La Vecchia et al. 2016. The global decrease in cancer mortality: Trends and disparities. *Annals of Oncology* 27, no. 5: 926–933. https://doi.org/10.1093/annonc/mdw027.

Hernán, M. A., S. Hernández-Díaz, and J. M. Robins. 2004. A structural approach to selection bias. *Epidemiology* 15, no. 6: 615–625. https://doi.org/10.1097/01.ede.0000135174.63482.43.

Hernán, M. A. and S. L. Taubman. 2008. Does obesity shorten life? The importance of well-defined interventions to answer causal questions. *International Journal of Obesity* 32: S8. https://doi.org/10.1038/ijo.2008.82. EP.

Hill, A. B. 1965. The environment and disease: Association or causation? *Proceedings of the Royal Society of Medicine* 58, no. 5: 295–300. https://doi.org/10.1177%2F003591576505800503.

Huo, D., Y. Feng, S. Haddad et al. 2016. Genome-wide association studies in women of African ancestry identified 3q26.21 as a novel susceptibility locus for oestrogen receptor negative breast cancer. *Human Molecular Genetics* 25: ddw305. https://doi.org/10.1093/hmg/ddw305.

Huo, D., F. Ikpatt, A. Khramtsov et al. 2009. Population differences in breast cancer: Survey in indigenous African women reveals over-representation of triple-negative breast cancer. *Journal of Clinical Oncology* 27: 4515–4521. https://doi.org/10.1200/JCO.2008.19.6873.

Kaplan, J. M. 2010. When socially determined categories make biological realities: Understanding black/white health disparities in the US. *The Monist* 93, no. 2: 281–297. https://doi.org/10.5840/monist201093216.

Krieger, N. 2008. Proximal, distal, and the politics of causation: What's level got to do with it? *American Journal of Public Health* 98, no. 2: 221–230. https://doi.org/10.2105/AJPH.2007.111278.

Krieger, N. 2017. Health equity and the fallacy of treating causes of population health as if they sum to 100. *American Journal of Public Health* 107, no. 4: 541–549. https://doi.org/10.2105/AJPH.2017.303655.

Krieger, N., J. T. Chen, B. A. Coull, and J. V. Selby. 2005. Lifetime socioeconomic position and twins' health: An analysis of 308 pairs of United States women twins. *PLOS Medicine* 2, no. 7: e162. https://doi.org/10.1371/journal.pmed.0020162.

Krieger, N., J. T. Chen, and P. D. Waterman. 2011. Temporal trends in the black/white breast cancer case ratio for estrogen receptor status: Disparities are historically contingent, not innate. *Cancer Causes Control* 22, no. 3: 511–514. https://doi.org/10.1007/s10552-010-9710-7.

Krieger, N. and G. Davey Smith. 2016. The tale wagged by the DAG: Broadening the scope of causal inference and explanation for epidemiology. *International Journal of Epidemiology* 45, no. 6: 1787–1808. https://doi.org/10.1093/ije/dyw114.

Krieger, N., J. L. Jahn, and P. D. Waterman. 2017. Jim Crow and estrogen-receptor-negative breast cancer: US-born black and white non-Hispanic women, 1992–2012. *Cancer Causes & Control* 28, no. 1: 49–59. https://doi.org/10.1007/s10552-016-0834-2.

Krieger, N., E. Wright, J. T. Chen, P. D. Waterman, E. R. Huntley, and M. Arcaya. 2020. Cancer stage at diagnosis, historical redlining, and current neighborhood characteristics: Breast, cervical, lung, and colorectal cancers, Massachusetts, 2001–2015. *American Journal of Epidemiology* 189, no. 10: 1065–1075. https://doi.org/10.1093/aje/kwaa045.

Linnenbringer, E., S. Gehlert and A. T. Geronimus. 2017. Black-white disparities in breast cancer subtype: The intersection of socially patterned stress and genetic expression. *AIMS Public Health* 4, no. 5: 526. https://doi.org/10.3934/publichealth.2017.5.526.

Lipton, P. 2003. *Inference to the best explanation.* New York: Routledge.

Livingston, J. 2012. *Improvising medicine: An African oncology ward in an emerging cancer epidemic.* Durham, NC: Duke University Press.

Mailankody, S. and V. Prasad. 2015. Five years of cancer drug approvals: Innovation, efficacy, and costs. *JAMA Oncology* 1, no. 4: 539–540. https://doi.org/10.1001/jamaoncol.2015.0373.

Marmot, M., G. Rose, M. Shipley, and P. Hamilton. 1978. Employment grade and coronary heart disease in British civil servants. *Journal of Epidemiology and Community Health* 32: 244–249. http://dx.doi.org/10.1136/jech.32.4.244.

McClintock, M. K., S. D. Conzen, S. Gehlert, C. Masi, and F. Olopade. 2005. Mammary cancer and social interactions: Identifying multiple environments that regulate gene expression throughout the life span. *Journals of Gerontology Series B: Psychological Sciences and Social Sciences* 60, no. 1: 32–41. https://doi.org/10.1093/geronb/60.Special_Issue_1.32.

NCI (National Cancer Institute). 2019. Funding allocated to major NCI program areas. https://www.cancer.gov/about-nci/budget/fact-book/data/program-structure (accessed December 23, 2021).

Neta, G., M. A. Sanchez, D. A. Chambers et al. 2015. Implementation science in cancer prevention and control: A decade of grant funding by the National Cancer Institute and future directions. *Implementation Science* 10, no. 1: 1–10. https://doi.org/10.1186/s13012-014-0200-2.

Oreskes, N. and E. M. Conway. 2011. *Merchants of doubt: How a handful of scientists obscured the truth on issues from tobacco smoke to global warming.* New York: Bloomsbury.

Park, S. L., I. Cheng, and C. A. Haiman. 2018. Genome-wide association studies of cancer in diverse populations. *Cancer Epidemiology, Biomarkers & Prevention* 27, no. 4: 405–417. https://doi.org/10.1158/1055-9965.EPI-17-0169.

Pearl, J. 2009. *Causality: Models, reasoning and inference.* 2nd edition Cambridge: Cambridge University Press.

Pearl, J. 2018. Does obesity shorten life? Or is it the soda? On non-manipulable causes. *Journal of Causal Inference* 6, no. 2. https://doi.org/10.1515/jci-2018-2001.

Phelan, J. and B. Link. 2015. Is racism a fundamental cause of inequities in health? *Annual Review of Sociology* 41: 311–330. https://doi-org.libproxy.wustl.edu/10.1146/annurev-soc-073014-112305.

Pilleron, S., E. Soto-Perez-de-Celis, J. Vignat et al. 2021. Estimated global cancer incidence in the oldest adults in 2018 and projections to 2050. *International Journal of Cancer* 148, no. 3: 601–608. https://doi.org/10.1002/ijc.33232.

Plutynski, A. 2011. Four problems of abduction: A brief history. *HOPOS: The Journal of the International Society for the History of Philosophy of Science* 1, no. 2: 227–248. https://doi.org/10.1086/660746.

Plutynski, A. 2021. How is cancer complex? *European Journal for Philosophy of Science* 11, no. 2: 1–30. https://doi.org/10.1007/s13194-021-00371-8.

Prasad, V. K. 2020. *Malignant: How bad policy and bad evidence harm people with cancer.* Baltimore, MD: Johns Hopkins University Press.

Proctor, R. N. 1994. *Cancer wars: How politics shapes what we know and don't know about cancer.* New York: Basic Books.

Reiss, J. 2015. A pragmatist theory of evidence. *Philosophy of Science* 82, no. 3: 341–362. https://doi.org/10.1086/681643.

Roberts, D. 2011. *Fatal invention: How science, politics, and big business re-create race in the twenty-first century.* New York: New Press/ORIM.

Robins, J. M., M. A. Hernán, and B. Brumback. 2000. Marginal structural models and causal inference in epidemiology. *Epidemiology* 11, no. 5: 550–560. https://doi.org/10.1097/00001648-200009000-00011.

Root, M. 2003. The use of race in medicine as a proxy for genetic differences. *Philosophy of Science* 70, no. 5: 1173–1183.https://doi.org/10.1086/377398.

Shrader-Frechette, K. 2007. Relative risk and methodological rules for causal inferences. *Biological Theory* 2, no. 4: 332–336. https://doi.org/10.1162/biot.2007.2.4.332.

Shrader-Frechette, K. 2008. Evidentiary standards and animal data. *Environmental Justice* 1, no. 3: 139–144. https://doi.org/10.1089/env.2008.0528.

Shrader-Frechette, K. 2010. Conceptual analysis and special-interest science: Toxicology and the case of Edward Calabrese. *Synthese* 177, no. 3: 449–469. https://doi.org/10.1007/s11229-010-9792-5.

Shrader-Frechette, K. 2012. *Risk analysis and scientific method: Methodological and ethical problems with evaluating societal hazards.* Dordrecht: Springer Science & Business Media.

Spencer, Q. 2016. Do humans have continental populations? *Philosophy of Science* 83, no. 5: 791–802. https://doi.org/10.1086/687864.

Spencer, Q. 2018. A racial classification for medical genetics. *Philosophical Studies* 175, no. 5: 1013–1037. https://doi.org/10.1007/s11098-018-1072-0.

Torre, L. A., F. Bray, R. L. Siegel, J. Ferlay, J. Lortet-Tieulent, and A. Jemal. 2015. Global cancer statistics, 2012. *CA: A Cancer Journal for Clinicians.* 65: 87–108. https://doi.org/10.3322/caac.21262.

Valles, S. A. 2012. Heterogeneity of risk within racial groups, a challenge for public health programs. *Preventive Medicine* 55, no. 5: 405–408. https://doi.org/10.1016/j.ypmed.2012.08.022.

Valles, S. A. 2018. *Philosophy of population health: Philosophy for a new public health era.* New York: Routledge.

Vandenbroucke, J. P., A. Broadbent, and N. Pearce. 2016. Causality and causal inference in epidemiology: The need for a pluralistic approach. *International Journal of Epidemiology* 45, no. 6: 1776–1786. https://doi.org/10.1093/ije/dyv341.

VanderWeele, T. J. 2012. Invited commentary: Structural equation models and epidemiologic analysis. *American Journal of Epidemiology* 176, no. 7: 608–612. https://doi.org/10.1093/aje/kws213.

VanderWeele, T. 2015. *Explanation in causal inference: Methods for mediation and interaction.* New York: Oxford University Press.

Verloop, J., F. E. van Leeuwen, T. J. Helmerhorst et al. 2017. Risk of cervical intra-epithelial neoplasia and invasive cancer of the cervix in DES daughters. *Gynecologic Oncology* 144, no. 2: 305–311. https://doi.org/10.1016/j.ygyno.2016.11.048.

Warner, M., P. Mocarelli, S. Samuels, L. Needham, P. Brambilla, and B. Eskenazi. 2011. Dioxin exposure and cancer risk in the Seveso Women's Health Study. *Environmental Health Perspectives* 119, no. 12: 1700–1705. https://doi.org/10.1289/ehp.1103720.

Wynder, E. L. and E. A. Graham. 1950. Tobacco smoking as a possible etiologic factor in bronchiogenic carcinoma: A study of six hundred and eighty-four proved cases. *Journal of the American Medical Association* 143, no. 4: 329–336. https://doi.org/10.1001/jama.1950.02910390001001.

Yudell, M., D. Roberts, R. DeSalle, and S. Tishkoff. 2016. Taking race out of human genetics. *Science* 351, no. 6273: 564–565. https://doi.org/10.1126/science.aac4951.

Zavala, V. A., P. M. Bracci, J. M. Carethers et al. 2021. Cancer health disparities in racial/ethnic minorities in the United States. *British Journal of Cancer* 124, no. 2: 315–332. https://doi.org/10.1038/s41416-020-01038-6.

26

PUBLIC HEALTH, HUMAN RIGHTS, AND PHILOSOPHY

Kristen Hessler

Introduction

In 1994, the inaugural issue of the journal *Health and Human Rights* introduced a broad, hopeful vision of collaboration between the fields of public health and human rights. In that issue, an interdisciplinary group of scholars, including Jonathan Mann, Sofia Gruskin, and Lawrence Gostin, presented the pioneering argument that the goals of public health and human rights were deeply aligned, contrary to received opinion at the time, which saw the two fields as inherently antagonistic. On the basis of revised and expanded views of both fields, they advocated for a partnership between them to advance their shared agendas. Public health (as opposed to medicine), they argued, "has a distinct, health-promoting goal," and its population-based (rather than individualistic) perspective includes "the mental and social dimensions of well-being" (Mann et al. 1994: 8–9). At the same time, human rights law was "expanding to include concerns about the environment and global socioeconomic development" and a growing recognition of how non-state actors and institutions might affect the enjoyment of human rights by individuals (1994: 11–12). Putting these developments together, the authors argued for the broad thesis that "promoting and protecting human rights is inextricably linked to the challenge of promoting and protecting health" because "health and human rights are complementary approaches to the central problem of defining and advancing human well-being" (1994: 19).

In this chapter, I unpack the case for a human rights approach to public health in more detail, highlighting the fact that it depends on a nontraditional understanding of both fields. I then argue for a greater role for the philosophy of human rights in interdisciplinary health and human rights scholarship. The philosophy of human rights is undergoing a similar expansion, including by developing novel ways of addressing methodological questions about its relationship to other disciplines and to international human rights law. As a result, philosophers of human rights are well placed to both contribute to and benefit from collaborative interdisciplinary scholarship that illuminates the moral basis of the human rights approach to public health.

DOI: 10.4324/9781315675411-31

From conflict to congruence: the case for the human rights approach to public health

As its early proponents were well aware, the vision of public health and human rights as "inextricably linked" requires challenging traditional and relatively narrow understandings of both fields. Regarding human rights, this vision reconsiders entrenched skepticism about the status of social, cultural, and economic human rights, such as rights to healthcare, an adequate standard of living, working conditions, and other material components of a good or at least decent life. The 1948 Universal Declaration of Human Rights (UDHR) included social, cultural, and economic rights (or, for ease of reference, simply "social rights") as well as civil and political rights, such as rights against torture or arbitrary imprisonment or rights to basic freedoms. Despite this early inclusiveness, efforts to implement human rights in international law ran into persistent debates about whether social rights are either less important than civil and political rights, or even whether they are really human rights at all. The international community was divided enough on this question that the unified set of rights proclaimed in the UDHR was translated into two separate, legally binding conventions: the International Convention on Civil and Political Rights and the International Convention on Social, Cultural, and Economic Rights (Nickel 2007: 137).

Philosophically, skepticism about the status of social rights is supported by the argument that human rights must be negative rights—that is, rights against interference in personal space, especially against being treated in certain ways, such as being subjected to torture or other violence (Cranston 1983; Lomasky 1987). By contrast, positive rights are rights to have something done for one, such as being provided with education, food, shelter, or medical care. A common line of argument identifies civil and political rights with negative ones, arguing that respecting civil and political rights requires only that the government and other individuals simply "leave a man alone" (Cranston 1983: 13). By contrast, realizing social rights generally requires implementing resource-intensive social programs. Therefore, while it is easy to agree that being subjected to torture is a violation of one's human rights, skepticism persists regarding whether lacking an adequate standard of living (being malnourished, ill, illiterate, and the like) can plausibly be considered a comparable human rights violation, especially in the absence of an identifiable agent who is in the wrong by not providing it (O'Neill 2002).[1]

For its part, public health has traditionally been concerned with government interventions, often coercive, that are designed to protect population health, especially with regard to preventing the outbreak of disease or improving sanitation. Mark Rothstein argues, for example, that public health is defined by the kinds of measures that governments are authorized to undertake in response to threats to the public's health (Rothstein 2002: 146). From this perspective, the objectives and animating values of public health seem antagonistic to, rather than synergistic with, human rights, understood as protections for individual freedoms and autonomy. Indeed, the traditional, narrow conception of public health invites the perception that the point of this kind of government-driven public health is to realize a form of "health utilitarianism" that aims to "advance the health of as many people as much as possible" (Wynia 2005: 6). On this view, coercive public health policies that restrict the rights and freedoms of individuals may be justifiable insofar as they are instrumental to achieving the aggregate social good of public health. By contrast, the narrow conception of human rights as protections of individuals' negative freedom and autonomy emphasizes the protection of individual liberty against government authority, even at the expense of an aggregate public benefit to population health.

Proponents of the human rights approach to public health have followed two distinct pathways to reveal underappreciated synergies between these two seemingly opposed fields. The first emphasizes that coercive public health measures, such as quarantine or mandatory testing and treatment, may infringe on civil and political human rights, and that developing public health measures that respect such rights may be more effective at protecting public and individual health. One example of this approach can be found in Mann and Gostin's proposal for a framework assessing the human rights impact of public health policies, which was published in a separate article in the inaugural issue of *Health and Human Rights*. Arguing that "economic, cultural, and social rights do not have the same standing in international law as civil and political rights," their proposal focused largely on how public health measures might burden civil and political rights like free movement, privacy, and the like (Gostin and Mann 1994: 71). In the same vein, some public health advocates have argued that "disease control methods blind to human rights" may be counterproductive, insofar as "insufficient attention has been devoted to assessing and monitoring the impact of such policies on the life of people whose rights were being restricted or denied, and to the negative consequences such impositions can have on their willingness to participate supportively in public health efforts that concern them" (Tarantola and Gruskin 2008: 480).

The argument here is that coercive public health policies may deter the most vulnerable from participating in various public health measures due to fears of having their freedom, autonomy, or privacy restricted. Conversely, the violation of traditional, negative human rights makes people more vulnerable to ill health. This may be most obvious when the human rights violation involves the direct imposition of physical or mental harm on the victim, such as torture or imprisonment under unhealthful conditions. However, human rights violations may impact public health in more complicated ways as well (Mann et al. 1994: 17–18). For example, restrictions on freedom of expression, access to information, or association can interfere with groups gathering and sharing relevant information that is needed to protect their health. In places where it is illegal to form an organization of sex workers, or where it is illegal or dangerous to identify publicly as LGBTQI, it is correspondingly difficult for these populations to share accurate and relevant information to protect them from serious disease. From this perspective, a concern for public health would, therefore, also entail a concern for the protection of civil and political human rights.

The second, more radical vision of the synergy between public health and human rights construes them as "not distinct but intertwined aspirations" (Tarantola and Gruskin 2008: 477). This model essentially reconceives the relationship between the two fields based on expanded views of both. On the human rights side, this vision is based on a broader conception of human rights that has developed within international human rights law. As is now widely recognized, protecting civil and political rights requires not only noninterference but also substantial social programs and investment, such as adequate training for police and military personnel to ensure the absence of torture, the funding of an adequate court system to recognize and redress rights violations, and the like (Holmes and Sunstein 2000). More importantly, international human rights law has not confined itself to the promotion and protection of civil and political rights, but rather has developed an extensive jurisprudence devoted to realizing and protecting social, cultural, and economic rights as well, including rights to health, education, and the material requirements of a decent life.

This version of the human rights approach also relies on an expanded conception of public health, insofar as it emphasizes the underlying social factors influencing public health. These include (for example) food insecurity, structural racism and other forms of discrimination and inequality, and violence—including violent crime, armed conflict, and domestic or intimate partner violence.[2] As Mann argues, "The vast majority of research into the health of populations identifies so-called 'societal factors' as the major determinants of health status" (Mann 1997b: 7). In turn, the broad scope of the "social" challenges the traditional, narrower definition of public health as government intervention in the face of a distinct threat to the health of the population. The early advocates of the human rights approach to public health were among the first to emphasize what by now is becoming increasingly clear and widely accepted: that the health of individuals and populations is affected not only by proximal exposures such as viruses and germs, or their individual behaviors. Rather, these proximal exposures and other disease pathways are created and distributed across populations by broader social, economic, and political factors such as economic development, access to education, levels of social inclusion and provision, or the prevalence of violence and political unrest. And under the expanded conception of human rights, these are all just as much concerns for and about human rights as they are relevant to health.

As the health and human rights pioneers argued, these more expansive views of public health and human rights suggest that the two fields are less fundamentally opposed (as they first appear to be based on narrow reading of both fields), and more like congruent pursuits of the same overall goal—namely, human health and well-being, not only individually but in social contexts as well—via different means. As a result, as Mann presciently argues: "Despite uncertainty and in the midst of profound changes in the two fields, health and human rights are increasingly understood and felt to be—actually—two entirely complementary ways of speaking about—and working to ameliorate—human suffering in all its forms and wherever it occurs" (Mann 1997a: 120).

Public health and human rights, international law and philosophy

Much of the scholarship on public health and human rights focuses on human rights as they are articulated in international human rights law, rather than on philosophical accounts of human rights morality. From the perspective of public health advocates, this makes pragmatic sense, for several reasons. The first is that public health has traditionally focused on the coercive exercise of governmental power, which, if it is to be legitimate, must be authorized and justified, but also constrained.[3] From that perspective, legal human rights are relevant for public health because they specify determinate legal standards for "what governments can do to us, cannot do to us, and should do for us" (Gruskin 2004: 319). International human rights law is, therefore, instrumentally valuable insofar as its provisions constitute binding obligations on governments, rather than "mere" moral obligations. Second, and relatedly, the emphasis on international human rights law allows public health and human rights advocates to bypass moral argument about human rights, pointing instead to positive legal standards. Finally, invoking international human rights law empowers public health advocates to appeal to human rights standards in criticizing existing public health measures, whether the government in question recognizes those standards or not.

At the same time, scholarship on the human rights approach to public health frequently emphasizes the status of human rights as especially important moral principles, as distinct from their status as legally binding norms of international law. For example, Mann describes "the language of human rights" as "extremely useful for expressing, considering, and incorporating values into public health analysis and response" (Mann 1997b: 10). Similarly, in her analysis of how public health can contribute to a better understanding of human rights violations during the armed conflicts in the former Yugoslavia, Alicia Yamin describes human rights in explicitly philosophical terms: "In embracing the idea that human beings possess inalienable rights by virtue of their unique capacities of reason and conscience, international human rights instruments reflect a rationalist and fundamentally modernist philosophy" (Yamin 1999: 83).

For the health and human rights pioneers, at least part of the original impetus for looking to human rights was to articulate and defend a system of globally shared values that would help support and guide the field of public health. As Mann put this point: "Public health, at least in its contemporary form, is struggling to define and articulate its core values" (Mann 1997b: 8) What the field needed, he thought, was a "more useful framework, vocabulary, and form of guidance for public health efforts to analyze and respond directly to the societal determinants of health than any inherited from the past biomedical or public health tradition" (1997b: 8–9). Perhaps most importantly, proponents of the human rights approach to public health emphasize its potential to guide and empower both fields in the pursuit of their most ambitious and revolutionary goals: challenging the status quo of society, and within each field, wherever necessary. Indeed, Mann describes public health professionals and human rights advocates as "seeking to change the 'givens' of personal and social life, the inherited so-called 'natural' order of things, the assumed 'inevitable.' Thus we continually call the status quo into question—and we have learned, slowly over time, that calling the larger societal status quo into question is the true task" (Mann 1997a: 119). Insofar as this goal is not the pursuit of change for its own sake, but rather the pursuit of changing the status quo in a morally progressive direction, it is clear that human rights are functioning in this vision as moral standards, not just legal ones.

In these and similar ways, proponents of a human rights approach to public health often deploy human rights as a moral concept, as distinct from a legal one. It is therefore important for them to address philosophical questions about human rights morality, and the relationship between moral and legal human rights, if only to make good on the implicit, and sometimes explicit, references to human rights morality that they often deploy. In addition, even proponents who see this approach as relying only on positive international human rights law would be well served to be able to address moral challenges to international human rights law itself. One reason is that legal standards can always be questioned from a moral perspective: the fact that a particular human right has been incorporated into international law by itself does not answer the question whether this incorporation was justified, all things considered. Another reason is that some skeptics question whether the system of international human rights law has really functioned to advance justice (Ignatieff 2001). For example, in response to Mann's assertion that public health and human rights are "'powerful, modern approaches to defining and advancing human well-being," Lynn Freedman argues that "public health and human rights have also, at times, been powerful tools for maintaining the status quo, reinforcing hierarchies of power and domination based on race, gender, and class" (Freedman 1999: 227). For all these reasons, a justification and defense of a human rights approach to public health requires at least some kind of moral justification for relying on international human rights law in the first place, as well as for defending particular norms within it.

Over the last twenty years, a vibrant literature has developed in the philosophy of human rights that squarely addresses these questions. There is, therefore, an important role for this branch of philosophy in interdisciplinary scholarship articulating and justifying a human rights approach to public health. However, philosophy faces challenges of its own. One is that, while philosophy is well suited for questioning received ideas and value structures, it has also (like both public health and human rights) been guilty at times of upholding status quo values and unjust forms of subordination and inequality. Second, many philosophers often choose to work at a high level of abstraction suitable for the development and defense of systematic theories of value, without contributing to the work needed to connect these theories to pressing problems and issues in the real world. To contribute productively to interdisciplinary scholarship on the human rights approach to public health, then, philosophers should be willing to question the social and philosophical status quo, and to do the work necessary to ensure the practical relevance of their philosophical contributions.

Happily, like both public health and international human rights law, philosophy as an academic field is also evolving and expanding. It is becoming more inclusive of a wider range of perspectives, more sensitive to the impacts of various forms of unjust power hierarchies on the production of knowledge, and more sophisticated in its analysis of how to do normative theorizing that is responsive to and engaged with real-world practices and problems. These developments-in-progress have improved philosophers' abilities to collaborate with other fields, and in a synergistic process, these collaborations are themselves contributing to philosophy's further evolution in these directions. In the remainder of the chapter, I review two ways in which the philosophy of human rights might contribute to, and benefit from, a constructive partnership with the fields of public health and human rights.

Human rights morality and law

One of the primary preoccupations of philosophers of human rights in recent years has been the relationship between moral human rights and international human rights law. Two camps have emerged.[4] The so-called orthodox approaches to the philosophy of human rights are primarily concerned with human rights understood as a subset of moral rights. To the extent that such approaches are concerned with human rights law or activism, they generally assume that the idea of human rights as it appears in such practices is derived from a preexisting (or pre-legal) philosophical concept. Making this explicit, John Tasioulas argues for what he calls the "formative aim thesis," which holds that international human rights law "is primarily concerned with giving effect to universal moral rights" (Tasioulas 2017). Orthodox theorists, therefore, take their primary task to be developing a philosophically sound theory of moral human rights, both for its own sake and on the further assumption that such a theory is needed to guide and/or reform international human rights law and its application.

In contrast, political or "practical" approaches argue that international human rights law and activism should have "a certain authority in guiding our thinking about the nature of human rights" (Beitz 2009: 10). This kind of approach rejects the idea that the best way to make sense of international human rights law is to understand it as attempting to give effect to a preexisting philosophical conception of moral human rights. Instead, such approaches assume that the point of philosophical reasoning is to make normative sense of international human rights law and activism as they have in fact developed. Practical or political approaches therefore allow existing human rights law and activism to set the agenda for theorizing moral human rights (at least to some extent), leaving room for considerations about how human rights actually function in the world to play a role in theorizing about what moral human rights are, which moral human rights exist, and similar questions.

The most important methodological difference between the two approaches is that orthodox theorists see their philosophical project as giving an account of human rights as a subset of pre-legal moral rights, on the assumption that the point of international human rights law and practice is is to provide a legal structure that "gives effect to" those moral rights. By contrast, political theorists take the real-world practice of international human rights law as itself the object of theorizing, and their goal is to provide a systematic account of the normative aims of that extant practice.

Importantly, rejecting the hypothesis that international human rights law aims to give effect to moral human rights does not entail abandoning a critical moral perspective on human rights law. As Allen Buchanan has argued, a moral assessment of international legal human rights need not proceed according to the standards of a philosophical theory of pre-existing, universal moral rights. For example, the recognition of a legal human right may "promote social utility, contribute to social solidarity, help to realize the ideal of a decent or a humane society, increase productivity and to that extent contribute to the general welfare, and provide an efficient and coordinated way for individuals to fulfill their obligations of beneficence" (Buchanan 2013: 53). Each item on this list describes a morally valuable social or political end, to which international legal human rights may contribute (or for which certain international legal human rights may be constitutive). What political approaches are united in rejecting, then, is not a critical moral analysis of international human rights law, but rather the assumption that such an analysis must be given in terms of a prior philosophical conception of moral human rights.

As discussed earlier, much of the scholarship on public health and human rights explicitly looks to existing international human rights law, even while many of these theorists at the same time appeal to human rights as moral or pre-legal ideas. For example, Brigit Toebes and Karien Stronks express a view that clearly refers to a background conception of human rights morality, and a conception of the relationship between morality and law:

> Human rights law consists of an authoritative, recognisable and universally applicable legally binding international value system. As such it is an important tool for addressing public health concerns that raise matters of social justice. Human rights law translates such injustices into concrete individual or collective claims towards governments; which again translate into concrete legal governmental obligations.
>
> *(Toebes and Stronks 2016: 512)*

While these authors do not offer a theory about the relationship between human rights morality and law, passages like this one at least at first glance seem to endorse something like Tasioulas's view that international human rights law aims to realize or give effect to a system of moral human rights. However, this view is deeply contested in the philosophical literature. The main criticisms of orthodox views focus on the absence of a convincing explanation for why philosophical theories about moral human rights should be considered normatively authoritative for human rights law and activism. For example, Joseph Raz argues that orthodox philosophical theories of moral human rights are frequently of only questionable relevance to international human rights law or activism (or collectively, human rights practice). As Raz puts it, such theories "derive their human rights from concerns which do not relate to the practice of human rights, and they provide no argument to establish why human rights practice should be governed by them" (Raz 2010: 327).

At least on paper, practical or political approaches to theorizing human rights are more grounded in human rights law, and consequently may be more responsive to moral ideas and concepts at play in the field, and to the pressing issues and problems on the ground regarding public health and human rights. However, some of the most prominent political theories of human rights do not actually live up to their promise to engage substantively with international human rights law. For example, John Rawls and Joseph Raz's theories of human rights posit that the primary role of human rights in international politics is that their violation provides at least prima facie grounds for disabling a country's right to noninterference on the international stage (Rawls 1999; Raz 2010). As very many commentators have noted, this is an artificially narrow and even misleading account of the role of human rights in international politics (Beitz 2009: 100–101). This shows that even political theorists, despite their commitment to theorizing human rights as they appear in the real world, may nonetheless fall prey to the familiar philosophical tendency to work at a level of abstraction extremely removed from the relevant practice, relying on overly idealized and potentially misleading accounts of the practice in constructing their theories.

On the one hand, then, I have argued that proponents of the human rights approach to public health would be well served to engage with the philosophical issues relevant to human rights morality, and the relationship between human rights morality and law. On the other hand, I have also argued that philosophers of human rights from both the orthodox and political camps have an unfortunately persistent tendency to rest content with work that aims to be normatively coherent and explanatory at an abstract level, but without exploring its practical implications for real-world contexts. Some philosophers assume that the distinctive work of philosophy ends when a coherent value system is developed, apparently assuming that others with distinct expertise can bridge the gap to apply the value theory to the real world.[5] It is therefore understandable that scholarship on the human rights approach to public health might find such philosophical work needlessly abstract and of questionable relevance to its agenda.

One mutually beneficial way out of this impasse is for philosophers of human rights to engage more closely and collaboratively with international human rights law and public health to build a collaborative interdisciplinary scholarship. This partnership should aim to address the relevant moral and philosophical issues at a more empirically informed and less abstract level, with the aim of clarifying the moral and philosophical commitments of such an approach. In turn, such engagement would provide welcome opportunities for philosophers to assess the adequacy of their moral theories in real-world contexts.

Theories of moral human rights

As discussed in the previous section, orthodox theories of human rights see the moral point of human rights law as giving legal effect to the pre-legal concept of moral human rights. The most prominent version of this approach explicates that pre-legal concept in terms of an interest-based conception of moral rights.[6] On this view, moral rights are grounded in the interests or well-being of rights-holders, and human rights are a subset of moral rights.[7] For example, Raz's influential account of moral rights holds that "'X has a right' if and only if X can have rights, and, other things being equal, an aspect of X's well-being (his interest) is a sufficient reason for holding some other person(s) to be under a duty" (Raz 1986: 166). The basic idea is that some interests constitute sufficient reasons for assigning duties to others regarding the satisfaction or realization of those interests, including negative duties not to set back those interests. Holding others to be under a duty establishes a moral claim on the part of the right-holder against the duty-bearers to meet these obligations. This moral claim constitutes a moral right.

Interest-based accounts of *human* rights argue that there are common interests, shared among all or most human beings, that ground moral human rights. For example, Pablo Gilabert argues that, at least in their abstract (rather than specific, legal) instantiations, moral human rights "are general claims based in extremely important interests shared by all (or most) human beings, and whose protection involves responsibilities for anyone who can affect their fulfillment" (Gilabert 2018: 18). Importantly, even some political accounts of human rights also refer to interests as an important moral ground for human rights (Beitz

2009: 137). This demonstrates the relevance of interest-based accounts of rights for a broad range of philosophical accounts of the moral significance of human rights law and practice.

Following the lead of Mann and his collaborators, public health and human rights theorists frequently identify the congruence between the two fields in terms of the shared aim of promoting human interests, flourishing, or well-being. For example, they argue that "health and human rights are complementary approaches to the central problem of defining and advancing human well-being" (Mann et al. 1994: 19). Similarly, George Annas and Wendy Mariner argue that "public health should welcome and promote the human rights framework. In almost every instance, this will make public health more effective in the long run, because the goals of public health and human rights are the same: to promote human flourishing" (Annas and Mariner 2016: 136). In describing human rights as fundamentally concerned with human well-being, the human rights approach to public health (perhaps unintentionally) aligns itself with an interest-based conception of moral human rights. In turn, this alignment points to one potentially fruitful way for the human rights approach to public health to avail itself of a well-developed and compatible moral framework.

Importantly, an interest-based conception of rights requires substantive moral reasoning to determine which specific rights may be grounded in which interests and under what conditions. Depending on the answers they give to these questions, interest-based accounts of human rights may be narrower or more capacious. For example, according to some more minimalist views, only certain particularly important interests, such as the interest in having basic needs met, or in avoiding torture or other inhumane treatment, can ground human rights (Shue 1996). The reasoning behind such restrictive views most often cites the role of human rights as especially urgent or universal moral rights, or the idea that human rights are conceptually linked with the justification for cross-border interventions, which should only take place in response to grievous wrongs (Rawls 1999; Raz 2010).

On the face of it, the human rights approach to public health might be well served by adopting a rich and capacious account of the interests that ground human rights. This would enable the justification of a broad range of human rights relevant to public health, in turn providing a moral rationale for expanding the concerns of public health to include the wide range of social conditions that a human rights approach argues are relevant to population health. However, such a broad account is vulnerable to the charge that it might allow trivial or overly demanding rights to be categorized as human rights, as long as they serve some interest of the right-holder (Nickel 2007: 95–98). Without addressing this controversy in any detail, much less resolving it, the point is that to the extent that proponents of a human rights approach to public health favor an interest-based conception of moral human rights, it would be advantageous for them to be able to provide some account of which interests ground human rights. Again, then, interdisciplinary scholarship that engages with the philosophy of human rights might better enable proponents of the human rights approach to public health to both justify this approach and defend it against familiar criticisms.

Finally, given the fact that substantive moral reasoning is needed to provide an account of which interests ground what moral human rights and why, it follows that it is important for a progressive account of moral human rights to be unbiased in its account of that reasoning. Unfortunately, mainstream thinking about human rights, both in philosophy and in law, has often neglected or downplayed the moral significance of the interests of marginalized groups, such as the poor, persons with disabilities, women, refugees, and indigenous peoples. For example, in critiquing mainstream accounts of human rights that privilege civil and political rights, Tom Campbell has criticized the widespread perspective according to which "torture is held to be unacceptable, poverty merely unfortunate" (Campbell 2007:

56). Similarly, in his analysis of the human rights implications of maternal mortality, Jonathan Wolff asks, "Why has the world been so slow to think of maternal mortality as a health crisis, and so ineffective in dealing with it?" In part, his answer is that "sexism and fatalism have a powerful numbing effect" (Wolff 2012: 125).

Or consider the Convention on the Rights of Persons with Disabilities (CRPD). Importantly, civil society organizations advocating for persons with disabilities played a significant role in developing the CRPD. Perhaps for this reason, among its other innovations, the CRPD imposes strong and clear duties on the part of governments to work proactively to dismantle negative stereotypes about persons with disabilities. For example, the United Nations emphasizes the role of the CRPD in championing

> the movement from viewing persons with disabilities as 'objects' of charity, medical treatment and social protection towards viewing persons with disabilities as 'subjects' with rights, who are capable of claiming those rights and making decisions for their lives based on their free and informed consent as well as being active members of society.
> *(United Nations Department of Economic and Social Affairs 2006)*

The key point here is that the same biases that explain the real-world social disadvantages of persons with disabilities also explain the failure in mainstream law and theory to see such people as paradigmatic rights-holders. The CRPD therefore insists that respect for the human rights of persons with disabilities requires actively dismantling prevalent misconceptions about the interests of persons with disabilities.

These examples demonstrate the widespread and potentially profound influence of various forms of bias in everyday thinking about human well-being. For that reason, an interest-based conception of rights would only function in a progressive way—one that overturns rather than supporting existing forms of social hierarchy and discrimination—if status quo conceptions of which interests ground human rights are questioned and reexamined. Given that each of the relevant fields—public health, international law, and philosophy—is still expanding beyond its own history of narrowly understanding its own aims and potential impacts, it seems clear that collaborative, interdisciplinary work could be mutually beneficial to each field. This work should engage with real-world problems, while also soliciting the input of those whose human rights are impacted, in order to contribute to the continued expansion of each field, and to further develop the moral vision of a human rights approach to public health.

Conclusion

Mann and his collaborators recognized the potentially transformative impact of deploying a human rights-based focus on social and political injustices to improve public health, especially including the health of marginalized populations. Their vision emphasized the potential of this approach for reconceptualizing both human rights and the purposes of public health. In this chapter, I have traced the conceptual expansions within public health and human rights law that inform this synergistic vision. I have also argued for a greater role for the philosophy of human rights in interdisciplinary health and human rights scholarship. The standard preoccupations of this branch of philosophy—including questions about human rights morality and its relationship to human rights law—could provide additional conceptual resources and perspectives to help illuminate the moral basis of the human rights approach to public health. At the same time, the recent focus on methodological questions has highlighted the importance of philosophical work that is relevant to other disciplines and to problems and issues facing people in the real world. For all these reasons, interdisciplinary scholarship emphasizing collaboration among philosophers, international human rights lawyers and activists, and public health professionals promises to foster cutting-edge research and methodologies within each field, while fostering greater effectiveness of human rights approaches to public health in the real world.

Acknowledgement

Many thanks to the editors for inviting me to be a part of this project. I am particularly grateful to Sridhar Venkatapuram for detailed comments on an earlier draft.

Notes

1 See the helpful discussion of this conception of rights in Powers and Faden (2006: 45–49).
2 For examples of public health and human rights research, see Johns Hopkins Bloomberg School of Public Health, Publications and Reports, https://www.jhsph.edu/research/centers-and-institutes/center-for-public-health-and-human-rights/resources/scientific-publications-reports/ (accessed August 14, 2021), or FXB Center for Health and Human Rights at Harvard University, FXB Center Publications, https://fxb.harvard.edu/reports/ (accessed August 14, 2021).
3 See, for example, Ronald Bayer's discussion of "public health officials who endorsed authoritarian attitudes in the name of public health" (Bayer 2007: 1099).
4 There is some disagreement about how to classify different views, however, as well as about whether the two camps can be reconciled or are simply pursing different projects (see Gilabert 2011; Hessler 2017; Liao and Etinson 2012).
5 For a broader critique of philosophers' traditional assumptions about their role in a disciplinary division of labor, see Anderson (1998).
6 Interest-based theories of moral human rights include Griffin (2008), Tasioulas (2015), Gilabert (2018), and Nickel (2007).
7 Will theories of rights, by contrast, emphasize the power or "sovereignty" of the right-holder over certain states of affairs, including whether others bear a moral duty to the right-holder (which the right-holder is free to waive according to her own discretion). See the discussion of will and interest theories of rights in Wenar (2020).

References

Anderson, E. 1998. Pragmatism, science, and moral inquiry. In *In face of the facts: Moral inquiry in American scholarship*, ed. R. W. Fox and R. Westbrook, 10–39. Cambridge: Cambridge University Press.

Annas, G. and W. Mariner. 2016. (Public) health and human rights in practice. *Journal of Health Politics, Policy and Law* 41, no. 1: 129–139. https://doi.org/10.1215/03616878-3445659.

Bayer, R. 2007. The continuing tensions between individual rights and public health. *European Molecular Biology Organization* 8, no. 12: 1099–1103. https://doi.org/10.1038/sj.embor.7401134.

Beitz, C. 2009. *The idea of human rights*. New York: Oxford University Press.

Buchanan, A. 2013. *The heart of human rights*. Oxford: Oxford University Press.

Campbell, T. 2007. Poverty as a violation of human rights: Inhumanity or injustice? In *Freedom from poverty as a human right: Who owes what to the very poor?* ed. T. Pogge, 55–74. Oxford: Oxford University Press.

Cranston, M. 1983. Are there any human rights? *Daedalus* 112, no. 4: 1–17.

Freedman, L. 1999. Reflections on emerging frameworks of health and human rights. In *Health and human rights: A reader*, ed. J. Mann, S. Gruskin, M. Grodin, and G. Annas, 227–252. New York: Routledge. Reprinted from *Health and Human Rights* 1, no. 4 (1995).

Gilabert, P. 2011. Humanist and political perspectives on human rights. *Political Theory* 39, no. 4: 439–467. https://doi.org/10.1177/0090591711408246.

Gilabert, P. 2018. *Human dignity and human rights*. Oxford: Oxford University Press.

Gostin, L. and J. Mann. 1994. Towards the development of a human rights impact assessment for the formulation and evaluation of public health policies. *Health and Human Rights* 1, no. 1: 58–80. https://doi.org/10.2307/4065262.

Griffin, J. 2008. *On human rights.* Oxford: Oxford University Press.

Gruskin, S. 2004. Is there a government in the cockpit: A passenger's perspective of global public health—the role of human rights. *Temple Law Review* 77: 313–334. https://www.academia.edu/2729063/Is_there_a_government_in_the_cockpit_a_passengers_perspective_or_global_public_health_the_role_of_human_rights (accessed December 23, 2021).

Hessler, K. 2017. Theory, politics, and practice: Methodological pluralism in the philosophy of human rights. In *Moral and political approaches to human rights: Implications for theory and practice*, ed. J. K. Schaffer and R. Maliks, 15–32. Cambridge: Cambridge University Press.

Holmes, S. and C. Sunstein. 2000. *The cost of rights: Why liberty depends on taxes.* New York: W. W. Norton.

Ignatieff, M. 2001. *Human rights as politics and idolatry.* Princeton, NJ: Princeton University Press.

Liao, S. M. and A. Etinson. 2012. Political and naturalistic conceptions of human rights: A false polemic? *Journal of Moral Philosophy* 9, no. 3: 327–352. https://doi.org/10.1163/17455243-00903008.

Lomasky, L. 1987. *Persons, rights, and the moral community.* New York: Oxford University Press.

Mann, J. 1997a. Health and human rights: If not now, when? *Health and Human Rights* 2, no. 3: 113–120. https://dx.doi.org/10.2105%2Fajph.96.11.1940.

Mann, J. 1997b. Medicine and public health, ethics and human rights. *Hastings Center Report* 27, no. 3: 6–13. https://doi.org/10.2307/3528660.

Mann, J., L. Gostin, S. Gruskin, T. Brennan, Z. Lazzarini, and H. Fineberg. 1994. Health and human rights. *Journal of Health and Human Rights* 1, no. 1: 7–23. https://dx.doi.org/10.1136%2Fbmj.312.7036.924.

Nickel, J. 2007. *Making sense of human rights.* 2nd edition. Malden, MA: Blackwell Publishing.

O'Neill, O. 2002. Public health or clinical ethics: Thinking beyond borders. *Ethics and International Affairs* 16, no. 2: 35–45. https://doi.org/10.1111/j.1747-7093.2002.tb00395.x.

Powers, M. and R. Faden. 2006. *Social justice: The moral foundations of public health and health policy.* Oxford: Oxford University Press.

Rawls, J. 1999. *The law of peoples.* Cambridge, MA: Harvard University Press.

Raz, J. 1986. *The morality of freedom.* Oxford: Clarendon Press.

Raz, J. 2010. Human rights without foundations. In *The philosophy of international law*, ed. S. Besson and J. Tasioulas, 321–337. New York: Oxford University Press.

Rothstein, M. 2002. Rethinking the meaning of public health. *Journal of Law, Medicine, and Ethics* 30: 144–149. https://doi.org/10.1111/j.1748-720x.2002.tb00381.x.

Shue, H. 1996. *Basic rights.* 2nd edition. Princeton, NJ: Princeton University Press.

Tarantola, D. and S. Gruskin. 2008. Human rights approach to public health policy. In *International encyclopedia of public health*, ed. S. R. Quah, 477–486. Amsterdam: Elsevier.

Tasioulas, J. 2015. On the foundations of human rights. In *Philosophical foundations of human rights*, ed. R. Cruft, S. M. Liao, and M. Renzo, 45–69. Oxford: Oxford University Press. https://doi.org/10.1093/acprof:oso/9780199688623.001.0001.

Tasioulas, J. 2017. Exiting the hall of mirrors: Morality and law in human rights. In *Political and legal approaches to human rights*, ed. T. Campbell and K. Bourne. London: Routledge.

Toebes, B. and K. Stronks. 2016. Closing the gap: A human rights approach towards social determinants of health. *European Journal of Health Law* 23: 510–524. https://doi.org/10.1163/15718093-12341402.

United Nations Department of Economic and Social Affairs, Disability. 2006. Convention on the rights of persons with disabilities. https://www.un.org/development/desa/disabilities/convention-on-the-rights-of-persons-with-disabilities.html (accessed December 23, 2021).

Wenar, L. 2020. Rights. In *The Stanford encyclopedia of philosophy*, ed. E. N. Zalta. https://plato.stanford.edu/archives/spr2021/entries/rights/ (accessed December 23, 2021).

Wolff, J. 2012. *The human right to health.* New York: W. W. Norton.

Wynia, M. 2005. Oversimplifications II: Public health ethics ignores individual rights. *American Journal of Bioethics* 5, no. 5: 6–8. https://doi.org/10.1080/15265160500244942.

Yamin, A. E. 1999. Ethnic cleansing and other lies: Combining health and human rights in the search for truth and justice in the former Yugoslavia. In *Health and human rights: A reader*, ed. J. Mann, S. Gruskin, M. Grodin, and G. Annas, 83–105. New York: Routledge. Reprinted from *Health and Human Rights* 2, no. 1 (1996).

INDEX

Note: **Bold** page numbers refer to tables; *italic* page numbers refer to figures and page numbers followed by "n" denote endnotes.